Study Guide to Accompany

Drug Therapy in Nursing

THIRD EDITION

Study Guide to Accompany

Drug Therapy in Nursing

THIRD EDITION

Diane S. Aschenbrenner, MS, APRN, BC
Course Coordinator
Johns Hopkins University
School of Nursing
Baltimore, Maryland

Samantha J. Venable, MS, RN, FNP
Professor
Saddleback College
Mission Viejo, California

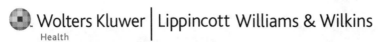
Wolters Kluwer | Lippincott Williams & Wilkins
Health

Philadelphia · Baltimore · New York · London
Buenos Aires · Hong Kong · Sydney · Tokyo

Development Editor: Betsy Gentzler
Managing Editor: Season Evans
Senior Production Editor: Sandra Cherrey Scheinin
Director of Nursing Production: Helen Ewan
Senior Managing Editor / Production: Erika Kors
Manufacturing Manager: Karin Duffield
Compositor: Spearhead

3rd Edition

9 8 7 6 5 4 3

ISBN-13: 978-0-7817-7029-3
ISBN-10: 0-7817-7029-7

Care has been taken to confirm the accuracy of the information presented and to describe generally accepted practices. However, the authors, editors, and publisher are not responsible for errors or omissions or for any consequences from application of the information in this book and make no warranty, expressed or implied, with respect to the currency, completeness, or accuracy of the contents of the publication. Application of this information in a particular situation remains the professional responsibility of the practitioner; the clinical treatments described and recommended may not be considered absolute and universal recommendations.

The authors, editors, and publisher have exerted every effort to ensure that drug selection and dosage set forth in this text are in accordance with the current recommendations and practice at the time of publication. However, in view of ongoing research, changes in government regulations, and the constant flow of information relating to drug therapy and drug reactions, the reader is urged to check the package insert for each drug for any change in indications and dosage and for added warnings and precautions. This is particularly important when the recommended agent is a new or infrequently employed drug.

Some drugs and medical devices presented in this publication have Food and Drug Administration (FDA) clearance for limited use in restricted research settings. It is the responsibility of the health care provider to ascertain the FDA status of each drug or device planned for use in his or her clinical practice.

Introduction

This study guide has been carefully designed to complement the third edition of *Drug Therapy in Nursing*. Each chapter in the study guide opens with the Top Ten Things to Know about the drugs in the chapter. This is a synthesis of the most important points that were made in the chapter. You will note that each of the other headings in the study guide focuses on one type of knowledge presented in each chapter, not on each drug presented. Thus, Key Terms are the key terms identified at the beginning of each chapter. Physiology and Pathophysiology: The Body Human represents pertinent physiology and pathophysiology relevant to the drugs presented in the chapter. Core Drug Knowledge: Just the Facts details the facts that comprise the core drug knowledge about each drug. Core Patient Variables: Patients, Please highlights the core patient variables relevant to each drug. Nursing Management: Every Good Nurse Should…, Case Study, and Critical Thinking Challenge are opportunities to apply knowledge to patient scenarios and practice intergrating the core drug knowledge with the core patient variables.

The study guide is also organized around how students learn a new, complex subject; that is, by starting to learn the basics and then moving on to harder material. In nursing, students start by memorizing some key points and then moving to understanding those points. As students become comfortable with this new knowledge, they begin to see how these new facts may have a bearing on or relationship with other facts they have learned. Students begin to realize that these two pieces of knowledge, which previously stood alone, mean something different when considered together. Students then continue to piece other facts together to draw conclusions. This is much like doing a jigsaw puzzle. At first it may seem that the 500 pieces have no relationship to each other, but as you sort them out you begin to see similarities. "These pieces together make the sky. These pieces together make the tree top." Eventually, it no longer looks like pieces of a puzzle, but one big picture.

Students advance from remembering facts to applying knowledge. They must be able to do this if they are to be competent nurses and care for patients. In pharmacotherapy, the facts about the drug (core drug knowledge) remain the same for every patient who takes that drug. But the relevancy of those facts depends on factors that are unique to that patient (core patient variables).

To help the student advance through these tiers of learning, each chapter in the study guide is arranged from the easiest concept to the most difficult learning tasks. The sections of Key Terms, Physiology, and Pathophysiology: The Body Human essentially require memorization, recognition, and understanding of some facts. Matching, essays, true/false, sentence completion, crossword puzzles, and word searches make up this level of learning, which may be time-consuming, but is not complex. All of the answers can easily be found in each chapter of the textbook. The sections on Core Drug Knowledge: Just the Facts, and Core Patient Variables: Patients, Please are somewhat harder. Multiple choice questions are offered that encourage students to begin to compare and make basic judgments. The section Nursing Management: Every Good Nurse Should… asks students to recognize what the nurse does specific to the drug therapy. Some application of knowledge is needed here. This is a somewhat more complex process. Multiple choice and decision trees make up this level of learning. Finally, the Case Study and the Critical Thinking Challenge require students to synthesize the knowledge presented and apply it to patient scenarios. To do so, students must be able to interpret the possible interaction of core drug knowledge and core patient variables presented in the case. Short answers are asked for the problems posed. This requires a much higher level of thinking than simple memorization. Some students will have great difficulty doing this. If you are having trouble with this level of thinking, don't despair, don't give up, and don't stop trying to do the case studies. The way you get proficient at a new task is to practice, practice, practice. Critical Thinking Challenge is designed to require the most thinking. Here, additional questions related to the case study are posed. To answer the question, students may need to apply knowledge not necessarily from this chapter or from the text. Some of the information may not be strictly "pharmacology" information. It may be knowledge learned from other fields of study. This is because in the practice of nursing, patients are multidimensional, and to meet their needs you will need to know varied types of information.

We hope this study guide is helpful to you in your quest to master facts about pharmacology and to learn how to apply those facts in nursing management. And we hope we have helped you to "see the whole picture."

Diane S. Aschenbrenner
Samantha J. Venable

Contents

Nursing Management of Drug Therapy

TOP TEN THINGS TO KNOW ABOUT NURSING MANAGEMENT IN DRUG THERAPY

1. Core drug knowledge consists of pharmacotherapeutics, pharmacokinetics, pharmacodynamics, contraindications and precautions, adverse effects, and drug interactions.
2. Core patient variables consist of health status; life span and gender; lifestyle, diet, and habits; environment; and culture and inherited traits.
3. Nursing management in drug therapy identifies potential interactions between core drug knowledge and core patient variables.
4. The nurse uses the nursing process and interactions of core drug knowledge and core patient variables to maximize therapeutic effects, minimize adverse effects, provide patient and family education, and evaluate effectiveness of the drug therapy.
5. *Pharmacotherapeutics* is why the drug is prescribed; *pharmacokinetics* is what the body does to the drug; and *pharmacodynamics* is what the drug does to the body.
6. *Contraindications and precautions* indicate restrictions in use or need for close monitoring during therapy; *adverse effects* are undesired effects of the drug, which range from minor to severe; *drug interactions* are effects that may be harmful or beneficial. They occur when a drug is coadministered with another drug, food, or substance.
7. *Health status* includes assessment of acute and chronic conditions, medication history, potential organ dysfunction, allergies, drug history, and diminished memory or mental status.
8. *Life span and gender* refer to age, physiologic development, reproductive stage, ability to read and write, and sex; *lifestyle, diet, and habits* are

the amount of activity and exercise, sleep–wake patterns, occupation, ability to pay for drug therapy, use or abuse of substances, use of over-the-counter drugs, use of alternative health practices, and eating preferences and patterns.
9. *Environment* includes the setting where drug therapy will be administered, the physical factors that may influence aspects of drug therapy, and exposure to potentially harmful substances; *culture and inherited traits* describe the religious, ethnic, racial, and genetic background of the patient.
10. Nursing assessment in drug therapy includes a health and drug history, physical assessment, and examination of the medical record, including current laboratory and other diagnostic findings.

KEY TERMS

Define the following terms.

1. pharmacotherapeutics
2. pharmacokinetics
3. pharmacodynamics
4. contraindications and precautions
5. adverse effects
6. drug interactions
7. core drug knowledge
8. core patient variables
9. health status
10. life span and gender
11. lifestyle, diet, and habits
12. environment
13. culture and inherited traits
14. drug response
15. nursing management in drug therapy
16. prototype drug

CORE DRUG KNOWLEDGE: JUST THE FACTS

Multiple Choice
Circle the option that best answers the question or completes the statement.

1. Administration of theophylline to a patient with acute asthma is an example of
   a. pharmacodynamics.
   b. pharmacokinetics.
   c. pharmacotherapeutics.
   d. adverse effects.

2. Your patient has hypertension and is administered minoxidil, an antihypertensive drug. Three months later, the patient notices an increase in the growth of his/her hair, which is an *expected effect* of the drug. This is an example of the _____ of minoxidil.
   a. pharmacodynamics
   b. pharmacokinetics
   c. pharmacotherapeutics
   d. adverse effects

3. Your patient, who is 2 months' pregnant, has just received a diagnosis of pneumonia. Which of the following areas of core drug knowledge would be most relevant to the selection of drug therapy for this patient?
   a. pharmacodynamics
   b. contraindications and precautions
   c. pharmacotherapeutics
   d. adverse effects

4. Which of the following is an example of an adverse effect of a drug?
   a. lowered white blood cell count after drug therapy for cancer
   b. lowered blood pressure after drug therapy for hypertension
   c. increased urinary output after drug therapy for edema
   d. increased cardiac output after drug therapy for chronic heart failure

CORE PATIENT VARIABLES: PATIENTS, PLEASE

Multiple Choice
Circle the option that best answers the question or completes the statement.

1. Which of the following statements/questions would be included in the nurse's assessment of health status?
   a. "Have you ever had any reactions to medications in the past?"
   b. "Will your insurance cover the cost of this prescription?"
   c. "When is your baby due?"
   d. "Tell me about your diet."

2. Your patient works from midnight to 8 AM and experiences insomnia during the day. This is an example of which of the following core patient variables?
   a. health status
   c. environment
   c. life span and gender
   d. lifestyle, diet, and habits

3. A history of smoking cigarettes is included in which of the following core patient variables?
   a. health status
   b. environment
   c. life span and gender
   d. lifestyle, diet, and habits

4. In assessing the patient care variable of environment, the nurse might include
   a. where the patient keeps his/her medication at home.
   b. what the patient's diet is.
   c. the last time the patient had a chest x-ray.
   d. the allergies of the patient.

NURSING MANAGEMENT: EVERY GOOD NURSE SHOULD …

Study Tools

Students may use grids like the ones below to help them see the relationship between the core drug knowledge and the core patient variables. Use them as you wish to meet your learning needs. Some suggestions: base the grid on one prototype or one class of a drug; use different colors to fill in the blocks if there is an interaction that occurs (e.g., if the pharmacotherapeutics of the drug include use for chronic heart failure, the block under pharmacotherapeutics and next to health status would be filled in because the nurse would need to assess the cardiovascular system); or use key words in the blocks. Make flash cards or large charts of the grids. To compare multiple drugs in a class, use the second chart. These tools can be used in every drug chapter. Edit the grids to match the requirements of your specific pharmacology course.

Drug name _____

	Pharmaco-therapeutics	Pharmaco-kinetics	Pharmaco-dynamics	Contraindications/ precautions	Adverse effects	Drug interactions
Health status						
Life span and gender						
Lifestyle, diet, and habits						
Environment						
Culture and inherited traits						

Drug class _____

	Pharmaco-therapeutics	Pharmaco-kinetics	Pharmaco-dynamics	Contraindications/ precautions	Adverse effects	Drug interactions
Drug 1						
Drug 2						
Drug 3						
Drug 4						

Drug class _____

	Relevant Core Patient Variables	Actions to Maximize Therapeutic Effect	Actions to Minimize Adverse Effects	Patient and Family Education Needed	Evaluating Effectiveness
Drug 1					
Drug 2					
Drug 3					
Drug 4					

CASE STUDY

1. Your patient is a 60-year-old woman who is a retired schoolteacher. She has just started drug therapy with sulfamethoxazole-trimethoprim (Bactrim, Septra) for a urinary tract infection. List the questions you would ask to assess her patient care variables.

   Health status
   Life span and gender
   Lifestyle, diet, and habits
   Environment
   Culture and inherited traits

2. Your assessment of this patient indicates that she has normal renal and liver function, has no chronic disease, and does not take any other medications. Another nurse walks by and, recognizing the patient, asks her about her garden. This information would lead you to further assess the patient's environment. What questions might you ask? (Are you lost? See Chapter 41 for information concerning the importance of environment with this drug.)

CRITICAL THINKING CHALLENGE

Essay

1. How would your assessment of this patient's environment influence your nursing interventions?

2. How can you minimize potential adverse effects?

CHAPTER 2

Pharmaceuticals: Development, Safeguards, and Delivery

TOP TEN THINGS TO KNOW ABOUT PHARMACEUTICALS: DEVELOPMENT, SAFEGUARDS, AND DELIVERY

1. Sources of drugs include plants, animals, synthetic chemicals, and genetically engineered chemicals (omics technology).
2. Drugs have three names: chemical, generic, and trade.
3. A drug's chemical name describes the drug using exact chemical nomenclature to show atomic and molecular structure.
4. A drug's generic name is derived from the chemical name; the first letter of the generic name is not capitalized.
5. A drug's trade name, provided by the drug manufacturer, is usually easy to say and remember. It is protected by trademark, and the first letter is capitalized.
6. Drugs that are grouped by similar characteristics are called a drug class, or classification. Classification may be chemical, physiologic, or therapeutic. Drugs may belong to more than one class.
7. Drug regulations and legislation have been developed to control drug use and promote consumer safety with drug products.
8. The Food and Drug Administration (FDA) approval process for a new drug is lengthy and expensive.
9. The FDA MedWatch program and the USP Practitioners' Reporting Network rely on all health care providers to report all problems or suspected problems with drug products to provide postmarketing surveillance of drugs.
10. Nurses administer drugs to patients, assess response to therapy, monitor for effectiveness, educate patients and their families about all aspects of drug therapy, and, in some settings, adjust drug regimens according to protocols. Nurse practitioners may prescribe drug therapy. Nursing management in drug therapy may be considered an applied science.

KEY TERMS

Matching
Match each key term with its definition.

1. _____ chemical name
2. _____ generic name
3. _____ trade name
4. _____ chemical classification
5. _____ physiologic classification
6. _____ therapeutic classification
7. _____ *National Formulary/United States Pharmacopeia*
8. _____ preclinical trials
9. _____ Canadian Food and Drug Act
10. _____ clinical trials
11. _____ controlled substance
12. _____ drug classification
13. _____ legend drugs
14. _____ Federal Food, Drug, and Cosmetics Act of 1938
15. _____ pharmacogenomics
16. _____ placebo response
17. _____ Practitioners' Reporting Network
18. _____ Pure Food and Drug Act of 1906
19. _____ pharmacogenetics

a. Drug listed according to its abuse potential
b. Classifies the drug by its use in therapy
c. Group of drugs that share similar characteristics
d. Documents that contain the official name for each drug
e. Positive response to any therapeutic intervention

f. The study of how genetic variables affect the pharmacodynamics of a drug in a specific patient

g. Designated the USP and NF as the official standards

h. Studies carried out on animal subjects in a laboratory

i. Laws maintained by the Health Protection Branch of government

j. Predicts the sensitivity or resistance of an individual patient's disease to a specific drug or group of drugs

k. Classifies the drug by its chemical base

l. System that allows testing of potential new drugs

m. Nonproprietary name of the drug

n. Another term for a prescription drug

o. Classifies the drug by its effects on a body system

p. Postmarketing forum to report problems with prescribed drugs

q. Exact chemical name of a drug

r. Brand name of a drug

s. Established the Food and Drug Administration (FDA) as the agency for monitoring and controlling drug manufacturing and marketing

CRITICAL THINKING CHALLENGE

Your 40-year-old patient tells you that he ordered his prescription medication from an online pharmacy, but it has not yet arrived. He wants to know if he can get some free samples until his medications arrive.

1. What assessments would you make?

2. What patient teaching would you do?

CHAPTER 3

Drug Administration

TOP TEN THINGS TO KNOW ABOUT DRUG ADMINISTRATION

1. The three routes of drug administration are enteral, parenteral, and topical.
2. Oral administration is the most frequently used method for the enteral route.
3. Coatings on oral drugs, food, fluids, and other drugs may affect the absorption and onset of action of oral drugs.
4. Oral drugs are easy to administer, may be self-administered, and are less expensive than other forms of drug administration.
5. Parenteral drug administration methods that are most frequently used are intramuscular (IM), subcutaneous (SC), intradermal (ID), and intravenous (IV).
6. Onset of action is more rapid with the parenteral than enteral route.
7. Consider the patient and drug characteristics when selecting a needle, syringe, and intramuscular site for IM drug administration.
8. Intravenous administration of drugs may be through continuous drip, intermittent infusion, or IV push methods.
9. Topical drugs are applied to skin and mucous membranes. Because they bypass the enteric route, they are technically parenteral drugs, but they are most commonly considered a unique form of drug administration.
10. Topical drugs primarily produce a localized effect, although some systemic effects are possible.

KEY TERMS

Fill in the Blank

Complete the following sentences using the correct key term.

1. Drugs administered into the GI tract are given via the _____ route.

2. A good example of a _____ injection is a PPD test.

3. The _____ route circumvents the GI tract.

4. Drugs applied directly on the skin are administered via the _____ route.

5. Drugs applied topically to the skin or mucous membranes exert a _____.

6. Drugs that distribute throughout the body exert a _____.

7. Drugs that come as a _____ must be shaken well before administration.

8. An _____ resists the acid environment of the stomach.

9. A solid drug dispersed within a liquid is called a _____.

10. Administration of a drug into the cerebrospinal fluid uses the _____ route.

11. _____ tablets are placed underneath the tongue.

12. A tablet placed between the cheek and gum in the mouth is an example of _____ administration.

13. A _____ is also known as a pastille or lozenge.

14. A drug compressed or molded into a specific shape is called a _____.

15. An _____ drug is administered directly into the bloodstream.

16. A _____ tablet is formulated to release a drug slowly over an extended period.

17. A drug encased in a hard or soft gelatin container is known as a _____.

18. A _____ is a concentrated solution of sugar in water.

19. The technique of instilling drugs into a muscle uses the _____ route.

20. An _____ is a clear hydroalcoholic mixture that is usually sweetened.

21. An _____ medication is administered over a few minutes, whereas a _____ medication is administered over 20 to 60 minutes.

22. _____ drugs are administered under the skin into the fat and connective tissues.

23. Drugs administered into a joint space are called _____.

24. An _____ drug is administered directly into an artery.

CORE DRUG KNOWLEDGE: JUST THE FACTS

Multiple Choice
Circle the option that best answers the question or completes the statement.

1. Absorption of enteral drugs occurs most frequently in the
   a. mouth.
   b. stomach.
   c. esophagus.
   d. small intestine.

2. What type of enteral medications should be avoided in children?
   a. syrups
   b. elixirs
   c. capsules
   d. tablets

3. The onset of action is rapid after IM administration because
   a. the drug is always in solution.
   b. the drug bypasses the vasculature.
   c. the muscle has a good blood supply.
   d. the drug reaches the GI system quickly.

4. A saline lock is an example of
   a. subcutaneous administration.
   b. intradermal administration.
   c. peripheral access device.
   d. central access.

5. Which of the following would be affected if an enteric-coated tablet were cut in half?
   a. absorption
   b. drug interactions
   c. adverse effects
   d. elimination

Essay

1. List the advantages and disadvantages of IV administration of drugs.

2. List three miscellaneous parenteral delivery routes.

3. What is the purpose of an enteric coating on a drug?

4. How do sustained-released capsules slow the delivery of medication?

5. Name five types of topical drugs.

CORE PATIENT VARIABLES: PATIENTS, PLEASE

Essay

1. Which is the preferred site for IM administration of drugs to an infant?

2. List five reasons enteral drugs may be contraindicated for a patient.

3. An 83-year-old patient is admitted to your unit after having a CVA (stroke). The patient has difficulty swallowing. Develop three strategies to administer enteral medications to this patient.

4. Describe the administration of medication to a patient with a nasogastric tube.

5. List three reasons topical absorption of a drug may occur.

6. Lists three nursing interventions to maximize therapeutic effects and minimize adverse effects when administering topical drugs.

7. List the six rights of medication administration.

8. Your patient is admitted to the hospital for an exacerbation of asthma. The patient has been receiving theophylline syrup for 9 months at home. Name three assessments you should make.

9. How would the nurse position a patient to administer an IM injection in the right vastus lateralis?

10. Your patient has received a diagnosis of leukemia and will receive chemotherapy for the next 6 months. What type of medication administration would be most appropriate for this patient?

NURSING MANAGEMENT: EVERY GOOD NURSE SHOULD ...

State the appropriate injection site(s) based on the following situations.

Situations

a. Thin 24-year-old man requiring 3 cc of a viscous drug (antibiotic) IM _____

b. Average-size 60-year-old woman requiring 0.5 cc of thin drug (vaccine) IM _____

c. Obese 40-year-old man requiring 2.5 cc of thin drug (narcotic) IM _____

d. Newborn requiring 0.5 cc of thin drug (vitamin K) IM _____

e. Average-size 16-year-old girl requiring 0.2 cc thin solution (insulin) SC _____

CASE STUDY

Your patient is 63 years old and has dysphagia (trouble eating and swallowing) because of muscle weakness in his mouth and throat associated with a neuromuscular disorder. He is receiving oral drug therapy for his neuromuscular disorder, hypertension, gastric ulcer, and an infection in his chest. The drug therapy that he receives daily includes the following oral forms: a tablet, an enteric-coated tablet, a capsule, a sustained-release capsule, and a suspension.

1. What assessment is indicated for this patient?

2. What questions regarding drug preparations might you discuss with the pharmacist and the prescriber of the drug therapy?

3. What patient and family education might be indicated?

CRITICAL THINKING CHALLENGE

Your patient's dysphagia progresses until he can no longer swallow food, fluids, or his drug therapy. A gastrostomy tube is placed. Describe the (a) assessments and (b) teaching that might be needed now regarding administration of his drug therapies.

CHAPTER 4

Pharmacotherapeutics, Pharmacokinetics, and Pharmacodynamics

TOP TEN THINGS TO KNOW ABOUT PHARMACOTHERAPEUTICS, PHARMACOKINETICS, AND PHARMACODYNAMICS

1. Pharmacotherapeutics is the therapeutic or desired effects of the drug. Pharmacokinetics is the effects of the body on the drug. There are four phases of pharmacokinetics: absorption, distribution, metabolism (biotransformation), and elimination. Pharmacokinetics is influenced by health status, life span, gender, and culture. Pharmacodynamics is the biologic, chemical, and physiologic actions of a particular drug within the body and the study of how those actions occur. Essentially, it is how the drug affects the body.

2. Drug absorption is dependent on route of administration, solubility and concentration of the drug, circulation, surface conditions, contact time and pH at the absorption site, and cell membrane transport mechanisms. Drugs are distributed throughout the body to the cells via the cardiovascular system. Distribution is dependent on drug flow to the tissues, the drug's ability to leave the vascular system and enter cells, the drug's lipid affinity (lipophilic) or water affinity (hydrophilic), and the drug's ability to bind with protein (usually albumin) in the blood.

3. Drugs cannot create new responses in the body; they can only turn on, turn off, promote, or block a response that the body is inherently capable of producing. Most drugs produce their effects from drug-receptor interactions (agonist/antagonist effects). Receptors are areas on a cell wall that, when activated by a particular chemical, cause the cell to respond in a certain, preprogrammed way. Drugs are designed to fit certain receptors. If the drug activates the response when it is on the receptor, it is said to be an agonist or stimulant of the receptor. If the drug blocks another chemical from activating the receptor, the drug is called an antagonist or blocker of the receptor.

4. Drugs have different affinities for binding with serum proteins. Drug particles that are not bound to protein (i.e., are "free") are active and exert an effect by attaching to a receptor or working in another way. An increase in the number of free drug particles (from low protein levels) increases the drug's effect, even though the dose of the drug is unchanged.

5. The potency of a drug refers to how many particles of a drug (measured in milligrams or grams) are needed to produce a desired effect. Efficacy is the innate ability of the drug to produce a desired effect. Two drugs may have the same efficacy but different potencies. Usually the potency of a drug is less important than the efficacy (i.e., it doesn't matter if it requires a 10-mg pill or a 20-mg pill, as long as it is effective in achieving the therapeutic effect).

6. The therapeutic index relates to the drug's margin of safety (ratio of effective dose to lethal dose). The closer the therapeutic index is to 1 (i.e., the more narrow the therapeutic index), the more dangerous the drug is and the more closely the patient must be monitored. Drug literature does not report the therapeutic index as a number; instead, the index is said to be "narrow." No mention of the therapeutic index indicates the margin of safety is wide.

7. Metabolism changes the drug from its pharmacologically active form to a more water-soluble form so that it can be more easily excreted. Most metabolism occurs in the liver. The percentage of drug metabolized each time the drug is circulated to the liver varies from drug to drug. When drugs are highly metabolized during the first circulation to the liver (first pass), little or no active drug is sent to the general circulation.

8. Most drugs are metabolized by at least one CYP isoenzyme (P-450 system). Drugs that are

metabolized by a specific isoenzyme are called substrates of that isoenzyme. A drug that is a CYP inducer increases the amount or activity of the isoenzyme. More active isoenzyme means that metabolism of the substrates occurs more rapidly, and circulating drug levels are decreased. A drug that is a CYP inhibitor decreases the activity of the isoenzyme; this decreases the metabolism of the isoenzyme's substrates. Less metabolism of a drug increases its blood level and pharmacologic action.

9. A drug's half-life is the time it takes the body to process and eliminate half of the molecules of the drug from an administered dose. The steady state usually occurs in five half-lives of the drug. A drug may be in steady state and still not produce the full therapeutic effect. These two processes are pharmacologically unrelated.

10. Elimination or excretion of drugs occurs primarily in the kidneys. The liver, GI tract, lungs, sweat and salivary glands, skin, and breast milk also have the ability to excrete some drugs. Pathology of these systems (e.g., renal failure) will decrease excretion of the drug. Decreased excretion increases circulating blood levels of the drug even though the dose is unchanged.

KEY TERMS

Matching
Match each key term with its definition.

1. _____ biotransformation

2. _____ blocker

3. _____ blood–brain barrier

4. _____ clearance

5. _____ distribution

6. _____ excretion

7. _____ first-pass effect

8. _____ half-life

9. _____ intrinsic activity

10. _____ metabolism

11. _____ metabolites

12. _____ P-450

13. _____ placebo

14. _____ prodrug

15. _____ pharmacotherapeutics

16. _____ steady state

17. _____ therapeutic index

a. Enzyme system to metabolize drugs

b. The time needed for the plasma concentration of a drug to be reduced by 50%

c. Rate of disappearance of the drug molecules from the circulation

d. Another term for antagonist

e. The delivery of the drug into any and all body compartments it can penetrate

f. Conversion of the drug into another substance or substances

g. Reason the drug is prescribed

h. Administration rate of a drug equals its elimination rate

i. Relation of ED_{50} to LD_{50}

j. Drug that requires conversion into its active form

k. Removal of a drug (or its metabolites) from the body

l. A combination of affinity and efficacy

m. Another term for metabolism

n. End product of a chemical change of one drug into another

o. Selective mechanism that opposes the passage of most ions and large molecular compounds from the blood to the brain tissue

p. Inactive substance

q. Drugs entering the body by the enteral route first go through the portal circulation to the liver before reaching the general circulation

TRUE OR FALSE

Mark true or false for the following statements. If the statement is false, replace the underlined word with the correct word to make a true statement.

1. _____ <u>Pharmacokinetics</u> is what the drug does to the body.

2. _____ An <u>enzyme</u> is a specialized area on the cell wall or within the cellular cytoplasm.

3. _____ An <u>antagonist</u> is a drug that has the ability to initiate the desired therapeutic effect by binding to a receptor.

4. _____ An <u>agonist</u> is a drug that has affinity for a receptor but does not achieve a response.

5. _____ The tendency of a drug to attach to a specific receptor site is called <u>efficacy</u>.

6. _____ The power of a drug to produce a therapeutic response is known as <u>affinity</u>.

7. _____ The term <u>potency</u> means the drug's ability to initiate a biologic activity at its maximum therapeutic ability.

8. _____ An increased rate or dose of a drug to achieve faster steady state is called a <u>maintenance</u> dose.

9. _____ The amount of drug needed to sustain a therapeutic effect is called the <u>loading dose</u>.

10. _____ <u>Pharmacodynamics</u> is what the body does to the drug.

11. _____ Movement from the site of administration to the bloodstream is called <u>absorption</u>.

CORE DRUG KNOWLEDGE: JUST THE FACTS

Multiple Choice

Circle the option that best answers the question or completes the statement.

1. Which of the following routes of administration provides the greatest control over the actual dose of the drug delivered to the patient?
   a. enteral
   b. sublingual
   c. parenteral
   d. rectal

2. _____ administration is the most common parenteral route.
   a. intravenous
   b. subcutaneous
   c. intramuscular
   d. intradermal

3. Which of the following is most likely to be affected by ischemia?
   a. absorption
   b. distribution
   c. metabolism
   d. excretion

4. Which of the following statements regarding the blood–brain barrier is correct?
   a. All drugs pass freely from the vasculature into the brain
   b. Drugs must be lipid soluble or have a transport system to be effective in the brain.
   c. Most antimicrobial agents cross the blood–brain barrier without difficulty.
   d. Benzodiazepines have difficulty diffusing through the blood–brain barrier.

5. Which of the following organs of the body is the primary site for metabolism?
   a. lungs
   b. kidneys
   c. liver
   d. skin

6. The attraction of certain molecules to specific sites is called
   a. solubility.
   b. efficacy.
   c. potency.
   d. affinity.

7. Biotransformation is also known as
   a. absorption.
   b. distribution.
   c. metabolism.
   d. excretion.

8. Which of the following is incorrect concerning the common characteristics of drugs?
   a. Drugs do not create responses.
   b. Drugs exert multiple, rather than single, effects on the body.
   c. Drug action results from a physiochemical interaction between the drug and a molecule or structure in the body.
   d. Drugs developed in the last 5 years have the ability to target a subtype receptor to create a single response.

Essay

1. In addition to the kidneys, what other routes of excretion are available?

2. Describe the difference between the therapeutic index and the therapeutic range.

CORE PATIENT VARIABLES: PATIENTS, PLEASE

Multiple Choice
Circle the option that best answers the question or completes the statement.

1. Which of the following patients would most likely receive a drug by the rectal route?
   a. patient A, age 63, with a history of diverticulitis
   b. patient B, age 9, with nausea and vomiting
   c. patient C, age 36, with peptic ulcer disease
   d. patient D, age 11, with irritable bowel syndrome

2. Your patient takes metoclopramide (Reglan), a drug that stimulates the upper GI tract. Which of the following pharmacokinetics would be affected?
   a. absorption
   b. distribution
   c. metabolism
   d. excretion

3. Your patient has both liver and kidney disease. The patient takes several enteral medications. You would expect the duration of action of these medications to
   a. increase.
   b. decrease.
   c. be absent.
   d. stay the same.

4. Your patient takes Drug A, which is 85% protein bound. Today the patient began to take Drug B, which is 90% protein bound. What is mostly likely to occur?
   a. Drug A becomes less pharmacologically active.
   b. Drug B becomes less pharmacologically active.
   c. Drug A becomes more pharmacologically active.
   d. Drug B becomes more pharmacologically active.

5. Your patient has renal and liver dysfunction. Which of the following nursing interactions is most appropriate for this patient?
   a. Monitor frequently and carefully for signs of adverse effects or toxicity.
   b. Refuse to administer any medications that are metabolized solely by the liver.
   c. Decrease the dose of medication by 1/3 should signs of toxicity occur.
   d. Decrease the dose but increase the frequency of drug administration.

NURSING MANAGEMENT: EVERY GOOD NURSE SHOULD …

Multiple Choice
Circle the option that best answers the question or completes the statement.

1. Before starting a patient on an oral drug therapy regimen, the nurse should assess for
   a. dysphagia.
   b. circulatory impairment.
   c. skin integrity.
   d. visual acuity.

2. Your patient has chronic renal failure. He is receiving medication that is renally excreted. You should expect that he needs
   a. a larger dose than normal to achieve the desired effect.
   b. a smaller dose than normal to achieve the desired effect.
   c. more frequent dosing than normal to achieve the desired effect.
   d. no changes in the normal dose to achieve the desired effect.

3. Your patient has liver disease and receives medication that is metabolized in the liver. A toxic effect from this drug is thrombocytopenia. Based on this information, a nursing diagnosis appropriate for this patient is

   a. ineffective individual coping related to liver disease.

   b. risk for injury related to potentially high drug serum levels.

   c. anxiety related to adverse effects of medication.

   d. risk for altered skin integrity related to poor liver function.

4. Your patient's blood work shows a low serum albumin level. She is receiving medication that is normally 95% protein bound. You should monitor for signs of

   a. hyperalbuminemia.

   b. drug toxicity.

   c. hypokalemia.

   d. CNS depression.

5. Your patient has been taking a drug (Drug A) that is highly metabolized by the cytochrome P-450 system. He has been taking this medication for 6 months. At this time he is hospitalized and begins taking a second medication (Drug B) that is an inducer of cytochrome P-450. You should monitor for

   a. increased therapeutic effect of Drug A.

   b. increased adverse effects of Drug B.

   c. decreased therapeutic effect of Drug A.

   d. decreased therapeutic effects of Drug B.

6. Your patient is asking you about over-the-counter analgesics (pain relievers). She says, "The commercials say this one is more potent. Is the most potent drug the best drug?" You should respond:

   a. "Yes, you always want to take the drug that is most potent."

   b. "Yes, a more potent drug has a more rapid effect."

   c. "No, a more potent drug is dangerous."

   d. "No, you want to take a drug that is more effective, not necessarily more potent."

7. Your patient has liver disease and is receiving a drug that is highly metabolized by the liver. To achieve the usual pharmacodynamic response of the drug, you would expect

   a. the drug's dose to be greater than a "standard" dose.

   b. the drug's dose to be smaller than a "standard" dose.

   c. the drug's dose to be the same as a "standard" dose.

   d. the drug's dose to be the same as a "standard" dose but given more frequently.

8. Your patient is 70 years old. She has peripheral vascular disease and a history of surgical removal of part of her stomach and small intestine. She has started taking a medication to treat her peripheral vascular disease. What aspects of pharmacokinetics may be altered because of her pathologies? *Mark all that apply.*

   a. absorption

   b. distribution

   c. metabolism

   d. elimination

CASE STUDY

Your patient has atrial fibrillation and an increased ventricular rate (150–160 beats per minute). She is to begin taking digoxin (a drug that slows the heart rate). Digoxin has a very long half-life of about 30 to 40 hours. The onset of action is 30 to 120 minutes if given orally and 5 to 30 minutes if given intravenously. The orders are as follows:

Digoxin 0.375 mg IV now
Digoxin 0.188 mg IV 4 hours from now and repeat again in another 4 hours
Digoxin 0.25 mg PO every day, starting tomorrow morning

1. Explain why IV doses were chosen to be given today but oral doses tomorrow.

2. Explain why the combined IV dose today (all three doses) is larger (more milligrams) than the oral dose ordered for tomorrow.

3. Digoxin is a drug with a narrow therapeutic index. What are the risks to this patient while receiving the loading dose of digoxin? What actions of the nurse are important now?

CRITICAL THINKING CHALLENGE

Your patient begins a regimen of heparin drip solution for a deep venous thrombosis. The half-life of heparin is 1.5 hours. The physician writes these orders:

Heparin drip solution 1,000 units per hour.
Check clotting time (aPTT) every 4 hours until patient's clotting time is two times the normal.
Titrate the heparin drip by increasing it 500 units per hour until aPTT is two times the normal.

Four hours after the heparin infusion is started, the aPTT is one and one-half times the normal. The nurse increases the infusion rate by 500 units per hour. Eight hours after the heparin infusion is started, the aPTT is two and one-half times the normal.

Use the principles of pharmacokinetics to determine what contributed to the excessively high aPTT 8 hours after initiation of the infusion.

CHAPTER 5

Adverse Effects and Drug Interactions

TOP TEN THINGS TO KNOW ABOUT ADVERSE EFFECTS AND DRUG INTERACTIONS

1. An adverse effect of drug therapy is any nontherapeutic response to the drug therapy; its consequences may be minor or significant.
2. A drug interaction is the action of one drug on a second drug or other element creating increased or decreased therapeutic effect of either or both drugs, a new effect, or an increase in the incidence of an adverse effect.
3. Allergic responses are altered physiologic reactions to a drug because a previous exposure to the drug stimulated the immune system to develop antibodies. Anaphylaxis is the most serious allergic response.
4. Specific patterns or groups of symptoms related to drug therapy that carry risk for permanent damage or death are called toxicities. The organ or system that is affected is used to name the toxicity (as in neurotoxicity, nephrotoxicity, cardiotoxicity).
5. Drug toxicities are a type of adverse effect from a drug. When two or more drugs can produce the same toxicity, the risk of that toxicity occurring increases.
6. Common drug toxicities are neurotoxicity, hepatotoxicity, immunotoxicity, cardiotoxicity, nephrotoxicity, and ototoxicity.
7. Drug interactions may affect the pharmacokinetics of a drug (absorption, metabolism [primarily through the P-450 system]), excretion, distribution, or the pharmacodynamics of a drug.
8. Pharmacodynamic interactions of drugs may produce additive effects (similar to 1 + 1 = 2), synergistic effects (similar to 1 + 1 = 3), potentiation effects (similar to $\frac{1}{2}$ + 1 = 2), and antagonistic effects (similar to 1 + 1 = 0).
9. The core patient variables may predispose a patient to adverse effects and drug interactions.
10. Collecting a thorough drug history before a new drug therapy is begun helps minimize the occurrence of adverse effects and drug interactions.

KEY TERMS

Using the Following Definitions, Unscramble Each of the Sets of Letters to Form a Word. Write Your Response in the Spaces Provided.

1. When a drug and a second drug or element (e.g., food) have an effect on each other

A C T E I N N R T O I
☐ ☐ ☐ ☐ ☐ ☐ ☐ ☐ ☐ ☐ ☐

2. An effect other than the desired effect

E S E V D A R
☐ ☐ ☐ ☐ ☐ ☐ ☐

3. The most serious type of allergic reaction

H N A A P A X Y L S I
☐ ☐ ☐ ☐ ☐ ☐ ☐ ☐ ☐ ☐ ☐

4. An unusual, abnormal, or peculiar response to a drug

Y C D I S I C A O T R I N
☐ ☐ ☐ ☐ ☐ ☐ ☐ ☐ ☐ ☐ ☐ ☐

5. An interacting effect in which 1 + 1 = 2

D D I V I T A E
☐ ☐ ☐ ☐ ☐ ☐ ☐ ☐

6. An interacting effect in which 1 + 1 = 3

G E I T S N I C R Y S
☐ ☐ ☐ ☐ ☐ ☐ ☐ ☐ ☐ ☐ ☐

7. The effect if only one of the two interacting drugs is increased

N O A N P E T O I T I T
☐☐☐☐☐☐☐☐☐☐☐☐

8. Injury to the nervous system related to drug therapy

T N O E X U I R C O I T Y
☐☐☐☐☐☐☐☐☐☐☐☐☐

9. Injury to the immune system related to drug therapy

M T I O X M I C U I N T O Y
☐☐☐☐☐☐☐☐☐☐☐☐☐☐

10. Injury to the liver related to drug therapy

E H T O P X A I C T O T I Y
☐☐☐☐☐☐☐☐☐☐☐☐☐☐

11. Injury to the kidneys related to drug therapy

C R T Y E O P O N X H I I T
☐☐☐☐☐☐☐☐☐☐☐☐☐☐

12. Injury to the 8th cranial nerve related to drug therapy

T C O I O I T X T Y O
☐☐☐☐☐☐☐☐☐☐☐

13. Injury to the heart related to drug therapy

R T C Y I T D C O I A O I X
☐☐☐☐☐☐☐☐☐☐☐☐☐☐

CORE DRUG KNOWLEDGE: JUST THE FACTS

1. Drug A and Drug B, given in combination, increase the incidence of thrombocytopenia. This is an example of _____.

2. List the common signs and symptom of an allergic reaction.

3. Identify the classic symptoms of anaphylaxis.

4. How is anaphylaxis treated?

5. Identify potential signs and symptoms of neurotoxicity.

6. Identify potential signs and symptoms of hepatotoxicity.

7. Identify potential signs and symptoms of ototoxicity.

8. List four potential interactions involving GI absorption.

9. Write an example of a beneficial additive drug–drug interaction.

10. What is the difference between potentiation and synergism?

11. You have just hung an IV piggyback of phenytoin (Dilantin) using the primary line of D5W. Ten minutes later you return and note that the tubing has a cloudy precipitant. What do you suspect has occurred?

CORE PATIENT VARIABLES: PATIENTS, PLEASE

Multiple Choice
Circle the option that best answers the question or completes the statement.

1. Your patient is allergic to several antibiotic agents. The patient has received a diagnosis of acute bilateral pneumonia, and an antimicrobial agent that he/she has never taken before has been prescribed. Which of these interactions would you do?
   a. Place an emesis basin next to the bed in easy reach of the patient.
   b. Obtain an order for calamine lotion in case of rash.
   c. Monitor the patient's vital signs every 4 hours.
   d. Have epinephrine available for quick access.

2. Your patient is given chloral hydrate for insomnia. Two hours later, as you are doing your routine rounds, you see the patient sitting in bed, anxious and hypervigilant. This is an example of a(n)
   a. adverse effect.
   b. allergic reaction.
   c. idiosyncratic response.
   d. drug toxicity.

3. Your patient is experiencing drowsiness, restlessness, and nystagmus since beginning drug therapy. You suspect the patient may be experiencing
   a. neurotoxicity.
   b. hepatotoxicity.
   c. nephrotoxicity.
   d. cardiotoxicity.

4. Your patient is receiving penicillin G and probenecid (Benemid) for a systemic infection. Why would the health care provider give these two drugs in combination?
   a. Probenecid and penicillin G, in combination, have a synergistic effect.
   b. Probenecid interacts with the kidneys and prevents renal excretion of penicillin G, thus prolonging its duration.
   c. Probenecid and penicillin G have a drug–drug interaction, which binds them together, resulting in an antagonistic effect.
   d. Penicillin G is destroyed in the acidic environment of the stomach. Probenecid inhibits its destruction.

5. Your patient takes nitroglycerin (NTG) for chest pain. Because the patient has arthritis, he places the NTG in a larger pill container for easier access. The patient states, "I've noticed that I do not feel that burning sensation under my tongue, and it takes longer for the chest pain to go away." This is an example of a(n)
   a. health status interaction.
   b. life span and gender interaction.
   c. environment interaction.
   d. cultural interaction.

NURSING MANAGEMENT: EVERY GOOD NURSE SHOULD …

Multiple Choice
Circle the option that best answers the question or completes the statement.

1. When a patient is receiving drug therapy that has the known adverse effect of causing nephrotoxicity, the nurse should monitor the patient's
   a. ALT and AST levels.
   b. intake and output levels.
   c. balance when standing.
   d. cognitive level.

2. Your patient has liver disease. He is receiving a drug that is metabolized by the liver. The nurse needs to *most* carefully monitor this patient for signs of
   a. therapeutic effects.
   b. allergic effects.
   c. adverse effects.
   d. idiosyncratic effects.

3. Your patient has hypertension and receives two different types of medications (a diuretic and a beta blocker drug) as drug therapy for this condition. They are both prescribed to be taken twice a day. The nurse knows that these two drugs
   a. should never be given at the same time.
   b. should only be given 1 hour apart.
   c. may be given at the same time.
   d. may have antagonistic effects.

4. A patient, before being discharged from a hospital on a new drug regimen, should receive education about
   a. possible adverse effects of the drug therapy.
   b. how to cope with possible adverse effects.
   c. foods that may interact with the drug therapy.
   d. all of the above.

5. In assessing the patient's core patient variables, you learn that the patient is 75 years old and is receiving oral drug therapy for asthma. The nurse recognizes that this patient is likely to have an altered response to drug therapy and should closely monitor the patient for
   a. increased adverse effects.
   b. decreased therapeutic effects.
   c. decreased pharmacodynamics.
   d. increased allergic response.

CASE STUDY

Your patient is 70 years old and has rheumatoid arthritis and hypertension. She is receiving aspirin and furosemide, a loop diuretic, as drug therapies for these conditions. Describe the patient education you, the nurse, would provide to minimize the serious adverse effects associated with these therapies. (Need help? See Chapters 24 and 27.)

CRITICAL THINKING CHALLENGE

The patient continues to take aspirin and furosemide for 6 months, at which time she returns to the clinic for follow-up. She complains that the aspirin is upsetting her stomach. She states her stomach feels too acidic and burns. What aspects of core patient variables should the nurse assess at this time? What strategies might the nurse suggest to minimize the adverse effects of aspirin?

CHAPTER 6

Life Span: Children

TOP TEN THINGS TO KNOW ABOUT LIFE SPAN: CHILDREN

1. Children are different from adults in many ways, and safe, appropriate drug therapy must reflect these differences. Many drugs administered to children are "off-label" because adequate clinical trials involving children have not been done. The pediatric patient is usually defined as someone younger than 16 years of age and weighing less than 50 kilograms.

2. Pediatric drug dosages must be accurate to reduce risk of adverse effects and prevent overdosage. Most drugs for children are based on the weight of the child in kilograms or the body surface area of the child. Two nurses should always check drug dosage calculations to prevent overdosage from math errors. Dosages often must be lowered to account for immature or impaired body systems in neonates and infants.

3. A child's age, growth, and maturation affect the core drug knowledge of drug therapy. Absorption of drugs in children may be altered by decreased gastrointestinal (GI) acidity, immature peripheral vascular systems, changes in body surface area, and skin permeability. Infants to 1 year of age have less acidic GI tracts than do older children and adults. This may affect absorption of some drugs. The erratic blood flow associated with immature peripheral vascular systems (especially in neonates) may alter absorption from the intramuscular (IM) and subcutaneous (SC) routes. Increased absorption of topical drugs is common in pediatric patients, especially infants, because of greater body surface area. The infant's skin is also more permeable, additionally increasing absorption of topical agents; this may result in adverse effects that usually do not occur in the adult patient.

4. Distribution of drugs in children can be altered because of differences in body water and fat, immature liver function, and an immature blood–brain barrier. Compared with adults, children, especially infants, have a higher concentration of water in their bodies and a lower concentration of fat. The infant's (especially neonate's) immature liver produces fewer plasma proteins, especially albumin, allowing for a higher percentage of free and active drugs. Drug binding to serum proteins reaches adult levels by 6 months of age. At birth, the blood–brain barrier is not fully developed. Newborns are particularly vulnerable to central nervous system (CNS) toxicity, intensified effects of drugs that act on the CNS, and exaggerated CNS adverse effects in response to other drug therapy.

5. Immaturity of the neonatal and infant liver results in decreased or incomplete metabolism of many drugs, which may necessitate lower drug dosages or an increased interval between doses to achieve appropriate blood levels.

6. The neonate, especially the preterm infant, has immature kidneys, and renal excretion of drugs is slow. Thus, drug dosages and therapeutic drug levels must be monitored closely to prevent toxicity. During the first 6 months of life, infants have a reduced glomerular filtration rate and decreased tubular secretion and reabsorption; both of these extend the half-life of many drugs.

7. Adverse effects of some drugs are more severe and more likely to occur in children because of the immature body systems of children. Newborns and young children may experience serious adverse effects from direct administration of a drug or through their mother's use of a medication.

8. The child's stage of growth and development must be considered when assessing core patient variables and the interaction of core drug knowledge and core patient variables.

9. Choice of appropriate route or site of drug administration varies by the child's age and size and the drug therapy. Special techniques may be needed when administering drug therapy to minimize traumatic effects to the child (e.g., use of EMLA cream to numb an area before an injection, use of Popsicle or ice chips to numb taste buds before unpleasant oral drugs, and not mixing drug therapy into infant formula).

10. The parent is an important source of information about the child and comfort for the child as well as a partner in the care of the child requiring drug therapy. Education about drug therapy should be provided to the patient, at a developmentally appropriate level, and to the family.

KEY TERMS

Matching
Match the following words or terms with the correct definition.

1. _____ body surface area

2. _____ play therapy

3. _____ kernicterus

4. _____ pediatric patient

5. _____ nomogram

a. Measuring device, such as a chart or graph

b. Younger than 16 years and weighing less than 50 kg

c. External surface of the body expressed in square meters

d. Effective technique to prepare a child for drug therapy

e. Life-threatening condition resulting from an accumulation of bilirubin

CORE DRUG KNOWLEDGE: JUST THE FACTS

1. In the pediatric patient, what physiologic differences affect core drug knowledge?

2. In pharmacotherapeutics for a pediatric patient, what is the major difference between a child and an adult?

3. What is the standard formula for calculating body surface area (BSA)?

4. For the absorption of drugs, at what age will a child's pH equal an adult's pH of the stomach?

5. How is distribution of drugs different in children than in adults?

6. List initial education for parents of children receiving drug therapy.

Matching
Match the following developmental levels with strategies for drug administration.

1. _____ have parent in room during administration

2. _____ allow to choose which medication to take first

3. _____ use ventrogluteal site for IM injections

4. _____ place liquid medication in buccal fold of mouth

5. _____ remember privacy and patient control when administering medication

a. Infant

b. Toddler

c. Preschooler

d. School-age child

e. Adolescent

CORE PATIENT VARIABLES: PATIENTS, PLEASE

Multiple Choice
Circle the option that best answers the question or completes the statement.

1. Your patient, age 14 months, is to receive penicillin V. She weighs 11.9 kg. The order reads: administer 50 mg/kg in 4 divided doses. Using the body weight method, how much penicillin V will you give this patient in one dose?

    a. 595 mg

    b. 150 mg

    c. 100 mg

    d. 1 gram

2. A patient has three children: two boys ages 5 and 8 years, and a daughter age 9 months. All of the children have been prescribed hydrocortisone cream for heat rash.. Which of the following instructions is most accurate?

    a. Apply the same amount of hydrocortisone for all the children.

    b. Use less of the hydrocortisone for the boys.

    c. Use less of the hydrocortisone for the girl.

    d. Do not use cream for any of the children.

3. The use of water-soluble drugs in children may result in an increased risk for

    a. toxicity.

    b. rapid elimination of drugs.

    c. subtherapeutic levels of drugs.

    d. enhanced pharmacodynamics.

4. Your patient, age 6 years, is hospitalized for seizures. He has been prescribed phenobarbital (Luminal), a lipophilic drug. In comparison with the dosage for an adult, the dosage for this pediatric patient should be

    a. increased.

    b. decreased.

    c. the same.

5. Your patient, age 4 years, is hospitalized with appendicitis. Which of the following should be done to reduce this patient's anxiety about receiving an intramuscular injection?

    a. Use parents to restrain child when giving an injection.

    b. Explain the pharmacodynamics of each drug and the rationale for therapy.

    c. Tell the patient she will be a "good girl" if she allows you to administer her medications.

    d. Demonstrate drug therapy to the patient using a rag doll.

NURSING MANAGEMENT: EVERY GOOD NURSE SHOULD ...

Multiple Choice
Circle the option that best answers the question or completes the statement.

1. You are preparing to give intramuscular vitamin K to a newborn. You should

    a. use the ventrogluteal site.

    b. select a needle longer than 5/8 inch.

    c. use a fine-gauge needle.

    d. avoid aspirating before injecting.

2. You are going to administer multivitamin drops to an infant. You should

    a. use a calibrated measuring cup to measure the dose.

    b. mix the measured dose into the infant's formula.

    c. explain the rationale for the drug to gain the child's cooperation.

    d. gently squeeze the infant's mouth open and place the drops in the buccal pouch.

3. An active 2-year-old patient is receiving an intravenous (IV) infusion of heparin, an anticoagulant. To minimize adverse effects from the drug therapy the nurse should

    a. run the IV solution by way of gravity.

    b. activate the lock feature on the pump's infusion rate.

    c. place enough volume in the microdrip calibrated chamber to last 4 hours.

    d. check the IV infusion site once a shift.

4. Which of the following statements made by the nurse would most likely gain cooperation from the preschooler during drug administration?

   a. "Would you like to take the liquid medicine or the pill first?"

   b. "Take your medicine pills or I will have to give you a shot."

   c. "Do you want to take your medicine for me?"

   d. "Only bad children don't want to take their medicine."

5. When administering drug therapy to an adolescent, the nurse should

   a. direct all questions to the parents.

   b. provide stickers and prizes for taking drug therapy.

   c. offer explanations and teaching directly to the patient.

   d. maintain tight control over all aspects of drug administration.

6. Which of the following nursing actions would be **most significant** when administering medication to a pediatric patient?

   a. Take the blood pressure and pulse.

   b. Weigh the child.

   c. Check the most recent lab results.

   d. Mix the medication in applesauce to mask the taste.

CASE STUDY

An 11-year-old child is to be discharged from the hospital on a regimen of oral theophylline, a bronchodilator, for his asthma. Core drug knowledge of theophylline includes the following: theophylline is similar to caffeine in chemical structure; cigarette and marijuana smoking will decrease the effectiveness of theophylline.

To maximize the therapeutic effect of the theophylline therapy, the nurse should assess what aspect of the child's core patient variables?

To minimize the adverse effects of the theophylline therapy, the nurse should assess what aspect of the child's core patient variables?

CRITICAL THINKING CHALLENGE

You are caring for a newborn infant who was born by cesarean section. The mother receives morphine for pain after the cesarean section and is breastfeeding the infant. What are the major risks to the infant and why?

CHAPTER 7

Life Span: Pregnant or Breast-Feeding Women

TOP TEN THINGS TO KNOW ABOUT LIFE SPAN: PREGNANT OR BREAST-FEEDING WOMEN

1. Drug therapy may be indicated for pregnant or breast-feeding women to manage pre-existing conditions or those that are newly developed.
2. The normal physiologic changes that occur during pregnancy may alter absorption, distribution, and elimination of drugs.
3. Drug therapy may produce therapeutic effects in the pregnant woman but adverse effects, including teratogenic effects, in the fetus or infant.
4. Potential fetal risks must be compared with maternal benefits when drug therapy is required.
5. The minimum therapeutic dose should be used for as short a time period as possible to minimize adverse effects in the fetus. If possible, drug therapy should be delayed until after the first trimester, especially if the drug has teratogenic effects.
6. FDA pregnancy categories for safety of use of drugs in pregnancy include five divisions, A through D and X. Categories A and B most likely carry no or little risk to the fetus, C and D most likely carry some risk to the fetus, and X is contraindicated in pregnancy.
7. Health status of the woman may indicate the need for drug therapy because of chronic conditions (e.g., epilepsy, diabetes) or conditions that develop secondary to pregnancy (e.g., hyperemesis gravidarum, preeclampsia and eclampsia, and thrombus formation).
8. Adverse effects of drug therapy may be misinterpreted as discomforts commonly associated with pregnancy.
9. Many drugs also cross into breast milk, although the dosage that reaches the infant is very small. Nursing mothers need to be educated about possible risks to the infant.
10. Nonpharmacologic alternatives to drug therapy should be used if possible.

KEY TERMS

Fill in the Blank
Complete the following sentences using the correct key term.

1. Hypertension, edema, and proteinuria are classic signs of _____.

2. The first trimester is the critical period of _____.

3. _____ is another term for pernicious vomiting of pregnancy.

4. Severe growth retardation, mental retardation, and microencephaly are signs of _____.

5. The secretion of breast milk is called _____.

6. Preeclampsia may lead to _____, characterized by cerebral edema and convulsions.

7. _____ is caused by secretion of placental hormones.

8. A(n) _____ effect causes physical defects in the developing fetus.

9. Craniofacial abnormalities, limb defects, and growth deficiency are signs of _____.

CORE DRUG KNOWLEDGE: JUST THE FACTS

Multiple Choice
Circle the option that best answers the question or completes the statement.

1. Which of the following pharmacokinetics is unaffected by pregnancy?
   a. absorption
   b. distribution
   c. metabolism
   d. excretion

2. During pregnancy, the pharmacodynamics of a drug must be carefully considered because of changes in the
   a. integumentary system.
   b. cardiovascular system.
   c. renal system.
   d. GI system.

3. Distribution of drugs is altered during pregnancy because of
   a. hemodynamic changes.
   b. increased hormone secretion.
   c. decreased renal function.
   d. increased attachment to plasma proteins.

4. Which of the following type of drugs most readily enter circulation in a breast-fed infant?
   a. highly protein-bound drugs
   b. ionized drugs
   c. lipophilic drugs
   d. large molecular drugs

5. What percentage of a drug taken by the mother passes into the infant during breast-feeding?
   a. 5%
   b. 10%
   c. 2%
   d. 20%

Matching
Match the following pregnancy categories with the correct clue.

1. _____ category A
2. _____ category B
3. _____ category C
4. _____ category D
5. _____ category X

a. Used in life-threatening situations
b. Drugs are given if benefit justifies the risk to the fetus
c. Human studies fail to demonstrate a risk to the fetus
d. Fetal risk outweighs potential benefit
e. Animal studies do not indicate a risk, but no human studies confirm lack of risk to fetus

CORE PATIENT VARIABLES: PATIENTS, PLEASE

Multiple Choice
Circle the option that best answers the question or completes the statement.

1. Which of the following patients is most likely to experience teratogenic effects of drug therapy?
   a. the patient in her first trimester of pregnancy
   b. the patient in her second trimester of pregnancy
   c. the patient in her third trimester of pregnancy
   d. All three patients have equal potential for teratogenic effects.

2. Your patient has preeclampsia. Which of the following classes of drugs would you expect to be prescribed?
   a. alpha-adrenergic blocking agent
   b. angiotensin-converting enzyme inhibitor
   c. benzodiazepine
   d. direct vasodilator

3. Your patient comes to the clinic with suspected pregnancy. She is concerned because she has multiple pre-existing health problems and takes furosemide (Lasix), atenolol (Tenormin), insulin, and phenytoin (Dilantin). Her urine pregnancy test is positive. Which of her current medications may need to be changed or discontinued?
   a. furosemide (Lasix)
   b. atenolol (Tenormin)
   c. insulin
   d. phenytoin (Dilantin)

4. Your pregnant patient has recurrent headaches. She states she has tried nonpharmacologic interventions but is unable to obtain relief. Which of the following analgesics would be best during your patient's pregnancy?
   a. acetaminophen
   b. aspirin
   c. ibuprofen
   d. codeine

NURSING MANAGEMENT: EVERY GOOD NURSE SHOULD …

Multiple Choice

Circle the option that best answers the question or completes the statement.

1. Your patient is in the first trimester of her pregnancy and has gestational diabetes. The physician has ordered a regimen of NPH insulin daily. You should

   a. contact the physician and request that oral hypoglycemics be ordered instead of NPH insulin.

   b. verify that blood glucose levels remain at levels above normal (>120) while the patient is taking insulin.

   c. teach the patient that she will need to take the insulin even after delivery.

   d. teach the patient that the insulin dose may need to be changed throughout the pregnancy.

2. Your pregnant patient has hyperemesis gravidarum. She is now in week 12 of the pregnancy. Antiemetic therapy of meclizine (piperazine) has been prescribed. She expresses concern to you about taking a drug while pregnant. Your patient education should include

   a. the risks of taking medicine during the second trimester.

   b. that piperazines have not been found to be teratogenic.

   c. the importance of taking this drug as frequently as possible.

   d. the benefits of hyperemesis gravidarum.

3. Your patient is 22 weeks' pregnant and is experiencing cardiac arrhythmia. Drug therapy has been prescribed. Before administering the first dose of the prescribed drug, you should

   a. verify the FDA pregnancy category of the drug.

   b. determine if the patient is allergic to the prescribed drug.

   c. verify if the dose is appropriate for the patient's age, weight, and health status.

   d. all of the above.

4. Your patient in the second trimester of pregnancy is experiencing some swelling of the ankles, feet, and hands. To minimize adverse effects from drug therapy, you should first

   a. consult with the physician or nurse midwife about ordering a mild diuretic.

   b. recommend a diet high in sodium.

   c. suggest the patient consume large amounts of coffee with caffeine for diuresis.

   d. instruct the patient to rest with her feet elevated several times a day.

5. Your patient in a postpartum care unit is a 17-year-old new mother who is an admitted abuser of heroin and cocaine. She is considering breast-feeding because it would be cheaper than bottle feeding. However, she is not sure that she wants to breast-feed. In your teaching with this patient, it is most important that you include information on

   a. the value to the infant from commercial formulas.

   b. heroin and cocaine being contraindicated with breast-feeding because of the effects on the infant.

   c. the importance of postpartum rest for the mother.

   d. positions for effective breast-feeding.

CASE STUDY

In the middle of January, a woman who is 26 weeks' pregnant comes to the emergency room having difficulty breathing. She is having bronchial constriction from bronchitis that developed after a bad cold. The physician orders aminophylline, a bronchodilator, administered by IV drip infusion. Aminophylline is a pregnancy category C drug. What assessments should be made while she receives IV aminophylline? When should use of the aminophylline be discontinued?

CRITICAL THINKING CHALLENGE

After delivery of a full-term, healthy baby, this same patient experiences continuing problems with bronchitis and is started on a regimen of ipratropium (Atrovent) via inhaler. This is a pregnancy category B drug and is an anticholinergic bronchodilator. The patient is breast-feeding. Should you be concerned about the patient breast-feeding while taking this drug? Are there other core patient variables that should be assessed with this patient?

CHAPTER 8

Life Span: Older Adults

TOP TEN THINGS TO KNOW ABOUT LIFE SPAN: OLDER ADULTS

1. Older adults share common age-related changes and risk factors that alter drug administration, dosage, and expected response to drug therapy.
2. Aging alters all of the pharmacokinetic processes, placing older adults at higher risk for adverse drug effects.
3. It is likely that disease processes alter the older adult's absorption patterns more than changes related to aging.
4. Decreased body mass, reduced levels of plasma albumin, and a less effective blood–brain barrier alter the older adult's distribution of drugs.
5. Hepatic metabolism is slowed and renal efficiency is decreased because of aging changes. Serum creatinine levels remain normal, even though kidney function is impaired.
6. Pharmacodynamics of drug therapy may be decreased in the older adult because of changes in the receptor systems.
7. Many of the signs and symptoms of health problems in older adults are attributable to the normal age-related decline in organ or system function. These symptoms of health problems often mimic the adverse effects of drug therapy.
8. Polypharmacy in older adults increases the risk for drug interactions and adverse effects.
9. Lifestyle of the older adult may affect the pharmacokinetics of drug therapy. Likewise, the adverse effects of drug therapy may affect the quality of life for the older adult.
10. To increase adherence, simplify the therapeutic regimen, give memory aids (if necessary), give written instructions, determine financial access to drug therapies, assess cultural barriers, and titrate the dose upward slowly to minimize adverse effects.

KEY TERMS

True or False

Mark true or false for the following statements. If the statement is false, replace the underlined word with the correct word to make a true statement.

1. _____ The margin between desired therapeutic effects and adverse consequences of drug therapy is called the <u>therapeutic index</u>.

2. _____ <u>Nonadherence</u> is the inability to follow a recommended drug therapy regimen.

3. _____ A patient who responds with hyperactivity to a drug that normally causes sedation has an adverse effect known as <u>idiosyncratic</u> excitement.

4. _____ A geriatric patient is also known as an <u>older adult</u>.

5. _____ The practice of one patient taking several drugs simultaneously is called <u>drug abuse</u>.

6. _____ An <u>older adult</u> is any patient older than 65 years with a debilitating medical problem.

PHYSIOLOGY AND PATHOPHYSIOLOGY: THE BODY HUMAN

Essay

1. Summarize the normal physiologic changes with age that affect absorption in an elderly patient receiving drug therapy.

2. Summarize the normal physiologic changes with age that affect distribution in an elderly patient receiving drug therapy.

3. Summarize the normal physiologic changes with age that affect metabolism in an elderly patient receiving drug therapy.

4. Summarize the normal physiologic changes with age that affect excretion in an elderly patient receiving drug therapy.

CORE DRUG KNOWLEDGE: JUST THE FACTS

Multiple Choice
Circle the option that best answers the question or completes the statement.

1. Because of age-related changes of the body, absorption of drugs in the elderly
   a. delays the onset of action.
   b. enhances the intensity of the peak response.
   c. is minimal compared with that in a younger adult.
   d. increases the risk for toxicity.

2. In the elderly patient, the dosage of fat-soluble drugs may need to be _____ to avoid toxicity.
   a. increased
   b. decreased
   c. neither of the above

3. Which of the following may occur as a result of physiologic changes in the elderly patient's metabolism?
   a. increased half-life
   b. decreased half-life
   c. decreased potential for adverse effects
   d. decreased potential for drug–drug interactions

4. Because of the reduction of creatinine production in the elderly patient, the creatinine clearance test may be normal. This is an indication of
   a. normal renal function.
   b. impaired renal function.
   c. more information concerning renal status being needed to make an assessment.
   d. impaired metabolism.

5. Which of the following is the least likely effect of drug therapy in the elderly?
   a. subtherapeutic drug regimens
   b. overdose or toxicity
   c. increased drug–drug interactions
   d. increased incidence of adverse effects

CORE PATIENT VARIABLES: PATIENTS, PLEASE

Multiple Choice
Circle the option that best answers the question or completes the statement.

1. Your patient, age 87 years, has been admitted to your unit with deep vein thrombosis of the left leg. The patient is receiving a heparin drip at the standard rate according to the standing protocol of the unit. Because of the patient's age, how may the aPTT be affected?
   a. It will not be affected.
   b. It may be 2 to $2^1/_2$ times the control.
   c. It may be more than 2 to $2^1/_2$ times the control.
   d. It may be less than the control.

2. Your patient has taken ibuprofen for arthritis for the past 5 years. As the patient advances with age, you would expect the onset of action to be
   a. delayed.
   b. shortened.
   c. the same, despite the age.

3. Your patient, age 89 years, is taking chloral hydrate, a hypnotic, for insomnia. The patient has an increased risk for which of the following adverse effects?
   a. sedation
   b. rash
   c. nausea
   d. paradoxical excitement

4. Which of the following questions should be included in an assessment of an elderly patient before drug therapy is initiated in an outpatient setting?
   a. "Do you have stairs in your home?"
   b. "Do you have difficulty opening the medication bottle?"
   c. "Do you have difficulty swallowing or chewing?"
   d. all of the above

Essay

Identify strategies that may decrease nonadherence to drug therapy in the elderly.

NURSING MANAGEMENT: EVERY GOOD NURSE SHOULD …

Multiple Choice

Circle the option that best answers the question or completes the statement.

1. Your patient, a 75-year-old man, tells you he needs to have his food cut finely because of trouble chewing and swallowing large pieces. What are the implications for his drug therapy?
   a. Drugs will not be absorbed as easily.
   b. The oral route cannot be used.
   c. Drugs will not be eliminated as easily.
   d. Oral drugs should be crushed or in a liquid form.

2. Your patient is an 80-year-old widow who lives alone. To assess potential problems with adherence to a prescribed drug regimen, you should determine
   a. whether the patient has friends that visit during the week.
   b. how the patient usually obtains refills on her prescriptions.
   c. the amount of fluid that she drinks in a day.
   d. whether she has renal or hepatic disease.

3. A 68-year-old patient is receiving gentamicin IV for a severe infection. Gentamicin has the adverse effect of causing renal toxicity. The nurse would expect that the ordered dose of gentamicin for this patient would be
   a. larger than the average adult dose.
   b. smaller than the average adult dose.
   c. the same as the average adult dose.
   d. larger than the average adult dose but given less frequently.

4. A 70-year-old man is started on a regimen of phenytoin, an antiepileptic, for a new onset of seizures. When he returns to the clinic for his 3-week checkup after starting the drug therapy, his daughter confides that she thinks her father is getting old. He falls asleep during the daytime frequently now and seems to have difficulty following conversations. The best response for the nurse is:
   a. "Yes, it's a shame to get older, isn't it?"
   b. "You need to expect these changes with aging."
   c. "These are signs that he is not getting enough drug therapy."
   d. "These are signs of adverse effects associated with the drug therapy."

5. An 84-year-old woman had surgery to repair a broken hip. Morphine, a narcotic, has been ordered for her for pain relief. The order states that she may have 4 to 10 mg every 4 hours as needed. If giving the first dose of the pain medication to this patient, the nurse should select
   a. 4 mg.
   b. 6 mg.
   c. 8 mg.
   d. 10 mg.

CASE STUDY

A 68-year-old man is admitted to your unit with uncontrolled hypertension. He also has a history of COPD and CHF. He was recently in the hospital for exacerbation of his COPD. In your assessment, you ask him about his drug therapies and if he takes them as prescribed. He replies that he is always taking some pill or other. He admits that he might forget sometimes to take some of his doses because there are so many. You write down what he says he takes and compare it with his discharge orders for drug therapy, written at the end of his last hospitalization.

Patient's List	Discharge Orders for Drug Therapy
"fluid pill" 2 × day	furosemide (Lasix) 40 mg BID
"pressure pill" 2 or 3 × day	captopril (Capoten) 100 mg TID
"heart pill" every day	nicardipine (Cardene) 30 mg BID
potassium 2 × day	potassium (K-Dur) 10-mg tablet BID
"breathing pill" 2 × day	theophylline (TheoDur) 100 mg q12 h

Is the patient receiving all of the prescribed drug therapy? Determine what times this patient should be taking drug therapy at home. What can you do to help him remember to take his drug therapy when it is due?

CRITICAL THINKING CHALLENGE

What other issues should you explore with this patient to determine whether nonadherence with the prescribed drug therapy is contributing to frequent hospitalizations?

CHAPTER 9

Lifestyle: Substance Abuse

TOP TEN THINGS TO KNOW ABOUT LIFESTYLE: SUBSTANCE ABUSE

1. Substance abuse is a problem occurring throughout the life span and in all socioeconomic, ethnic, and cultural groups.

2. Three components must be present for drug addiction to have occurred: psychological dependence, physical dependence, and tolerance. Physical dependence and tolerance may occur independently without psychological dependence (behavioral changes and cravings). When this happens, addiction has not occurred.

3. Genetic disposition, developmental and environmental influences, personality traits, mood disorders, availability of drugs, cultural attitudes, and socioeconomic factors may all contribute to substance abuse in an individual.

4. Most abused drugs affect the central nervous system as stimulants, depressants, or hallucinogens.

5. Alcohol is the most widely abused central nervous system (CNS) depressant. Nicotine is the most widely abused CNS stimulant.

6. Prescription drugs may be abused for their own effects, for a combined effect that is similar to that obtained from an illegal drug, to increase the duration or "high" of an illegal drug, or to prevent withdrawal from an illegal drug.

7. Cocaine, a CNS stimulant, increases neurotransmitter (dopamine, norepinephrine, and serotonin) activity, leading to ease of addiction; prolonged, intense craving during withdrawal; and high rates of relapse.

8. Abused substances have significant adverse effects on developing fetuses, infants, and children. The effects from substance abuse may be misinterpreted as signs of aging in the older adult.

9. Substance abuse may create health problems requiring drug therapy, require drug therapy to prevent or treat withdrawal, or interact with drug therapy for another physiologic problem.

10. Nurses need to assess patients for substance abuse, act to prevent life-threatening or debilitating effects from a substance or its withdrawal, administer drugs to treat withdrawal or its symptoms, and provide education about the substance, addiction, drug therapy, and rehabilitation.

KEY TERMS

Crossword Puzzle

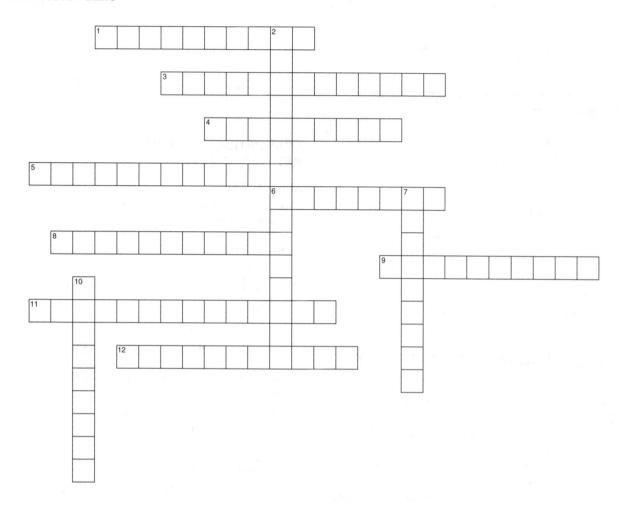

ACROSS

1. A syndrome caused by sudden cessation of drug ingestion
3. A type of dependence that results from the influence of drugs on brain chemistry
4. A type of abuse involving self-administration of drug substance for nonmedical purposes
5. Another term for CNS stimulants
6. A type of dependence that occurs when the body "needs" the drug for homeostasis
8. Another term for addiction
9. Another name for abstinence syndrome
11. Tolerance to a drug in a particular class transfers to another drug in the same class
12. Another term for hallucinogens

DOWN

2. Use of a drug in the same class as the dependent drug keeps the patient from experiencing withdrawal syndrome

7. The state of having a physical or psychological need for a drug
10. The body develops a natural resistance to a drug's physical or euphoric effects

PHYSIOLOGY AND PATHOPHYSIOLOGY: THE BODY HUMAN

Matching
Match the drug with the correct physiologic effects during intoxication.

1. _____ inhalants

2. _____ amphetamines

3. _____ opioids

4. _____ alcohol

a. Motor incoordination, nystagmus, slurred speech

b. Motor agitation, papillary dilation, tachycardia

c. Pinpoint pupils, euphoria, apathy

d. Distorted perceptions, light-headedness, euphoria

Matching
Match the drug with the correct physiologic effects during withdrawal.

1. _____ inhalants

2. _____ amphetamines

3. _____ opioids

4. _____ alcohol

a. Myalgia, piloerection, yawning

b. Fatigue, nightmares, depression, increased appetite

c. None, appreciably

d. Nausea, vomiting, tremors, seizures

CORE DRUG KNOWLEDGE: JUST THE FACTS

True or False
Mark the following statements true or false.

1. _____ Psychological dependence occurs because the patient has a pre-existing mental health disorder.

2. _____ Chronic stress is an environmental factor that may influence a person's substance abuse.

3. _____ There is a clearly identified addictive personality.

4. _____ Drug abuse occurs most frequently in lower socioeconomic groups.

5. _____ Individuals with a personality disorder may use drugs initially to become socially acceptable.

6. _____ The three main categories of abusable drugs are CNS stimulants, CNS depressants, and hallucinogens.

7. _____ Designer drugs are difficult to develop but are very popular because of their safety profile.

8. _____ Common adverse effects to anabolic-androgenic steroids include sex hormone imbalances, permanent sterility, and hepatic cancer.

9. _____ Alcoholism may induce hypertension.

10. _____ Cocaine has a very long half-life and can sustain a "high" for 12 hours.

CORE PATIENT VARIABLES: PATIENTS, PLEASE

Multiple Choice
Circle the option that best answers the question or completes the statement.

1. In the alcoholic patient, liver damage may be attributed to the
   a. mechanism by which alcohol is metabolized.
   b. increased absorption of alcohol.
   c. interference of nerve impulses.
   d. utilization of the P-450 enzyme system.

2. Your patient is admitted to the hospital for acute anemia. He has received a diagnosis of esophageal varices. Knowing this information, you would monitor for symptoms of
   a. opiate withdrawal.
   b. alcohol withdrawal.
   c. cocaine withdrawal.
   d. hallucinogen withdrawal.

3. In the patient who abuses cocaine, which of the following vital signs would you expect to see?
   a. BP 100/90; P 88; R 22
   b. BP 122/88; P 60; R 16
   c. BP 150/100; P 100; R 22
   d. BP 140/90; P 82; R 12

4. In the patient who abuses heroin, which of the following would you expect?
   a. frequent bronchitis
   b. abscess formation
   c. pruritus
   d. renal failure

5. You notice that your patient has very labile moods: one minute he is quiet, and the next he is yelling loudly. Which of the following is most likely the substance that has been abused?
   a. heroin
   b. cocaine
   c. glue
   d. LSD

6. Your patient, age 16 years, comes to the school nurse with a complaint of decreased mental and physical abilities. With your knowledge of substance abuse, which of the following drugs do you think may be responsible for these symptoms?
   a. PCP
   b. cannabis
   c. inhalants
   d. CNS stimulants

7. Your 32-year-old patient has just delivered a baby with microencephaly and craniofacial abnormalities. What drug of abuse may be responsible?
   a. alcohol
   b. heroin
   c. cocaine
   d. marijuana

8. Your patient confides to you that she had been unable to stop her use of heroin during her pregnancy and is concerned about her newborn. You should expect the baby to demonstrate which of these behaviors?
   a. microencephaly
   b. cleft palate
   c. tremor, increased muscle tone, or hyperirritability
   d. weak cry, lethargy, decreased muscle tone

NURSING MANAGEMENT: EVERY GOOD NURSE SHOULD …

Multiple Choice
Circle the option that best answers the question or completes the statement.

1. When the nurse is performing a complete drug history and health assessment, the patient should be questioned about use of which of the following substances?
   a. cigarettes
   b. alcohol
   c. street or recreational drugs
   d. all of the above

2. Your patient is a recovered alcoholic and has started a regimen of disulfiram (Antabuse). Which of the following should be included in the teaching about this drug?
   a. Take this drug whenever you have a desire to drink.
   b. This drug has no adverse effects at all.
   c. If you drink any alcohol while you are taking this drug, you will feel ill.
   d. Moderate drinking is allowed while taking this drug.

3. A 17-year-old girl is brought to a busy emergency room by some friends. The girl is screaming, covering her ears and eyes with her hands, and appears to be having hallucinations. Her friends say she used some LSD at a party. An initial nursing action should include
   a. placing her on a stretcher in the middle of the emergency room to observe her.
   b. administering phenothiazines if ordered.
   c. staying with her and speaking calmly and soothingly.
   d. referring her to an inpatient psychiatric facility.

4. As a middle-school nurse, you are called to a classroom to help a 12-year-old boy who is short of breath after sniffing correction fluid. An item of priority that you should bring with you from the health suite is
   a. a syringe of epinephrine.
   b. portable oxygen.
   c. an emesis basin.
   d. a defibrillator.

5. Your patient is an alcoholic who has completed a detoxification program. The patient has been prescribed naltrexone (Vivitrol). Which of the following nursing actions would be appropriate for this patient?

   a. Advise the patient to take the medication at the same time each day.

   b. Coordinate a clinic appointment in 1 month for the patient to receive the next dose of medication.

   c. Arrange for periodic blood alcohol testing.

   d. Refer the patient to a psychiatrist to obtain additional treatment for alcoholism.

CASE STUDY

A 35-year-old successful lawyer is admitted to your unit on a Monday morning after surgery, with general anesthesia, to repair a torn rotator cuff. He received the narcotic morphine in the recovery room for complaints of pain. It is now 2 hours after surgery and 1 hour after the morphine injection. He is somewhat more difficult to arouse than most patients after surgery. His history states that he drinks "socially on weekends." When asked to clarify this, his wife states that he usually has one or two drinks before dinner, a bottle of wine with dinner, one or two drinks after dinner, and then usually another drink or two later in the evening on Friday, Saturday, and Sunday nights.

What factors might be contributing to the difficulty in arousing this patient after surgery?

CRITICAL THINKING CHALLENGE

On Tuesday, this same patient is somewhat irritable and anxious. You note a very fine tremor in his hands when he offers you his arm to take his pulse. His pulse is 90 beats per minute.

1. What assessment might you make from these data? What actions should you take?

2. Assessment of a patient's physical condition may be influenced by bias or stereotypical thinking of the health care provider. What factors may lead a nurse or other health care provider to overlook alcohol abuse and possible withdrawal in this patient?

CHAPTER 10

Lifestyle, Diet, and Habits: Nutrition and Complementary Medications

TOP TEN THINGS TO KNOW ABOUT LIFESTYLE, DIET, AND HABITS: NUTRITION AND COMPLEMENTARY MEDICATIONS

1. The use of dietary supplements, herbs, and other botanicals to promote wellness is considered a complementary therapy.
2. A well-balanced diet may prevent chronic illness, indirectly decreasing the need for drug therapy.
3. Nutritional deficiencies may occur because of chronic illness or as an adverse effect of drug therapy.
4. Malnutrition, with decreased protein stores, can alter the effectiveness of many drug therapies. Low serum protein levels can cause significantly elevated serum levels of drugs that are normally highly protein bound.
5. Some foods, beverages, and dietary supplements can affect the pharmacokinetics of a drug. Grapefruit and grapefruit juice interact with many drugs via the P-450 system.
6. Some foods, beverages, and dietary supplements can alter the effectiveness of some drugs or produce an adverse effect.
7. Adverse drug–nutrient interactions are most likely to occur with medications taken for chronic conditions, if several medications are taken, or if nutrition status is poor or deteriorating.
8. The nurse should encourage the patient to inform all health care providers about all dietary supplements (including herbs) used.
9. Drug interactions can occur with many herbs. The nurse should teach the patient and family about any potential interactions of drug therapy with herbal preparations.
10. The nurse should always ask if the patient uses dietary supplements because patients may not realize the importance of mentioning this use.

KEY TERMS

1. Differentiate between the terms alternative therapy and complementary therapy.

2. Define herbal and botanical preparations.

3. Identify the major mineral cations.

4. Define phytomedicinals.

5. Identify the most important trace elements.

6. Define the word vitamin.

CORE DRUG KNOWLEDGE: JUST THE FACTS

Multiple Choice
Circle the option that best answers the question or completes the statement.

1. Which of the following should encompass approximately 50% to 60% of a healthy diet per day?
   a. protein
   b. fats
   c. carbohydrates
   d. dietary fiber

2. Which of the following major mineral cations plays a role in the transmission of nerve impulses, contraction of cardiac, skeletal, and smooth muscle, acid-base balance, and the maintenance of normal renal function?
   a. calcium
   b. magnesium
   c. potassium
   d. sodium

3. Which of the following types of vitamins requires frequent consumption to maintain adequate body levels?
   a. water-soluble vitamins
   b. lipid-soluble vitamins
   c. both of the above

4. Which of the following trace elements is essential for the formation of red blood cells?
   a. chromium
   b. copper
   c. iron
   d. selenium

CORE PATIENT VARIABLES: PATIENTS, PLEASE

Multiple Choice
Circle the option that best answers the question or completes the statement.

1. Your patient has taken an overdose of a vitamin/mineral supplement. You assess central nervous system changes, hypotension, and an abnormal electrocardiogram. Which of the following minerals is most likely to cause these symptoms?
   a. calcium
   b. magnesium
   c. potassium
   d. sodium

2. Your patient has hypertension and is prescribed furosemide (Lasix) 40 mg QD. In this patient, it is important to monitor
   a. trace elements.
   b. protein.
   c. dietary fiber.
   d. major mineral cations.

3. Your patient is admitted to the medical-surgical unit for management of a deep vein thrombosis (DVT). During your admission assessment, you find that the patient is homeless and consumes alcohol on a daily basis. For therapy to be successful, which of the following nutritional states should be further evaluated?
   a. vitamin consumption
   b. use of dietary fiber
   c. protein intake
   d. carbohydrate intake

NURSING MANAGEMENT: EVERY GOOD NURSE SHOULD …

Multiple Choice

Circle the option that best answers the question or completes the statement.

1. Which of the following should be included in a drug history?
   a. Do you use any vitamin or nutritional supplements?
   b. Do you use any herbal supplements?
   c. Who recommended that you use this supplement?
   d. all of the above
   e. none of the above

2. You are caring for a patient who is 94 years old. He has a history of hypertension, cardiac arrhythmias, hyperlipidemia, and an enlarged prostate. He takes five different prescription drugs for these problems. You should assess for
   a. nutritional deficiencies.
   b. typical daily diet.
   c. the time of day prescribed medications are taken.
   d. all of the above.
   e. none of the above.

3. A patient who has chronic obstructive pulmonary disease (COPD) and takes prednisone as an immune suppressant as part of her drug therapy is returning to the clinic for follow-up. She tells you, the nurse, that because the weather is getting colder, she is going to start taking Echinacea to keep her from getting pneumonia. Your best response is:
   a. "That's a good idea. You should also take vitamin C."
   b. "Echinacea will be beneficial to your COPD and make you feel better."
   c. "Echinacea may counteract the immunosuppressant effect of the prednisone, and you might actually have more respiratory problems."
   d. "Be sure you buy your Echinacea from a reputable source."

Case Study

Your patient is malnourished because of a history of alcohol abuse. He is hospitalized with a deep vein thrombosis in his left leg and is prescribed intraveinous heparin as treatment. Heparin is an anticoagulant and highly protein bound. After 24 hours of heparin therapy, the patient's coagulation time is much longer (i.e., he bleeds longer) than would be expected from the heparin infusion. What might be contributing to his altered coagulation time? How would you confirm your assessment?

CRITICAL THINKING CHALLENGE

The patient described above is discharged home on warfarin, an oral anticoagulant, also highly protein bound. His coagulation times at discharge are lengthened appropriately to be therapeutic from the warfarin. When he returns to the clinic for follow-up in 4 weeks, he tells you he has been trying to improve his health by cutting down on his drinking and using herbs. He tells you he has been drinking chamomile tea several times a day as a substitute for some of the alcohol that he drank. He thinks the chamomile tea soothes his stomach pain from a gastric ulcer that flared up from alcohol use. He also tells you that he is taking garlic tablets to bring down his cholesterol levels. His laboratory results show that his coagulation time is excessively elevated. What might be contributing to his altered laboratory values?

Environment: Influences on Drug Therapy

TOP TEN THINGS TO KNOW ABOUT ENVIRONMENT: INFLUENCES ON DRUG THERAPY

1. The environment where drug therapy may occur is diverse. It may be the acute care hospital, acute rehabilitation unit, transitional care unit, outpatient center, long-term care facility, or the patient's home. Medication reconciliation is completed each time the patient transfers from one environment to another.

2. Each type of environment has limitations as to which drug may be given or which route of drug administration may be used. These limitations are related to the need for close monitoring of the patient, specialized equipment, life-saving equipment and drugs, and specialized personnel.

3. Environmental conditions, such as pollutants, heat, light, moisture, and temperature, can alter a drug's pharmacokinetics or a drug's pharmacodynamics.

4. Environmental factors may make the patient more susceptible to adverse effects from drug therapy (such as sunlight and photosensitivity).

5. Environmental factors of the home may place the patient at increased risk of injury if a drug adverse effect does occur (such as falls from dizziness when there are no stair railings).

6. The patient's occupation, part of his/her personal environment, may place him/her at added risks for some adverse effects associated with drug therapy.

7. Environmental pollutions or toxins in the home or place of employment may create a specific disease or an alteration in the health status, necessitating drug therapy.

8. The nurse should assess the environment where drug therapy will occur for potential influences on pharmacotherapy.

9. The nurse should consider environmental factors that can maximize the therapeutic effect and minimize the adverse effects of some drug therapies. (For example, some drugs deteriorate if exposed to light, so keeping the drug out of the light will maximize the therapeutic effect.)

10. Providing patient and family education about the potential interactions of drug therapy and the patient environment is an important nursing action.

KEY TERMS

Matching
Match the following words or terms with the correct definition.

1. _____ hepatic drug-metabolizing enzymes

2. _____ environment

3. _____ industrial chemicals

4. _____ medication reconciliation

5. _____ pollutants

a. Physical setting in which a drug is given

b. Contaminated or noxious substances

c. Compounds that may influence pharmacologic properties of drugs

d. Used to biotransform drugs

e. The process of identifying potential omissions or errors in patient orders

CORE DRUG KNOWLEDGE: JUST THE FACTS

1. Identify the major environmental settings in which drugs are administered.

2. In addition to the setting, what other concepts are important to the safe administration of medications?

3. Identify possible environmental influences on drug stability.

4. List environmental chemicals that may induce hepatic drug-metabolizing enzymes in susceptible patients.

5. What two environmental factors are most frequently associated with the development of cancer?

CORE PATIENT VARIABLES: PATIENTS, PLEASE

Multiple Choice
Circle the option that best answers the question or completes the statement.

1. Your patient is a heavy cigarette smoker who has bronchitis and takes a bronchodilator. Because cigarette smoke is an active inducer of hepatic enzymes, this patient should be monitored for
   a. continued symptoms of bronchitis.
   b. adverse effects because of drug toxicity.
   c. both of the above.
   d. neither of the above.

2. A patient has been given instructions about taking opioid medications at home. Which of these statements, if made by the patient, would indicate that the patient needs additional teaching?
   a. "I will change positions slowly."
   b. "I will not drink any alcohol while I take these drugs."
   c. "I will take only one pill when I drive."
   d. "I will hold onto the handrail when I go upstairs."

3. Your patient had total knee replacement surgery today. At 10 PM the nurse administers a sedative-hypnotic agent to help the patient fall asleep. When doing rounds at 1 AM, you find the patient still awake. Which of the following would be appropriate at this time?
   a. Use this time to teach the patient leg-strengthening exercises.
   b. Close the patient's door to decrease external stimuli.
   c. Contact the physician for additional orders.
   d. Offer the patient a snack.

4. Your patient is being discharged from the hospital later today. What is the primary role of the nurse regarding drug therapy at this time?
   a. consultation with a pharmacy
   b. patient advocacy with the billing department
   c. patient education
   d. referral

NURSING MANAGEMENT: EVERY GOOD NURSE SHOULD…

Multiple Choice
Circle the option that best answers the question or completes the statement.

1. It is May and your patient is being sent home with a prescription for tetracycline, an antibiotic that is known to cause photosensitivity reactions. In your assessment of her learning needs related to environmental concerns, you should ask the patient
   a. if she can refrigerate the drug at home.
   b. where she normally stores medications.
   c. how many people live in the house.
   d. how much time she spends outdoors.

2. Your patient has started taking a vasodilator for hypertension. He tells you he can't wait to get home and take a long soak in his hot tub. The best response to this patient is:

 a. "Soaking in hot tubs will be helpful with this drug therapy. Do it every day."

 b. "Excessive heat from hot tubs will cause additional vasodilation and may cause problems for you. Please avoid using them now."

 c. "Hot tubs will not have any effect on this drug therapy. Use them if you wish."

 d. "I'm envious. Can I make a home visit and use the hot tub with you?"

3. Your patient works in the insulation industry and handles polychlorinated biphenyls as part of his job activities. When doing patient education about his prescribed drug therapy (a drug that is highly metabolized in the liver), you would want to emphasize

 a. that he should contact the physician if he has any of the adverse effects that you describe.

 b. that he cannot go to work while he is on this drug therapy.

 c. that adverse effects are less likely to occur in him than in other patients.

 d. none of the above.

4. You have just received a new patient from the step-down unit of your hospital. Your supervisor asks if you have completed medication reconciliation for this patient. The purpose of medication reconciliation is to

 a. comply with a regulating agency's requirement.

 b. obtain a medication history from the patient.

 c. improve patient outcomes.

 d. review the health care provider's orders.

CASE STUDY

A 20-year-old woman is 42 weeks' pregnant with her first child, and the obstetrician wishes to administer oxytocin to induce her labor. The obstetrician has a nurse who works with her in the office, and he can stay with the patient. Would the obstetrician start the oxytocin infusion in her office?

CRITICAL THINKING CHALLENGE

You are a nurse working on a general medical surgical unit. The admitting department calls and tells you that your unit will receive the above-mentioned patient because the labor and delivery suite is currently full, and there are no beds on the postpartum floor. The admitting department says the patient can be transferred to the delivery room at the time of delivery but will return to your floor after giving birth. What would you do in this situation?

CHAPTER **12**

Culture and Inherited Traits: Considerations in Drug Therapy

TOP TEN THINGS TO KNOW ABOUT CULTURE AND INHERITED TRAITS: CONSIDERATIONS IN DRUG THERAPY

1. The five major cultures in the United States are white American, black American, Asian/Pacific Islander American, Hispanic American, and Native American Indian/Alaskan Native.

2. Many cultural groups in the United States have beliefs that reflect both their original ethnic culture and the dominant culture of the United States. Although members of a culture share certain beliefs and practices, individual variations still occur. Each patient needs to be considered an individual.

3. Pharmacogenetics is the study of individual inherited differences in response to clinical drug therapy. Pharmacogenes are those genes involved in the response to a drug. People with variations of genetically carried traits can have alterations in many drug processes resulting in an increased or decreased drug level; or increased or decreased effectiveness of a drug's dose. These changes place these patients at risk for developing adverse effects or clinical failure from drug therapy

4. White Americans (e.g., European Americans) have a linear sense of time, are future oriented, are predominantly Christian, share bioscientific views of disease and health management, and rely primarily on traditional Western medical practices.

5. Black Americans (e.g., African Americans) have a circular view of time, are present oriented, are more relaxed about time than European Americans, tend to be spiritual, are predominantly Christian, may use folk medicine, and, in general, have different responses to some drugs than do white Americans.

6. Asian/Pacific Islander Americans (e.g., Chinese Americans) have a concept of time related to the natural cycles of birth, life, and death; believe time is to be integrated into life; may or may not value punctuality; may or may not belong to a formal religion; believe that the body and spirit must be maintained through harmony with nature and yin and yang; have health care practices that include traditional Chinese medicine and Western medicine; and may be affected differently than white Americans by herbal medicines and Western drugs.

7. Hispanic Americans (e.g., Mexican Americans) are more present than future oriented. They may or may not value punctuality, may believe that life is ruled by chance or luck or be deeply religious, are primarily Catholic, believe that disease occurs when there is an imbalance between opposing life forces (hot, cold, wet, dry), and may metabolize some drugs differently from those in other cultural groups.

8. Native American Indians (e.g., Navaho Indians) are present oriented; attach little value to planning for the future; view time as nonimportant; are spiritual but do not practice formalized religions; believe good health depends on maintaining a balance among the elements of the body, mind (or spirit), and environment; and use herbal remedies to treat disease. Younger Native American Indians are more accepting of Western medical practices than are older Native American Indians. Responses to drug therapy may vary by tribe, but this has not been studied adequately.

9. The nurse should consider the patient's cultural backgrounds, religious preferences, personal practices, and ethnic background when providing nursing care in drug therapy.

10. Patient education related to drug therapy needs to consider cultural variations to be effective.

KEY TERMS

Use the following anagrams to define the key terms:

1. Study of inherited differences in response to clinical drug therapy

N I M H O S A G T C A E C R P E

☐☐☐☐☐☐☐☐☐☐☐☐☐☐☐☐

2. Specific physical, biologic, and psychosocial variations in ethnic and racial groups

O I B L R A T L U C U
L O Y G C O E

☐☐☐☐☐☐☐☐☐☐☐
☐☐☐☐☐☐☐

3. Assumption that all members of a particular ethnic or cultural group will have the same response

G S Y R P E E T I T O N

☐☐☐☐☐☐☐☐☐☐☐☐

4. Shared customs and traditions of a group

T E U C U L R

☐☐☐☐☐☐☐

5. The inability to accept the culture of others

N E S T E T C R H O M I N

☐☐☐☐☐☐☐☐☐☐☐☐☐

6. Group that shares common cultural heritage linked by race, nationality, and/or language

I I Y C T T N H E

☐☐☐☐☐☐☐☐☐

7. Awareness of one's own values and beliefs without letting it have undue influence on those of other backgrounds

T L C L U U A R
E C N E T E M P C O

☐☐☐☐☐☐☐☐☐
☐☐☐☐☐☐☐☐☐

8. Inability to recognize differences between groups or individuals within a group

T L U C R U L A
D N I L N S B S E

☐☐☐☐☐☐☐☐
☐☐☐☐☐☐☐☐☐

9. Study of patterns of human genome variations known to influence drug action

G M C A N A O S O R H E P M I C

☐☐☐☐☐☐☐☐☐☐☐☐☐☐☐☐

CORE DRUG KNOWLEDGE: JUST THE FACTS

Multiple Choice
Circle the option that best answers the question or completes the statement.

1. Despite cultural differences, the goal of the nurse is to
   a. provide appropriate nursing care.
   b. "normalize" patient behaviors.
   c. integrate all cultural customs into drug therapy.
   d. be aware of each culture's acceptable practices.

2. A nurse with cultural competence
   a. is able to provide care for an individual from a particular culture.
   b. understands the difference between cultural beliefs that coincide with Western medicine and those that do not.
   c. accepts and respects cultural and ethnic differences.
   d. is able to assist patients of different cultures to attain acculturation.

3. Biocultural ecology
   a. integrates commonalities among different cultures to the care of a patient.
   b. examines physical, biologic, and psychological variations in ethnic or racial groups.
   c. predicts common behavior patterns of a particular culture or ethnic group.
   d. categorizes cultures according to geographic locality.

4. The philosophy of yin and yang is prevalent in which of the following groups?

   a. Chinese Americans

   b. African Americans

   c. European Americans

   d. Native Americans

5. In planning drug therapy for a Chinese-American patient, which of the following drugs does *not* need consideration for a lower dose?

   a. amitriptyline (Elavil), a tricyclic antidepressant

   b. diazepam (Valium), a benzodiazepine

   c. penicillin (Pen-VEE K), an antibiotic

   d. propranolol (Inderal), a beta-adrenergic antagonist

Essay

1. List the 12 domains of Purnell's model for cultural competence.

2. What is the difference between mutation and polymorphism?

3. What is the potential role for pharmacogenomics in drug therapy?

CORE PATIENT VARIABLES: PATIENTS, PLEASE

Multiple Choice
Circle the option that best answers the question or completes the statement.

1. Which of the following influences may be associated with a white-American patient?

   a. They tend to place little emphasis on the importance of obtaining medications.

   b. Primarily, they have a magicoreligious view of disease and health management.

   c. They are usually future oriented and have a strong work ethic.

   d. They tend to be late for appointments or meetings.

2. Which of the following influences may be associated with an African-American patient?

   a. They have a linear view of time.

   b. Most families have a nuclear family with the father being the head of the family.

   c. They are very religious and are accepting of medical treatment unless it is viewed contrary to their religious beliefs.

   d. The drug response and adverse effects profile of drug therapy are the same as those for white Americans.

3. Which of the following influences may be associated with a Chinese-American patient?

   a. Time is of little value and can be mastered for their benefit.

   b. Harmony with nature is essential for spiritual and physical well-being.

   c. They rarely use herbal medications.

   d. They metabolize drugs the same as do patients of other cultures.

4. Which of the following influences may be associated with a Hispanic-American patient?

   a. They tend to seek medical attention rather than use self-care practices.

   b. They believe an imbalance of hot, cold, wet, and dry may induce disease.

   c. The families tend to be matriarchal.

   d. They metabolize drugs the same as do patients of other cultures.

5. Which of the following influences may be associated with a Native-American patient?

   a. They believe good health depends on maintaining a balance among the elements of the body, mind or spirit, and environment.

   b. The families tend to be patriarchal.

   c. They tend to be very punctual for appointments.

   d. Frequency of disease is the same for all tribal groups.

6. In order to be an effective culturally competent nurse, it is important to

   a. develop cultural blindness when giving patient care.

   b. integrate all cultural practices into patient care.

c. remember that cultural patterns are helpful, but a wide range of responses is possible within each group.

d. assist the patient to acculturation.

NURSING MANAGEMENT: EVERY GOOD NURSE SHOULD …

Multiple Choice
Circle the option that best answers the question or completes the statement.

1. Why is it important to assess the patient's cultural background before beginning drug therapy?

   a. Patients may respond to drug therapy differently depending on their cultural and racial background.

   b. Patients' attitudes about the value of drug therapy may contribute to their adherence to the drug therapy regimen.

   c. Patients may use folk or herbal remedies based on their cultural background that may interact with the prescribed drug therapy.

   d. All of the above are important reasons.

2. You have worked with a patient who is a Mexican American for several days. You have come to learn that he is generally present-time oriented. He has been hospitalized for osteomyelitis, a severe infection of the bone. He has received antibiotic therapy intravenously and is to be discharged on a regimen of oral antibiotics for 6 more weeks. In your teaching about the drug, you most likely want to emphasize

   a. failure to take all of the prescription will cause him to be hospitalized again.

   b. evenly spaced daily doses will help to keep the drug levels up to treat the infection.

   c. skipping doses eventually may cause permanent damage to the bone.

   d. all of the above.

3. An elderly Chinese American was hospitalized for a heart attack. He tells you he did not come to the hospital sooner because he thought he had only indigestion. He had treated himself for the "indigestion" with ginseng. To minimize adverse effects from the currently prescribed drug therapy, the most effective response of the nurse would be to

   a. tease the patient about his use of herbs.

   b. tell the patient that he is foolish to use herbs.

   c. emphasize to the patient that Western medicine is much safer than using herbs.

   d. ask the patient to describe other herbs that he uses regularly.

4. Three patients have been admitted to your unit for treatment of tuberculosis. One is a Native American Indian, one is a white American, and one is an Asian/Pacific Islander American. They are all to be started on isoniazid for tuberculosis. The nurse would expect that the ordered interval between doses might be longer for which of these patients?

   a. the white American

   b. the Native American Indian

   c. the Asian/Pacific Islander American

   d. The interval would be the same for all three.

5. Your patient is known to be an ultra-rapid metabolizer of certain P-450 drugs. Which of the following nursing actions would be most appropriate for this patient?

   a. Monitor for the patient more closely for adverse effects.

   b. Monitor the patient for continued symptoms of the disorder being treated.

   c. Monitor the drug levels daily.

   d. Refuse to administer this medication to the patient.

CASE STUDY

Two patients, one a Chinese-American woman and the other an African-American man, both begin a regimen of the same sulfonamide antibiotic for a urinary tract infection. At a 3-week follow-up appointment, the woman is found to be anemic, but the man has normal hemoglobin levels.

What factors might be contributing to this different response to the identical drug therapy?

CRITICAL THINKING CHALLENGE

What other core patient variables might have placed the Chinese-American woman at increased risk for anemia?

CHAPTER 13

Drugs Affecting Adrenergic Function

TOP TEN THINGS TO KNOW ABOUT DRUGS AFFECTING ADRENERGIC FUNCTION

1. Norepinephrine is the terminal neurotransmitter in the sympathetic nervous system (SNS); the receptors are alpha-1, alpha-2, beta-1, and beta-2. Drugs that stimulate the receptors are called agonists; those that block are antagonists or blockers. Most drugs are nonselective as they stimulate or block more than one receptor at a time, although some drugs are relatively selective in their stimulation or blockade.

2. Stimulation of alpha-1 receptors causes vasoconstriction, increased peripheral resistance, increased blood pressure, pupil dilation (mydriasis), and increased closure of the internal sphincter of the bladder. Blocking alpha-1 receptors causes the opposite effects. Stimulation of alpha-2 receptors decreases release of norepinephrine, reducing sympathetic outflow from brain, and produces vasodilation with a resultant decrease in blood pressure. Currently, there are no alpha-2 blocking agents approved in the United States.

3. Stimulation of beta-1 receptors causes tachycardia, increased myocardial contractility, and increased lipolysis. Blocking beta-1 receptors causes the opposite effects.

4. Stimulation of beta-2 receptors causes bronchodilation, vasodilation, slightly decreased peripheral resistance, increased muscle and liver glycolysis, increased release of glucagon, and relaxation of uterine smooth muscle. Blocking beta-2 receptors causes the opposite effects.

5. Epinephrine is a nonselective adrenergic agonist that stimulates all alpha and beta receptors. It has many uses, primarily to treat cardiopulmonary arrest, ventricular fibrillation, anaphylactic shock, and asthma. Adverse effects are related to stimulation of all receptors. Central nervous system (CNS) and cardiac adverse effects are most common and may be the most serious.

6. Phenylephrine is an alpha-1 stimulant and a potent vasoconstrictor used to treat vascular failure, hypotension, and related shock. It also is used as a nasal decongestant and to cause pupil dilation (mydriasis). Avoid intravenous (IV) extravasation.

7. Prazosin, an alpha-1 blocker, is used to treat hypertension and benign prostatic hypertrophy (BPH). The first dose may cause syncope.

8. Dopamine, the precursor to norepinephrine, affects three types of receptors. Low-dose dopamine stimulates the dopaminergic receptors, producing an increase in renal blood flow, glomerular filtration rate, and urinary output. Moderate-dose dopamine is a beta-1 stimulant used to correct hemodynamic imbalances present in shock; it increases cardiac output, the force of contraction, and heart rate, and it dilates vessels in the cerebral, cardiac, renal, and mesenteric vascular beds. High-dose dopamine stimulates alpha-1 receptors, increasing peripheral resistance and blood pressure.

9. Propranolol is a nonspecific beta blocker used primarily for cardiovascular disorders. Adverse effects occur most frequently in the cardiac and respiratory systems. Use of this drug should be discontinued slowly to prevent rebound tachycardia, leading to angina and possibly myocardial infarction.

10. Fenoldopam stimulates the dopaminergic and alpha-2 receptors. It is used to rapidly reduce severe hypertension. It is also used to prevent radiocontrast dye-induced renal impairment in high-risk patients.

KEY TERMS

Fill in the Blank
Complete the following sentences using the correct key term.

1. The _CNS_ is comprised of the brain and spinal cord.

2. The _PNS_ consists of all neurons that are found outside the brain and spinal cord.

3. The _ANS_ has been identified as an involuntary system responsible for the control of smooth muscle (e.g., bronchi, blood vessels, and GI tract), cardiac muscle, and exocrine glands (e.g., gastric, sweat, and salivary glands).

4. Adrenergic _Agonist_ are drugs that mimic the action of the sympathetic nervous system.

5. Drugs that block the receptor's ability to respond to a stimulus are known as a(n) _Antagonist_.

6. Norepinephrine and epinephrine are the major _Neurotransmitter_ in the sympathetic nervous system.

7. _Synaptic transmission_ initially involves the synthesis of neurotransmitters in the nerve terminal, with subsequent storage of the neurotransmitter awaiting an action potential that allows the neurotransmitter to be released.

8. Agents that stimulate multiple adrenergic subtype receptors are called _Nonselective drugs_.

9. A(n) _Selective_ targets a specific subtype receptor.

10. The autonomic nervous system is divided into the _SNS_ and the _PSNS_.

11. Another term for the sympathetic nervous system is the _Adrenergic nervous syst_.

12. A potential result of inadequate tissue perfusion is _Shock_.

PHYSIOLOGY AND PATHOPHYSIOLOGY: THE BODY HUMAN

Matching
Match the following body response with the correct adrenoceptor.

1. _beta 1_ tachycardia

2. _Alpha_ vasoconstriction

3. _beta 2_ relaxed uterine smooth muscle

4. _Alpha 1_ mydriasis

5. _Alpha 2_ inhibition of norepinephrine

6. _beta 1_ increased myocardial contractility

7. _Alpha 1_ increased blood pressure

8. _Alpha 1_ increased peripheral resistance

9. _beta 2_ bronchodilation

10. _beta 2_ increased glucagon release

a. Alpha-1   c. Beta-1
b. Alpha-2   d. Beta-2

CORE DRUG KNOWLEDGE: JUST THE FACTS

Multiple Choice
Circle the option that best answers the question or completes the statement.

1. Phenylephrine (Allerest) works by stimulating which of the following receptors?
   a. alpha-1
   b. alpha-2
   c. beta-1
   d. beta-2
   e. all of the above

2. Which of the following is *not* a contraindication or precaution to phenylephrine (Allerest) therapy?
   a. hypertension
   b. pregnancy
   c. hypothyroidism
   d. closed-angle glaucoma

3. Epinephrine works by stimulating which of the following receptors?
   a. alpha-1
   b. alpha-2
   c. beta-1
   d. beta-2
   e. all of the above

4. Which body systems are most affected by epinephrine therapy?
   a. renal and respiratory
   b. respiratory and cardiovascular
   c. cardiovascular and integumentary
   d. CNS and respiratory

5. Dopamine (Inotropin), a vasopressor, is used in the management of
   a. hypertensive crisis.
   b. rebound tachycardia.
   c. shock.
   d. acute respiratory failure.

6. Dopamine (Inotropin) works by
   a. stimulation of alpha-2, beta-2, and dopamine receptors.
   b. inhibition of alpha-1, beta-1, and dopamine receptors.
   c. stimulation of alpha-1, beta-1, and dopamine receptors.
   d. inhibition of alpha-2, beta-2, and dopamine receptors.

7. Prazosin (Minipress), an alpha-1 antagonist, is used in the treatment of
   a. COPD.
   b. hypertension.
   c. hypotension.
   d. urinary frequency.

8. Which drug is similar to prazosin?
   a. doxazocin (Cardura)
   b. yohimbine
   c. propranolol (Inderal)
   d. isoproterenol (Isuprel)

9. Which of the following disorders *cannot* be managed by beta-adrenergic antagonists such as propranolol (Inderal)?
   a. tachycardias
   b. essential tremor
   c. bradycardia
   d. migraine headaches

10. Which of the following adverse effects is not associated with propranolol (Inderal) therapy?
    a. hallucination and psychosis
    b. hypoglycemia
    c. hyperthyroidism
    d. weight loss

11. Fenoldopam (Corlopam) may be useful in which of the following patients? The patient having
    a. an ECG
    b. a radiocontrast diagnostic exam
    c. a bronchoscopy
    d. a chest x-ray

CORE PATIENT VARIABLES: PATIENTS, PLEASE

Multiple Choice

Circle the option that best answers the question or completes the statement.

1. Your patient has chronic allergies and takes phenylephrine (Allerest) on a daily basis. What potential adverse effects may this patient experience?
   a. hypotension
   b. hypoglycemia
   c. hyperglycemia
   d. hypertension

2. Your 78-year-old patient in the coronary intensive care unit has a diagnosis of cardiogenic shock. What is the goal of epinephrine therapy for this patient?
   a. control arrhythmias
   b. reduce intraocular pressure
   c. treat hypotension
   d. increase circulating glucose

3. The teaching plan for a patient with a severe allergy to bees should include self-administration of epinephrine by which route?
   a. inhalation
   b. sublingual
   c. intramuscular
   d. subcutaneous

4. Your patient who has just self-administered epinephrine calls and states, "I feel like I am going to jump out of my skin." What is the best response for this patient?
   a. "These are expected effects from the dose of epinephrine."
   b. "You should drive to your doctor's office right away."
   c. "You need to call 911 immediately and come to the hospital."
   d. "Take another dose of medication to stop the symptoms."

5. Patient A uses an albuterol (Proventil) metered-dose inhaler for asthma. Patient B uses an isoproterenol (Isuprel) metered-dose inhaler for the same condition. Which of these two patients has a higher risk for cardiovascular adverse effects?

   a. Patient A

   b. Patient B

   c. They have the same risk.

   d. Neither has a risk.

6. Your patient, age 55 years, has been prescribed prazosin (Minipress) for hypertension. What instructions should you give this patient to safely self-administer the first dose?

   a. "It is important for you to void before taking your medication so that your bladder will be empty."

   b. "Take your dose with a small amount of food at bedtime, then lie down."

   c. "Take three deep breaths then cough forcefully before you take the medication."

   d. "After you have taken the medication, do not eat for 2 hours."

7. Which of the following patient instructions is inappropriate for the patient receiving prazosin (Minipress) therapy?

   a. "It is OK to drink beer, but you should stay away from the hard stuff."

   b. "You should have your blood pressure and pulse checked periodically."

   c. "It would be best not to drive or do anything that requires alertness until you see how the medication affects you."

   d. "You should change positions slowly to avoid getting dizzy."

8. Your patient is prescribed propranolol (Inderal) for migraine headaches. In the past, the patient has been noncompliant because the patient prefers narcotic analgesics. Which of the following physical findings would indicate the patient has not been taking propranolol?

   a. BP 132/88

   b. respirations 20

   c. temperature 98.2

   d. pulse 110

9. Your patient has just received a diagnosis of migraine headaches. After reviewing the patient's medical history, you note that the patient uses an albuterol (Proventil) metered-dose inhaler intermittently for asthma. Why would propranolol (Inderal) be an inappropriate drug for migraine prophylaxis in this patient?

   a. It is not inappropriate; she may use it without problems.

   b. It may increase her blood pressure, which may result in increased headaches.

   c. It may induce bronchospasm, which may result in an asthma attack.

   d. It may induce cerebral hypotension and hypoperfusion, thus increasing the intensity of her headache.

10. Which of these findings, if identified in a patient who is being treated with fenoldopam (Corlopam), would indicate that the drug is having the desired effect?

    a. increased respiratory rate

    b. decreased abdominal distension

    c. decreased blood pressure

    d. increased heart rate

NURSING MANAGEMENT: EVERY GOOD NURSE SHOULD …

Multiple Choice

Circle the option that best answers the question or completes the statement.

1. Your patient is receiving IV phenylephrine, an alpha-1 agonist, to treat drug-induced hypotension. The drug is infusing into a vein in the antecubital space of the left arm. The IV infusion infiltrates, and the drug extravasates into the tissues. Your first action should be to

   a. check the blood pressure.

   b. turn off the IV infusion.

   c. lower the left arm below heart level.

   d. place a tourniquet around the left forearm.

2. To treat this patient's extravasation, you should use

   a. epinephrine SC.

   b. epinephrine IV.

   c. phentolamine SC.

   d. phentolamine IV.

3. A patient is brought to the emergency room after a severe allergic response to a newly prescribed drug therapy. He is having difficulty breathing and is in anaphylactic shock. He receives epinephrine, a mixed adrenergic stimulator, intravenously. The nurse should monitor him for

   a. hypotension.

   b. ECG changes.

   c. decreased urinary output.

   d. fever.

4. Your patient is showing signs of shock after hemorrhaging after surgery. The new resident wants you to administer dopamine. However, you know that something needs to be administered before the dopamine. You should request an order to administer (pick the best answer)

   a. D5W solution.

   b. D5.9NS solution.

   c. platelets.

   d. whole blood.

5. Your patient is to start a regimen of prazosin, an alpha-1 blocker, for treatment of his blood pressure. Patient education regarding this drug therapy should include:

   a. "It is important to come to a standing position quickly after lying flat."

   b. "Alcohol may be consumed without concerns."

   c. "Avoid driving for about 4 hours after the first dose."

   d. "Take the first dose in the morning after a hot shower."

6. A 60-year-old man is receiving propranolol, a beta blocker, for his angina. However, he has developed depression while taking the drug and wishes to stop taking propranolol. Education for this patient should include that

   a. the depression will stop after he adjusts to taking the propranolol.

   b. use of the drug should not be abruptly stopped.

   c. depression is not related to beta blocker use.

   d. the dose needs to be increased if he is depressed.

CASE STUDY

You are working in a critical care unit caring for a patient who is receiving an IV infusion of dopamine to treat shock that followed acute renal failure. Currently her blood pressure is 84/70 and output is 20 cc/hour. You are to adjust the dose of the dopamine until the patient's systolic blood pressure rises to between 110 and 120 and her urinary output is at least 30 cc per hour. You are measuring this patient's urinary output every hour.

1. Why does the order specify to titrate the dose of the dopamine in response to the blood pressure and the urine output? *Dopamine increase blood Pressure and urinary o/put*

2. On assessment you find that the systolic blood pressure is 108 and the hourly urinary output is 28 cc. You increase the dose of the dopamine per protocol twice. In 2 hours, the patient's blood pressure is 150/90 and urinary output is 40 cc/hour. What would account for these findings? What would you do next? *Reduce the dopamine level (titrate) Monitor for pt's vital*

CRITICAL THINKING CHALLENGE

As a nursing student, you are preparing to send your patient to the operating room for an inguinal hernia repair. He is expected to be in the operating room and recovery room a total of $2^1/_2$ hours. He is NPO now, but he should be able to receive oral fluids after he has fully awakened from anesthesia. The patient takes propranolol, a beta-blocker, for hypertension. His blood pressure is currently 126/80. Another dose of propranolol is due now, but the patient cannot have it because he is NPO. His last dose was last night. Your instructor asks you if you think the patient will experience adverse effects from skipping this dose. How should you respond? Can you safely withhold this dose?

CHAPTER 14

↓ BP ↑ saliva
↓ HR

Drugs Affecting Cholinergic Function

Tx Myasthenia Gravis

TOP TEN THINGS TO KNOW ABOUT DRUGS AFFECTING CHOLINERGIC FUNCTION

1. The parasympathetic neurotransmitter is acetylcholine; the receptors are muscarinic or nicotinic.
2. Muscarinic receptors are concentrated in the heart, smooth muscle, and exocrine glands. Nicotinic receptors are found in the central nervous system (CNS), the neuromuscular junction, autonomic ganglia, and the adrenal medulla.
3. Cholinergic stimulants are also known as cholinergic agonists or, simply, cholinergics; cholinergic blockers are known as cholinergic antagonists or anticholinergics.
4. Cholinergic agonist drugs cause decreased intraocular pressure, miosis (pupil constriction), sweating, increased salivation and bronchial secretions, bronchial constriction, increased GI tone, diarrhea, decreased blood pressure, slowed heart rate, and contraction of bladder detrusor muscle.
5. Anticholinergic drugs cause increased intraocular pressure, mydriasis (pupils dilate), photophobia, decreased sweating, dry mouth, decreased bronchial secretions, respiratory depression, decreased GI motility, constipation, decreased then increased blood pressure, tachycardia and possibly palpitations, urinary retention, vasodilation, and drowsiness, confusion, and agitation.
6. Anticholinergic crisis (overdose) is characterized by the phrase "mad as a hatter (CNS psychotic effect), dry as a bone (salivary), red as a beet (peripheral vasodilation), and blind as a bat (mydriasis)."

   Psychotic
   dry saliva
   periph
   vasodilat
   dilating
   pupil
7. Pilocarpine is a direct-acting cholinergic used topically to treat simple and acute glaucoma, pre- and postoperative elevated intraocular pressure, and drug-induced mydriasis.
8. Nicotine stimulates the CNS. Its use as a drug is limited to preparations to assist in smoking cessation. Adverse effects are related to its effects on the cardiovascular and central nervous systems.
9. Neostigmine is an indirect-acting cholinergic drug that acts by reversibly inhibiting postsynaptic cholinesterase. Because acetylcholine is not broken down as quickly, it has more opportunity to stimulate cholinergic receptors and create an effect. It is used in the treatment of myasthenia gravis to minimize muscle fatigue. Cholinergic crisis is the most serious adverse effect.
10. Atropine is an anticholinergic drug. It is the antidote for cholinergic poisoning. It is used preoperatively to dry secretions, in acute cardiac emergencies, topically (homatropine) to treat ophthalmic disorders, and to treat motion sickness and diarrhea. Adverse effects are related to loss of acetylcholine stimulation on receptors; the most serious adverse effect is anticholinergic overdose (or poisoning).

KEY TERMS

Matching
Match the key term with its definition.

1. __H__ autonomic nervous system
2. __F__ cholinergic agonist
3. __C__ cholinergic antagonist
4. __E__ cholinergic crisis
5. __I__ miosis
6. __A__ muscarinic receptors
7. __G__ nicotinic receptors
8. __B__ parasympathetic nervous system
9. __D__ sympathetic nervous system

a. Cholinergic receptor with subtypes M_1–M_5
b. Division of the ANS with acetylcholine as the terminal neurotransmitter

c. Drugs that block the action of acetylcholine

d. Division of the ANS with norepinephrine as the terminal neurotransmitter

e. Caused by cholinergic toxicity and results in medullary paralysis

f. Drugs that mimic the action of acetylcholine

g. Cholinergic receptors found in the CNS, neuromuscular junction, autonomic ganglia, and adrenal medulla

h. Involuntary system controlling smooth muscle, cardiac muscle, and exocrine glands

i. Constriction of the pupil in the eye

PHYSIOLOGY AND PATHOPHYSIOLOGY: THE BODY HUMAN

True or False

Mark true or false for the following statements. If the statement is false, replace the underlined word with the correct word to make a true statement.

1. _f_ Cholinergic stimulation of the eye results in <u>dilation</u> of the pupil. *constrict*

2. _f_ The heartbeat <u>increases</u> when stimulated by the cholinergic system. *Decrease*

3. _T_ Digestion <u>increases</u> with cholinergic stimulation.

4. _f_ Cardiovascular effects of cholinergic stimulation include <u>hypertension</u>. *hypotension*

5. _f_ In the respiratory system, cholinergic drugs may <u>decrease</u> bronchial secretions. *increase*

6. _f_ Blocking cholinergic stimulation may induce urinary <u>frequency</u>. *retention*

7. _T_ Constipation is a potential effect of blocking cholinergic stimulation.

8. _f_ To dilate the bronchioles, drugs that <u>mimic</u> the cholinergic nervous system may be used. *antagonist*

9. _f_ Nicotinic receptors respond to acetylcholine and have a <u>low</u> affinity for nicotine. *high*

10. _T_ <u>Muscarinic</u> receptors are concentrated in the heart, smooth muscle, and exocrine glands.

CORE DRUG KNOWLEDGE: JUST THE FACTS

Multiple Choice

Circle the option that best answers the question or completes the statement.

1. Which of the following is not a contraindication to the use of pilocarpine?
   a. glaucoma
   b. hypersensitivity
   c. acute iritis
   d. uncontrolled asthma

2. Ophthalamologic pilocarpine should be instilled
   a. directly over the pupil.
   b. in the inner canthus of the eye.
   c. at the lateral edge of the eye.
   d. in the conjunctival sac.

3. Nicotine replacement is used primarily
   a. in patients with hypoactive states.
   b. for smoking cessation programs.
   c. for patients with adrenal insufficiency.
   d. in alcohol recovery programs.

4. Which of the following adverse effects may be induced by nicotine replacement therapy?
   a. constipation
   b. hyperactivity
   c. sedation
   d. headache

5. Some indirect-acting cholinergic agonists are also known as
   a. cholinesterase inhibitors.
   b. cholinesterase agonists.
   c. anticholinergics.
   d. cholinergic blockers.

6. Myasthenia gravis, a neuromuscular disorder, may be treated with
   a. pilocarpine.
   b. neostigmine.
   c. atropine.
   d. nicotine.

7. The antidote for neostigmine overdose is
   a. pilocarpine.
   b. atropine.
   c. nicotine.
   d. oxygen.

8. Pralidoxime (PAM) is used in the treatment of
   a. myasthenia gravis.
   b. urinary hesitancy.
   c. overexposure to irreversible anticholinesterase drugs.
   d. acetaminophen overdose.

9. In the preoperative patient, atropine is used to
   a. diminish bronchial secretions.
   b. prevent dysentery.
   c. treat muscarinic excess.
   d. decrease cardiac stimulation.

Essay

1. Identify the principal actions of atropine.
   Dry secretion in preop
   ↑ Heart Rate
   mydriasis, contraction of bladder detrusor muscle

2. List the potential symptoms of a cholinergic crisis.
   nausea/vomiting
   Diarrhea, increase salivation
   Sweating, peripheral vasodilation
   bronchial constriction,
   respiratory arrest

CORE PATIENT VARIABLES: PATIENTS, PLEASE

Multiple Choice
Circle the option that best answers the question or completes the statement.

1. In the patient with____ C ____, pilocarpine should be used with caution.
   a. cancer
   b. AIDS
   c. cardiovascular disease
   d. depression

2. Which of the following patients would benefit most from nicotine replacement therapy?
   a. A 46-year-old man with cardiac dysrhythmias
   b. A 35-year-old woman with chronic bronchitis
   c. A 50-year-old woman with angina
   d. A 67-year-old man with acute myocardial infarction

3. Which of the following strategies may be *ineffective* for patients using nicotine replacement therapy?
   a. encourage participation in stop-smoking programs
   b. when cravings occur, have just one cigarette to abate the symptoms
   c. advise the patient to adhere to the recommended dosage and frequency to minimize craving
   d. encourage the patient to avoid exposure to others who smoke

4. Your patient has myasthenia gravis and is in crisis. To differentiate between a myasthenic crisis and a cholinergic crisis, the patient is given edrophonium (Tensilon). What effect from edrophonium would indicate this patient is in cholinergic crisis?
   a. increase in muscle weakness
   b. decrease in muscle weakness
   c. sedation
   d. cough

5. Which of the following may predispose a patient to psychogenic effects of neostigmine?
   a. pregnancy status
   b. gender
   c. culture
   d. age

6. Your 68-year-old patient has symptomatic bradycardia and is being transported to the hospital by paramedics. On the way to the hospital the patient's heart rate drops to 38. As the mobile intensive care nurse on the radio, what drug would you order?
   a. neostigmine
   b. pralidoxime
   c. atropine
   d. digoxin

7. Your 60-year-old male patient takes an anticholinergic agent for pronounced motion sickness. Because of this therapy, as well as the patient's age and gender, what adverse effect would you anticipate?
   a. constipation
   b. urinary retention
   c. blurred vision
   d. dry mouth

8. Your patient takes a medication that contains atropine for peptic ulcer disease. The patient states, "Sometimes my heart is beating really fast." Which of the following may interact with atropine to induce this symptom?
   a. over-the-counter or herbal medications
   b. ice cream
   c. fat-soluble vitamins
   d. green leafy vegetables

Essay

List important ongoing assessments to make for the patient receiving neostigmine for myasthenia gravis.

NURSING MANAGEMENT: EVERY GOOD NURSE SHOULD …

Multiple Choice
Circle the option that best answers the question or completes the statement.

1. Your patient is to begin therapy with pilocarpine eye drops to treat simple glaucoma. As part of your patient education on this drug therapy, you should include which of the following instructions?
   a. "Avoid or be very cautious with night driving."
   b. "Drink additional fluids."
   c. "Place the drop directly over the eyeball."
   d. "Suck on sugar-free hard candy to relieve a dry mouth."

2. You are working with a patient who wants to stop smoking, and nicotine patches have been prescribed. The patient says to you, "I think I should skip the first few patches that have the higher nicotine dosage and start with the patches that have the lowest dose of nicotine possible. That way I can stop smoking sooner." Appropriate patient education would include:
   a. "You should start with the lowest dosage of nicotine and use the higher doses last. This will prevent tolerance."
   b. "You should start with the highest dosage of nicotine and then decrease the dose. This will decrease withdrawal symptoms."
   c. "That's a good idea. And whenever you have an urge to smoke, place a patch on your skin."
   d. "If you want to do that, then you should smoke while using the nicotine patch."

3. Your patient has just received a diagnosis of myasthenia gravis and is to begin taking neostigmine 45 mg every 8 hours. You have looked up the time of onset and duration of action of neostigmine and learned that onset is 45 to 75 minutes, with duration being 2 to 4 hours. The patient wants to take the drug at 7 AM, 3 PM, and 11 PM. When would be the best times for the patient to perform daily activities that are the most tiring?
   a. 6 AM, 2 PM, and 10 PM
   b. 7 AM, 3 PM, and 11 PM
   c. Between 8:30 AM and noon, and between 4:30 PM and 8 PM
   d. Between 1 PM and 3 PM, and between 9 PM and 11 PM

4. A 1-year-old child is rushed to the emergency room by the child's grandmother. The grandmother reports finding the child playing with her pilocarpine drops and believes the child swallowed some of the pilocarpine. The child is sweating, drooling, flushed, and has vomited. Based on the history and the current symptoms, the nurse suspects
   a. nicotinic poisoning.
   b. cholinergic poisoning.
   c. anticholinergic overdose.
   d. parasympathetic blockage.

5. To treat the child in the scenario described above, the nurse would expect to administer

   a. pilocarpine.

   b. atropine.

   c. ipecac.

   d. neostigmine.

CASE STUDY

One of your patients in the outpatient clinic, a 60-year-old man, tells you he would like medication to help prevent motion sickness because he is going on a fishing trip. You know that the scopolamine transdermal patch, an anticholinergic drug, is often prescribed to prevent motion sickness. What other information should be assessed before requesting that the nurse practitioner or physician write an order for scopolamine?

CRITICAL THINKING CHALLENGE

The patient described above is found to be a suitable candidate and is given a prescription for scopolamine patches. He returns to the clinic 2 days later reporting blurred vision. His pupils are dilated. He tells you he removed the scopolamine patch this morning. Shortly after that he began to have blurred vision and photosensitivity. What could have caused these eye problems?

CHAPTER 15

Drugs Producing Anesthesia and Neuromuscular Blocking

TOP TEN THINGS TO KNOW ABOUT DRUGS PRODUCING ANESTHESIA AND NEUROMUSCULAR BLOCKING

1. Isoflurane is an inhaled anesthetic. As part of balanced anesthesia it is used to induce and maintain anesthesia. It can also be used for sedation and analgesia.
2. As with all inhaled anesthetics, respiratory depression occurs with isoflurane, and the patient requires mechanical ventilation. Prolonged hypotension during induction of anesthesia may occur. Postoperative respiratory depression and cardiovascular problems are possible and are more likely if the patient has ongoing chronic respiratory or cardiac problems before surgery or is significantly obese.
3. After surgery, the nurse minimizes the adverse effects of isoflurane by monitoring blood pressure, pulse, and temperature; supporting respiratory function; preventing aspiration; keeping the patient warm; and assessing for return of normal bowel sounds and urinary output.
4. Propofol is a nonbarbituate hypnotic used as a parenteral anesthetic as part of balanced general anesthesia. Propofol is used to induce anesthesia, and loss of consciousness occurs rapidly after IV administration, although the effects are short lived. Thus, the drug is administered as a continuous infusion.
5. Lidocaine is a local anesthetic with multiple uses, creating anesthesia in a confined area without loss of consciousness. It works by diminishing the permeability of the nerve membrane to sodium; this reversibly blocks nerve conduction.
6. Neuromuscular blockade occurs at acetylcholine receptors in the neural muscular joint (NMJ), where the neurotransmitter acetylcholine reacts with the muscle cell membrane, causing depolarization and subsequent muscle relaxation.
7. Nondepolarizing drugs prevent the muscle from contracting (muscle stays relaxed). Depolarizing drugs cause depolarization (muscle contraction) but then prevent the muscle from being stimulated again (contraction followed by flaccid paralysis).
8. Tubocurarine, a nondepolarizing neuromuscular blocker, is used as an adjunct to general anesthesia to facilitate endotracheal intubation, and with mechanically ventilated patients to conserve energy and prevent "fighting" the respirator. Neuromuscular blockade can be reversed with anticholinesterases (neostigmine, pyridostigmine, and edrophonium).
9. Tubocurarine does not depress the central nervous system (CNS). Although the patient cannot speak, move, or breathe unassisted, hearing, thought processes, and sensation are not affected. General anesthetics should be administered before tubocurarine is administered for surgical intubation. The nurse should provide reassurance to ventilated patients receiving tubocurarine.
10. Succinylcholine is a depolarizing neuromuscular blocker used in endotracheal intubation and short procedures such as endoscopy or electroconvulsant therapy (ECT). It is not used as an adjunct to anesthesia. A small amount of a nondepolarizing neuromuscular blocker is used before succinylcholine administration to prevent or decrease muscle fasciculations.

KEY TERMS

True or False
Mark true or false for the following statements. If the statement is false, replace the underlined word with the correct word to make a true statement.

1. _F_ The use of sedating drugs to help uncover unconscious material during psychoanalysis is called neuroleptanesthesia.

neuroanalysis

2. _false_ non depolarizing Depolarizing drugs prevent neural communication by depolarizing the muscle.

3. _false_ Local General anesthesia is the condition that results when sensory transmission from a local area of the body to the CNS is blocked.

4. _f_ The inability to move or function is called anesthesia. _Paralysis_

5. _T_ The site of communication between a nerve and a muscle is called the end plate.

6. _f_ anastesia Paralysis is a loss of feeling or sensation.

7. _f_ neuroleptenalia Narcoanalysis is also known as conscious sedation.

8. _f_ depolarzing Nondepolarizing drugs cause muscle depolarization and prevent repolarization.

9. _f_ balanced Local anesthesia is a combination of drugs to produce a lighter stage of anesthesia.

10. _T_ Dissociative anesthesia is a loss of perception of certain stimuli while that of others remains intact.

11. _f_ general Balanced anesthesia is characterized by a state of unconsciousness, analgesia, and amnesia.

PHYSIOLOGY AND PATHOPHYSIOLOGY: THE BODY HUMAN

Matching
Match the clue with the stage of anesthesia.

1. _d_ Unless rapid intervention and support occur, coma and death follow.

2. _a_ The patient remains conscious.

3. _c_ Contains four planes or levels

4. _b_ Systolic pressure rises, and the patient may experience excitation.

a. Stage I
b. Stage II
c. Stage III
d. Stage IV

CORE DRUG KNOWLEDGE: JUST THE FACTS

Multiple Choice
Circle the option that best answers the question or completes the statement.

1. The onset of action of isoflurane (Forane) is
   a. 30 to 60 minutes.
   b. 2 to 3 minutes.
   c. 20 to 30 seconds.
   d. 7 to 10 minutes.

2. Isoflurane (Forane) is contraindicated for use in patients with
   a. hyperthyroidism.
   b. head trauma.
   c. orthopedic injuries.
   d. glaucoma.

3. Ketamine (Ketalar) is contraindicated for adult patients with a history of psychiatric disorders because it may induce
   a. nausea and vomiting.
   b. anaphylaxis.
   c. emergence reaction.
   d. syncope.

4. An unusual potential adverse effect associated with long-term or high-dose propofol (Diprivan) therapy is
   a. headache.
   b. bright green urine.
   c. decreased albumin levels.
   d. amnesia.

5. To minimize potential bacterial growth, propofol (Diprivan) should be discarded after _____ hours.
   a. 6   c. 24
   b. 2   d. 12

6. Local anesthetics such as lidocaine (Xylocaine) are *not* useful in the management of
   a. laceration repair.
   b. regional blocks.
   c. ophthalmic anesthesia.
   d. general anesthesia.

7. What is the anticipated onset of action of tubocurarine (Tubarine) when given intravenously?

    a. 90 minutes

    b. 20 to 30 minutes

    c. 2 minutes

    d. 60 minutes

8. During tubocurarine (Tubarine) therapy, release of histamine may result in

    a. hypertension.

    b. hypotension.

    c. pasty white complexion.

    d. bronchospasm.

9. Succinylcholine (Anectine) is used during _____ because of its rapid and complete neuromuscular blockade.

    a. electroconvulsive therapy

    b. long and protracted surgeries

    c. anaphylaxis

    d. mechanical ventilation

10. What is the major difference between the mechanism of action of tubocurarine (Tubarine) and that of succinylcholine (Anectine)?

    a. Tubocurarine produces paralysis by excitation of muscles, and succinylcholine produces paralysis by relaxation of muscles.

    b. Tubocurarine produces paralysis by relaxation of muscles, and succinylcholine produces paralysis by excitation of muscles.

    c. Tubocurarine has a slower onset and shorter duration than succinylcholine.

    d. Succinylcholine has a slower onset and longer duration than tubocurarine.

Essay

Identify important differences between the local anesthetic agent groups: esters and amides.

CORE PATIENT VARIABLES: PATIENTS, PLEASE

Multiple Choice

Circle the option that best answers the question or completes the statement.

1. Which of the following patients has an increased risk for adverse effects from isoflurane (Forane)?

    a. A man, age 70, with COPD

    b. A woman, age 66, with hypothyroidism

    c. A girl, age 16, with anorexia

    d. A woman, age 80, with Parkinson disease

2. Your patient has just returned to your unit after having surgery. Which of the following should be documented?

    a. vital signs

    b. bowel sounds

    c. urine output

    d. all of the above

3. Your patient was involved in a severe motor vehicle accident and sustained a closed head injury. To keep your patient in a protective coma, the nurse administers propofol (Diprivan). Which of the following laboratory tests should be done before and during administration of propofol?

    a. triglycerides

    b. hemoglobin

    c. urinalysis

    d. arterial blood gas

4. Which of the following nursing interventions is important during the administration of propofol (Diprivan)?

    a. Because of paralysis, turn the patient frequently.

    b. Because of the potential for diarrhea, place the patient on plastic sheets.

    c. To enhance propofol's effects, keep environmental stimulus to a minimum.

    d. To enhance propofol's effects, keep the patient on a ventilator.

5. Your patient came to the emergency department with a full-thickness laceration. The physician anesthetized the area with lidocaine (Xylocaine) before suturing. The patient asks, "When will that wear off?" Which of the following is correct?

   a. 30 to 40 minutes

   b. 2 to 5 minutes

   c. 1 to 3 hours

   d. 12 hours

6. Your patient has just received viscous lidocaine to treat an ulceration in her throat. Which of the following nursing interventions should you do?

   a. Withhold food and fluids for 1 hour.

   b. Take her blood pressure every 15 minutes.

   c. Give an antacid to decrease stomach acids.

   d. Place an ice bag over her neck.

7. Your patient has a history of COPD. Why would tubocurarine (Tubarine) be a poor choice for surgery?

   a. Patients with COPD may experience decreased efficacy of tubocurarine.

   b. Tubocurarine releases histamine, which may exacerbate COPD.

   c. Tubocurarine induces electrolyte disturbances, which may induce bronchospasm.

   d. Drugs used in the treatment of COPD inactivate tubocurarine.

8. Your patient is receiving mechanical ventilation and tubocurarine (Tubarine) therapy. Her family has come to visit. Which of the following statements by the nurse is most appropriate?

   a. "Stroke her arm; she will be able to feel your touch although she cannot move."

   b. "Talk to her; she may be afraid because she cannot move but can still hear what is going on around her."

   c. "She can hear what you are saying but will not understand because the drug has made her unconscious."

   d. "She cannot feel your touch below the neck, but you can touch her head and she will feel it."

9. Your patient is scheduled for surgery and administration of tubocurarine (Tubarine). After reviewing your patient's health status, you note a history of COPD and renal insufficiency. Which of the following interventions would be most appropriate?

   a. Call the surgical suite and cancel the surgery.

   b. Contact the anesthesiologist and advise him/her of the patient's history.

   c. Write a note on a sticky pad and place it on the progress notes in the chart.

   d. Call the patient's family and advise them of the risks of anesthetic agents for this patient.

10. Your 66-year-old patient has a history of cardiac arrhythmias. Why would succinylcholine (Anectine) be a poor choice for this patient's surgery? Succinylcholine

   a. produces profound CNS obtundation, so the patient could not tell the staff he was experiencing chest pain.

   b. slows the conduction of the heart and may induce CHF.

   c. releases potassium from intense muscle contraction, which may induce cardiac arrhythmias.

   d. requires pseudocholinesterase for degradation, which is enhanced by cardiac insufficiency.

NURSING MANAGEMENT: EVERY GOOD NURSE SHOULD …

Multiple Choice
Circle the option that best answers the question or completes the statement.

1. You are the nurse responsible for admitting patients into the operating room holding area and performing the final checks and preparation for surgery. You anticipate that a patient will receive isoflurane, an inhaled anesthetic. To help maximize the therapeutic effect of the isoflurane, you would

   a. involve the patient in an active conversation about politics or sports to distract him.

   b. place the patient in a busy hallway so that he can be easily observed.

   c. tell the patient as little as possible about the events that will occur during induction of anesthesia in order not to frighten him.

   d. keep the holding room as quiet as possible with subdued lighting to promote relaxation.

2. You are the nurse working in the recovery room of an outpatient surgical center. Your patient has received general anesthesia with isoflurane, an inhaled anesthetic. Before discharging him from the recovery room and allowing him to go home, you should verify

   a. that his vital signs are stable and have returned to baseline.

   b. that he has voided.

   c. that he has someone to drive him home.

   d. all of the above.

3. Your patient is intubated and is on mechanical ventilation. He is receiving tubocurarine, a nondepolarizing NMJ blocker. Which of the following should be included in the nursing care for this patient?

   a. turn and reposition every 1 to 2 hours

   b. keep skin clean and dry

   c. explain all activity and care that will be performed

   d. all of the above

   e. none of the above

4. Your patient received succinylcholine before receiving electroconvulsant therapy (ECT) yesterday. Today the patient states to you, the nurse, that "My muscles hurt all over." The most appropriate nursing action would be to

   a. administer another dose of succinylcholine.

   b. contact the anesthesiologist immediately.

   c. explain that these feelings may be expected.

   d. complete an incident sheet.

5. Your emergency room patient has sustained a full-thickness laceration to the first finger on the right hand. Which of the following nursing actions is most appropriate when preparing the laceration repair tray for the physician?

   a. Determine the correct size of suture material.

   b. Open a fresh bottle of betadine.

   c. Explain the procedure to the patient.

   d. Verify the lidocaine does not contain epinephrine (adrenalin).

CASE STUDY

You are caring for a patient who requires lidocaine as a local anesthetic before having a chest tube inserted. You are to prepare the lidocaine for use. Through what route would you expect the lidocaine to be administered? Do you need any other information to prepare the medication?

CRITICAL THINKING CHALLENGE

The patient described above requires several doses of lidocaine before adequate anesthesia has occurred. As the physician prepares to proceed with inserting the chest tube, the patient begins to act confused and disoriented. You check his vital signs and his pulse is 55 and irregular, and his blood pressure is 86/50. What could account for these findings?

CHAPTER 16

Drugs Affecting Muscle Spasm and Spasticity

TOP TEN THINGS TO KNOW ABOUT DRUGS AFFECTING MUSCLE SPASM AND SPASTICITY

1. A muscle spasm is a sudden violent involuntary contraction of a muscle or group of muscles. When a muscle goes into spasm, it freezes in contraction and becomes a hard knotty mass, rather than normally contracting and relaxing in quick succession. Spasm is usually related to a localized skeletal muscle injury from acute trauma. Muscle spasms are treated with centrally acting muscle relaxants.

2. Spasticity is a condition in which certain muscles are continuously contracted. This contraction causes stiffness or tightness of the muscles and may interfere with gait, movement, or speech. Damage to the portion of the brain or spinal cord that controls voluntary movement usually causes spasticity. Spasticity is treated with either centrally acting spasmolytics or peripherally acting spasmolytics.

3. Cyclobenzaprine, the prototype centrally acting muscle relaxant, is used to manage muscle spasms associated with acute musculoskeletal disorders, such as low back strain. It relieves muscle spasms through a central action, possibly at the level of the brain stem, with no direct action on the neuromuscular junction or the muscle involved. It reduces pain and tenderness and improves mobility. Cyclobenzaprine is ineffective for treating spasticity associated with cerebral or spinal cord disease or in children with cerebral palsy. In addition to its central nervous system (CNS) depressant effects, cyclobenzaprine has anticholinergic effects.

4. The most common adverse effects of cyclobenzaprine are drowsiness, dizziness (both from CNS depression), and dry mouth (from anticholinergic effect). Older adults are more susceptible to these adverse effects. Caution patients to avoid driving and hazardous activities until the effect of the drug is known.

5. Interactions between cyclobenzaprine and CNS depressants or antimuscarinic drugs may be extensive.

6. Baclofen, a centrally acting spasmolytic, is a derivative of the neurotransmitter gamma-aminobutyric acid (GABA). It acts at the spinal end of the upper motor neurons at GABA receptors to cause hyperpolarization; this reduces excessive reflex spasms and spasticity, allowing muscle relaxation.

7. Baclofen relieves some components of spinal spasticity—involuntary flexor and extensor spasms and resistance to passive movements. It is useful in MS and traumatic lesions of the spinal cord that result in paralysis. Baclofen is not useful in treating spasms that follow a cerebrovascular accident (CVA, or stroke) or those that occur in Parkinson disease or Huntington chorea.

8. CNS adverse effects from baclofen, especially sedation, are the most common. Older adults are more susceptible to baclofen-induced sedation and psychiatric disturbances, including hallucinations, excitation, and confusion. Teach patients to avoid alcohol and other CNS depressants while taking baclofen.

9. Dantrolene, a peripherally acting spasmolytic, acts directly on the muscle cells by reducing the amount of calcium released from the sarcoplasmic reticulum, resulting in muscle relaxation. It does not interfere with neuro-muscular communication or have CNS effects. It may decrease hyperreflexia, muscle stiffness, and spasticity in patients with upper motor neuron disorders.

10. Dantrolene is used to treat or prevent malignant hyperthermia and to treat upper motor neuron disorders. The most common adverse effect is muscle weakness. Fatal hepatitis is possible, especially in women older than 35 years who take estrogens.

KEY TERMS

Matching
Match the key term with its definition.

1. ___G___ spasm
2. ___C___ spasticity
3. ___f___ centrally acting
4. ___e___ peripherally acting
5. ___d___ spasmolytic
6. ___b___ tonic spasm
7. ___a___ clonic spasm

a. Contractions of the affected muscles take place repeatedly, forcibly, and in quick succession, with equally sudden and frequent relaxations.

b. Characterized by an unusually prolonged and strong muscular contraction, with relaxation taking place slowly

c. A condition in which certain muscles are continuously contracted

d. Drugs that work in the CNS to reduce excessive reflex activity and allow muscle relaxation

e. Drugs that relax a muscle by a direct action within the skeletal muscle fiber

f. Drugs that act in the CNS to reduce the perception of pain induced from muscle spasm

g. A sudden violent involuntary contraction of a muscle or a group of muscles

PHYSIOLOGY AND PATHOPHYSIOLOGY: THE BODY HUMAN

Essay

1. What two contractile proteins are integral to muscle contraction?

2. Describe the sliding filament theory.

3. List potential etiologies of muscle spasm.

4. List potential etiologies of muscle spasticity.

5. List symptoms of spasticity.

CORE DRUG KNOWLEDGE: JUST THE FACTS

Multiple Choice
Circle the option that best answers the question or completes the statement.

1. Optimal effects of cyclobenzaprine (Flexeril) therapy should occur within
   a. 1 week.
   b. 12 hours.
   c. 1 to 2 days.
   d. 2 hours.

2. Cyclobenzaprine (Flexeril) is *ineffective* in the management of
   a. tonic spasms.
   b. clonic spasms.
   c. strained muscles.
   d. cerebral palsy.

3. Cyclobenzaprine (Flexeril) is structurally similar to
   a. tricyclic antidepressants.
   b. lithium.
   c. phenothiazines.
   d. selective-serotonin reuptake inhibitors.

4. Serious adverse effects of cyclobenzaprine (Flexeril) therapy affect the
   a. GI system.
   b. cardiovascular system.
   c. CNS.
   d. integumentary system.

5. The pharmacotherapeutics for baclofen (Lioresal) include
   a. Huntington chorea.
   b. Parkinson disease.
   c. cerebral vascular accidents.
   d. multiple sclerosis.

6. Which of the following symptoms is *not* associated with abrupt withdrawal of baclofen (Lioresal)?
   a. agitation
   b. hyperglycemia
   c. exacerbation of spasticity
   d. seizure

7. Which drug is similar to baclofen?
   a. carisoprodol (Soma)
   b. tizanidine (Zanaflex)
   c. dantrolene (Dantrium)
   d. orphenadrine (Norflex)

8. Malignant hyperthermia is treated with which of the following drugs?
   a. baclofen (Lioresal)
   b. dantrolene (Dantrium)
   c. orphenadrine (Norflex)
   d. cyclobenzaprine (Flexeril)

9. Dantrolene works by
   a. reducing the amount of calcium from the sarcoplasmic reticulum.
   b. interfering with pseudocholinesterase.
   c. increasing cellular potassium.
   d. interrupting cerebral recognition of pain stimulus.

10. Which of the following disorders is *not* a precaution to dantrolene therapy?
    a. active liver disease
    b. cardiac disease
    c. pulmonary dysfunction
    d. increased intraocular pressure

CORE PATIENT VARIABLES: PATIENTS, PLEASE

Multiple Choice

Circle the option that best answers the question or completes the statement.

1. Which of the following patients has the highest risk for increased anticholinergic and CNS depressant effects of cyclobenzaprine (Flexeril)?
   a. Abby, age 45, with asthma
   b. Ben, age 56, with musculoskeletal back pain
   c. Carey, age 68, with hypothyroidism
   d. David, age 17, with chronic sinus infections

2. Your 45-year-old patient was involved in a motor vehicle accident 1 year ago. The patient has been taking cyclobenzaprine (Flexeril) and ibuprofen (Motrin) since the accident. The patient is scheduled for back surgery in the morning. The nurse should review the physician's orders to ensure
   a. physical therapy has been ordered.
   b. cyclobenzaprine has been ordered as a continuous or tapered medication.
   c. ibuprofen has been ordered as a continuous or tapered medication.
   d. occupational therapy has been ordered.

3. Your patient is being discharged from the hospital with a prescription for cyclobenzaprine (Flexeril). Discharge instructions should include:
   a. "Assess your level of sedation before driving a car."
   b. "Take this medication only at bedtime."
   c. "Be sure to eat lots of vegetables."
   d. "Limit your alcohol intake to three glasses of wine a day."

4. Elderly patients taking baclofen (Lioresal) therapy have an increased risk for
   a. hallucinations.
   b. hyperglycemia.
   c. urinary frequency.
   d. rash.

5. Your 28-year-old patient is taking baclofen (Lioresal) for muscle spasms in his back. What assessment of lifestyle, diet, and habits should you do?

   a. sugar intake

   b. smoking history

   c. alcohol ingestion

   d. all of the above

6. Your patient takes dantrolene (Dantrium) for multiple sclerosis. Which of the following adverse effects may occur?

   a. rash

   b. drooling

   c. aplastic anemia

   d. all of the above

NURSING MANAGEMENT: EVERY GOOD NURSE SHOULD …

Multiple Choice
Circle the option that best answers the question or completes the statement.

1. Your patient is 75 years old and was in a car accident, which caused strained back muscles. The patient started a regimen of cyclobenzaprine to treat the painful back spasms. Five days after starting treatment, the patient calls the clinic and reports a severely dry mouth. As the nurse in the clinic, your best response would be:

   a. "This is a sign of a significant drug interaction. Stop taking the cyclobenzaprine."

   b. "This is a common adverse effect from cyclobenzaprine. Try sucking on sugarless hard candies to relieve your dry mouth."

   c. "This indicates that you are allergic to cyclobenzaprine. Come into the clinic today to be checked."

   d. "This is the desired effect of the drug and indicates that cyclobenzaprine is working effectively."

2. Your patient has been taking cyclobenzaprine, 10 mg TID, for the last 4 months to treat severe back spasms. At this time, the back spasms have decreased, and the patient would like to stop taking the cyclobenzaprine. The physician has ordered to discontinue baclofen therapy when the spasms are no longer painful. In providing the patient education, you should teach this patient to:

   a. "Stop the drug completely tomorrow."

   b. "Take only 1 pill today and tomorrow and then stop drug therapy."

   c. "Take 2 pills a day for the next month, then 1 pill a day for a month, and then stop drug therapy."

   d. "Take 2 pills a day for the next 7 days, then 1 pill a day for 7 days, and then stop drug therapy."

3. Yesterday your patient started a regimen of baclofen, a centrally acting spasmolytic, for the treatment of multiple sclerosis. Which of the following is appropriate to minimize adverse effects from the baclofen?

   a. Assist the patient in ambulating.

   b. Encourage the patient to stand up and touch his toes.

   c. Offer the patient a glass of wine with dinner.

   d. Provide the patient with large, full meals.

4. You are making a home visit to a patient who has progressing multiple sclerosis and is receiving dantrolene, a peripherally acting spasmolytic. The family tells you that the patient is not eating well because of difficulty in swallowing and that there are periods of choking. They ask if use of the medication should be discontinued. Your best response is:

   a. "Continue giving the dantrolene capsule as long as it can be swallowed."

   b. "Mix the contents of the capsule with a small amount of fruit juice."

   c. "Administer half of the capsule, instead of a whole capsule."

   d. "Stop administering the dantrolene."

5. In the acute care setting, nursing care for a patient who is receiving muscle relaxants or antispasmodic agents should be directed toward preventing

   a. adverse effects.

   b. injury.

   c. anorexia.

   d. overstrain of muscles.

CASE STUDY

Your patient has amyotrophic lateral sclerosis (ALS) and is receiving baclofen to treat the spasms associated with the disease. The patient also has diabetes and takes miglitol, an oral antidiabetic drug. At the follow-up clinic visit 1 month after starting therapy, the patient states, "I'm feeling so fatigued and weak. I also have to urinate all the time."

1. What questions should be asked to determine the exact cause of the symptoms?

2. What lab work should be done to assess for other complications of therapy? (Hint: See the discussion in Chapter 17 regarding ALS for more information.)

CRITICAL THINKING CHALLENGE

The patient described above adjusts to baclofen therapy and reports that the sedative effects have diminished greatly. However, after 6 months of baclofen therapy, the patient becomes depressed. Amitriptyline (Elavil), a tricyclic antidepressant, is prescribed once a day in the morning. After the patient receives the amitriptyline for 1 week, the family calls to report the patient is very lethargic all day and can barely keep his eyes open.

1. What explanation for these effects can you offer to the family?

2. What nursing interventions can you suggest to help minimize these adverse effects?

CHAPTER 17

Drugs Treating Parkinson Disease and Other Movement Disorders

TOP TEN THINGS TO KNOW ABOUT DRUGS FOR TREATING PARKINSON DISEASE AND OTHER MOVEMENT DISORDERS

1. Movement disorders are chronic, severe, and debilitating. None of the currently available drug therapies cure movement disorders.
2. The relative lack of dopamine combined with the relative excess of excitatory acetylcholine cause the symptoms of Parkinson disease. Drugs used to treat Parkinson's disease either increase dopamine levels (dopaminergics), stimulate dopamine receptors (dopamine agonists), extend the action of dopamine in the brain (dopa decarboxylase [DDC] or catecholamine O-methyl transferase [COMT] inhibitors), or prevent the activation of cholinergic receptors (anticholinergics).
3. Carbidopa-levodopa is a dopaminergic drug that diffuses levodopa into the central nervous system (CNS), where it is converted to dopamine. The resulting change in dopamine-acetylcholine balance is believed to improve nerve impulse control and to form the basis of the drug's antiparkinsonian activity. Carbidopa does not cross the blood–brain barrier.
4. The most common adverse effects of carbidopa-levodopa are gastrointestinal (GI) (nausea and vomiting, anorexia, and weight loss) and orthostatic hypotension. Serious adverse effects of carbidopa-levodopa include abnormal movements resulting from the increased dopamine in the brain and bradykinetic (on-off) episodes that place the patient at risk for injury. Neuroleptic malignant syndrome can occur if use of carbidopa-levodopa is stopped suddenly; it is more common if the patient is also receiving antipsychotic drugs.
5. Continuous therapy with carbidopa-levodopa causes the drug to lose its overall effectiveness in controlling symptoms of Parkinson disease.

Administering a higher dose may control symptoms but also increases the patient's risk for adverse effects.
6. Anticholinergic drugs work by blocking the access of acetylcholine to cholinergic receptors in the striatum. Anticholinergic drugs are less effective than carbidopa-levodopa in treating the symptoms of Parkinson disease. They can be used as monotherapy in early Parkinson disease or in combination with dopaminergic drugs in later stages. They are used with caution in older patients because of the potential for severe CNS effects. The anticholinergics used most frequently in treating Parkinson disease are benztropine (Cogentin), diphenhydramine (Benadryl), and trihexyphenidyl (Artane).
7. The goal of riluzole drug therapy for amyotrophic lateral sclerosis (ALS) is to delay respiratory compromise and the need for tracheostomy or mechanical ventilation, but it is not a cure.
8. Riluzole is believed to work in ALS by inhibiting glutamate release, inactivating voltage-dependent sodium channels, or interfering with intracellular events that follow transmitter binding at excitatory amino acid receptors.
9. Adverse effects of riluzole are CNS (fatigue, dizziness, vertigo, somnolence) and GI (nausea, diarrhea, anorexia). Riluzole increases levels of hepatic enzymes in 50% of patients. Women and native Japanese patients are at a higher risk for adverse effects from riluzole because of mechanisms of drug metabolism.
10. Drug treatment for multiple sclerosis (MS) includes interferon beta-1a, interferon beta-1b, and glatiramer. Glatiramer acetate is a synthetic chemical that is similar in structure to myelin basic protein. It is thought to modify immune processes that cause MS by acting as a decoy to locally generated autoantibodies. This effect results in decreased tissue destruction.

Glatiramer is given by SC injection. The most common adverse effects include lumps, pain, or redness at the site of injection.

KEY TERMS

Anagrams
Use the following anagrams to explain the key terms in the chapter.

1. Idiopathic parkinsonism

L	S	P	R	A	Y	A	S	I

G	A	N	A	I	T	S

2. Clenching of the teeth associated with forceful lateral or protrusive jaw movement

X	B	M	S	U	R	I

3. On–off effect

K	D	B	R	C	N	A	E	I	Y	I	T

P	D	S	O	E	S	E	I

4. Loss of voluntary movement

A	A	N	I	E	K	S	I

5. Jerking, flinging movements of an extremity

S	L	A	B	L	S	M	I	U

6. Group of darkly pigmented cells in the midbrain

T	B	S	A	I	A	U	S	N	T

G	I	A	N	R

7. Drugs that promote activation of dopamine receptors

P	E	G	C	D	O	M	R	I	N	I	A

8. Characterized by an abrupt onset of marked rigidity, akinesia, tremor, and hyperpyrexia

O	C	R	I	U	T	E	P	N	E	L

G	T	I	N	L	A	A	N	M

D	E	N	M	Y	O	S	R

9. A drug class that stimulates dopamine receptors, but does not require conversion

0	A	M	N	P	D	I	E

G	T	A	N	I	S	O

10. Abnormal slowness of movement

K	Y	E	A	I	B	A	S	I	N	D	R

11. Disorder that ceases with withdrawal of the offending drug

S	M	N	S	I	I	K	N	R	O	A	P

12. Another term for bradykinetic episodes

N	O	F	F	O	F	F	E	C	T	E

PHYSIOLOGY AND PATHOPHYSIOLOGY: THE BODY HUMAN

Essay

1. Why does the basal ganglia produce the neurotransmitters dopamine and acetylcholine?

2. Parkinson disease is called a "naturally occurring disease." What does this mean?

3. List the symptoms that result from the imbalance between dopamine and acetylcholine.

4. What is the difference between parkinsonism and Parkinson disease?

5. What is the usual progression of amyotrophic lateral sclerosis (ALS)?

CORE DRUG KNOWLEDGE: JUST THE FACTS

Multiple Choice
Circle the option that best answers the question or completes the statement.

1. Carbidopa-levodopa (Sinemet) works by
   a. blocking the action of acetylcholine.
   b. blocking the action of dopamine.
   c. increasing activation of dopamine receptors in the brain.
   d. increasing activation of acetylcholine receptors in the brain.

2. Carbidopa-levodopa (Sinemet) is preferred over plain levodopa in drug treatment of Parkinson disease because it
   a. is better absorbed from the GI tract.
   b. induces fewer CNS adverse effects.
   c. allows more dopamine to reach the brain.
   d. can be administered once a day.

3. Which of the following adverse effects is *not* associated with the use of carbidopa-levodopa (Sinemet)?
   a. thrombocytopenia
   b. suicidal tendencies
   c. ballismus
   d. bruxism

4. Drug interactions with carbidopa-levodopa (Sinemet) include
   a. most antibiotics.
   b. thiazide diuretics.
   c. hydantoins.
   d. cardiac glycosides.

5. Centrally acting anticholinergic drugs are used in the management of Parkinson disease to
   a. inhibit the release of dopamine.
   b. increase the release of dopamine.
   c. inhibit the release of acetylcholine.
   d. increase the release of acetylcholine.

6. Tolcapone (Tasmar) is used in the management of Parkinson disease to
   a. increase the amount of levodopa that reaches the brain.
   b. decrease the amount of levodopa that reaches the brain.
   c. block the conversion of levodopa to dopamine.
   d. increase the rate of conversion of levodopa to dopamine.

7. Dopamine agonists such as pramipexole (Mirapex) and ropinirole (Requip) are used to
   a. block the adverse effects of carbidopa-levodopa.
   b. decrease the amount of carbidopa-levodopa needed to control the symptoms of Parkinson disease.
   c. block the action of acetylcholine in the periphery of the body.
   d. increase the conversion of levodopa to dopamine.

8. A therapeutic indication for riluzole (Rilutek) is
   a. Parkinson disease
   b. multiple sclerosis.
   c. amyotrophic lateral sclerosis.
   d. Alzheimer disease.

9. When given concurrently with riluzole, inhibitors of CYP1A 2, such as caffeine or theophylline, may induce
   a. an increased risk for toxicity.
   b. subtherapeutic blood levels of riluzole.
   c. delayed absorption.
   d. increased elimination.

10. Which of the following drugs would be *inappropriate* for use in the management of multiple sclerosis (MS)?
    a. bromocriptine (Parlodel)
    b. interferon beta
    c. glatiramer acetate (Copaxone)
    d. oxybutynin (Ditropan)

CORE PATIENT VARIABLES: PATIENTS, PLEASE

Multiple Choice
Circle the option that best answers the question or completes the statement.

1. You are assessing the patient's health status for contraindications for carbidopa-levodopa therapy. Which of the following statements would you report to the provider?
   a. "My ophthalmologist says my glaucoma is getting worse."
   b. "I have recurrent urinary tract infections."
   c. "I've been taking amitriptyline (Elavil) for my depression."
   d. "I haven't had a migraine in 6 months."

2. Your patient is taking carbidopa-levodopa. In your assessment of lifestyle, diet, and habits, which of the following statements by the patient would you need to address?
   a. "I just love avocados! I could eat them every day."
   b. "I tend to watch my meat intake because it bothers my stomach."
   c. "I eat bran flakes every morning."
   d. "I drink at least 8 glasses of water a day."

3. Which of the following cultural groups may need dosing adjustments for symptom management of Parkinson disease?
   a. Hispanic
   b. African American
   c. Chinese
   d. Caucasian

4. Your patient has Parkinson disease and has been taking carbidopa-levodopa (Sinemet) for several years. Because of many adverse effects, the patient wishes to stop the drug. What should you tell this patient?
   a. "Drink lots of water in the next week to flush the drug out of your system."
   b. "You really need to see the doctor before making that decision."
   c. "Just decrease your dose to only once a day and see how you feel."
   d. "That should be fine; I'll make an appointment for you to see the doctor next month."

5. Your patient is taking carbidopa-levodopa (Sinemet) and ropinirole (Requip) for Parkinson disease. The patient asks, "Why do I need to take both of these drugs?" How would you respond?
   a. "Taking these drugs together decreases the potential for adverse effects."
   b. "That is just the way this disease is treated."
   c. "Why don't you ask the doctor that question?"
   d. "Taking these drugs together stops the progression of the disease."

6. Before the initiation of therapy with riluzole, the nurse should assess all of the following laboratory data *except*
   a. renal function.
   b. complete blood count.
   c. arterial blood gases.
   d. hepatic function.

7. Which of the following should be assessed related to the core patient variable of environment for the patient taking riluzole therapy? The ability to
   a. climb stairs.
   b. refrigerate the drug.
   c. cover the cost of the drug.
   d. store in a warm environment.

8. Your patient is prescribed riluzole (Rilutek) for ALS. Patient teaching should include:

   a. "Don't worry about your diet; you need all the calories you can get."

   b. "Limit caffeine and high-fat foods."

   c. "Decrease the amount of green leafy vegetables."

   d. "Be sure to drink at least 10 glasses of water a day."

NURSING MANAGEMENT: EVERY GOOD NURSE SHOULD …

Essay

Devise a plan of care to maximize therapeutic effects and minimize adverse effects for the patient taking combination therapy benztropine with carbidopa-levodopa.

CASE STUDY

1. Your patient is 65 years old and has just received a diagnosis of Parkinson disease. He has not begun pharmacotherapy. The patient returns to your clinic for the first visit since the diagnosis was made.

   a. What assessments should you make at this time?

   b. Why was drug therapy not started at this time?

2. Nine months later, the patient returns to the clinic. The patient states, "I can't dress myself anymore. My hands shake too much." The nurse practitioner prescribes benztropine (Cogentin) and requests a return visit in 1 month.

   What assessments would you make at that visit 1 month after the initiation of therapy?

3. A year after starting drug therapy, the patient is experiencing an increase in tremors, a mildly ataxic gait, and muscular rigidity in the face and extremities. The patient now begins taking carbidopa-levodopa (Sinemet).

   What patient teaching should you do at this time?

4. Two years later, the patient comes to the clinic and expresses concern that this medication is not as effective as before.

   What patient teaching should be done at this time?

CRITICAL THINKING CHALLENGE

You are caring for a patient who has ALS, and the neurologist has prescribed riluzole. Blood work is drawn before the patient is discharged to check the ALT and AST levels. After 1 month of therapy, the patient has a follow-up outpatient visit, at which time the ALT and AST levels are found to be elevated to approximately twice normal levels. The neurologist instructs the patient to continue to take the riluzole and return for more follow-up blood work in 2 months. The patient asks you, the nurse, to explain the need for more blood work.

CHAPTER 18

Drugs Relieving Anxiety and Promoting Sleep

TOP TEN THINGS TO KNOW ABOUT DRUGS RELIEVING ANXIETY AND PROMOTING SLEEP

1. Central nervous system (CNS) depression causes multiple effects in the body. Some drugs that depress the CNS, such as the benzodiazepines, can produce multiple effects, depending on the dose and the route of administration. Two of those effects are relieving anxiety and promoting sleep.

2. Anxiety is a feeling of unease that something bad or undesirable may happen. Some anxiety is normal; it is a protective mechanism that has evolved to help people recognize danger and take action for self-preservation. However, anxiety becomes pathologic when it is severe and chronic and interferes with an individual's ability to function in normal life. Anxiety is actually several related disorders. Drugs that reduce anxiety are called anxiolytics.

3. Insomnia is the perception or complaint of inadequate or poor-quality sleep. Transient and intermittent insomnia can be related to stress, environmental noise, extreme temperatures, change in the surrounding environment, sleep/wake schedule problems such as jet lag, or adverse effects of drug therapy. Chronic insomnia often results from more than one cause, including underlying physical or mental disorders, such as depression.

4. Lifestyle changes can prevent insomnia in most people with transient or intermittent insomnia; short-term drug therapy to help induce sleep may be indicated for some patients. The use of drug therapy to treat chronic insomnia is a matter of great controversy. Generally, drug therapy to promote sleep is considered best if used for the shortest duration possible. The best treatment for chronic insomnia is diagnosing and treating any underlying medical or psychological cause.

5. The benzodiazepines (prototype lorazepam) potentiate the effect of GABA, an inhibitory CNS

neurotransmitter. This results in CNS depression. However, none of the benzodiazepines acts like GABA or increase the amount of GABA present. The intrinsic amount of GABA is limited, so the effects from benzodiazepines are also limited. Tolerance to lorazepam and the other benzodiazepines can occur if they are used long term, requiring larger doses to achieve a therapeutic effect.

6. Benzodiazepines are used to treat anxiety disorders and insomnia, as well as seizures, muscle spasms and tension, and acute alcohol withdrawal symptoms. Lorazepam has a labeled indication for treating anxiety. It is used off label for treatment of status epilepticus, chemotherapy-induced nausea and vomiting, the symptoms of acute alcohol withdrawal, and psychogenic catatonia. Oral lorazepam is also used in treating chronic insomnia.

7. Lorazepam, like other benzodiazepines, is generally well tolerated, with few adverse effects; those that occur are from CNS depression. Mild drowsiness is common but transient; ataxia and confusion may also occur, especially in older adults and in debilitated patients. Dose adjustments should be made if these effects persist. Respiratory disturbances and partial airway obstruction may occur if excessive lorazepam is given intravenously before a procedure. Paradoxical excitatory reactions are possible. The risk for fatal overdose is small with benzodiazepines because of their wide therapeutic index unless it is taken with other CNS depressants, especially alcohol.

8. The major nursing consideration is to ensure the safety of the patient. Caution patients to avoid taking other CNS depressants when taking a benzodiazepine because of additive CNS depression that may occur. Caution patients not to drive or do potentially hazardous activities until the effects of the benzodiazepine on them are known.

9. Some benzodiazepines have long half-lives; some have short half-lives. When benzodiazepines are used to promote sleep, a drug with a short half-life will produce less daytime drowsiness and sedation than a drug with a longer half-life. Lorazepam is not approved for treating insomnia but is used off label for this condition.

10. There are many non-benzodiazepine agents to promote sleep. They include zolpidem (Ambien), zaleplon (Sonata), eszopiclone (Lunesta), ramelteon (Rozerem), and trazodone (Desyrel). With the exception of ramelteon, these drugs interact with the GABA or benzodiazepine receptor complexes. Ramelteon stimulates melatonin receptors.

KEY TERMS

Crossword Puzzle

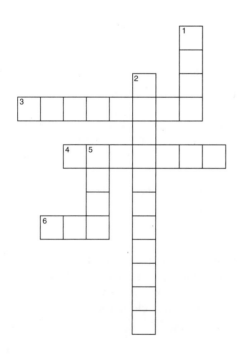

ACROSS

3. The inability to fall or stay asleep
4. A feeling of unease that something bad or undesirable may happen
6. A stage of sleep in which eye movement occurs

DOWN

1. An inhibitory neurotransmitter
2. Drugs that ease the sensation of anxiety
5. A stage of sleep in which eye movement does not occur

Essay

List the most common pathologic anxiety disorders.

PHYSIOLOGY AND PATHOPHYSIOLOGY: THE BODY HUMAN

Essay

1. What is the function of the amygdala?

2. What is the function of the hippocampus?

3. What is the importance of stages 3 and 4 sleep?

CORE DRUG KNOWLEDGE: JUST THE FACTS

Multiple Choice

Circle the option that best answers the question or completes the statement

1. For the management of seizure disorders, benzodiazepines affect the
   a. spinal cord.
   b. cerebellum.
   c. limbic area.
   d. brain stem.

2. Lorazepam (Ativan) is a pregnancy category _____ drug.
   a. A
   b. C
   c. D
   d. X

3. Paradoxical reactions with lorazepam are most likely to occur in patients with
   a. psychiatric disorders.
   b. hepatic insufficiency.
   c. renal failure.
   d. seizure disorders.

4. CNS effects of lorazepam (Ativan) may be potentiated when given concurrently with
   a. phenytoin (Dilantin).
   b. flumazenil (Romazicon).
   c. alcohol.
   d. levodopa (Dopar).

5. Acute cessation of long-term benzodiazepine therapy may induce
   a. increased sedation.
   b. withdrawal symptoms.
   c. diarrhea.
   d. blurred vision.

6. Which of the following groups of patients should receive a lower dose of lorazepam?
   a. children and elder patients
   b. children and Asian patients
   c. elder and Native-American patients
   d. children, elder, and Asian patients

Essay

1. In addition to benzodiazepines, what other drugs or drug classes are useful in the management of anxiety?

2. How do benzodiazepines for anxiety differ from those used for insomnia?

CORE PATIENT VARIABLES: PATIENTS, PLEASE

Multiple Choice
Circle the option that best answers the question or completes the statement.

1. Which of the following patients should avoid the use of lorazepam (Ativan)?
   a. Malcom, with a history of mitral valve prolapse
   b. Christy, with a history of peptic ulcer disease
   c. Tyler, age 45
   d. Myrna, 18 weeks' pregnant

2. Your patient has been taking lorazepam (Ativan) for an anxiety disorder for the past year. The patient is now admitted to your unit for appendicitis. What nursing intervention related to the patient's long-term use of lorazepam would you do? Obtain an order for
   a. restraints as needed
   b. liver function tests
   c. a benzodiazepine taper
   d. vital sign checks every half hour

3. Your 70-year-old Asian patient has been ordered benzodiazepine for sleep during the patient's hospitalization. You would expect the dose of benzodiazepine to be
   a. higher than normal.
   b. lower than normal.
   c. the same as for any adult.

4. Your patient with anxiety has been taking benzodiazepine for the past year. Which of the following laboratory tests should you coordinate at the patient's next clinic visit?
   1. 24-hour urine
   2. CBC
   3. liver enzymes
   4. BUN
   5. creatinine
      a. 1, 3, 5
      b. 2, 3
      c. 1, 2, 3,
      d. 1, 2, 3, 4, 5

5. Your patient is being discharged home with a prescription for lorazepam. The patient states, "Boy, that was a lot of information you gave me. What is the bottom line–what should I really look out for?" Which of the following is your best response?

   a. "Assess how much sedation you experience before you attempt anything that requires mental alertness."

   b. "Try to take the medication on an empty stomach."

   c. "Just let me know if you need a refill on your prescription."

   d. "Take your medication as frequently as you feel you need it."

NURSING MANAGEMENT: EVERY GOOD NURSE SHOULD ...

Multiple Choice
Circle the option that best answers the question or completes the statement.

1. Your patient is a 33-year-old woman who has been prescribed lorazepam, a benzodiazepine, as an anxiolytic. What would you include in your teaching for this patient regarding drug therapy?

   a. "Avoid activities requiring mental alertness initially."

   b. "Avoid drinking alcohol."

   c. "Avoid becoming pregnant while taking this drug."

   d. all of the above

2. Your patient is 70 years old and is to receive lorazepam as a sedative tonight before surgery tomorrow morning. You would expect to administer

   a. an average adult dose.

   b. a dose larger than the average adult dose.

   c. a dose smaller than the average adult dose.

   d. none of this drug because it is contraindicated in older adults.

3. Your patient is a 60-year-old woman who was seen today in the outpatient department. She is to begin a regimen of lorazepam to treat anxiety she has had since her husband died suddenly a month ago. She is to take the drug twice a day. She has told you, the nurse, that she has a two-story house, with her bedroom and bathroom upstairs. To minimize adverse effects, teach this patient to

   a. use the handrail when going down the stairs.

   b. take the evening dose at bedtime.

   c. take the larger portion of the day's dose at night.

   d. do all of the above.

   e. do none of the above.

4. Your patient received lorazepam nightly for the last 6 months to treat a sleep disorder secondary to depression. Counseling has helped lift the patient's mood, and the patient would like to stop taking the lorazepam. The best way for the patient to do this would be to

   a. stop taking the drug tonight.

   b. take half of the usual dose tonight with a glass or two of wine, then stop the drug tomorrow.

   c. take half of the usual dose tonight, then stop taking the drug starting tomorrow.

   d. taper the dose of the drug slowly before discontinuing it.

5. Your patient experiences intermittent panic attacks. The prescriber has ordered sertraline (Zoloft). The patients states, "What's with this doctor? My friend takes this drug for depression. I am not depressed." What is the nurse's best response?

   a. "You may not feel depressed, but your behavior indicates that you are."

   b. "This drug keeps the neurotransmitter serontonin working longer. People with panic disorders have a decreased amount of this neurotransmitter."

   c. "This drug will sedate you so that you will not respond to your feeling of panic."

   d. "This drug stops your anxiety by blocking the release of a neurotransmitter called serotonin."

6. Your patient had a surgical repair of a fractured arm earlier today. The patient states, "I cannot fall asleep—I am going home in the morning and my mind is just racing." After reviewing the medication order sheet, you note the patient has orders for morphine IV push every 4 to 6 hours as needed for pain, zaleplon (Sonata) as needed for sleep, and lorazepam (Ativan) as needed for anxiety. Which of these medications would be most appropriate for your patient?

a. zaleplon

b. morphine

c. lorazepam

d. none of the above

CASE STUDY

Your patient is 68 years old, has CHF, and takes digoxin, hydrochlorothiazide, and captopril daily. He is scheduled for an inguinal hernia repair this morning. He receives IV lorazepam before being anesthetized. After surgery, he confides in you, the nurse, that he "must be getting old" because he can't remember anything that happened from before surgery until he was back in his bed. What would you say to this patient?

CRITICAL THINKING CHALLENGE

The morning after surgery the patient described above reports feeling very weak, lethargic, nauseated, and does not feel like eating. What is your assessment of a possible cause of these complaints? What lab work would confirm your assessment?

CHAPTER 19

Drugs Treating Mood Disorders

TOP TEN THINGS TO KNOW ABOUT DRUGS TREATING MOOD DISORDERS

1. The two major mood disorders are depression and bipolar disorder (mania and depression alternating). Mood disorders are believed to be caused by an imbalance or dysregulation in neurotransmitters or the function of neurotransmitter receptors.

2. Antidepressants are divided into the selective serotonin reuptake inhibitors, tricyclic, and monoamine oxidase inhibitors. They bring about long-term changes in norepinephrine (NE) and serotonin (5-HT) receptor symptoms. This may be why the full therapeutic (antidepressant) effect from drug therapy may take several weeks to occur.

3. Sertraline is the prototype selective serotonin reuptake inhibitor (SSRI) antidepressant, meaning it has little effect on other neurotransmitters. This accounts for the few adverse effects. Some symptoms of depression, such as loss of energy, may be corrected before the mood is fully elevated. Patients receiving these drugs must be closely watched during the initial phases of therapy because they may be more likely to attempt suicide during this period. Sertraline and other SSRIs may actually induce suicidal thoughts and suicide, especially in children and adolescents, although this is not known positively.

4. Adverse effects that do occur tend to be mild and usually transient. Disturbances of sexual functioning can be problematic for many patients taking the drug long term and are the primary reason drug therapy is discontinued. Anticholinergic effects, cardiovascular effects, and weight gain are possible but not common.

5. Nortriptyline, the prototype tricyclic antidepressant, specifically blocks reuptake of norepinephrine (NE) into nerve terminals, thereby allowing increased concentration at postsynaptic effector sites. Three major pharmacologic actions of nortriptyline are

blocking of the amine pump, sedation, and peripheral and central anticholinergic actions.

6. The most frequently occurring adverse effects of nortriptyline are sedation and anticholinergic effects, although tolerance develops to these adverse effects. Serious adverse effects include ventricular arrhythmias, torsades de pointes, AV block, and QT prolongation.

7. Phenelzine is a monoamine oxidize inhibitor (MAOI) used for depression that does not respond to other antidepressants. Phenelzine increases the concentrations of dopamine, norepinephrine, and serotonin within the neuronal synapse. Common adverse effects of phenelzine and other MAOIs are anticholinergic effects and CNS depression effects. Severe drug–drug interactions (mixed acting sympathomimetics) or drug–food interactions (tyramine or tryptophan-rich foods) will produce severe hypertensive crisis because of excessive norepinephrine stimulation. These interactions have limited the use of phenelzine.

8. Lithium is a mood stabilizer (prevents mood swings) used in bipolar affective disorder; its effectiveness is believed to be caused by increased norepinephrine uptake and increased serotonin receptor sensitivity.

9. Lithium toxicity is dose related, and there is a narrow therapeutic index. Because the body perceives lithium ions to be sodium ions, the two compete for resorption in the proximal tubule. Decreased sodium intake causes the body to resorb more lithium, which increases the risk for toxicity. Signs of lithium toxicity include serious CNS effects, ranging from coarse hand tremor and vertigo to seizures and coma. Minimize adverse effects by monitoring drug blood levels and maintaining consistent sodium intake and blood levels.

10. Selective antiepileptic agents, such as carbamazepine, valproic acid, and lamotrigine, demonstrate antimanic effectiveness in patients who do not respond or are intolerant of lithium. Several antipsychotic drugs such as

olanzapine/fluoxetine, risperidone, aripiprazole, and ziprasidone are used for either the depressive or manic episodes in bipolar disorder.

KEY TERMS

Anagrams

Use the following anagrams to explain the key terms in the chapter.

1. Drugs used to treat depressive disorders

S S T N A S E R P E D T I N A

2. Often associated with decreased productivity, work absenteeism, unemployment, alcohol and drug abuse, and risk for suicide

E N R O P I E S D S

3. An elevated or irritable mood lasting at least 1 week

A A N M I

4. Drugs to manage or prevent mood swings in patients with bipolar disorder

O O M D
L S A E S R B I T Z I

5. Agents that affect the mind, emotions, or behavior

O C T P I C Y H S O R P S

6. A conscious state of mind or predominant emotion

D O M O

7. Characterized by recurrent episodes of depression, mania, or mixed states

R B A I L P O
O R D E I D S R

8. An imbalance of neurotransmitters that affect mood

O G Y S L I N D R E T U A

9. Depression may be caused by dysregulation of these

S N R E E U T R T O I T M R S A N

10. Overactivation of serotonin receptors

O O N N R E S T I R M
E O Y S N D

PHYSIOLOGY AND PATHOPHYSIOLOGY: THE BODY HUMAN

Essay

1. Identify the four defining symptoms of major depressive disorders.

2. Identify the defining symptoms of the manic phase of bipolar disorder.

3. Identify the symptoms that characterize serotonin reuptake inhibitor withdrawal syndrome.

CORE DRUG KNOWLEDGE: JUST THE FACTS

Multiple Choice

Circle the option that best answers the question or completes the statement.

1. Which of the following classes of antidepressants is the first choice for treating depression?
   a. selective serotonin reuptake inhibitors (SSRIs)
   b. tricyclic antidepressants (TCAs)
   c. monoamine oxidase inhibitors (MAOIs)
   d. any of the above

2. Which of the following is *not* a disorder treated with sertraline (Zoloft)?
   a. post-traumatic stress disorder
   b. bulimia
   c. panic disorder
   d. obsessive-compulsive disorder

3. The optimal therapeutic effect of sertraline (Zoloft) takes
   a. 4 to 7 days.
   b. 3 days.
   c. 1 to 2 weeks.
   d. 10 days to 4 weeks.

4. Which of the neurotransmitters are inhibited by sertraline (Zoloft)?
   1. serotonin (5-HT)
   2. acetylcholine (Ach)
   3. dopamine (DA)
   4. histamine (H1)
   5. norepinephrine (NE)
   6. epinephrine (Epi)
      a. 1, 2, 6
      b. 2, 4, 6
      c. 1, 3, 5
      d. 3, 5, 6

5. Precautions for the use of sertraline (Zoloft) include patients
   1. with compromised liver function.
   2. with compromised renal function.
   3. with chronic heart failure.
   4. with seizure disorders.
   5. who are of pediatric/adolescent age.
      a. 1, 4, 5
      b. 1, 2, 4
      c. 2, 3, 5
      d. 3, 4, 5

6. Which of the following adverse effects is associated with bupropion (Wellbutrin)?
   a. headache
   b. renal failure
   c. blood dyscrasias
   d. seizure activity

7. Because of its ability to block alpha-1 and alpha-2, trazodone (Desyrel) may induce
   a. hypertension.
   b. bronchospasm.
   c. orthostatic hypotension.
   d. nervousness.

8. The most serious potential adverse effect of tricyclic antidepressants is
   a. migraine headache.
   b. hyperpyrexia.
   c. metabolic acidosis.
   d. cardiovascular toxicity.

9. The unlabeled pharmacotherapeutics of nortriptyline (Pamelor) include
   a. enuresis in children.
   b. chronic pain syndromes.
   c. bipolar disorder.
   d. atypical psychoses.

10. The most frequently occurring adverse effects of nortriptyline (Pamelor) are
    a. anticholinergic effects and headache.
    b. hypertension and bronchospasm.
    c. sedation and anticholinergic effects.
    d. diarrhea and GI distress.

11. Phenelzine (Nardil), a monoamine oxidase inhibitor, is used in the treatment of

    a. enuresis in children.

    b. manic phase of bipolar disease.

    c. schizophrenia.

    d. depression unresponsive to other therapies.

12. The most serious potential adverse effect with phenelzine (Nardil) is

    a. anticholinergic effects.

    b. hypertensive crisis.

    c. blood dyscrasias.

    d. sexual dysfunction.

13. In the treatment of bipolar affective disorder, _____ is the drug of choice.

    a. lithium carbonate (Eskalith)

    b. carbamazepine (Tegretol)

    c. valproic acid (Depakene)

    d. gabapentin (Neurontin)

14. Contraindications for lithium (Eskalith) therapy include

    a. hepatic and renal insufficiency.

    b. cardiovascular and renal disease.

    c. seizure disorders.

    d. peptic ulcer disease.

15. The therapeutic range of lithium (Eskalith) is

    a. 5 to 12 mEq/L.

    b. 10 to 20 mEq/L.

    c. 0.5 to 2.0 mEq/L.

    d. 0.5 to 1.2 mEq/L.

CORE PATIENT VARIABLES: PATIENTS, PLEASE

Multiple Choice
Circle the option that best answers the question or completes the statement.

1. After 1 week of sertraline (Zoloft) therapy, your patient states, "I still feel so depressed." Your response is based on the fact that

    a. the dose should be increased.

    b. it takes at least 10 days of drug therapy before effects are noted.

    c. the dose should be decreased.

    d. the patient is probably being noncompliant.

2. Your 12-year-old patient is taking sertraline (Zoloft) for depression. This patient may have an increased risk for which of the following adverse effects?

    a. suicidal tendencies

    b. orthostatic hypotension

    c. blood dyscrasias

    d. weight gain

3. Your 40-year-old male patient comes to the clinic and states "I'm just not going to take sertraline (Zoloft) anymore." The patient refuses to discuss the decision to discontinue use of the medication. With your knowledge of sertraline, which adverse effect do you suspect he may be experiencing?

    a. weight gain

    b. sexual dysfunction

    c. blood dyscrasias

    d. headache

4. Your patient has been transferred from the medical surgical unit to the CICU because of a suspected myocardial infarction (MI). You note that the orders state to continue previous medications, which include nortriptyline (Pamelor). Before giving this medication, you would

    a. take the patient's blood pressure.

    b. measure a capillary blood glucose.

    c. assure adequate urine output.

    d. verify the order with the prescribing health care professional.

5. Your patient is being discharged home with a prescription for nortriptyline (Pamelor). Discharge instructions should include:

    a. "Be sure to drink lots of fluids to avoid dehydration."

    b. "Be sure to keep this medication out of the reach of your children."

    c. "Watch your intake of foods that contain tyramine."

    d. "This drug may keep you awake; use an over-the-counter sleep preparation if needed."

6. Your patient is being discharged from the hospital with a prescription for phenelzine (Nardil). Which of the following patient instructions is *incorrect*?

    a. "You must monitor your diet for foods that contain tyramine."

    b. "You should limit your exposure to sunlight."

    c. "Refrain from drinking alcohol."

    d. "This drug may make you gain weight; try using an over-the-counter weight-loss medication."

7. When performing a nursing assessment, which of these observations would be the most significant finding of a patient who takes lithium (Eskalith)?

    a. coarse hand tremor, severe GI distress, and blurred vision

    b. photophobia, weight loss, and blurred vision

    c. headache, sedation, and anxiety

    d. fatigue, irritability, and increased blood pressure

8. Your clinic patient has been taking lithium (Eskalith) for 2 years and comes to the clinic for a routine recheck. For which of the following laboratory assessments should you prepare?

    1. serum glucose
    2. cholesterol level
    3. EKG
    4. cardiac enzymes
    5. thyroid function
    6. renal function

    a. 1, 2, 6

    b. 3, 5, 6

    c. 1, 5, 6

    d. 3 only

NURSING MANAGEMENT: EVERY GOOD NURSE SHOULD …

Multiple Choice

Circle the option that best answers the question or completes the statement.

1. Your patient has started a regimen of phenelzine, an MAO inhibitor to treat depression that has not responded to other drug therapy. To minimize adverse effects, you should teach the patient to avoid

    a. aged, cured meats and cheeses.

    b. semolina pasta.

    c. apples.

    d. orange juice.

2. Your patient is taking nortriptyline, a tricyclic antidepressant, and reports a severe dry mouth after 1 week of drug therapy. The patient states, "My depression isn't better. I want to stop taking the nortriptyline." Your best response to her would be:

    a. "The dry mouth is a sign of an allergic response. You should stop taking the drug now."

    b. "Dry mouth can occur when you take this drug, but it often goes away after you are on the drug awhile. You will need to stay on the drug for a few weeks until the full antidepressant effect occurs."

    c. "Dry mouth can be bothersome with use of this drug. But the drug should have relieved your depression by now. Contact the doctor."

    d. "A dry mouth is an unusual occurrence from nortriptyline. Are you sure you are taking the drug as prescribed?"

3. A 40-year-old man has been treated for depression with sertraline, an SSRI antidepressant, for the last 6 months. At his last two visits, he reported that his depression had improved. Today he reports beginning to feel worse and more depressed again. When you ask if he is still taking the drug regularly, he admits he is not. Which of the following may have contributed to his lack of adherence? *Mark all that apply.*

    a. adverse effects of drug affecting sexuality

    b. improved mood while on the drug

    c. cost of medication

    d. no refills on the prescription

4. A 15-year-old patient who was severely depressed started a regimen of sertraline. After 2 weeks of the drug therapy, the patient's parent reports that the child is no longer spending all of her time lying on the couch, but the child's mood seems unimproved. The nurse should be certain to educate the parent that

   a. the full therapeutic effect of sertraline should be evident by now; another drug may be needed.

   b. the child may be at increased risk of suicide at this time and should be monitored closely for any changes.

   c. the child is unlikely to commit suicide because of her age.

   d. the increase in energy is a sign that the depression has fully lifted.

5. Your patient is severely depressed and tells you: "Life isn't worth living. I wish I could just end it all." He has been prescribed nortriptyline, a tricyclic antidepressant. To maximize therapeutic effects and minimize adverse effects, you should

   a. instruct the patient to discontinue use of the drug if he is still depressed after 1 week of therapy.

   b. verify that the prescription is for only a limited number of pills.

   c. discourage the patient from continuing with psychotherapy now that he is receiving drug therapy.

   d. do all of the above.

6. To minimize adverse effects from lithium, you should monitor

   a. blood lithium levels.

   b. blood potassium levels.

   c. tyramine intake.

   d. dairy intake.

CASE STUDY

Your patient was started on a regimen of lithium as drug therapy for bipolar affective disorder about 2 weeks ago. The patient tells you, "I don't feel any different than before I started this drug." The patient reports having one manic episode, although it was not quite as severe as the ones experienced before starting lithium therapy. The patient's major complaint today is an upset stomach after taking the lithium in the morning. What patient-related variables should you assess to obtain more information related to this patient's comments?

CRITICAL THINKING CHALLENGE

The patient described above returns to the clinic for follow-up 3 months later. At this time, the patient reports blurred vision and vertigo. You note a hand tremor in the left hand. Blood lithium levels are 2 mEq/L. You ask if there have been any other recent changes. The patient replies, "Well, I've cut my salt intake to practically zero because I heard that salt wasn't good for my 'pressure.'"

What is your assessment of the patient's current condition? What factors contributed to the current blood lithium levels? Explain how these factors contributed to the condition.

CHAPTER 20

Drugs Treating Psychotic Disorders and Dementia

TOP TEN THINGS TO KNOW ABOUT DRUGS TREATING PSYCHOTIC DISORDERS AND DEMENTIA

1. **Psychosis** is the inability to perceive and interpret reality accurately, think clearly, respond correctly, and function in a socially appropriate manner. Disordered thoughts can produce speech and behavior patterns that are confusing and even frightening to the individual and those around him.

2. **Dementia** is a clinical syndrome of progressive, degenerative loss of memory and one or more of these abilities: language skills, judgment, comprehension, problem solving, ability to recognize or identify objects despite intact sensory function, and ability to perform motor skills. Mood and behavior may also be affected in dementia. There are many types of dementia, including Alzheimer disease.

3. **Delirium** is a sudden disruption in cognitive functioning that is most often caused by a physical change in the body, as opposed to changes within the brain. Disturbance in the level of consciousness will come and go (waxing and waning) throughout the day(s) that delirium is present. Psychotic-like symptoms (hallucinations and delusions) can occur with delirium. Delirium has an underlying cause, which must be identified and treated, or delirium may be fatal. Use of an antipsychotic or sedative will calm the patient but not resolve the cause of the delirium.

4. Antipsychotic drugs are used in the treatment of acute and chronic psychotic illnesses, such as schizophrenia. Antipsychotics are divided into two groups: the typical and the atypical.

5. Typical antipsychotic drugs block dopamine receptors. In addition, these drugs block some nondopamine receptors (histamine, alpha-1 adrenergic, and cholinergic). Many of the adverse effects from these drugs are from binding to these other receptor sites. Typical antipsychotic drugs typically cause extrapyramidal (EPS) adverse effects. They vary in their potency, although all are similarly effective in controlling psychotic symptoms. More potent drugs tend to have more EPS adverse effects; less potent drugs tend to have more anticholinergic adverse effects.

6. Haloperidol, the prototype typical antipsychotic, is used in the treatment of psychotic disorders such as schizophrenia. The full therapeutic effect can take several days to be achieved. Haloperidol produces its effects by blocking dopamine, alpha, serotonin, and histamine receptors. It has minimal blocking effects at cholinergic receptors. Blockade of dopaminergic receptors produces a decrease in movement disorders, relief of hallucinations and delusions, relief of psychosis, worsening of negative symptoms, and a release of prolactin. Dopamine blockade also quiets the chemoreceptive trigger zone in the brain that produces nausea and vomiting. Blockade of alpha receptors produces many of the cardiac adverse effects of haloperidol treatment.

7. The most common adverse effect of haloperidol is extrapyramidal symptoms (akinesia, dystonia, pseudoparkinsonism) in the first weeks of therapy and, with long-term use, tardive dyskinesia (abnormal involuntary movements of mouth, tongue, and face). Tardive dyskinesia is irreversible. The cause of these symptoms is the relative lack of dopamine stimulation and relative excess of cholinergic stimulation. The risk for EPS increases if drug therapy is repeatedly and abruptly stopped and then restarted. A potentially fatal adverse effect called neuroleptic malignant syndrome can occur from haloperidol and other typical antipsychotics. It is more likely to occur if large doses are used. Adverse effects may limit a patient's acceptance of and adherence with drug therapy. Teach the patient how to manage or deal with these adverse effects.

8. Atypical antipsychotics differ from the typical antipsychotics in that they target specific dopamine receptors instead of all of them. This creates a much lower adverse effect profile. Another major advantage of the atypical antipsychotics is that they treat both the negative and positive symptoms of schizophrenia. Atypical antipsychotics have significant attraction for serotonin receptors, alpha adrenergic receptors, histamine receptors, and muscarinic receptors and produce a blockade at these sites. Atypical antipsychotics are unlikely to cause the extrapyramidal symptoms that are common with the typical antipsychotics.

9. Olanzapine, an atypical antipsychotic drug, is used for treatment of psychotic symptoms in schizophrenia and short-term treatment of bipolar mania. Full therapeutic effects can take several weeks of treatment to achieve. The most common adverse effects affect the CNS, although the drug is usually well tolerated. Hyperglycemia, which can be severe, can occur from olanzapine and other atypical antipsychotics. Patients with diabetes are at most risk of hyperglycemia and require frequent blood glucose monitoring.

10. Rivastigmine is used in the treatment of mild to moderate dementia associated with Alzheimer disease. It enhances memory, language and orientation, and improves the ability to perform activities of daily living. Rivastigmine inhibits acetylcholinesterase (an enzyme that degrades acethycholine) and thus increases the concentration of acetylcholine. The most common adverse effects of rivastigmine are gastrointestinal ones (nausea, vomiting, anorexia, weight loss).

KEY TERMS

Fill in the Blank
Complete the following sentences using the correct key term.

1. A clinical syndrome of progressive, degenerative loss of memory and one or more of these abilities: language skills; higher-level skills such as judgment, comprehension, and problem solving; ability to recognize or identify objects despite intact sensory function; and ability to perform motor skills is called _____.

2. Pseudoparkinsonism, akathisia, acute dystonia, and tardive dyskinesia are types of _____.

3. Symptoms of _____ include involuntary lip smacking, chewing, mouth movements, tongue protrusion, blinking, grimacing, and involuntary muscle twitching of the limbs.

4. _____ is characterized by fever, sweating, tachycardia, muscle rigidity, tremor, incontinence, stupor, leukocytosis, elevated creatinine phosphokinase (CPK) levels, and renal failure.

5. A sudden disruption in cognitive functioning that is most often caused by a disturbance within the body, as opposed to within the brain, is known as _____.

6. For people older than 65 years, _____ is the most common cause of dementia.

7. _____ is the inability to perceive and interpret reality accurately, think clearly, respond correctly, and function in a socially appropriate manner.

8. A psychosis that is characterized mainly by a clear sensory apparatus but a marked disturbance in thinking is known as _____.

9. _____ results from damage to brain tissue caused by cerebrovascular events, such as transient ischemic attacks.

PHYSIOLOGY AND PATHOPHYSIOLOGY: THE BODY HUMAN

Essay

1. What are the functions of the frontal lobes of the brain?

2. Identify the other CNS functional systems and their responsibilities.

3. What role do the brain neurotransmitters play in the treatment of psychosis?

4. Describe the results of neurotransmitter blockade with haloperidol (Haldol).

5. Compare and contrast the "positive," "negative," and disorganized symptoms of schizophrenia.

CORE DRUG KNOWLEDGE: JUST THE FACTS

Multiple Choice
Circle the option that best answers the question or completes the statement.

1. Haloperidol (Haldol) is commonly used in the treatment of
   a. schizophrenia.
   b. bipolar affective disorder.
   c. major depression.
   d. all of the above.

2. The most common adverse effect associated with haloperidol (Haldol) is
   a. hypertension.
   b. blurred vision.
   c. extrapyramidal syndromes.
   d. photosensitivity.

3. Antipsychotic drugs, such as haloperidol (Haldol), work by
   a. blocking neurotransmitter receptor sites.
   b. increasing the excretion of neurotransmitters.
   c. increasing the metabolism of neurotransmitters.
   d. decreasing the metabolism of neurotransmitters.

4. Haloperidol (Haldol) is contraindicated in patients with pre-existing
   a. chronic heart failure.
   b. asthma.
   c. Parkinson disease.
   d. myasthenia gravis.

5. A potentially fatal adverse effect associated with the administration of clozapine (Clozaril) is
   a. neuroleptic malignant syndrome.
   b. agranulocytosis.
   c. hepatotoxicity.
   d. hypothyroidism.

6. Which of the following statements concerning olanzapine (Zyprexa) is incorrect?
   a. It is efficacious in treating the symptoms of schizophrenia.
   b. It causes fewer EPS adverse effects than do typical antipsychotic drugs.
   c. It blocks dopamine, serotonin, muscarinic, histamine-1, and alpha-1 receptors.
   d. It has no serious adverse effects.

7. Adverse effects to olanzapine (Zyprexa) occur most commonly in the _____ system.
   a. central nervous
   b. gastrointestinal
   c. cardiovascular
   d. integumentary

8. Olanzapine (Zyprexa) is given cautiously to patients with
   a. asthma.
   b. seizures.
   c. hyperthyroidism.
   d. diabetes mellitus.

9. Alzheimer disease may be treated with
   a. clozapine (Clozaril).
   b. rivastigmine (Exelon).
   c. haloperidol (Haldol).
   d. olanzapine (Zyprexa).

10. Rivastigmine (Exelon) works by
    a. stimulating cholinergic activity.
    b. blocking cholinergic activity.
    c. stimulating sympathetic activity.
    d. stimulating dopaminergic activity.

11. Rivastigmine (Exelon) should be used cautiously in patients with
    a. diabetes mellitus.
    b. hypertension.
    c. asthma.
    d. chronic heart failure.

12. Adverse effects to rivastigmine (Exelon) occur most commonly in the _____ system.

    a. central nervous

    b. gastrointestinal

    c. cardiovascular

    d. integumentary

13. Which of the following statements regarding memantine (Namenda) is accurate?

    a. It has the same mechanism of action, adverse effects, and drug interactions as rivastigmine (Exelon).

    b. It is used for the management of schizophrenia.

    c. It can be used in combination with rivastigmine (Exelon) to manage Alzheimer disease.

    d. It is similar to clonazepam (Clozeril) and may cause serious blood dyscrasias.

Matching

Match the symptoms with the type of EPS or adverse effect associated with haloperidol.

1. _____ neuroleptic malignant syndrome

2. _____ pseudoparkinsonism

3. _____ akathisia

4. _____ acute dystonia

    a. Constant feeling of restlessness

    b. Cog-wheeling, muscle rigidity, fine tremor

    c. Prolonged muscular contractions and spasms

    d. Fever, sweating, tachycardia, muscle rigidity

CORE PATIENT VARIABLES: PATIENTS, PLEASE

Multiple Choice
Circle the option that best answers the question or completes the statement.

1. Your 66-year old female patient is taking haloperidol (Haldol) for schizophrenia. You note that the patient is smacking her lips and has muscle twitching of the limbs. You suspect the patient is experiencing

    a. akathisia.

    b. neuroleptic malignant syndrome.

    c. tardive dyskinesia.

    d. acute dystonia.

2. Your patient comes to the clinic today for a refill of haloperidol (Haldol). The patient reports nausea, fatigue, rash, and yellow skin. You understand that

    a. these are expected adverse effects because of the anticholinergic and antidopaminergic properties of the drug.

    b. the nausea is an expected adverse effect, but the yellow skin may mean the dose needs to be increased.

    c. these are annoying symptoms, but nothing needs to be done.

    d. these are symptoms of adverse effects, and use of the drug should be stopped immediately.

3. Which of the following patients has the highest risk for adverse effects from haloperidol (Haldol) therapy?

    a. Louise, age 36, with asthma

    b. Malcolm, age 65, with cardiovascular disease

    c. Terry, age 17, with seizures

    d. Stephanie, age 27, with hyperthyroidism

4. Your patient takes haloperidol (Haldol) for schizophrenia. He is very excited about a new horticulture class he is taking. What assessment should you make related to this patient's new class?

    a. "Are you taking precautions to keep away from pesticides?"

    b. "Do you use tools that can be used to injure someone else?"

    c. "How much time do you need to spend in the sunlight?"

    d. "Are you able to handle the increased movement OK?"

5. Your patient has been taking chlorpromazine (Thorazine) for 2 months and states, "My mouth feels like cotton." What is your best response?

    a. "This is very common. Let me give you some suggestions to make it better."

    b. "This is very rare. Stop taking the drug immediately."

    c. "This happens once in a while. I will make an appointment for you."

    d. "I will call the doctor; this sounds serious."

6. Your patient has been taking olanzapine (Zyprexa) for 1 year. The patient comes to the clinic today and is excited about installing a hot tub in the back yard. What important patient teaching should be done with this patient?

    a. "Soaking for too long can damage your skin."

    b. "Be sure that there is no chlorine in the water."

    c. "You should not get in the hot tub."

    d. "Be sure to always have someone with you."

7. Your diabetic patient takes olanzapine (Zyprexa) for schizophrenia. Patient teaching for this patient should include

    a. foods that will help the patient gain weight.

    b. nonpharmacologic ways to manage constipation.

    c. relaxation techniques for headaches.

    d. the need for frequent glucose monitoring.

8. Your patient has been hospitalized after an automobile accident and subsequent seizure. The health care provider plans to prescribe an antiepileptic drug for the patient. You note that the patient has been taking olanzapine (Zyprexa) for the past year. Which of the following antiepileptics could be problematic for this patient?

    a. phenytoin (Dilantin)

    b. valproic acid (Depakene)

    c. carbamazepine (Tegretol)

    d. gabapentin (Neurontin)

9. Your patient has Alzheimer disease. He begins a regimen of rivastigmine (Exelon). Patient teaching for him should include

    a. cessation of smoking.

    b. low-fat foods to avoid weight gain.

    c. methods to manage constipation.

    d. the need to avoid caffeine products.

10. Your patient takes rivastigmine (Exelon) for Alzheimer disease. Her caregiver should monitor her

    a. breath sounds.

    b. heart rate.

    c. weight.

    d. for all of the above.

11. To assess the efficacy of rivastigmine (Exelon) therapy, the nurse should assess for

    a. occurrence of adverse effects.

    b. increased cognition.

    c. weight gain.

    d. control of bladder and bowel.

NURSING MANAGEMENT: EVERY GOOD NURSE SHOULD …

Multiple Choice

Circle the option that best answers the question or completes the statement.

1. Your patient has recently started treatment with haloperidol, a typical antipsychotic. The patient reports that her mouth is dry all of the time. The nurse should recommend

    a. rinsing the mouth with hydrogen peroxide.

    b. sucking on sugarless hard candies.

    c. increasing dietary intake of sodium.

    d. discontinuation of use of haloperidol.

2. Your patient works as a brick mason. He is currently being treated with haloperidol, a typical antipsychotic. Education about his drug therapy should include

    a. the importance of wearing sunscreen or protective clothing while working outside.

    b. the importance of needing daily exposure to sunlight.

    c. that he should not be working while he is taking this drug.

    d. that his urine may turn blue while he is taking this drug.

3. Your patient has been receiving a daily maintenance dose of olanzapine for 3 weeks. The patient returns to the clinic voicing the following complaints: "I'm dizzy when I first get out of bed and stand up. I'm also sleepy all the time during the daytime." To minimize these adverse effects, the nurse should recommend that the patient

    a. increase the dose of olanzapine.

    b. stand up quickly when getting out of bed.

    c. eat six large meals a day.

    d. take the drug at bedtime.

4. You are caring for a patient with schizophrenia who also has type 1 diabetes. He is receiving olanzapine, an atypical antipsychotic. To minimize adverse effects, the nurse should closely monitor

   a. SGOT and SGPT levels.

   b. BUN levels.

   c. glucose levels.

   d. sodium levels.

5. Your patient is being treated for a psychotic illness with haloperidol, a typical antipsychotic. He is experiencing akathisia, which he finds annoying and embarrassing. Which suggestion would best help him deal with this adverse effect?

   a. play quiet music on headphones during the day

   b. try to sleep more

   c. get up and move around frequently

   d. get used to these feelings

6. A patient taking haloperidol, a typical antipsychotic, has been brought to the emergency room by his family. The patient has a temperature of 102°F and a pulse of 110 bpm. He is lethargic and sweating, and his muscles seem rigid, with a tremor noted. He has had an episode of urinary incontinence. His white blood cell count is 14.0 $10^3/mm^3$ (normal range, 3.2–9.8 $10^3/mm^3$), and his creatinine phosphokinase (CPK) level is 250 mcg/L (normal range, is 0–150 mcg/L). Which actions would you, as the nurse, expect to implement? *Mark all that apply.*

   a. give another dose of the haloperidol STAT

   b. infuse large volumes of 0.9 NS solution IV

   c. administer acetaminophen by rectal suppository

   d. place patient on a stretcher in the middle of the ER to be easily observed

7. To maximize the therapeutic effect of rivastigmine given for Alzheimer disease, the nurse should do which of the following before initiating the drug therapy?

   a. confirm that there are no current, uncorrected hearing problems

   b. take away the patient's glasses to prevent injury

   c. confirm that the patient is reliable enough to administer his own medications

   d. all of the above

8. Your patient has Alzheimer disease and is being treated with rivastigmine. A family member who cares for the patient tells you that the patient is eating very little and has lost a great deal of weight. To minimize the adverse effects of rivastigmine, you should suggest the family member

   a. encourage a greater daily intake of water.

   b. withhold all solid food.

   c. supplement meals with Boost or Ensure beverages.

   d. provide a diet with high fiber and roughage content.

CASE STUDY

Your patient has been receiving haloperidol, a typical antipsychotic, for 6 weeks. Today you notice that he appears to shuffle some when he walks. He appears somewhat stiff and rigid. His hand shakes slightly when he tries to use his arm. He is somewhat expressionless, without facial expression.

What do you think is the patient's problem?
What do you think is the cause of these findings?
Would you seek any changes in the drug therapy that is ordered?

CRITICAL THINKING CHALLENGE

The patient described above stops taking his haloperidol for a few weeks. When the psychotic symptoms return, he resumes taking the haloperidol. Two weeks later he is rushed to the ER. He demonstrates arching and twisting of the neck, arching of the back, rolling of the eyes up toward the back of the head, and spasms of the laryngeal-pharyngeal muscles. What do you think is the patient's problem now? What do you think has caused these symptoms? What drug would you be likely to administer? By what route? What other nursing actions would be necessary?

CHAPTER 21

Drugs Treating Seizure Disorders

TOP TEN THINGS TO KNOW ABOUT DRUGS TREATING SEIZURE DISORDERS

1. Most antiepileptic drugs (AED) control seizures through one of three ways: decreasing the rate that sodium flows into the cell, inhibiting calcium flow rate into the cell via specific channels, and increasing the effect of the neuroinhibitor GABA. Some drugs work in more than one way.

2. The choice of AED depends on the type of seizures and on patient-related variables, such as age and health status. Monotherapy is the desired goal, although combination therapy may be necessary. Insufficient dosage of an AED or sudden withdrawal of an AED may precipitate seizures or status epilepticus.

3. AEDs are all central nervous system (CNS) depressants, and CNS depressant adverse effects are common. Other CNS depressants, such as alcohol, will cause additive CNS depression and should be avoided.

4. All AEDs carry risks of teratogenicity. Stopping drug therapy also carries the risk of inducing seizures, which is risky to the mother and the fetus. Most babies born to epileptic mothers receiving drug therapy are unaffected.

5. Nursing management for AEDs includes having patients take prescribed drug at regular intervals, monitoring blood drug levels to determine therapeutic or toxic levels, instructing in the importance of wearing a Medic Alert bracelet stating they have epilepsy, encouraging good oral hygiene (with use of phenytoin), teaching to avoid sudden cessation of AED, teaching safety precautions relevant to CNS depression, and teaching to avoid simultaneous use of other CNS depressants.

6. Phenytoin, a hydantoin, reversibly binds to sodium channels while they are in the inactive state. This delays the return of the channel to an active state, preventing sodium from entering the cells, lengthening the time between action potentials, and preventing excessive muscle contractions that occur in grand mal-type seizures. Phenytoin selectively binds to sites where there is hyperactivity of the neurons; it does not affect cells that have normally firing neurons. Phenytoin is the drug of choice for most seizures, except absence seizures. The half-life of phenytoin increases as the dose increases.

7. Phenytoin has numerous drug interactions because phenytoin induces some of the P-450 isoenzymes; these drug interactions usually alter metabolism of either drug. Drug absorption will be decreased if given within 2 hours of an antacid or if given via NG or GT concurrently with tube feedings.

8. The most common adverse effects of phenytoin are related to CNS depression. A fairly common adverse effect is gingival hyperplasia, which may be disfiguring. If given too rapidly intravenously, cardiovascular collapse, hypotension, and significant CNS depression may occur. A known syndrome of fetal teratogenic effects occurs when phenytoin is used in pregnancy.

9. Ethosuximide is used in managing and controlling absence seizures. Ethosuximide works by inhibiting the influx of calcium ions when they travel through a special set of channels (T-type calcium channels). This decreases the electric current generated by calcium movement and decreases the frequency of an action potential. This effect is evident only in the hypothalamus neurons, which are responsible for absence seizures. Common adverse effects of ethosuximide are drowsiness, dizziness, and lethargy.

10. Diazepam, a benzodiazepine, is the first-line treatment for status epilepticus; lorazepam is also used, but it is an off-label use. Both drugs work by potentiating the effects of the inhibitory neurotransmitter GABA.. They are not used for maintenance of a seizure disorder. Clonazepam and clorazepate are also benzodiazepines; however, they are not used for status epilepticus, rather, they are used as maintenance drugs for specific types of seizures.

KEY TERMS

Fill in the Blank
Complete the following sentences using the correct key term.

1. A(n) _____ occurs when the muscles alternate between contracting and relaxing.

2. A(n) _____ is caused by disturbances of nerve cells in more diffuse areas and both hemispheres of the brain.

3. The _____ phase of a seizure is when abnormal movements cease.

4. A petit mal seizure is also known as a(n) _____ seizure.

5. A(n) _____ is a paroxysmal involuntary alteration of behavior, movement, or sensation, triggered by an abnormal electric discharge in the brain.

6. A(n) _____ is subdivided into simple, complex, and secondarily generalized seizures.

7. A grand mal seizure is also called _____.

8. A chronic condition characterized by recurrent, unprovoked seizures is labeled _____.

9. _____ is the main inhibitory neurotransmitter in the mammalian central nervous system.

10. A patient who experiences seizure after seizure is said to have _____.

11. _____ is an excitatory neurotransmitter balanced by GABA.

PHYSIOLOGY AND PATHOPHYSIOLOGY: THE BODY HUMAN

Essay

1. Uncontrolled electrical impulses and excessive neuronal firing are prevented by:

2. How do seizures occur?

3. What are the subdivisions of generalized seizures?

CORE DRUG KNOWLEDGE: JUST THE FACTS

Multiple Choice
Circle the option that best answers the question or completes the statement.

1. Phenytoin (Dilantin) inhibits seizure activity by
   a. decreasing calcium influx from the neurons in the motor cortex of the brain.
   b. decreasing sodium influx from the neurons in the motor cortex of the brain.
   c. increasing the effectiveness of GABA.
   d. none of the above.

2. Which of the following statements concerning phenytoin (Dilantin) is *incorrect*?
   a. widely used AED for tonic-clonic seizure activity
   b. most effective AED for absence seizures
   c. used as prophylaxis for postoperative neurologic patients
   d. may also be used in the treatment of trigeminal neuralgia

3. The therapeutic margin (index) for phenytoin (Dilantin) is
   a. 10 to 20 mcg/mL.
   b. 2 to 10 mcg/mL.
   c. 40 to 100 mcg/mL.
   d. 4 to 12 mcg/mL.

4. Which of the following adverse effects would necessitate cessation of phenytoin (Dilantin) therapy?
   a. acne
   b. urine discoloration
   c. gingival hyperplasia
   d. blistered skin rash

5. The most common adverse effects to phenytoin (Dilantin) occur in which body system?

    a. gastrointestinal

    b. integumentary

    c. CNS

    d. hematopoietic

6. Which of the following patients would be a poor candidate for phenytoin (Dilantin) therapy?

    a. a 60-year-old man with bradycardia

    b. an 18-year-old woman with asthma

    c. a 40-year-old woman with migraine headaches

    d. a 42-year-old man with benign prostatic hypertrophy

7. Pharmacotherapeutics for carbamazepine (Tegretol) include

    a. bipolar disorder.

    b. migraine headache.

    c. restless leg syndrome.

    d. parkinsonism.

8. Serious adverse effects to carbamazepine (Tegretol) therapy include

    a. Stevens-Johnson syndrome.

    b. blood dyscrasias.

    c. nephrotoxicity.

    d. cardiotoxicity.

9. Serious adverse effects to valproic acid (Depakene) therapy include

    a. liver toxicity.

    b. photosensitivity.

    c. tremors.

    d. renal toxicity.

10. Serious adverse effects to topiramate (Topamax) therapy include

    a. psychomotor slowing.

    b. decreased sweating and hyperthermia.

    c. renal toxicity.

    d. liver toxicity.

11. Serious adverse effects to levetiracetam (Keppra) therapy include

    a. hepatitis.

    b. arrhythmias.

    c. asthenia.

    d. headache.

12. Serious adverse effects to felbamate (Felbatol) therapy include

    a. arrhythmias.

    b. aplastic anemia.

    c. respiratory infections.

    d. renal toxicity.

13. The drug of choice for the treatment of absence seizures is

    a. valproic acid (Depakene).

    b. ethosuximide (Zarontin).

    c. diazepam (Valium).

    d. carbamazepine (Tegretol).

14. The therapeutic margin (index) for ethosuximide (Zarontin) is

    a. 10 to 20 mcg/mL.

    b. 40 to 100 mcg/mL.

    c. 2 to 10 mcg/mL.

    d. 4 to 12 mcg/mL.

15. Serious adverse effects to ethosuximide (Zarontin) therapy include

    a. Parkinson-like symptoms.

    b. sedation.

    c. headache.

    d. blood dyscrasias.

16. The drug of choice for status epilepticus is

    a. clonazepam (Klonopin).

    b. clorazepate (Tranxene).

    c. diazepam (Valium).

    d. phenytoin (Dilantin).

17. A benefit of gabapentin (Neurontin) therapy is

    a. minimal drug–food interactions.

    b. extensive pharmacotherapeutic profile.

    c. once-a-day dosing.

    d. all of the above.

18. One of the most serious potential adverse effects of phenobarbital (Luminal) therapy is

    a. bone marrow depression.

    b. Stevens-Johnson syndrome.

    c. respiratory depression.

    d. migraine headaches.

19. In the elderly, phenobarbital (Luminal) therapy may induce
    a. excitement and confusion.
    b. lethargy and hypertension.
    c. headache and tachypnea.
    d. suicide ideation.

20. Which of the following adverse effects may occur with *all* antiepileptic drugs?
    a. blood dyscrasias c. hepatic injury
    b. nosocomial   d. teratogenic effects
       infections

Short Answer

Identify which AED drugs are used for partial seizures, generalized seizures and status epilepticus. Drugs may be used in more than one column.

Partial Seizures	Generalized Seizures (except status epilepticus)	Status Epilepticus

CORE PATIENT VARIABLES: PATIENTS, PLEASE

Multiple Choice
Circle the option that best answers the question or completes the statement.

1. Your patient has been prescribed phenytoin (Dilantin) for a seizure disorder. Which of the following should be included in this patient's discharge instructions?
   a. "Be sure to use precautions when you are in the sunlight."
   b. "Brush and floss your teeth at least twice a day."
   c. "Have your cholesterol level checked once a year."
   d. "Be sure to increase your intake of carbohydrates."

2. Your patient who takes phenytoin (Dilantin) tells you that another physician has prescribed several new drugs. What is your best response?
   a. "I am sure that your other doctor knows what he is doing."
   b. "Most medications are fine to take with phenytoin."
   c. "Before you start any new drugs, be sure both doctors know what the other doctor is prescribing."
   d. "I would not take those."

3. Your patient who takes phenytoin states, "I'm ready to get pregnant." What is your best response?
   a. "Phenytoin will not interfere with your ability to conceive."
   b. "Just stop taking the medication before you try to conceive."
   c. "That is not such a good idea."
   d. "Before you stop your medication, let's get you an appointment with the doctor."

4. Your patient has been prescribed ethosuximide (Zarontin) for absence seizures. The patient tells you of an episode of hepatitis in the past. Which of the following laboratory tests should be completed before the initiation of therapy?
   a. CBC
   b. arterial blood gas
   c. AST, ALT
   d. BUN, creatinine clearance

5. Your patient, who is taking ethosuximide, reports a sore throat and easy bruising. Which of the following diagnostic tests should you coordinate?
   a. liver function
   b. thyroid function
   c. complete blood count
   d. chest x-ray

6. Your patient is in status epilepticus, and the health care provider has ordered IV diazepam (Valium). How will you administer this drug?
   a. 5 mg/minute, undiluted
   b. 2 mg/minute, undiluted
   c. 50 mg/minute, mixed with normal saline
   d. 10 mg/minute, mixed with sterile water

7. A patient, age 18, calls the clinic and tells the advice nurse, "My friends all make fun of me because I have to take clonazepam (Klonopin). I'm not coming for my appointment, and I'm just going to stop taking this medication." The best response would be:

   a. "It doesn't matter what your friends think, but if you want to stop the medication, just go ahead."

   b. "I understand your problem. I'll cancel your appointment."

   c. "Sounds like you are upset. Would you like to see the psychiatrist?"

   d. "If you stop your medication abruptly you may have seizures again."

8. Your patient takes carbamazepine (Tegretol). She calls the clinic and reports a sore throat and easy bruising. You would advise her to

   a. stop taking the drug and make an appointment to be seen next week.

   b. continue taking the drug and make an appointment to be seen next week.

   c. come to the clinic to be seen today.

   d. increase her intake of green leafy vegetables and call if the symptoms continue.

9. Your patient, age 22, calls the clinic and states she is having trouble swallowing her topiramate (Topamax) tablets. You would advise her to

   a. continue to swallow the medication whole and make an appointment to discuss the problem with her provider.

   b. crush the tablet and place it in a glass of water.

   c. chew the tablet.

   d. break the tablets in half and chew them.

10. Your patient was brought to the emergency department after having a seizure. The patient states, "I've taken my primidone (Mysoline) twice a day. I never miss." Which of the following STAT tests would be indicated for this patient?

    a. primidone level

    b. phenobarbital level

    c. liver function tests

    d. renal function tests

NURSING MANAGEMENT: EVERY GOOD NURSE SHOULD …

Multiple Choice
Circle the option that best answers the question or completes the statement.

1. Your patient is receiving phenytoin for seizures. There are new orders for the patient to start a regimen of cimetidine, an H_2-receptor blocker, for a gastric ulcer. You should

   a. administer both drugs as ordered.

   b. administer cimetidine one day and phenytoin the next day.

   c. verify if drug interactions exist between the drugs.

   d. obtain an order for an oral antacid to be given with both drugs.

2. Your patient has been stabilized with a regimen of phenytoin and is to begin taking theophylline, a drug known to increase the metabolism of phenytoin. The nurse should expect to

   a. monitor blood phenytoin levels for a drop compared with before theophylline therapy.

   b. monitor blood phenytoin levels for an increase compared with before theophylline therapy.

   c. monitor blood theophylline levels; they may remain below therapeutic levels because of phenytoin.

   d. monitor blood theophylline levels; they may become toxic because of phenytoin.

3. Your patient is a 22-year-old woman who receives phenytoin for seizures. Her disease is well controlled, and she has not had a seizure for 5 years. During her routine follow-up visit, she tells you she is getting married and would like to have children. She asks if she should stay on the phenytoin if she becomes pregnant. Your best response would be that

   a. phenytoin is safe to use during pregnancy.

   b. she should stop using the phenytoin as soon as she becomes pregnant.

   c. before she attempts to become pregnant, she should consult with her provider to see if she could be weaned from the phenytoin.

   d. she may continue to take the phenytoin as long as her blood levels remain in the therapeutic range.

4. Your patient receives nutrition through continuous tube feeding (30 cc/hour). He also is to receive phenytoin suspension via gastrostomy tube every 8 hours. To maximize the therapeutic effects of phenytoin, you should

    a. mix the phenytoin with 200 cc of tube feeding and administer at 30 cc/hour.

    b. mix the phenytoin with 100 cc of tube feeding and administer as a bolus.

    c. turn the tube feeding off for 1 hour before and 1 hour after administering phenytoin.

    d. turn the tube feeding off for 8 hours, then administer all three daily doses of phenytoin as one bolus.

5. You are to administer phenytoin IV to your patient, who is experiencing status epilepticus and who did not experience response to IV diazepam, a benzodiazepine. To minimize the risk of serious adverse effects to this patient, you should

    a. provide good oral hygiene.

    b. administer the drug slowly.

    c. obtain a blood phenytoin level before administering the drug.

    d. warn the patient that he may be drowsy.

6. You are caring for a 6-year-old child who is to begin a regimen of ethosuximide for absence seizures. What information should be included in teaching for the child and his parents?

    a. Drowsiness may occur initially, but this should go away after the child has been on drug therapy for awhile.

    b. Fever is a common and nonserious adverse effect.

    c. If a dose is missed, it may be made up by doubling the dose the next time.

    d. Avoid eating fried foods because this may produce a drug–food interaction.

7. Your patient has begun a regimen of carbamazepine for grand mal seizures that have not been controlled by several other AEDs. To minimize adverse effects, the nurse should teach the importance of

    a. returning for lab appointments and follow-up.

    b. increasing fluid intake.

    c. driving a car, to maintain independence.

    d. all of the above.

    e. none of the above

CASE STUDY

An 8-year-old child begins a regimen of phenytoin suspension 125 mg BID (125 mg/5 cc) for seizures. At the first visit after drug therapy was initiated, the mother reports that the seizures have not improved. The blood phenytoin level is 4 (therapeutic levels are usually 10 to 20 mcg/mL). Based on these findings, the daily dose of phenytoin is increased. Two weeks later, the child is rushed to the emergency room. The child's eyes are moving in unusual patterns (nystagmus) and speech is slurred. The blood phenytoin level is now 24 mcg/mL.

1. What is your assessment of the patient's condition?

2. What questions should you ask the mother to gain understanding regarding what may have contributed to the patient's current condition?

CRITICAL THINKING CHALLENGE

An adult is receiving phenytoin for seizures. At a follow-up visit to the clinic, the patient reports that his seizures are well controlled by the drug therapy. The blood phenytoin level is 8 mcg/mL. The physician increases the dose so that the blood level will be in the range of normal. The patient returns in a week reporting his eyes are bothering him, he has an awkward gait, and confusion. The blood phenytoin level is now 14 mcg/mL. What is your assessment of his current findings? What explanation can be made for this assessment?

CHAPTER 22

Drugs Stimulating the Central Nervous System

TOP TEN THINGS TO KNOW ABOUT DRUGS STIMULATING THE CENTRAL NERVOUS SYSTEM

1. Central nervous system (CNS) stimulants may provoke an increased release of neurotransmitters, a decreased reuptake of neurotransmitters, and/or inhibition of postsynaptic enzymes. The net result of these actions is increased stimulation at the receptor and increased arousal.
2. CNS stimulants are used in the treatment of narcolepsy, attention deficit hyperactivity disorder (ADHD), obesity, and respiratory depression.
3. All of the drugs currently used for the treatment of ADHD increase the risk for serious cardiovascular and psychiatric adverse effects. Sudden death may occur in patients with underlying serious heart problems or defects, and stroke and heart attack in adults with certain risk factors.
4. Dextroamphetamine, used primarily for the treatment of narcolepsy and ADHD, causes the release of norepinephrine, the release of dopamine in adrenergic nerve terminals (in high doses), and interferes with the reuptake of dopamine.
5. Adverse effects of dextroamphetamine (similar to all CNS stimulants) are signs of CNS overstimulation. They include restlessness, dizziness, insomnia, agitation, tachycardia, palpitations, and elevated blood pressure.
6. Dextroamphetamine, like all amphetamines, has the potential to be abused. Assess the patient for a history of substance abuse.
7. Sibutramine is used in the treatment of obesity, by increasing weight loss. Sibutramine inhibits the central reuptake of dopamine, norepinephrine, and serotonin. It is thought that the serotonin mechanism enhances satiety, whereas the norepinephrine mechanism raises the metabolic rate.
8. The nurse should assess the patient's diet and suggest appropriate modifications because sibutramine is most effective when combined with a low-calorie diet and behavior changes.
9. Caffeine is a mild, direct stimulant at all levels of the CNS. It stimulates the cardiovascular system and the medullary respiratory center, although it relaxes bronchial smooth muscle.
10. Caffeine is used in the management of neonatal apnea, asthma, drowsiness, and fatigue, and in combination with other drugs to treat headache and migraine. When used for neonatal apnea, the nurse should monitor the patient's vital signs carefully.

KEY TERMS

Fill in the Blank

Complete the following sentences using the correct key term.

1. In the disorder ADHD, dextroamphetamine has a paradoxical effect.

2. A brief, sudden loss of motor control is known as cataplexy

3. Irresistible bouts of rapid-eye movement sleep during nonsleep cycles are characteristic of Narcolepsy, a neurologic condition.

4. Sleep paralysis is characterized by being unable to speak or move before the onset of sleep.

5. An excessive accumulation of adipose is termed Obesity

6. Hypercapnia is a buildup of carbon dioxide in the body.

7. Substances used to stimulate the CNS are called ___Analeptic___

8. To suppress the appetite, a(n) ___Anorectic___ drug may be ordered.

9. During the transition period between wakefulness and sleep, the appearance of auditory, visual, or kinesthetic sensations in the absence of stimuli is called ___Hypnagogichalucination___

10. ___overweight___ refers to an excess of body weight compared with set standards.

PHYSIOLOGY AND PATHOPHYSIOLOGY: THE BODY HUMAN

Multiple Choice
Circle the option that best answers the question or completes the statement.

1. What part of the brain mediates appetite and satiety?
   a. pituitary
   b. pons and medulla
   c. hypothalamus
   d. reticular activating system

2. What part of the brain controls respiration?
   a. pituitary
   b. pons and medulla
   c. hypothalamus
   d. reticular activating system

3. What part of the brain is associated with sleep and arousal?
   a. pituitary
   b. pons and medulla
   c. hypothalamus
   d. reticular activating system

4. Attention deficit hyperactivity disorder may be associated with a decrease of _____ in the brain.
   a. acetylcholine
   b. dopamine
   c. carbon dioxide
   d. glucose

CORE DRUG KNOWLEDGE: JUST THE FACTS

Essay

1. List five contraindications for dextroamphetamine (Dexedrine) therapy.

2. Name the most common CNS adverse reactions to dextroamphetamine (Dexedrine).

3. Summarize the potential adverse effects of dextroamphetamine (Dexedrine) in relation to the cardiovascular system.

4. Dextroamphetamine (Dexedrine) may lead to cachexia or hypoproteinemia. Why is this a potential problem for drug therapy?

5. What diet considerations must be considered for the patient taking dextroamphetamine (Dexedrine)?

6. How does sibutramine (Meridia) decrease appetite?

7. What are the most common adverse effects associated with sibutramine (Meridia) therapy?

8. What signs and symptoms may be present when sibutramine (Meridia) is given concurrently with selective serotonin reuptake inhibitor (SSRI) medications?

CORE PATIENT VARIABLES: PATIENTS, PLEASE

Multiple Choice

Circle the option that best answers the question or completes the statement.

1. Your 14-year-old patient who has ADHD has been taking dextroamphetamine (Dexedrine) for the past 6 years. Last week the patient attempted suicide and was placed on the adolescent unit of your community mental health hospital. Which of the following antidepressants would be a poor choice for this patient?

   a. amitriptyline (Elavil)

   b. trazodone (Desyrel)

   c. bupropion HCl (Wellbutrin)

   d. phenelzine (Nardil)

2. Your 9-year-old patient has been taking dextroamphetamine (Dexedrine) for ADHD for the past 2 years. Because of the patient's age, you should evaluate _____ at each recheck.

   a. blood pressure

   b. height and weight

   c. glucose level

   d. liver function

3. Your patient taking dextroamphetamine (Dexedrine) states, "This drug is driving me crazy. I'm nervous all day long." Which of the following assessments may be helpful to identify the cause of these adverse effects?

   a. assess for diet changes

   b. assess for frequent headaches

   c. assess for tachycardia or palpitations

   d. assess for height or weight changes

4. Your patient's parents have agreed to their child starting a regimen of dextroamphetamine (Dexedrine) for ADHD. Which of the following statements would you include in your family teaching when initiating therapy?

   a. "Expect a 25-pound weight loss in the first 6 months."

   b. "Give your child the drug at bedtime to minimize the nausea."

   c. "Your child may experience a significant growth spurt after a couple of months."

   d. "This is the number for a support group that works with children to increase their self-esteem."

5. Your patient taking dextroamphetamine states, "I am having so many adverse effects to my medication." Which of the following adverse effects would concern you the most?

   a. decreased appetite and headache

   b. GI distress and anxiety

   c. decreased lacrimation and mydriasis

   d. jittery feeling and insomnia

6. Your 16-year-old patient is 60 pounds overweight. The patient's mother comes to the clinic with the patient and requests sibutramine (Meridia) for weight loss. Before beginning therapy with sibutramine, the patient should have

   a. testing to exclude organic causes of obesity.

   b. a fasting blood glucose test.

   c. triglyceride level determination.

   d. a CBC.

7. Your 25-year-old patient is beginning sibutramine (Meridia) therapy for her morbid obesity. For this patient, it is important to teach

   a. the need for diet and exercise.

   b. appropriate diet.

   c. the need for consistent birth control.

   d. the need for follow-up examinations.

8. Your patient is taking caffeine for chronic fatigue. This patient should be advised to avoid taking caffeine with

   a. milk.

   b. orange juice.

   c. water.

   d. grapefruit juice.

NURSING MANAGEMENT: EVERY GOOD NURSE SHOULD …

Multiple Choice

Circle the option that best answers the question or completes the statement.

1. Before initiating dextroamphetamine drug therapy for the treatment of narcolepsy, the nurse should assess the patient for
   a. symptomatic cardiovascular disease.
   b. hyperthyroidism.
   c. history of drug abuse.
   d. all of the above.
   e. none of the above.

2. An 8-year-old patient has been prescribed dextroamphetamine to treat attention deficit hyperactivity disorder. Patient and family education about the drug therapy should include instructions to
   a. take the drug in the evening to minimize adverse effects.
   b. avoid drinking caffeinated beverages, such as colas.
   c. chew the sustained-release capsules carefully before swallowing.
   d. take a double dose when a dose is skipped accidentally.

3. A patient calls the advice line at the HMO and speaks with you, the "answer nurse." The patient tells you that she recently began taking dextroamphetamine as an adjunct therapy for weight loss. The patient says, "I feel so restless, and I don't sleep well at night. Could I have a prescription for a sleeping pill?" Your best response would be that
   a. an over-the-counter sleep aid should be used.
   b. you will contact the prescriber regarding obtaining a prescription sleep aid.
   c. the dose of dextroamphetamine should be increased.
   d. she appears to be having adverse effects from the dextroamphetamine and you will contact the prescriber.

4. Sibutramine has been prescribed to assist your patient in weight loss. The patient confides to you, "I really hope this drug will help me lose weight." To maximize the therapeutic effect of sibutramine, you should emphasize
   a. that the drug should be taken on a full stomach, 1 hour after eating.
   b. that the current dietary pattern should be continued.
   c. that the patient should increase his activity level.
   d. that the drug should be taken at bedtime.

5. A patient has come to the clinic requesting a prescription for sibutramine. She states, "I have tried everything—even those over-the-counter diet pills. I've been so depressed since I gained all this weight." What information from the patient's history is *most* important?
   a. How long the patient has been overweight?
   b. What over-the-counter medication the patient is taking?
   c. How much exercise does the patient get during the week?
   d. Does the patient take prescription medication for her depression?

6. You are administering caffeine to a newborn with apnea. To minimize adverse effects, you should monitor for
   a. tachypnea.
   b. fever.
   c. hyperglycemia.
   d. all of the above.
   e. none of the above.

CASE STUDY

Your patient has come to the clinic for her 4-week postpartum checkup. She is eager to lose the extra 15 pounds she gained during the pregnancy. She states, "Breast-feeding is helping me to lose weight, but I'm not losing fast enough. I was thinking about trying some weight-loss pills. Would a prescription pill help me lose weight faster than the ones I can buy over the counter?" What should you advise this patient regarding the use of anorexics?

CRITICAL THINKING

What additional advice might you give this patient regarding weight loss?

CHAPTER 23

Drugs Treating Severe Pain

TOP TEN THINGS TO KNOW ABOUT DRUGS TREATING SEVERE PAIN

1. Pain can be classified by physiologic origin, duration, or pathologic source. Pain may be caused by injury, trauma, disease, diagnostic procedures, or therapy to treat disease or pathologies.
2. Pain is subjective, and the patient must be assessed with an appropriate tool to determine the extent of the pain being experienced. Pain levels should be reassessed after an analgesic is given.
3. Pain is best controlled when analgesics are given before pain becomes severe and when the doses are administered around the clock. Doses of narcotic analgesics should be titrated to obtain maximum efficacy with minimal adverse effects. Tolerance and cross-tolerance should be considered when titrating dosages.
4. Patients treated for pain should also have a prescribed rescue dose to manage any breakthrough pain. Patients who require more than three rescue doses in a day should have their analgesic dosage adjusted, either by increasing the baseline dose or maximizing the co-analgesics.
5. Patients and families should be educated about the facts concerning pain, pain management, and what will be done if and when they report pain.
6. Morphine, a narcotic agonist used to treat moderate to severe pain, stimulates at the opiate receptors (especially mu), decreasing the release of substance P in the spinal cord and altering pain perception.
7. The most common adverse effects of morphine are respiratory depression, decreased urinary output or urinary retention, delayed return of peristalsis, and constipation. Excessive respiratory depression is treated with naloxone (usually IV), a narcotic antagonist. The onset of naloxone is rapid, but the duration of action is quite short. Repeated doses may be necessary to prevent a relapse of the respiratory arrest or depression.
8. Codeine, a moderate narcotic, is used to treat mild to moderate pain and as a cough suppressant. Codeine and synthetic forms of codeine are often combined with nonsteroidal anti-inflammatory agents for increased pain control.
9. Adverse effects of codeine include drowsiness, dry mouth, nausea and vomiting, and constipation. Respiratory depression and cardiovascular effects are not as common as with morphine but can occur in higher doses. Avoid giving codeine to patients who require a cough reflex.
10. Pentazocine is a mixed agonist/antagonist narcotic, meaning it stimulates at some receptors but blocks at others. It produces analgesia in patients who have not taken other opioid narcotics but interrupts pain control in patients also receiving narcotic agonists (such as morphine) and produces withdrawal in patients who abuse narcotics.

KEY TERMS

Matching
Match the key term with its definition.

1. _d___ acute pain
2. _c___ addiction
3. _n___ adjunct analgesics
4. _a___ analgesics
5. _____ breakthrough pain
6. _____ chronic pain
7. _____ dependence
8. _____ narcotics
9. _____ neuropathic pain
10. _____ nociceptic pain
11. _____ opioid
12. _____ pain
13. _____ rescue doses
14. _____ tolerance

a. Drugs used to treat pain

b. Characterized by a withdrawal syndrome upon cessation of the drug

c. Compulsive use of a drug for a secondary gain

d. The immediate phase of response to an insult or injury

e. Drugs used to treat pain that work on the perception of pain by the brain

f. Pain that persists well beyond actual tissue injury

g. Transitory flare-ups of pain over baseline

h. Drugs used in the management of pain that have another primary pharmacotherapeutic action

i. An unpleasant sensory and emotional experience

j. Results from injury to the peripheral receptors, afferent fibers, or CNS

k. Caused by the activation of delta and C nociceptors in response to painful stimuli

l. The body becomes accustomed to the drug and needs a higher dose to relieve pain

m. Another name for a narcotic drug derived from opium

n. A dose of medication added to the standing doses for pain management

PHYSIOLOGY AND PATHOPHYSIOLOGY: THE BODY HUMAN

Essay

1. In general, what is the theory that explains how CNS depressants work?

2. What is the difference between myelinated delta fibers and unmyelinated C fibers in the perception of pain?

3. In addition to the pain stimulus, what other phenomena influence the perception of pain?

4. Identify specific areas of the brain involved in interpreting pain.

5. List potential sequelae to unresolved pain.

CORE DRUG KNOWLEDGE: JUST THE FACTS

Multiple Choice

Circle the option that best answers the question or completes the statement.

1. Equianalgesic dosages are compared with
   a. meperidine (Demerol).
   b. codeine.
   c. fentanyl (Sublimaze).
   d. morphine (Roxanol).

2. Morphine has many actions, including
   a. decreasing A-delta fibers.
   b. increasing C fibers.
   c. inhibiting release of substance P.
   d. inhibiting release of acetylcholine.

3. Morphine administration is contraindicated in which of the following disorders?
   a. head injury
   b. hepatic insufficiency
   c. renal impairment
   d. all of the above

4. The most hazardous adverse effects to the use of morphine occur to the
   a. integumentary system.
   b. cardiovascular system.
   c. respiratory system.
   d. gastrointestinal system.

5. In addition to pain relief, codeine is also frequently used as a
   a. decongestant.
   b. laxative.
   c. cough suppressant.
   d. sedative.

6. Codeine is used cautiously in patients with respiratory disorders because it may

   a. cause bronchoconstriction.

   b. cause bronchodilation.

   c. decrease respiratory secretions.

   d. lead to accumulation of secretions and a loss of respiratory reserve.

7. In addition to CNS depressants, codeine may have drug–drug interactions with

   a. antibiotics.

   b. anti-ulcer medications.

   c. bronchodilators.

   d. anticoagulants.

8. Which of the following statements about pentazocine (Talwin) is correct?

   a. It is a narcotic agonist.

   b. It is a narcotic antagonist.

   c. It is both a narcotic agonist and antagonist.

   d. It is none of the above.

9. Because of its pharmacodynamics, IV pentazocine (Talwin)

   a. increases the workload of the heart.

   b. decreases the workload of the heart.

   c. increases the workload of the lungs.

   d. decreases the workload of the lungs.

10. The most common adverse effects to pentazocine (Talwin) include

    a. respiratory depression.

    b. soft tissue induration, nodules, and cutaneous depression.

    c. nausea, vomiting, dizziness, and euphoria.

    d. excitement, tinnitus, disorientation, and confusion.

CORE PATIENT VARIABLES: PATIENTS, PLEASE

Multiple Choice

Circle the option that best answers the question or completes the statement.

1. Your patient has been given morphine 2 mg IV. She now has an increase in her BP and resting pulse and states she feels very anxious. You suspect

   a. an idiosyncratic reaction.

   b. an additive effect.

   c. a synergistic effect.

   d. an agonist response.

2. Your 77-year-old patient has just had surgery for a fractured ankle. The patient is in severe pain and has morphine sulfate ordered to control pain. With your knowledge of morphine, you would expect the dosage of morphine to

   a. be equal to the dose for a young adult.

   b. be higher than the dose for a young adult.

   c. be lower than the dose for a young adult.

3. Your 55-year-old patient has a fractured rib. She is being released from the emergency room with a prescription for a narcotic analgesic. Before discharging this patient, you assess the patient's lifestyle, diet, and habits. Which of the following questions should be included in this assessment?

   a. "Are you able to drink 3 liters of water a day?"

   b. "Do you drink alcoholic beverages?"

   c. "Do your take other medications?"

   d. "Do you have stairs in your home?"

4. Your patient is taking Tylenol with Codeine No. 3 to control the pain from a fractured arm. Five days later, the patient calls the clinic and states, "I'm having problems having a bowel movement since I started this drug." Which of the following is the most appropriate response?

   a. "This is an expected adverse effect to the use of codeine. Increase your fluid intake and take a bulk laxative such as Metamucil."

   b. "This is an additive effect of codeine. Stop taking the medication."

   c. "This is an expected adverse effect to the use of codeine. Double the dose, and it will clear out your bowel."

   d. "You are probably allergic to the codeine. Stop taking the medication."

5. Your patient is being discharged with a prescription for Tylenol with codeine. Which of these areas of assessment needs special attention?

   a. health status and environment

   b. culture and lifestyle, diet and habits

   c. health status, lifestyle, diet and habits, and environment

   d. health status and culture

6. Your patient was admitted for observation after a suicide attempt. Upon discharge the patient is prescribed a narcotic analgesic for an injury sustained during the suicide attempt. Which of the following narcotics would be *contraindicated* for this patient?

   a. propoxyphene (Darvon)

   b. hydrocodone (Vicodin)

   c. codeine

   d. none of the above

7. During a psychiatric intake interview with your patient, she states, "My mom put me here. She is concerned because of my use of 'Ts' and 'blues.'" With your knowledge of this drug combination, you carefully assess

   a. the heart and lungs.

   b. the lungs and CNS.

   c. kidney and liver function.

   d. the CNS and skin.

8. Your surgical patient's pain has been well controlled with the fentanyl iontophoretic transdermal system (Ionsys). The patient states, "I am so afraid of going home because I just know I am going to have a lot of pain." Prior to discharge the nurse should

   a. teach the patient how to clean the iontophoretic system.

   b. discontinue the iontophoretic system.

   c. fill the system with fentanyl to avoid opioid withdrawal.

   d. contact the home health department to ensure the home health nurse will monitor the system at the patient's home.

9. Your patient in the emergency department arrived non-responsive. The friend of the patient states, "I think he took an overdose of methadone, but I'm not sure." You administer IV naloxalone and the patient awakes. What is the *most* essential nursing action for this patient?

   a. Contact psychiatry services for an admit consult.

   b. Administer sodium bicarbonate to keep the patient's blood pH normal.

   c. Draw blood for a methadone level.

   d. Frequently monitor the patient's level of consciousness.

10. Which of the following adverse effects is *specifically* related to tramadol (Ultram)?

   a. seizure activity

   b. respiratory depression

   c. constipation

   d. vomiting

NURSING MANAGEMENT: EVERY GOOD NURSE SHOULD ...

Decision Tree

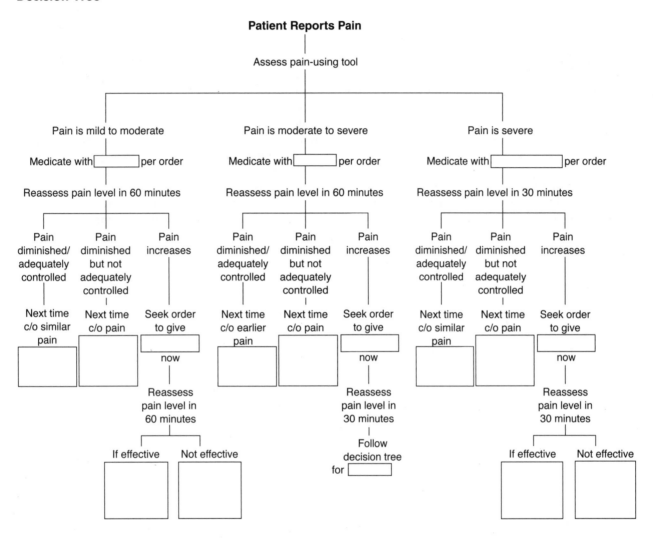

Patient Reports Pain

Assess pain-using tool

Pain is mild to moderate

Medicate with ⬚ per order

Reassess pain level in 60 minutes

Pain diminished/ adequately controlled — Next time c/o similar pain ⬚

Pain diminished but not adequately controlled — Next time c/o pain ⬚

Pain increases — Seek order to give ⬚ now — Reassess pain level in 60 minutes — If effective ⬚ / Not effective ⬚

Pain is moderate to severe

Medicate with ⬚ per order

Reassess pain level in 60 minutes

Pain diminished/ adequately controlled — Next time c/o earlier pain

Pain diminished but not adequately controlled — Next time c/o pain ⬚

Pain increases — Seek order to give ⬚ now — Reassess pain level in 30 minutes — Follow decision tree for ⬚

Pain is severe

Medicate with ⬚ per order

Reassess pain level in 30 minutes

Pain diminished/ adequately controlled — Next time c/o similar pain ⬚

Pain diminished but not adequately controlled — Next time c/o pain ⬚

Pain increases — Seek order to give ⬚ now — Reassess pain level in 30 minutes — If effective ⬚ / Not effective ⬚

You are the nurse on an orthopedic unit. You are caring for a patient who is 64 years old and fell on the ice this morning. The patient has a hip fracture, is in traction, and is awaiting surgical repair late today. The patient requests something for pain. The following orders are written for pain management:

Ibuprofen 400 mg PO q 4 hours PRN for mild pain
Percocet one tablet PO q 4 to 6 hours for moderate pain
Morphine sulfate 5 to 10 mg IM q 4 hours for severe pain

Complete the decision tree to show the steps you would take to assess and treat this patient's pain. (Hint: Ibuprofen is a nonsteroidal anti-inflammatory [NSAID]). See Chapter 24. Percocet is a trade name for a combination drug containing 5-mg oxycodone and 325-mg acetaminophen.)

CASE STUDY

You are caring for a patient hospitalized after surgical removal of a bullet from the leg today. You learn from your nursing assessment that this patient drinks four beers a day and uses cocaine. You assess for pain using a visual analogue scale, and the patient indicates that his pain is an 8 level on a 0 (no pain) to 10 (worst pain imaginable) scale. The patient lies quietly in bed while you talk with him and assess him. No analgesics have been given for the last 6 hours. The medication orders for this patient are: Percocet 1 to 2 tablets PO every 4 to 6 hours, and morphine 8 to 10 mg IM every 3 to 4 hours. He last received one Percocet for pain.

1. Does this patient have pain?

2. What information should be assessed regarding the pain and pain control in addition to the rating of pain on the pain scale?

3. Assuming that this patient reports minimal pain relief for 2 hours after receiving one Percocet, what is the most appropriate action to take?

CRITICAL THINKING CHALLENGE

The patient described above continues to report severe pain, with pain ratings of 8 or 9 using the visual analogue scale. You have switched to morphine 10 mg every 3 hours. This dose reduces the pain while maintaining wakefulness and alertness. The roommate of your patient is also under your care. That patient also has severe pain, rating it at 8 on the visual analogue scale. The roommate had surgery 2 hours ago for a ruptured appendix. The medication orders for this patient read morphine 8 to 15 mg IM q 4 hours PRN × 24 hours. You administer 10 mg of morphine to this patient also. Thirty minutes later, this second patient is very lethargic and hard to arouse. His pulse rate has dropped from 88 to 68 beats per minute. What can account for the difference in reaction to the same dose of analgesic?

CHAPTER 24

Drugs Treating Mild to Moderate Pain, Fever, Inflammation, and Migraine Headache

TOP TEN THINGS TO KNOW ABOUT DRUGS TREATING MILD TO MODERATE PAIN, FEVER, INFLAMMATION, AND MIGRAINE HEADACHE

1. Prostaglandins modulate some components of inflammation, body temperature, pain transmission, platelet aggregation, and many other body actions. Prostaglandins are converted from arachidonic acid by the enzyme cyclooxygenase (COX). There are two forms of the COX enzyme: COX-1 and COX-2. COX-1 synthesizes prostaglandins involved in the regulation of normal cell activity; COX-2 produces prostaglandins, mainly at sites of inflammation.

2. Nonsteroidal anti-inflammatory drugs (salicylates and prostaglandin synthetase inhibitors [NSAIDs, PSI]) and para-aminophenol derivatives (acetaminophen) work by inhibiting the synthesis of prostaglandins. Most NSAIDs indiscriminately target both COX-1 and COX-2 and deplete the prostaglandins needed for normal cell function and protection. This is the cause of many of these drugs' adverse effects.

3. Aspirin, a salicylate, is used for analgesic, antipyretic (fever reduction), anti-inflammatory, and antiplatelet effects. It irreversibly inhibits COX and therefore inhibits the synthesis of prostaglandins. Therapeutic and most adverse effects are related to the inhibition of COX 1.

4. Most common adverse effects of aspirin are gastrointestinal (GI); renal and hepatic toxicity are possible, although not common in normal dosage. Avoid use in children with flu-like illness, pregnant women (especially during the third trimester), and in patients with pathophysiologic conditions that would be adversely affected by the action or adverse effects of aspirin.

5. Ibuprofen, a prostaglandin synthetase inhibitor (PSI), is used for anti-inflammatory, analgesic, and antipyretic effects. It reversibly inhibits COX. Therapeutic and most adverse effects are related to the inhibition of COX 1.

6. Most common adverse effects of ibuprofen are GI; renal and hepatic toxicities are possible, although not common with normal use; long-term use increases the risk. Avoid use in third-trimester pregnancy (category D), patients with active GI disease, and patients with pathophysiologic conditions that would be adversely affected by the action or adverse effects of ibuprofen.

7. Acetaminophen, a para-aminophenol derivative, is used for its antipyretic and analgesic effects. Often grouped with the NSAIDs because of some similarities in actions, it has no anti-inflammatory effects and no effect on platelet aggregation. The exact mechanism of action is unknown. Hepatic and renal toxicities are possible from acetaminophen. Overdosage produces hepatic and renal failure and is fatal if not treated. The antidote is acetylcysteine.

8. The COX-2 inhibitor, celecoxib reduces inflammation without removing the protective prostaglandins in the stomach and kidney made by COX-1. It does not have the GI adverse effects of other anti-inflammatory agents. It is used in treating osteoarthritis and rheumatoid arthritis.

9. Sumatriptan is used to treat acute migraine headache with or without aura and to manage cluster headache. Sumatriptan is selective for serotonin receptors located on cranial blood vessels and sensory nerves of the trigeminal vascular system. Stimulation of these receptors results in vasoconstriction and inhibition of the release of proinflammatory neuropeptides. The end result is a decreased throbbing sensation in

the head that often accompanies migraine and cluster headaches, as well as decreasing vascular inflammation. Most common adverse effects of sumatriptan are: central nervous system (dizziness, weakness, drowsiness, fatigue), gastrointestinal (nausea), cardiovascular (flushing, feelings of tingling, heat), and stiffness.

10. Administer sumatriptan at the first sign of pain, rather than waiting until the pain is intolerable. Decrease the environmental stimuli during the migraine attack. Assess the patient for a history of cardiovascular or cerebrovascular disorders that might induce adverse effects during sumatriptan therapy. After administering sumatriptan, monitor for signs and symptoms of vasospasm and allergy.

KEY TERMS

Matching
Match the key term with its definition.

1. _____ cyclooxygenase

2. _____ NSAIDs

3. _____ para-aminophenol derivative

4. _____ prostaglandin synthetase inhibitor

5. _____ prostaglandins

6. _____ Reye syndrome

7. _____ salicylates

8. _____ salicylate poisoning

9. _____ salicylism

10. _____ triptans

a. Life-threatening toxicity of salicylic acid

b. Drugs containing a salt or ester of salicylic acid

c. Chemical mediator in the pain process

d. Toxicity of salicylic acid or any of its compounds

e. Another term used for the class of NSAIDs

f. Enzyme that produces prostaglandins from arachidonic acid

g. Acetaminophen is the only drug in this class

h. An acquired encephalopathy of young children that follows an acute febrile illness

i. Common term for antimigraine drugs

j. Umbrella term for anti-inflammatory drugs that are not steroids

PHYSIOLOGY AND PATHOPHYSIOLOGY: THE BODY HUMAN

Essay

1. What are the classic signs of local inflammation?

2. What occurs in the vascular response of acute inflammation?

3. What are the four phases of cellular response to acute inflammation?

4. Why are NSAIDs responsible for both decreasing inflammation and inducing adverse effects?

CORE DRUG KNOWLEDGE: JUST THE FACTS

Multiple Choice
Circle the option that best answers the question or completes the statement.

1. Which of the following is *not* an action of aspirin?
   a. analgesic
   b. anti-inflammatory
   c. antipyretic
   d. antihistamine

2. In which of the following patients would aspirin be contraindicated?
   a. Mary with hypertension
   b. Judy with migraine headaches
   c. Constance with peptic ulcer disease
   d. Clair with chronic constipation

3. What is the usual adult dosage of aspirin?

   a. 325 mg q 8 hours

   b. 650 mg q 4 to 6 hours

   c. 325 mg q 4 hours

   d. 650 mg q 12 hours

4. Salicylate poisoning may occur in adults with a dose of

   a. 5 to 8 grams.

   b. 10 to 30 grams.

   c. 50 to 100 grams.

   d. 40 to 60 grams.

5. Salicylism is a form of mild aspirin toxicity with symptoms such as

   a. headache, tinnitus, and GI distress.

   b. respiratory stimulation, constipation, and GI distress.

   c. GI distress, diarrhea, and respiratory depression.

   d. headache, hypervigilance, and confusion.

6. The most common adverse effects to most NSAIDs are _____ in nature.

   a. CNS

   b. respiratory

   c. GI

   d. cardiovascular

7. Analgesic effects of ibuprofen occur within

   a. 30 minutes.

   b. 24 hours.

   c. 2 to 4 hours.

   d. 12 hours.

8. Which of the following statements concerning NSAIDs is accurate?

   a. If one medication does not work, none will.

   b. A benefit of NSAIDs therapy is a longer duration of action than that provided by salicylates.

   c. There is a cross-sensitivity among all NSAIDs.

   d. Unlike salicylates, NSAIDs do not have antiplatelet activity.

9. Which of the following NSAIDs has both oral and IM administration?

   a. ketoprofen (Orudis)

   b. mefenamic acid (Ponstel)

   c. naproxen (Naprosyn)

   d. ketorolac (Toradol) *both oral/IM*

10. Which of the following NSAIDs has a decreased incidence of GI adverse effects?

   a. naproxen (Naprosyn, Anaprox)

   b. diclofenac sodium (Voltaren)

   c. celecoxib (Celebrex)

   d. mefenamic acid (Ponstel)

11. Which of the following statements concerning celecoxib is accurate?

   a. It does not have any antiplatelet activity.

   b. It has increased antiplatelet activity.

   c. It has an increased risk for CNS depression.

   d. It has a decreased risk for CNS depression.

12. Which of the following effects occur with acetaminophen therapy?

   a. analgesic and anti-inflammatory

   b. antipyretic and antiplatelet

   c. antiplatelet and anti-inflammatory

   d. analgesic and antipyretic

13. Which of the following adverse effects is associated with acetaminophen therapy?

   a. pulmonary edema

   b. urinary retention

   c. hepatotoxicity

   d. ototoxicity

14. Which of the following patients should *not* take acetaminophen?

   a. Kelly, age 30, who is pregnant

   b. Helen, age 16, who has a seizure disorder

   c. Mark, age 55, with a history of hepatitis

   d. John, age 40, who is an alcoholic

15. Sumatriptan (Imitrex) works by

   a. inhibiting prostaglandin synthesis.

   b. vasoconstriction and inhibiting the release of proinflammatory neuropeptides.

   c. enhancing the release of proinflammatory neuropeptides.

   d. stimulating prostaglandin synthesis.

16. Sumatriptan should not be given to patients with pre-existing _____ disorders.
    a. hematologic
    c. cardiovascular
    d. respiratory

17. The most frequently occurring adverse effects to sumatriptan most commonly affect the _____ system.
    a. cardiovascular
    b. integumentary
    c. respiratory
    d. immune

18. Which of the following should be included in patient teaching for the patient receiving sumatriptan?
    a. "Be sure to increase your intake of fluids."
    b. "Do not take sumatriptan for ordinary headaches." only migraine
    c. "You can take as many as 3 tablets in an hour for a really bad migraine."
    d. "Drink a caffeine product if your headache is not relieved in an hour."

CORE PATIENT VARIABLES: PATIENTS, PLEASE

Multiple Choice
Circle the option that best answers the question or completes the statement.

1. Your 60-year-old patient has arthritis. This patient smokes one pack of cigarettes per day and drinks at least six beers each evening. Which of the following statements would be most appropriate during patient teaching for this patient?
    a. "Take the aspirin at least four times a day. If there is no relief, take an additional dose."
    b. "Because of your age, you should limit your aspirin intake to only six times a day."
    c. "You have three predisposing factors for an increased risk to develop an ulcer with aspirin therapy. Let's start with trying to stop smoking."
    d. "You just can't take these pills because of your lifestyle. Get used to the discomfort."

2. Your patient takes aspirin for chronic arthritis pain. The patient is currently hospitalized for treatment of a deep vein thrombosis and is prescribed warfarin. Which of the following interventions should be done with this patient? Monitor
    a. daily PT/INR.
    b. urine output.
    c. respiratory rate.
    d. CBC every other day.

3. Your patient is a steroid-dependent asthmatic. The patient also takes aspirin for bursitis. You would anticipate this patient's aspirin dose may
    a. need to be increased.
    b. need to be decreased.
    c. remain unchanged.

4. Your patient has nasal polyps and asthma. Because of this health status history, the patient has an increased risk for aspirin-induced _____ with aspirin therapy.
    a. ototoxicity
    b. CHF
    c. GI bleeding
    d. bronchospasm

5. Your 54-year-old patient takes propranolol (Inderal) for hypertension. The patient has chronic tendonitis from playing tennis. Which of the following interventions should be done for this patient while the patient receives NSAIDs for tendonitis?
    a. monitor renal output
    b. monitor for CHF
    c. monitor for loss of hypertension control
    d. monitor for constipation

6. Your 55-year-old patient has bipolar disorder and takes lithium. The patient also has arthritis, and the provider has prescribed ibuprofen. The patient states, "I'm not sure I should be taking other drugs with my lithium." Which of the following statements would be most appropriate?
    a. "Taking these drugs together is not a problem."
    b. "We will monitor your lithium level closely and make any adjustments necessary."
    c. "Call us if you have any adverse reactions. You should be OK."
    d. "I'm not sure why your provider has prescribed this; it's pretty dangerous."

7. Your patient was prescribed ibuprofen for bursitis 1 week ago. The patient calls the clinic and states, "I just don't feel any better." Which of the following statements is most appropriate?

    a. "It may take up to 2 weeks to feel the benefit of this medication."

    b. "I guess you should make an appointment and get something else."

    c. "Your bursitis is obviously resistant to NSAIDs."

    d. "It might work better if you double the dose for a few days."

8. Your 60-year-old patient has been taking ibuprofen (Motrin) for 6 months. The physician has changed the patient's medication to celecoxib (Celebrex). Because of her age, the patient should be advised to

    a. increase the amount of fluids taken with the celecoxib.

    b. take an additional 81 mg of aspirin daily.

    c. monitor her blood pressure closely.

    d. add green leafy vegetables to her daily diet.

9. Patient teaching for acetaminophen therapy should include to

    a. take only the recommended dose.

    b. read the labels of OTC medications to avoid overdose.

    c. seek medical care immediately for accidental overdose.

    d. do all of the above.

10. Your patient takes acetaminophen daily for chronic headaches. The patient should have which of the following lab tests done periodically?

    a. CBC

    b. liver function tests

    c. kidney function tests

    d. all of the above

11. Which of the following patients with comorbid disorders would have an increased risk for adverse effects when taking sibutramine (Imitrex)? The patient with

    a. depression

    b. benign prostatic hypertrophy

    c. diabetes mellitus

    d. hypothyroidism

12. Your patient with migraines states, "I'm taking that sumatriptan, but my headaches just don't go away for a long time." Which of the following questions would be appropriate in response to this statement?

    a. "Have you tried doubling the dose?"

    b. "Are you taking the drug at the first sign of the headache?"

    c. "Are you still smoking?"

    d. "Do you take it with a glass of water?"

NURSING MANAGEMENT: EVERY GOOD NURSE SHOULD …

Multiple Choice
Circle the option that best answers the question or completes the statement.

1. A 70-year-old patient is prescribed aspirin for treatment of arthritis. Patient teaching should include to

    a. take aspirin on an empty stomach.

    b. store aspirin in the bathroom medicine chest.

    c. return for laboratory tests every 6 months.

    d. crush the extended-release tablets for easier swallowing.

2. Patients receiving ibuprofen on a regular basis should be told to contact the physician or nurse practitioner immediately if they note

    a. unusual bruising.

    b. slow heartbeat.

    c. upset stomach.

    d. slight dizziness.

3. A patient is brought to the emergency room after having attempted suicide by swallowing half of a bottle of acetaminophen. The nurse would expect to

    a. draw blood work for platelet count.

    b. administer acetylcysteine.

    c. administer acetylsalicylic acid.

    d. send the patient for an abdominal CT scan.

4. A mother calls the clinic to report that her 4-year-old has a sudden fever of 101.5°F orally, is listless, complains of muscle aches all over and a scratchy throat, and has loss of appetite. The mother asks what she should give her child to treat the fever and muscle aches. The medical record indicates the child has no allergies and no chronic medical problems. The nurse practitioner should recommend

   a. children's aspirin.

   b. children's acetaminophen.

   c. adult aspirin.

   d. adult acetaminophen cut in half.

5. A 67-year-old patient with a history of a gastric ulcer is to begin a regimen of celecoxib, a COX-2 inhibitor, for osteoarthritis. She asks you, "Why do I have to have a prescription for this? Can't I take something over the counter, like aspirin or ibuprofen?" Your best reply is

   a. either aspirin or ibuprofen can be substituted if the patient prefers.

   b. aspirin and ibuprofen don't relieve arthritis pain.

   c. celecoxib does not cause GI adverse effects as frequently as aspirin and ibuprofen.

   d. celecoxib is prescription-strength aspirin.

6. Your patient has received a diagnosis of migraine headaches and is to be sent home with a prescription for sumatriptan. Your patient teaching should include which of the following? *Mark all that apply.*

   a. Take the medication at the first sign of a migraine headache.

   b. Take the medication with a full glass of water.

   c. The medication may be crushed if the patient has difficulty swallowing.

   d. The medication may cause dizziness, weakness, or light-headedness.

CASE STUDY

You are caring for a 75-year-old patient who had a right hip replacement related to degeneration of the hip from arthritis. After surgery, the patient was given ibuprofen 400 mg every 6 hours and oxycodone (an opioid analgesic) 5 mg every 6 hours.

1. Describe why this patient was given ibuprofen postoperatively.

2. Is it safe for this patient to receive both ibuprofen and oxycodone? (Need help? See Chapter 23.)

3. Why were these drugs ordered to be given every 6 hours (around the clock) as opposed to PRN?

CRITICAL THINKING CHALLENGE

On the second postoperative day, the nurse notices that the patient's urine output, via a Foley catheter, has decreased to less than 30 cc of urine during each of the last 2 hours, although intake has been adequate. The blood pressure this morning is 150/90 mm Hg, compared with 136/84 mm Hg previously.

1. What is your assessment of the patient's current condition?

2. What core patient variables may have contributed to this current condition?

3. What actions would you take?

CHAPTER 25

Drugs Treating Rheumatoid Arthritis and Gout

methotrexate = RA
colchicine = acute Gout

TOP TEN THINGS TO KNOW ABOUT DRUGS TREATING RHEUMATOID ARTHRITIS AND GOUT

1. Disease-modifying antirheumatic drugs (DMARDs) are used in rheumatoid arthritis (RA) to reduce signs and symptoms of the disease and delay structural damage. They are called DMARDs because they are capable of arresting the progression of rheumatoid arthritis (RA) and can induce remission in some patients.

2. Methotrexate is often the first DMARD prescribed for RA. It is usually combined with a tumor necrosis factor inhibitor (TNF) or other biologic drug (combination therapy) because combination therapy is more effective than monotherapy and because, when used in combination therapy, lower doses of the individual drugs can be used, decreasing the risk for adverse effects.

3. Methotrexate exerts immunosuppressive effects by inhibiting the replication and function of T lymphocytes that stimulate the production of cytokines, in particular interleukin-1 (IL-1), IL-6, and IL-8, as well as tumor necrosis factor-alpha (TNF-alpha). It also induces folate depletion, which leads to inhibition of purine synthesis and results in the arrest of DNA, RNA, and protein synthesis. Because of its effects as a folate antimetabolite, methotrexate is also used in treating various malignancies.

4. Common adverse effects of methotrexate include headache, nausea, stomatitis, gingivitis, and alopecia. Methotrexate can suppress bone marrow function and induce gastrointestinal (GI) ulceration, hepatitic fibrosis, or pneumonitis. The risk for these serious adverse effects is small because of the relatively low doses used to manage RA.

5. Etanercept (Enbrel) is a TNF inhibitor drug that may be given as monotherapy or, more often, in combination with methotrexate. TNFs work by binding to circulating TNF, which prevents it from binding to TNF receptors on the cell membranes, and prevents the TNF-mediated cellular response.

6. Etanercept is contraindicated for patients with an active infection because of its ability to induce sepsis and fatal infections, especially in patients with predisposing diseases such as advanced diabetes mellitus and demyelinating disorders.

7. Common adverse effects of etanercept include injection-site reactions, upper respiratory infections, headache, nausea, and rhinitis. Less common but very serious adverse effects include severe infections, induction of demyelinating diseases, and blood dyscrasias.

8. Colchicine, an antigout drug, is used in treating acute gout attacks. It acts through inhibition of leukocyte migration, resulting in an interruption of the inflammatory response. It does not affect uric acid clearance and does not prevent gout attacks. Teach patients receiving colchicine to take the drug at the first sign of a gout attack.

9. Probenecid is used to prevent acute gout attacks. It prevents resorption of uric acid in the kidney, preventing the formation and deposit of urate crystals. Use of probenecid should be discontinued at the time of an acute attack because its use can prolong the inflammatory response. Probenecid should not be taken if an acute attack of gout occurs because it will prolong inflammation. An acute attack may occur when therapy is first started.

10. Advise patients who take either colchicine or probenecid to avoid alcohol because it can cause stomach problems and increase uric acid concentrations in the blood, making a gout attack more likely.

KEY TERMS

Matching
Match the key term with its correct definition.

1. _____ ankylosis

2. _____ antigout drugs

3. _____ chrysotherapy

4. _____ cytokine

5. _____ DMARDS

6. _____ monoclonal antibody

7. _____ nitritoid crisis

8. _____ pannus

9. _____ tophi

10. _____ tumor necrosis factor

11. _____ uricosuric drugs

a. Drugs that slow the progression of rheumatoid arthritis

b. Cell that recognizes and binds to a specific antigen

c. Drugs that increase the excretion of uric acid

d. Granular tissue that damages the articular cartilage

e. Administration of gold salts

f. Extreme stiffness or joint fusion

g. Severe reaction after administration of gold salts

h. Drugs that abate gout

i. Mediates inflammation and joint destruction

j. Type of cytokine

k. Lysosomal nodules found along the extensor surface of the forearm

PHYSIOLOGY AND PATHOPHYSIOLOGY: THE BODY HUMAN

Essay

1. How does rheumatoid arthritis destroy joint cartilage?

2. What clinical signs may indicate the presence of rheumatoid arthritis?

3. Explain the etiology of gout.

CORE DRUG KNOWLEDGE: JUST THE FACTS

Multiple Choice
Circle the option that best answers the question or completes the statement.

1. In addition to rheumatoid arthritis, methotrexate (Rheumatrex) is used to treat
   a. osteoarthritis.
   b. malignancies.
   c. gout.
   d. generalized inflammation.

2. The most serious adverse effects to methotrexate (Rheumatrex) therapy include
   a. bone marrow suppression, GI ulceration, hepatitic fibrosis, and pneumonitis.
   b. Stevens-Johnson syndrome and exfoliative dermatitis.
   c. cardiac arrhythmias.
   d. nephrolithiasis.

3. Contraindications to the use of methotrexate (Rheumatrex) include
   a. cardiac arrhythmias.
   b. malnutrition.
   c. renal dysfunction.
   d. pre-existing blood dyscrasias.

4. To monitor the patient receiving methotrexate (Rheumatrex), the nurse should coordinate which of the following tests every 2 weeks after the initiation of therapy?

   1. CBC
   2. EKG
   3. chest x-ray
   4. liver function tests
   5. renal function tests
   a. 1, 2, 4
   b. 1, 4, 5
   c. 2, 3, 5
   d. 1, 2, 3, 4, 5

5. Methotrexate (Rheumatrex) is a pregnancy category _____ drug.

   a. X
   b. D
   c. C
   d. B

6. Nursing care for a client who receives etanercept should be directed toward preventing

   a. injury.
   b. fatigue.
   c. infection.
   d. photo sensitivity reactions.

7. You just completed patient teaching for your patient who has been given a prescription for etanercept (Enbrel). Which of these statements, if made by the patient, would indicate that the patient correctly understood your instructions?

   a. "I will call my daughter before I visit the grandchildren to be sure they are not ill."
   b. "I will make an appointment to get my flu shot this week."
   c. "I am sure that my knees will stop hurting this week."
   d. "I will stop taking my infliximab (Remicade) when this drug starts working."

8. Which of the following lab tests must be completed before IM aurothioglucose (Solganal) therapy?

   a. CBC and renal function
   b. hepatic and renal function
   c. UA and hepatic function
   d. CBC and UA

9. Before administering aurothioglucose (Solganal), the nurse should

   a. warm blankets in case the patient feels cold after the injection.
   b. have an ice pack ready to place over the injection site.
   c. have resuscitation equipment available in the room.
   d. have an emesis basis at the bedside.

10. Which of the following medications used in the management of rheumatoid arthritis has a unique mechanism of action that allows for its use in combination with other DMARDs?

    a. leflunomide (Arava)
    b. aurothioglucose (Solganal)
    c. Penicillamine (Cuprimine)
    d. Methotrexate (Rheumatrex)

11. How do TNF-inhibitors such as etanercept (Enbrel) work?

    a. They decrease the amount of neutrophils that circulate in the serum.
    b. They block the ability of the cytokine TNF to attach to its receptor.
    c. They block the release of macrophages.
    d. They increase the number of neutrophils in the joint space.

12. Which of the following drugs is indicated for treatment of acute exacerbations of gout?

    a. acetaminophen (Tylenol)
    b. probenecid (Benemid)
    c. colchicine
    d. allopurinol (Zyloprim)

13. During colchicine therapy, patients may experience

    a. constipation, flatulence, or cramps.
    b. headache, flatulence, or constipation.
    c. nausea, vomiting, or diarrhea.
    d. foot cramps, headache, or blurred vision.

14. Allopurinol (Zyloprim) is used in the treatment of

    a. bursitis.
    b. chronic gout.
    c. rheumatoid arthritis.
    d. acute gout.

15. In addition to the treatment of gout, probenecid (Benemid) is used to
    a. enhance renal excretion of copper.
    b. enhance bioavailability of antiretroviral agents.
    c. delay renal excretion of antibiotics.
    d. enhance renal excretion of diuretics.

Essay

The patient taking methotrexate (Rheumatrex) should be instructed to inform the health care provider of what adverse effects or symptoms of potential toxicity?

CORE PATIENT VARIABLES: PATIENTS, PLEASE

Multiple Choice

Circle the option that best answers the question or completes the statement.

1. Your 60-year-old patient who takes methotrexate (Rheumatrex) calls the clinic and states, "I'm just so tired all the time. I never felt like this before." Which of the following responses would be appropriate?
    a. "Have you been doing more than usual lately?"
    b. "How much sleep are you getting each night?"
    c. "Have you noticed any bruising or bleeding?"
    d. "I am sure this is just a phase."

2. Your patient has received a diagnosis of RA and is prescribed methotrexate (Rheumatrex). While reviewing the patient's chart, you note that the patient is taking acetaminophen daily for back pain and headaches. Which nursing intervention is most appropriate?
    a. Continue with patient teaching; these two drugs may be safely given together.
    b. Contact the provider and report the information.
    c. Tell the patient to take only half as much acetaminophen.
    d. Tell the patient to take the methotrexate every other day.

3. Your 60-year-old patient has rheumatoid arthritis and is being prescribed etanercept (Enbrel) today. During your patient education session, the patient states, "I'm not coming back for all those tests. Just give me a year-long prescription." What is your best action?
    a. Administer the medication and schedule the lab tests anyway.
    b. Notify the health care provider of the potential for nonadherence.
    c. Administer the medication; then notify the health care provider of the patient's statement.
    d. Administer only half of the dose and tell the patient he can receive the other half after the lab tests are completed.

4. Your patient, age 70, has been receiving etanercept (Enbrel) for her arthritis for the past 2 weeks. She comes to the clinic today and states, "I just don't feel any better. Are you sure this drug works?" What is your best response?
    a. "You seem a little cranky today."
    b. "Are you sure you are taking the medication correctly?"
    c. "You are right. You should be feeling much better by now."
    d. "This drug can take up to 12 weeks for you to feel its effects."

5. Your patient is receiving aurothioglucose (Solganal) for rheumatoid arthritis. After administration, he complains of feelings of warmth and light-headedness. You note facial flushing and hypotension. You suspect
    a. anaphylaxis.
    b. drug interaction.
    c. nitritoid crisis.
    d. this is an expected reaction to IM therapy.

6. Your 6-year-old patient has been receiving methotrexate for juvenile rheumatoid arthritis. Today, the physician suggests that etanercept (Enbrel) be added to the treatment. Before the initiation of etanercept therapy, you should ensure that this patient
    a. does not have a history of migraine headaches.
    b. is up to date on all immunizations.
    c. understands the mechanism of action of the drugs.
    d. does not have an aversion to needles.

7. Your 26-year-old patient has been taking penicillamine (Cuprimine) for RA for the past year. The patient states, "I have this funny rash on my body. Is it from the drug?" Which of the following is your best response?

   a. "No, this drug does not have any problems with rash."

   b. "Let me fit you into the doctor's schedule today to have a look at it."

   c. "It might be. I will make an appointment for you next week."

   d. "If it does not go away in a couple of days, call me and I will make an appointment."

8. Patient teaching for the patient receiving anakinra (Kineret) should include

   a. instructions for self-administration of an intramuscular injection.

   b. instructions to decrease the amount of vitamin C ingested each day.

   c. the need to contact the provider at any sign of infection.

   d. all of the above.

9. Your 40-year-old patient has acute gout and is prescribed colchicine. The patient states, "My brother takes allopurinol (Zyloprim) for his gout. Why didn't I get that?" Which of the following is the best response?

   a. "At this time, allopurinol may make your attack worse."

   b. "Different providers use different drugs."

   c. "I'll see if your provider will change the prescription."

   d. "At your age, allopurinol is contraindicated."

10. Your 50-year-old patient is experiencing a first gout attack. The patient is prescribed colchicine. Which of the following is appropriate patient teaching?

    a. "Decrease your intake of spinach, asparagus, cauliflower, and mushrooms."

    b. "Decrease your alcohol intake to only 3 glasses of wine a day."

    c. "Decrease your fluid intake to only 4 glasses of water a day."

    d. "Decrease your intake of dairy products."

11. Your patient is receiving radiation therapy for a tumor. He has a history of hypertension, atrial fibrillation, and gout. His medications include clonidine, atenolol, digoxin, and probenecid (Benemid). The use of which of his medications should be discontinued while he is receiving radiation therapy?

    a. clonidine (Catapres)

    b. probenecid (Benemid)

    c. digitalis (Digoxin)

    d. atenolol (Tenormin)

12. Your patient has diabetes and gout. She takes probenecid (Benemid) for prophylaxis of her gout. What instructions should be given to her? Monitor

    a. for ketones in her urine.

    b. blood glucose with Clinitest strips.

    c. for dehydration from diarrhea.

    d. blood glucose with blood monitoring system.

NURSING MANAGEMENT: EVERY GOOD NURSE SHOULD ...

Multiple Choice
Circle the option that best answers the question or completes the statement.

1. Your patient is to begin a regimen of methotrexate, a DMARD drug, for rheumatoid arthritis. Teaching related to this drug therapy should include

   a. no serious adverse effects are possible.

   b. diarrhea may occur initially.

   c. full therapeutic effect is not seen immediately.

   d. all of the above.

   e. none of the above.

2. Your patient has been given a prescription for colchicine because he is experiencing periodic attacks of gout. Teaching regarding appropriate dosing of this drug includes taking the drug

   a. every day to prevent gout attacks.

   b. at the first sign of a gout attack.

   c. when the gout attack is resolving.

   d. when the gout attack is most severe.

3. Information regarding the patient's diet, lifestyle, and habits that should be emphasized during patient education about allopurinol include to

   a. take the allopurinol with cranberry juice.

   b. take the allopurinol after a meal

   c. drink two or three glasses of water a day.

   d. limit alcoholic drinks to 3 a day if desired.

4. Your patient is being treated with colchicine for acute gout. The patient asks you, the nurse, if there is anything that can be done to decrease the levels of uric acid. You recommend that the patient avoid eating, or minimize the consumption of

   a. meat products and seafood.

   b. lettuce and apples.

   c. chicken and wheat products.

   d. dairy products.

CASE STUDY

Your patient is a 22-year-old woman who recently received a diagnosis of rheumatoid arthritis. She has been prescribed ibuprofen and methotrexate to treat the rheumatoid arthritis.

Why is this patient prescribed both drugs?
What lab work will be needed while she receives this combination drug therapy?

CRITICAL THINKING CHALLENGE

After a year on therapy, the patient described above feels better and would like to become pregnant. What would you advise this patient about pregnancy and drug therapy?

CHAPTER 26

Drugs Affecting Lipid Levels

TOP TEN THINGS TO KNOW ABOUT DRUGS AFFECTING LIPID LEVELS

1. Hyperlipidemia is an elevation of serum lipid (fat) levels. The lipids include cholesterol, cholesterol esters (compounds), phospholipids, and triglycerides. They are transported in the blood as part of large molecules called lipoproteins. The low-density lipoproteins (LDLs) are considered the "bad" lipids; the high-density lipoproteins (HDLs) are considered the "good" lipids. Current guidelines recommend that total cholesterol levels be less than 200 mg/dL, LDL cholesterol levels optimally should be less than 100 mg/dL, and that HDL levels be between 40 and 59 mg/dL.

2. Many people receiving antilipid drugs are not receiving enough to successfully lower their lipid levels into the desired, targeted, therapeutic range; many more people with risk factors for cardiovascular disease who should be receiving antilipid therapy are not prescribed the drugs. Limiting dietary fat intake is an important part of reducing serum lipid levels. Diet modifications are started before drug therapy and should continue with the use of antilipid drugs.

3. The lipid-lowering class of the statins (prototype lovastatin) is highly effective in reducing lipid levels and is the most prescribed class of antilipid drug. The statins all increase HDL and decrease LDL, total cholesterol, very-low-density lipoprotein (VLDL), and plasma triglycerides.

4. Adverse effects of lovastatin are generally mild and transient. Two potentially serious adverse effects are myopathies (diseases of the muscles) and elevated liver enzymes. Nonspecific muscle aches or joint aches are common and usually are not associated with signs of muscle damage, but serious skeletal muscle effects, such as rhabdomyolysis, may occur. Rhabdomyolysis can lead to acute renal failure and death. Myopathy should be considered in any patient who receives this drug and has diffuse myalgia, muscle tenderness or weakness, and substantial elevation of creatine phosphokinase (CPK) levels. Adults older than 80 years, especially women, seem most at risk for statin-associated myopathy.

5. An elevated liver enzyme level is the other potentially serious adverse effect from lovastatin. Although mild and transient enzyme elevations are common, elevations of more than three times the normal limit may occur within 3 to 12 months of starting lovastatin therapy. If this elevation persists, the dose should be reduced or use of the drug discontinued. Hepatotoxicity and liver failure may occur from lovastatin (although this is rare). Avoid during pregnancy (category X).

6. Lovastatin is metabolized by the hepatic enzyme CYP3A4; all drugs and substances (such as grapefruit juice) that inhibit this pathway may decrease lovastatin's metabolism and raise blood levels of lovastatin. Drugs that are also metabolized by CYP3A4 may have their rate of metabolism altered when coadministered with lovastatin. Polypharmacy increases the risk of drug interactions.

7. Lovastatin is most effective when administered in the evening, possibly because evening is also when most cholesterol synthesis occurs. Immediate-release lovastatin should be administered after the evening meal; extended-release lovastatin is administered at bedtime without food to be most effective.

8. Fibric acid derivatives lower triglyceride levels and increase HDL cholesterol. Unlike lovastatin and other statins, their effect on LDL cholesterol can be either to lower it slightly or to increase it slightly. Nicotinic acid reduces triglycerides, reduces LDL cholesterol, and increases HDL cholesterol. The adverse effect of facial flushing often limits the ability to dose the drug appropriately to be completely therapeutic.

9. The bile acid sequestrants are not orally absorbed; they bind with the bile acids in the intestine to make them nonreabsorbable, and then they are excreted. The lowered bile acid level prompts cholesterol to be used to make more bile acid.

10. Ezetimibe, a cholesterol absorption inhibitor, localizes and appears to act at the brush border of the small intestine, where it inhibits the absorption of cholesterol, leading to a decrease in the delivery of intestinal cholesterol to the liver. This causes a reduction of hepatic cholesterol stores and an increase in the clearance of cholesterol from the blood.

KEY TERMS
ESSAY
Define the following key terms

1. atherosclerosis

2. arteriosclerosis

3. hyperlipidemia

4. lipids

PHYSIOLOGY AND PATHOPHYSIOLOGY: THE BODY HUMAN

Essay

1. Name the five major families of blood (plasma) lipoproteins.

2. Differentiate between the different types of cholesterol.

3. Why is an elevated triglyceride level an independent risk factor for coronary artery disease (CAD)?

4. What are the benefits of lowering serum lipid levels?

5. List the potential drug classes that may be beneficial in the management of hyperlipidemia.

CORE DRUG KNOWLEDGE: JUST THE FACTS

Matching
Match the following drugs with their mechanism of action.

1. _____ lovastatin

2. _____ gemfembrozil

3. _____ nicotinic acid

4. _____ ezetimibe

a. Inhibits lipolysis in adipose tissue to decrease esterification of triglyceride in the liver and increase lipoprotein lipase activity

b. Inhibits the absorption of cholesterol, leading to a decrease in the delivery of intestinal cholesterol to the liver.

c. Inhibits HMG-CoA reductase, which is the enzyme that catalyzes the early rate-limiting step in cholesterol biosynthesis

d. Inhibits peripheral lipolysis and reduces hepatic triglyceride production, decreases VLDL production, and increases HDL concentration

Multiple Choice
Circle the option that best answers the question or completes the statement.

1. Patients taking lovastatin (Mevacor) should have periodic
   a. chest x-rays.
   b. liver function tests.
   c. ophthalmology exams.
   d. complete blood count (CBC).

2. Lovastatin (Mevacor) is a pregnancy category _____ drug.
   a. A
   b. B
   c. D
   d. X

3. One of the most serious adverse effects associated with lovastatin (Mevacor) is
   a. myalgias.
   b. elevated liver enzymes.
   c. rhabdomyolysis.
   d. blood dyscrasias.

4. In addition to treating hyperlipidemia, cholestyramine (LoCHOLEST, Questran, Prevalite) is used to
   a. decrease peristalsis.
   b. increase peristalsis.
   c. relieve pruritus.
   d. relieve constipation.

5. The most common adverse effect to cholestyramine (LoCHOLEST, Questran, Prevalite) therapy is
   a. cough.
   b. constipation.
   c. headache.
   d. sedation.

6. Potential adverse reactions to gemfembrozil include
   a. liver failure and rhabdomyolysis.
   b. severe blood dyscrasias.
   c. Stevens-Johnson syndrome.
   d. ulcerative colitis.

7. Contraindications to the use of ezetimibe include
   a. diabetes mellitus.
   b. hypothyroidism.
   c. irritable bowel syndrome.
   d. active liver disease.

8. Which of the following statements regarding colesevelam is *incorrect*?
   a. It is contraindicated for patients with a bowel obstruction.
   b. GI effects occur less frequently than with cholestyramine and colestipol.
   c. It has the same indications as cholestyramine and colestipol.
   d. There are less drug–drug interactions with colesevelam than cholestyramine.

CORE PATIENT VARIABLES: PATIENTS, PLEASE

Multiple Choice

Circle the option that best answers the question or completes the statement.

1. Your patient takes lovastatin for hypercholesteremia. The patient has a history of alcohol and drug abuse. Which of the following interventions would be appropriate for this patient?
   a. baseline and serial liver function tests
   b. monthly CBC
   c. monthly urine drug screen
   d. baseline renal function tests

2. Your patient is being prescribed lovastatin (Mevacor). Patient teaching should include to contact the health care provider *immediately* for
   a. severe muscle pain.
   b. diarrhea.
   c. intermittent headaches.
   d. nausea.

3. Your patient has hyperlipidemia, despite an aggressive lifestyle change. The health care provider has prescribed extended-release lovastatin (Mevacor). Patient teaching should include instructions to
   a. take this medication at bedtime.
   b. take this medication 1 hour before or 2 hours after eating.
   c. take this medication immediately after eating in the morning.
   d. take this medication 4 times a day.

4. Which of the following patients receiving gemfibrozil (Gemcor, Lopid) needs special patient education?
   a. Kim, with hypertension
   b. Allison, with diabetes
   c. Nancy, with asthma
   d. Susan, with bipolar disease

5. Your patient is taking nicotinic acid (niacin or vitamin B₃) for hyperlipidemia. Today, she comes to the clinic and complains of facial flushing. With your knowledge of this drug, what is your best response?
   a. "Stop taking this drug right away."
   b. "This is very unusual, I'll have to speak to the doctor."
   c. "You must be taking way too much."
   d. "This is normal and it usually goes away."

6. A patient is receiving colesevelam (Welchol). The nurse should plan to teach the patient to take the medication
   a. at bedtime.
   b. 1 to 3 hours after a full meal.
   c. on an empty stomach first thing in the morning.
   d. before meals.

7. Which of these laboratory results would be most important for the nurse to assess for a patient taking lovastatin who has complaints of severe muscle pain and brownish urine?
   a. renal function
   b. liver function
   c. creatine kinase (CK)
   d. CBC

NURSING MANAGEMENT: EVERY GOOD NURSE SHOULD …

Multiple Choice
Circle the option that best answers the question or completes the statement.

1. Your patient has elevated LDL levels and low HDL levels. She has been on a fat-restricted diet for the last 6 months, but it has not significantly altered the blood lipid levels. The patient is to start taking lovastatin, a lipid-lowering statin, to treat her condition. The patient says to you, the nurse, "I won't mind starting a drug for my cholesterol. I was tired of following that diet." Your best response would be
   a. "Yes, this therapy will be much simpler for you."
   b. "If you choose not to follow the diet, you will need to take a larger dose of the lovastatin."
   c. "Lovastatin will be much more effective when combined with a low-fat diet."
   d. "A slight increase in your dietary fat intake will help to prevent adverse effects from lovastatin."

2. Your patient is 84 years old and takes medication for hypertension, diabetes, peripheral vascular disease, and asthma. The patient is to start taking lovastatin, an antilipid drug, to treat his elevated cholesterol levels and atherosclerosis. You know that this patient should be closely monitored for
   a. anaphylactic reactions.
   b. adverse effects.
   c. electrolyte imbalance.
   d. decreased therapeutic response.

3. Patient education for a patient who is to start taking lovastatin should include
   a. the need for periodic blood work to monitor liver enzymes.
   b. the importance of additional sun exposure while taking lovastatin.
   c. that muscle aches and weakness are part of the therapeutic effect.
   d. that constipation should be reported at once to the prescriber.

CASE STUDY

A patient with a family history of cardiovascular disease has an elevated LDL cholesterol level (160 mg/dL); lovastatin therapy is begun. The patient's baseline AST is 15 U/L (n = 7 – 27 U/L) and ALT is 10 U/L (n = 1 – 21 U/L). After 6 weeks, he returns for follow-up blood work. The LDL level is now 150 mg/dL; AST is now 54 U/L, and ALT is now 42 U/L. The patient is instructed to continue taking the same dose of lovastatin and return in 6 weeks.

1. Why was the same dose of lovastatin continued for this patient?

2. What is the rationale for having another return visit for more blood work in 6 weeks?

CRITICAL THINKING CHALLENGE

When the above-mentioned patient returns in 6 weeks, the LDL level is 128 mg/dL, the AST is 89 U/L, and the ALT is 66 U/L.

What actions of the nurse would be appropriate now?

CHAPTER 27

Drugs Affecting Urinary Output

TOP TEN THINGS TO KNOW ABOUT DRUGS AFFECTING URINARY OUTPUT

1. Diuretics are used to reduce fluid volume in the body. Reduction of fluid volume is useful in treating conditions such as hypertension, chronic heart failure (CHF), cirrhosis, renal disease, increased intracranial pressure, and increased intraocular pressure.

2. Diuretics work along the renal tubule of the nephron in the kidney to decrease reabsorption of sodium and water and, therefore, increase urine output. The degree of diuresis depends on which part of the tubule is affected by the drug.

3. Diuretics also affect the excretion and reabsorption of other electrolytes, especially potassium. The site of action in the tubule determines which electrolytes are lost and how great is the loss. Electrolyte imbalance is a major adverse effect of diuretic therapy. Thiazide and loop diuretics are the two classes of diuretics most frequently used.

4. Hydrochlorothiazide, a thiazide diuretic, acts in the distal tubule and increases the excretion of sodium, chloride, potassium, and water. It can reduce the glomerular filtration rate, so it should not be used if the patient has pre-existing renal disease. Hydrochlorothiazide is widely used alone or with other drugs to treat hypertension and edema.

5. Adverse effects of hydrochlorothiazide are related to fluid and electrolyte loss. Monitor the patient's blood pressure, pulse, weight, intake and output, and serum electrolyte levels during therapy.

6. Furosemide, a loop diuretic, works in the loop of Henle to promote the excretion of sodium, chloride, potassium, and water. It has a strong diuretic effect. It is used to treat edema from CHF, pulmonary edema, and hepatic and renal disease. It may be used to treat hypertension, especially if pre-existing renal disease is present.

7. Adverse effects of furosemide are related to fluid and electrolyte loss, especially potassium. Monitor the patient's blood pressure, edema, breath sounds, weight, intake and output, and serum electrolyte levels. Encourage a diet high in potassium or give supplements if indicated.

8. Triamterene, a potassium-sparing diuretic, works in the distal tubule to promote sodium and water excretion but promotes reabsorption of potassium. It has the weakest diuretic effect of the diuretics if given alone but works synergistically with other diuretics. The major electrolyte imbalance is hyperkalemia (high potassium); risk is highest in older adults.

9. Mannitol, an osmotic diuretic, is a sugar that draws water into the vascular space through osmosis. It is filtered in the kidney but not reabsorbed and thus allows diuresis. It is used to treat acute renal failure, increased intracranial pressure, and increased intraocular pressure. Adverse effects include serious fluid and electrolyte imbalances. Mannitol crystallizes easily; warm the drug in water before administering it to dissolve crystals. Acetazolamide, a carbonic anhydrase inhibitor diuretic, is used primarily in treating chronic, open-angle glaucoma because it prevents formation of aqueous humor and decreases intraocular pressure.

10. Tolterodine is used in treating overactive bladder, to help manage the symptoms of urinary frequency, urgency, and urge incontinence. Tolterodine is a competitive cholinergic muscarinic antagonist with relative selective preference for the muscarinic receptors in the bladder. Blockade of these muscarinic receptors decreases the ability of the bladder to contract. Men and women can achieve equal therapeutic effects from drug therapy. The most frequently occurring adverse effect of tolterodine is dry mouth (anticholinergic effect). Teach the patient or family to report the anticholinergic adverse effects of urinary retention, severe constipation, or blurred vision.

KEY TERMS

Anagrams

Using the following definitions, unscramble each of the following sets of letters to form a word. Write your response in the spaces provided.

1. Movement across capsular membrane

R L G M E R U L A O
T I F L A R T N I O

[ ][ ][ ][ ][ ][ ][ ][ ][ ][ ]

[ ][ ][ ][ ][ ][ ][ ][ ][ ][ ]

2. Molecules move from peritubular blood into tubule

L U B T A R U
C E S E N O I T R

[ ][ ][ ][ ][ ][ ][ ]

[ ][ ][ ][ ][ ][ ][ ][ ][ ]

3. Abnormally reduced renal output

A G I I R L U O

[ ][ ][ ][ ][ ][ ][ ][ ]

4. Fluid shifts into interstitial spaces

M E A D E

[ ][ ][ ][ ][ ]

5. Process of ridding the body of fluids

S I D U R E S I

[ ][ ][ ][ ][ ][ ][ ][ ]

6. Abnormal increase in circulating blood volume

P O L E R Y E H M A I V

[ ][ ][ ][ ][ ][ ][ ][ ][ ][ ][ ]

7. Molecules move into peritubular blood

R U B U L A T
P A E R S O B N O I T R

[ ][ ][ ][ ][ ][ ][ ]

[ ][ ][ ][ ][ ][ ][ ][ ][ ][ ]

8. Chronically elevated blood pressure

N Y E R N S O H P T E I

[ ][ ][ ][ ][ ][ ][ ][ ][ ][ ][ ][ ]

9. Abnormally low potassium level in the blood

P Y K A L E H O A I M

[ ][ ][ ][ ][ ][ ][ ][ ][ ][ ][ ]

10. Concentration of urine

L O M O S I A L Y T

[ ][ ][ ][ ][ ][ ][ ][ ][ ][ ]

11. Drug that causes diuresis

C D I R U E I T

[ ][ ][ ][ ][ ][ ][ ][ ]

12. Abnormally high potassium level in the blood

K E I M A P E Y H R A L

[ ][ ][ ][ ][ ][ ][ ][ ][ ][ ][ ][ ]

PHYSIOLOGY AND PATHOPHYSIOLOGY: THE BODY HUMAN

Essay

1. What are the functions of the renal system?

2. Name the components of the renal system.

3. What processes are required for the formation of urine?

4. How much urine is usually produced in 24 hours?

5. What action by the kidney influences regulation of acid-base balance?

6. What action by the kidney influences regulation of blood pressure?

7. What action by the kidney influences the production of red blood cells?

8. What action by the kidney influences calcium deposition in bones?

CORE DRUG KNOWLEDGE: JUST THE FACTS

Multiple Choice
Circle the option that best answers the question or completes the statement.

1. Maximum effect from hydrochlorothiazide (HCTZ) therapy occurs in
   a. 3 to 6 hours.
   b. 2 to 4 weeks.
   c. 1 to 2 days.
   d. 30 to 60 minutes.

2. Which of the following patients should refrain from HCTZ therapy?
   a. Julie, with CHF
   b. Anthony, with hypertension
   c. Justin, with renal impairment
   d. Stephanie, with kidney stones

3. Which of the following statements concerning HCTZ is correct?
   a. There are very few drug–drug interactions, and they are insignificant.
   b. There are numerous drug–drug interactions, but none are significant.
   c. There are numerous drug–drug interactions, and many are very significant.
   d. There are very few drug–drug interactions, and a couple may be significant.

4. Thiazide diuretics may cause hypersensitivity in patients with a known history of
   a. sulfa allergy.
   b. penicillin allergy.
   c. nasal polyps.
   d. asthma.

5. Loop diuretics, such as furosemide (Lasix), are called "high-ceiling" diuretics because
   a. the minimum dosage needed to affect diuresis is very high.
   b. the maximum dosage available for use is very high.
   c. the maximum diuretic effect is much higher than with other diuretics.
   d. all of the above.

6. In addition to diuresis, what effects does furosemide (Lasix) have on body processes?
   a. decreases blood glucose
   b. decreases low-density lipoprotein
   c. decreases excretion of uric acid
   d. decreases triglyceride levels

7. Long-term therapy with furosemide (Lasix) may
   a. increase glucose.
   b. decrease glucose.
   c. increase potassium.
   d. decrease uric acid.

8. Which of the following drugs should not be coadministered with drugs that may cause hyperkalemia?
   a. triamterene (Dyrenium)
   b. furosemide (Lasix)
   c. hydrochlorothiazide (HCTZ)
   d. ethacrynic acid (Edecrin)

9. Which of the following symptoms may indicate hyperkalemia?
   a. anorexia, nausea, diarrhea, constipation
   b. irregular pulse, muscle weakness, constipation
   c. nausea, diarrhea, weak pulse, cardiac arrhythmias
   d. elevated LDH and triglycerides, muscle cramps

10. Which of the following diuretics is the drug of choice in the treatment of cerebral edema?

    a. triamterene (Dyrenium)

    b. mannitol (Osmitrol)

    c. furosemide (Lasix)

    d. acetazolamide (Diamox)

11. Which of the following is a contraindication for the use of mannitol (Osmitrol)?

    a. pulmonary edema

    b. asthma

    c. hypertension

    d. diabetes

12. To maximize therapeutic effects of mannitol (Osmitrol), which of the following interventions may be done?

    a. refrigerate the solution until administration

    b. shield the medication from light

    c. warm the medication to 100°F

    d. infuse with an in-line filter

13. Chronic open-angle glaucoma is treated with

    a. bumetanide (Bumex).

    b. amiloride (Midamor).

    c. acetazolamide (Diamox).

    d. glycerin (glycerol).

14. Which of the following statements concerning the potential adverse effects of acetazolamide (Diamox) is correct?

    a. There are very few adverse effects, and they are insignificant.

    b. There are numerous adverse effects, but none are significant.

    c. There are numerous adverse effects, and many are very significant.

    d. There are very few adverse effects, and a couple may be significant.

15. Tolterodine (Detrol) is used in the management of

    a. peripheral edema.

    b. urinary incontinence.

    c. hypertension.

    d. head trauma.

CORE PATIENT VARIABLES: PATIENTS, PLEASE

Multiple Choice

Circle the option that best answers the question or completes the statement.

1. Your patient has hypertension and is being treated with hydrochlorothiazide (HCTZ). On the patient's next clinic visit, you would anticipate obtaining which of the following lab tests?

    a. CBC

    b. sed rate

    c. electrolyte panel

    d. hepatic enzymes

2. Your patient takes HCTZ for leg edema. The patient states, "I've been taking my medication every day, but my legs are still swollen." Which of the following assessments should be made?

    a. diet, especially sodium intake

    b. time of day medication is taken

    c. smoking history

    d. amount of water ingested each day

3. Your 88-year-old patient is admitted to your unit for CHF. The prescriber orders IV furosemide (Lasix). This patient has an increased risk for which of furosemide's many adverse effects?

    a. hyperuricemia

    b. vascular thrombosis

    c. headache

    d. photosensitivity

4. Your patient is prescribed IV furosemide (Lasix). You should administer this medication

    a. within 30 seconds.

    b. over 1 to 2 minutes.

    c. over 5 to 10 minutes.

    d. over 1 hour.

5. Your 50-year-old patient takes furosemide (Lasix) daily for hypertension. This patient should have which of the following tests done periodically?

    a. HbA_{1C}

    b. CBC

    c. ophthalmologic exam

    d. chest x-ray

6. Which of the following instructions should be given to a patient taking triamterene (Dyrenium), a potassium-sparing diuretic?

   a. "Be sure to eat lots of green leafy vegetables."

   b. "Drink at least 3 glasses of orange juice a day."

   c. "Eat liver at least twice a week."

   d. "Limit your intake of potassium-rich foods."

7. Your patient takes triamterene and HCTZ (Dyazide) daily. Instructions should include

   a. "Take at bedtime."

   b. "Take TID with meals."

   c. "Take in the morning."

   d. "Take every other day."

8. Your 72-year-old patient has been involved in an auto accident and has blunt head trauma. The patient is receiving IV mannitol (Osmitrol). When reviewing the patient's health status history, you note a history of chronic heart failure (CHF) and arthritis. Because of this history, you should monitor the patient's

   a. hearing.

   b. lung sounds.

   c. temperature.

   d. extremity movement.

9. Your patient has been admitted to your unit with a closed head injury and has an order for IV mannitol (Osmitrol). Before administration, you should

   a. insert an indwelling catheter.

   b. shield the medication from heat.

   c. dilute with lidocaine (Xylocaine).

   d. contact the on-call physician to insert a central line.

10. Which of the following patients should receive close monitoring when receiving acetazolamide (Diamox) for chronic open-angle glaucoma?

    a. Patty, with hypertension

    b. Susan, with migraine headaches

    c. Carole, with hypothyroidism

    d. Janice, with adrenal insufficiency

11. When taking a history from a patient who takes hydrochlorothiazide, which of these questions would be *most important* for the nurse to ask?

    a. "How long have you been taking this medication?"

    b. "Do you know the name of the provider who prescribes this medication for you?"

    c. "Why are you taking this medication?"

    d. "Do you take the generic or brand name medication?"

12. Your patient is admitted for an exacerbation of chronic heart failure (CHF) and is being administered IV furosemide (Lasix). Which of these responses should the nurse expect the patient to have if the furosemide is achieving the desired therapeutic effect?

    a. normalized blood pressure

    b. weight loss

    c. improved level of consciousness

    d. normalized blood glucose

13. The nurse should assess a patient receiving IV furosemide for symptoms of dehydration, which include

    a. hypertension, bradycardia, and GI disturbances.

    b. hypotension, oliguria, tachycardia, arrhythmia, and GI disturbances.

    c. hyperglycemia, oliguria, and hypertension.

    d. hypotension, bradycardia, and feeling of hunger.

14. Prior to administration of IV furosemide (Lasix), the nurse should check the medication administration record for other drugs that may cause

    a. nephrotoxicity.

    b. hepatotoxicity.

    c. ototoxicity.

    d. cardiotoxicity.

15. Which of the following patients receiving triemterene has the highest risk for the development of hyperkalemia?

    a. Jennifer, with a history of hypothyroidism

    b. Bobby, with a history of type 1 diabetes

    c. Noel, with a history of gastric bypass surgery

    d. Ben, with a history of chronic adrenal insufficiency

NURSING MANAGEMENT: EVERY GOOD NURSE SHOULD ...

Decision Trees

Complete the decision tree on this page based on the following information.

An 80-year-old patient is admitted to your unit with pulmonary edema. The patient is experiencing shortness of breath and labored breathing. Vital signs are: temperature, 98.6°F; heart rate, 98; respirations, 24; and blood pressure, 150/88. On auscultation, coarse rhonchi are heard throughout both lungs. The patient also has a history of diabetes and chronic renal failure. Her daily medication regimen at home includes furosemide 10 mg PO. Her admitting medication orders to treat the pulmonary edema are:

Furosemide 40 mg IV push STAT
Repeat furosemide 40 mg IV push 2 hours after
    STAT dose if needed
Start furosemide 10 mg IV push BID this evening

Two hours later, the total urinary output has been 200 cc. The patient still has rhonchi, although not as pronounced. The patient is complaining of feeling somewhat weak, dizzy, and nauseous. Vital signs are heart rate, 80 bpm; respirations, 22/minute; blood pressure, 140/80 mm Hg. You decide to administer the second dose of furosemide 40 mg IV push. After the second dose, an additional 800 cc of urine is excreted during the next 2 hours. The patient's lungs now have scattered fine rales. The patient reports ringing in her ears. The vital signs are now heart rate, 110; respirations, 24; blood pressure, 88/58

Complete the decision tree on page 127 based on the information provided above.

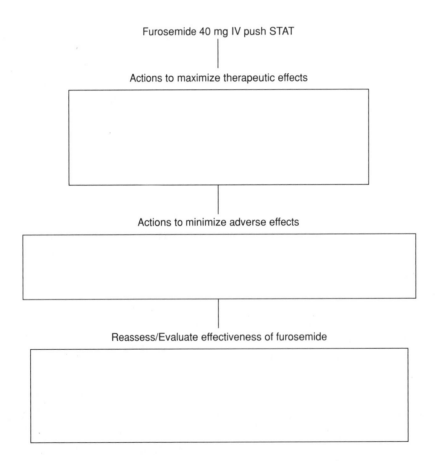

Furosemide 40 mg IV push STAT

Actions to maximize therapeutic effects

Actions to minimize adverse effects

Reassess/Evaluate effectiveness of furosemide

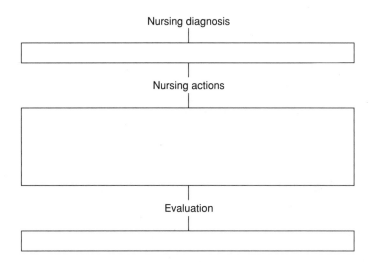

Nursing diagnosis

Nursing actions

Evaluation

CASE STUDY

You are caring for a 70-year-old patient who was in a car accident and hit his head on the interior side of the car. The patient is admitted to the hospital with increased intracranial pressure from cerebral edema. Mannitol 1.5 g/kg of weight, infused over 60 minutes, is ordered. When the vial of mannitol is taken from the medication cart, you notice many clear crystals in the solution.

1. What actions would be appropriate to prepare the mannitol for infusion?

2. Why is this drug administered by an IV route?

3. How will you determine whether the drug therapy is effective?

4. What adverse effects are most likely for this patient?

CRITICAL THINKING CHALLENGE

Before the mannitol infusion is started, you learn that this patient has an elevated creatinine level, a sign that renal impairment may be present.

1. How should you proceed?

2. What patient-related variables put this patient at risk for impaired kidney function?

CHAPTER 28

Drugs Affecting Blood Pressure

TOP TEN THINGS TO KNOW ABOUT DRUGS AFFECTING BLOOD PRESSURE

1. Blood pressure is the product of cardiac output multiplied by peripheral resistance (BP = CO × PR). Drug therapy to reduce hypertension is designed to reduce either cardiac output (by decreasing heart rate, decreasing force of contraction, or decreasing preload) or peripheral resistance (by decreasing afterload), or both.

2. Individuals with a systolic reading of 120 to 139 mm Hg or a diastolic blood pressure of 80 to 89 mm Hg are considered to be prehypertensive; they are at increased risk for becoming hypertensive later in life and should modify their lifestyle. Stage 1 hypertension is systolic pressure of 140 to 159 mm Hg or diastolic pressure of 90 to 99 mm Hg. Stage 2 hypertension is systolic pressure equal to or greater than 160 mm Hg or diastolic pressure equal to or greater than 100 mm Hg. Drug therapy should be started with every patient with a diagnosis of hypertension (stage 1 or stage 2). Drug therapy is also recommended in prehypertension if the patient has compelling indications.

3. Monotherapy, most commonly with a thiazide diuretic, may be used as the initial treatment of stage 1 hypertension. Combination therapy may also be used initially to treat stage 1 hypertension. Combination therapy of at least two drugs is indicated for stage 2 hypertension. Most patients with hypertension require two or more antihypertensive drugs to achieve blood pressure control. The exact combinations of drugs vary, based on whether or not the patient also has comorbidities. Drug classes used as first-line antihypertensives include: diuretics, beta blockers, calcium channel blockers, angiotensin-converting enzyme (ACE) inhibitors, angiotensin II receptor blockers (ARBs), and selective aldosterone blockers.

4. A thiazide diuretic should be used in drug treatment for most patients with uncomplicated hypertension, either alone or with drugs from other classes. Thiazide diuretics have been shown to be as effective as, but less expensive than, other drug classes. Thiazides may produce electrolyte imbalances.

5. Drugs affecting the renin-angiotensin-aldosterone (RAA) system include angiotensin-converting enzyme inhibitors (ACE inhibitors) (captopril), angiotensin-receptor blockers (ARB) (losartan), direct renin blockers (aliskiren), and selective aldosterone blockers (eplerenone). ACE and ARB drugs affect angiotensin-II; however, they have a different mechanism of action. Aliskiren and eplerenone affect different sites of the RAA. All of the antihypertensive drugs that affect the RAA are contraindicated for use during pregnancy, with the exception of selective aldosterone blockers.

6. Calcium channel blockers (CCB) (verapamil) inhibit the movement of calcium ions across cell membranes, resulting in decreased mechanical contraction of the heart, reduced automaticity, and decreased conduction velocity. In addition, they dilate coronary vessels and peripheral arteries, with a subsequent reduction in peripheral resistance and blood pressure. Despite their negative inotropic activity, cardiac output is unaffected, most likely because of the reflex tachycardia that occurs due to vasodilation. CCBs are generally a second-line drug unless the patient also has a history of atrial fibrillation or angina.

7. Alpha-beta blockers (Labetalol) are second-line therapy for hypertension. They are generally prescribed in combination with thiazide or loop diuretics. Alpha-beta blockers affect both beta-1 and beta-2 sites in addition to selective alpha-1 sites. Alpha blocking causes peripheral vasodilation that reduces blood pressure. Beta blocking prevents reflex tachycardia. The alpha-2 *agonist* or *stimulator* (Clonidine) is also second-line therapy used when other classes of drugs have been unsuccessful in controlling hypertension. Alpha-2 agonists are not generally used as monotherapy. Alpha-2 agonists inhibit

sympathetic nervous system response and reduce sympathetic outflow from the central nervous system (CNS). This decreases heart rate, blood pressure, vasoconstriction, and renal vascular resistance; these effects are why alpha-2 agonists can be used to control withdrawal symptoms from abused substances.

8. Hydralazine is a direct-acting vasodilator that causes peripheral vasodilation. Peripheral resistance and arterial blood pressure are then decreased. Hydralazine is also a second line of drug therapy used as an adjunct to other antihypertensive drugs. It is used with beta blockers (preferably) or clonidine to prevent reflex tachycardia from the peripheral vasodilation, and with diuretics to offset fluid retention from the increased production of angiotensin II.

9. A hypertensive crisis is when systolic blood pressure exceeds 210 mm Hg and diastolic blood pressure exceeds 120 mm Hg. Hypertensive crisis places the patient in danger of rapidly developing damage to one of the vital organs; it is an emergency. Nitroprusside is used to treat hypertensive crisis. It directly relaxes vascular smooth muscle, dilates veins more than arteries, thus decreasing preload and afterload, and lowers blood pressure dramatically. Administer nitroprusside by way of an infusion pump and monitor blood pressure constantly. Cyanide poisoning is possible from the metabolism of nitroprusside. Avoid overdosage.

10. Dopamine is a vasopressor used in treating shock. It increases cardiac output and peripheral resistance, thus increasing blood pressure. Because it increases renal perfusion, the drug's correct dose is often determined by the dose required to increase urinary output to adequate levels. The most common adverse effects involve the cardiovascular system. Administer dopamine by IV only in acute care settings where continuous monitoring of the patient's cardiovascular status can occur.

KEY TERMS

Fill in the Blank and Word Search
Read each statement carefully and, using the chapter's key terms, write the correct answer in the space provided.

1. Denoting mimicking of action of the sympathetic nervous system _Sympathemmetic_

2. Denoting antagonism to or inhibition of adrenergic nerve activity _Sympatholytic_

3. The highest blood pressure measured when the heart contracts and ejects blood into the circulation _Systolic blood pressure_

4. The lowest blood pressure measured when the heart relaxes _Diastolic blood pressure_

5. The type of hypertension responsible for 90% to 95% of all cases of hypertension _Primary_

6. Another term for primary hypertension _Essential hypertension_

7. Systolic blood pressure exceeding 210 and diastolic blood pressure exceeding 120 _Hypertensive crisis_

8. Defined as a blood pressure greater than 140/90 _Hypertension_

9. Characterized by a low blood pressure _hypotension_

10. A type of hypertension that occurs because of another condition _secondary hypertension_

11. A system controlled by the kidneys that increases blood pressure _Renin angiotensin-Aldosterone system_

PHYSIOLOGY AND PATHOPHYSIOLOGY: THE BODY HUMAN

Essay

1. Which phase of the cardiac cycle is occurring when you are able to palpate the patient's pulse?

Systolic

2. For a patient with a decreased cardiac output, what type of blood pressure would you expect?

3. In the adrenergic system, stimulation of alpha-1 would generate what type of response? Alpha-2? Beta-1? Beta-2?

```
E   T   H   T   X   J   N   C   I   T   Y   L   O   H   T   A   P   M   Y   S
A   S   E   A   T   P   T   S   F   O   Q   Y   R   A   M   I   R   P   C   S
H   S   S   Y   S   G   X   Z   X   O   G   E   X   K   S   N   V   I   Y   G
V   S   I   E   B   A   J   Q   B   Z   L   G   A   B   A   I   L   M   U   Y
O   M   P   S   N   Y   I   I   C   O   J   Y   O   D   F   O   P   O   R   R
R   O   Y   Q   I   T   T   U   Q   D   T   D   H   Y   T   A   B   P   H   F
I   V   C   S   O   R   I   Y   E   K   Y   Y   M   S   T   Y   B   O   I   D
N   B   V   V   Y   H   C   A   W   L   X   O   A   H   R   S   T   E   I   H
O   A   K   X   S   I   R   E   L   Y   G   I   O   F   D   A   N   G   I   R
I   X   N   T   I   I   G   H   V   B   D   M   Y   C   P   D   X   X   E   E
S   I   W   M   P   M   G   Q   G   I   I   T   E   P   D   V   A   Q   P   N
N   G   J   F   O   W   K   Z   S   M   S   S   Q   D   J   F   O   P   T   O
E   C   L   Q   V   K   S   E   E   I   U   N   Y   R   K   G   O   Y   E   R
T   K   X   L   T   A   C   T   E   K   J   J   E   S   D   F   V   T   B   E
R   C   U   L   E   O   I   D   K   A   X   X   S   T   T   F   R   B   R   T
E   O   R   V   N   C   S   V   F   M   U   O   M   H   R   O   R   M   V   S
P   H   C   D   R   G   N   N   K   Y   P   F   Q   G   S   E   L   Y   B   O
Y   S   A   Z   B   I   G   N   Y   S   U   F   C   J   V   N   P   I   V   D
H   R   R   E   N   I   N   O   M   W   Z   P   A   I   Z   J   Z   Y   C   L
Y   A   N   G   I   O   T   E   N   S   I   N   M   F   M   Z   B   F   H   A
```

4. What is the primary location of the adrenergic receptors?

5. What are the effects of the renin-angiotensin-aldosterone system?

CORE DRUG KNOWLEDGE: JUST THE FACTS

Multiple Choice
Circle the option that best answers the question or completes the statement.

1. Which of the following adverse reactions may occur with *all* antihypertensive medications?
   a. cardiac arrhythmias
   b. volume depletion
   c. hypokalemia
   d. orthostatic hypotension

2. In addition to hypertension, captopril (Capoten), an ACE inhibitor, may be useful in the treatment of
   a. chronic heart failure (CHF).
   b. cardiac arrhythmias.
   c. reentry phenomena.
   d. pulmonary emboli.

3. Because of the action of captopril (Capoten), which of the following electrolytes should be monitored?
   a. calcium and chloride
   b. chloride and sodium
   c. potassium and sodium
   d. magnesium and calcium

4. Which of the following adverse reactions is associated with ACE inhibitors?
   a. bradycardia
   b. cough
   c. hypertension
   d. ankle edema

5. Which of the following cultural groups may have a decreased response to captopril (Capoten) when used as monotherapy?
   a. black American
   b. white American
   c. Asian American
   d. Mexican American

6. Losartan (Cozaar), an angiotensin II blocking agent, works by blocking the
   a. conversion of angiotensin I to angiotensin II.
   b. release of renin.
   c. binding of angiotensin II to the AT 1 receptors.
   d. sympathetic response to alpha-1 receptors.

7. Patient education for female patients receiving ACE inhibitors or angiotensin II blocking agents *must* include
   a. dietary restrictions.
   b. potential harm to a fetus or infant child.
   c. need for supplemental potassium.
   d. risk for increased menstrual bleeding.

8. What is the mechanism of action of eplerenone (Inspra)? It binds to
   a. alpha-1 receptors, blocking norepinephrine.
   b. the mineralocorticoid receptors, blocking aldosterone.
   c. cholinergic receptors, blocking acetylcholine.
   d. beta-2 receptors, blocking epinephrine.

9. Serious potential adverse effects to eplerenone (Inspra) occur in the _____ system.
   a. respiratory
   b. hematopoietic
   c. cardiovascular
   d. skeletal

10. How does labetalol (Normodyne), an alpha-beta blocking agent, work?
    a. specifically blocks alpha-1 and nonspecifically blocks beta-1 and beta-2
    b. specifically blocks alpha-2 and specifically blocks beta-1
    c. specifically blocks alpha-1 and specifically blocks beta-2
    d. nonspecifically blocks alpha-1 and alpha-2 and specifically blocks beta-1

11. How does clonidine (Catapres), an alpha-2 agonist, work?
    a. Stimulation of alpha-2 inhibits the release of norepinephrine.
    b. Blocking alpha-2 inhibits the release of norepinephrine.
    c. Stimulation of alpha-2 inhibits the release of acetylcholine.
    d. Blocking alpha-2 inhibits the release of acetylcholine.

12. Pharmacotherapeutics for clonidine (Catapres) are derived from its
    a. parasympathetic inhibition effects.
    b. sympathetic stimulant effect.
    c. sympathetic inhibition effects.
    d. parasympathetic stimulant effect.

13. Abrupt discontinuation of the use of clonidine (Catapres) may result in
    a. increased drowsiness.
    b. rebound hypertension.
    c. orthostatic hypotension.
    d. constipation.

14. In addition to hypertension, alpha-1 blockers may be useful in the treatment of
    a. benign prostatic hypertrophy.
    b. diverticulitis.
    c. asthma.
    d. peptic ulcer disease.

15. Hydralazine (Apresoline), a direct-acting vasodilator, works by
    a. blocking the beta-1 receptors in the heart, decreasing cardiac output.
    b. interrupting the renin-angiotensin-aldosterone system.
    c. blocking the calcium channels, resulting in vasodilation.
    d. directing smooth muscle relaxation of the arterioles.

16. When administered as monotherapy, hydralazine (Apresoline) may induce
    a. decreased stroke volume.
    b. tachycardia.
    c. decreased cardiac output.
    d. hypertension.

17. In addition to hypertension, minoxidil is useful in the treatment of
    a. male pattern baldness.
    b. peptic ulcer disease.
    c. psoriasis.
    d. hyperaldosteronism.

18. Nitroprusside (Nitropress) is the drug of choice in the management of
    a. rebound hypotension.
    b. hypertensive crisis.
    c. rebound tachycardia.
    d. bradycardia.

19. Dopamine (Intropin), a vasopressor, is used in the management of
    a. hypertensive crisis.
    b. rebound tachycardia.
    c. shock.
    d. acute respiratory failure.

20. Major differences between dopamine (Intropin) and dobutamine (Dobutrex) include which of the following?
    a. Dobutamine is more effective than dopamine at increasing the rate at the sinoatrial (SA) node.
    b. Dobutamine increases blood pressure, whereas dopamine decreases blood pressure.
    c. Dopamine does not cause vasoconstriction or the release of endogenous norepinephrine.
    d. Dobutamine does not cause vasoconstriction or the release of endogenous norepinephrine.

CORE PATIENT VARIABLES: PATIENTS, PLEASE

Multiple Choice
Circle the option that best answers the question or completes the statement.

1. Your patient has received a diagnosis of hypertension and takes captopril (Capoten). The patient's blood pressure has remained elevated despite compliance with captopril and lifestyle changes. The provider decides to add a diuretic to this patient's drug regimen. Which of the following classes of diuretics would be *inappropriate* for this patient?
    a. thiazide
    b. loop
    c. potassium-sparing
    d. osmotic

2. Your 33-year-old female patient takes captopril for hypertension. Which of the following instructions should be given to this patient?
    a. "It is better to use a salt substitute containing potassium instead of adding salt to your food."
    b. "If you decide to become pregnant, please make an appointment and discuss your medications with your health care provider."
    c. "You may experience more adverse effects, such as constipation, if you exercise while taking this medication."
    d. "Cough is a common adverse effect to this medication, but you have less than 1% chance to develop it because you are female."

3. Your 55-year-old patient has hypertension and is to begin taking medication. When reviewing the patient's health status history, you note a history of asthma and arthritis. Which of the following drugs would be *inappropriate* for this patient?

   a. captopril (Capoten)

   b. clonidine (Catapres)

   c. hydralazine (Apresoline)

   d. labetalol (Normodyne)

4. Your 61-year-old patient is admitted to your unit with severe hypertension. The health care provider orders IV labetalol (Normodyne). Because this medication is being administered by the IV route, you should routinely evaluate this patient for the development of

   a. CHF.

   b. hemorrhage.

   c. constipation.

   d. sedation.

5. Your patient has been prescribed labetalol (Normodyne) at the clinic visit today. Which of the following instructions would be *inappropriate*?

   a. "You should change positions slowly to avoid hypotension."

   b. "Do not stop use of this medication abruptly because it may cause some severe problems."

   c. "Take this medication on an empty stomach to increase its absorption."

   d. "It is important to let us know if you become pregnant."

6. Your patient has hypertension, and clonidine (Catapres) has been prescribed. Which of the following comorbid states may contraindicate the use of clonidine?

   a. chronic renal failure

   b. Parkinson disease

   c. diverticulitis

   d. asthma

7. Your patient is prescribed clonidine for hypertension. Which of the following educational points should be made with patients taking this drug?

   a. "Stop taking the medication and make a new appointment if you are having adverse effects."

   b. "You need to stop taking the medication at least 4 weeks before you have any surgery."

   c. "It is very important that you do not stop taking this medication abruptly."

   d. "Take the full dose early in the morning."

8. Your 55-year-old male patient has hypertension and benign prostatic hypertrophy. Because of these comorbid states, he may benefit from

   a. clonidine (Catapres).

   b. prazosin (Minipress).

   c. losartan (Cozaar).

   d. captopril (Capoten).

9. Your patient takes hydralazine (Apresoline) and propranolol (Inderal) for his hypertension. Propranolol is given concurrently with hydralazine to decrease the possibility of reflex tachycardia. Because of this combination, the patient should be instructed to

   a. eat green leafy vegetables.

   b. monitor the blood pressure for efficacy of treatment.

   c. monitor weight for fluid retention.

   d. take the medication every other day.

10. Your 72-year-old patient is in the coronary care unit for hypertensive crisis. He is receiving nitroprusside (Nitropress). The patient reports abdominal pain, headache, and palpitations. You note that he appears apprehensive and restless. Which of the following actions would be appropriate?

    a. medicate with morphine

    b. call the health care provider to respond STAT

    c. slow the infusion rate

    d. administer thiosulfate according to hospital protocol

11. Your patient is experiencing a hypertensive crisis. The provider has ordered IV nitroprusside (Nitropress). Before administration, you should take action to
    a. protect the solution from light.
    b. use pressurized tubing for administration.
    c. administer by IV bolus only.
    d. use lidocaine as the diluent.

12. Your patient is admitted to your unit because of shock and has received fluid resuscitation. Dopamine (Intropin) is ordered to increase renal blood flow. With your knowledge of this drug, you expect the dopamine to be administered
    a. within the low dosage range.
    b. within the moderate dosage range.
    c. within the high dosage range.
    d. within any of the above ranges.

13. Throughout therapy with dopamine (Intropin), the nurse should carefully monitor all of the following *except*
    a. cardiac output.
    b. pulmonary capillary wedge pressure.
    c. urinary output.
    d. arterial blood gases.

14. Your patient has been prescribed eplerenone. Patient teaching should include:
    a. "Increase your intake of green leafy vegetables."
    b. "Do not use a salt substitute that contains potassium."
    c. "Do not drink any dairy products."
    d. "Increase your intake of vitamin B_{12}."

NURSING MANAGEMENT: EVERY GOOD NURSE SHOULD …

Multiple Choice
Circle the option that best answers the question or completes the statement.

1. You are working in the outpatient hypertension center today. You are working with a patient whose blood pressure is uncontrolled on hydrochlorothiazide, a thiazide diuretic alone, and is to begin taking captopril, an ACE inhibitor. The patient says, "I hate to take medicine because I always get side effects. Is there anything you can do to help me?" To minimize adverse effects that can occur with starting captopril, the nurse should recommend
    a. taking the drug with meals.
    b. taking the drug at bedtime.
    c. changing positions rapidly.
    d. increasing dietary sodium.

2. Your hypertensive patient is receiving a thiazide diuretic, a calcium channel blocker, and an ACE inhibitor. Labetalol, a mixed alpha and beta adrenergic-blocking agent, is now to be added to the drug therapy for hypertension. This patient also has diabetes and a history of ischemic heart disease. Patient teaching about labetalol for this patient should include advice to
    a. increase intake of dietary sugars.
    b. take hot baths or showers to promote pharmacotherapeutic effects.
    c. monitor blood glucose levels more closely.
    d. discontinue drug use immediately if orthostatic hypotension occurs.

3. Your patient's blood pressure remains 150/90 mm Hg even though he is taking a diuretic, a beta blocker, an ARB, and a calcium channel blocker. He is to begin taking transdermal clonidine, a centrally acting alpha-2 agonist, to treat hypertension. To maximize the therapeutic effect of the drug, you should
    a. apply a new patch every 7 days.
    b. apply the patch to a hairy area.
    c. always use the same application site.
    d. avoid using extra adhesives over the patch.

4. Your patient has uncontrolled hypertension. The new drug treatment plan includes atenolol, a beta blocker; hydrochlorothiazide, a diuretic; and hydralazine, a direct-acting vasodilator, for hypertension. The patient questions the need for three medicines. What would you include in your patient teaching? *Mark all that apply.*

   a. Most people with hypertension require two or more drugs to adequately treat their hypertension.

   b. These drugs work in different ways to lower your blood pressure.

   c. Hydralazine produces peripheral vasodilation, decreased peripheral resistance, and a decrease in blood pressure.

   d. Atenolol and hydrochlorothiazide reduce blood pressure but also offset adverse effects of the hydralazine.

   e. Three drugs are needed because you let your blood pressure get high before seeking treatment.

5. You are caring for a patient experiencing a hypertensive crisis. As his nurse, you are to prepare the nitroprusside ordered as treatment. You take a vial of nitroprusside out of the stock drug cabinet. After you reconstitute the powder with 3 mL of sterile water, the solution has a blue-green appearance. You should

   a. run the vial under warm water to clarify the solution.

   b. withdraw the solution and administer by IV push.

   c. further dilute in D5W and expose to sunlight.

   d. discard and use another vial of drug.

6. Your patient, a 30-year-old woman, is to begin taking losartan, an ARB, for hypertension. Patient education should include

   a. the need to prevent pregnancy while taking this drug.

   b. the importance of a high-sodium diet.

   c. that fluid loss is an adverse effect.

   d. that hypertension is an adverse effect.

CASE STUDY

A patient is admitted to the intensive care unit in a hypertensive crisis. The blood pressure is 220/170 mm Hg. A nitroprusside infusion is started. The orders read to start the infusion at 0.3 mcg per kilo-gram of weight per minute and titrate upward until blood pressure is no greater than 130/80 mm Hg, the patient's previous known blood pressure. After the first 15 minutes, the blood pressure is 200/160 mm Hg, and the nurse increases the rate of the infusion. After another 15 minutes, the blood pressure is 190/156 mm Hg. The nurse again increases the rate of infusion. In 15 minutes, the blood pressure is 126/70 mm Hg. The patient is now reporting abdominal pain and nausea.

1. What nursing actions would be most appropriate at this time?

2. Why?

CRITICAL THINKING CHALLENGE

The patient described above continues to require nitroprusside to keep his blood pressure under control. He remains on drug therapy of 7 mcg per kilogram per minute of nitroprusside for 6 hours. At this time, the nurse needs to start a second IV line so labetalol, another antihypertensive drug that is longer acting, can be administered. While inserting the line, the nurse notes that the venous blood appears brighter red than usual. The patient seems confused now as to why he is in the hospital; previously he knew his blood pressure was high.

1. What assessment would the nurse make?

2. What actions would be appropriate?

CHAPTER 29

Drugs Treating Heart Failure

TOP TEN THINGS TO KNOW ABOUT DRUGS TREATING HEART FAILURE

1. Cardiac output is the product of stroke volume and heart rate (CO = SV × HR). Stroke volume is affected by three factors: preload (amount of blood that has filled the ventricles by the end of diastole), contractility (force of squeezing achieved by ventricles), and afterload (amount of pressure ventricles must overcome to eject blood; pressure is controlled by peripheral resistance).

2. In chronic heart failure (CHF), there is increased preload, increased afterload, and decreased cardiac output from the left ventricle. Drug therapy for CHF alters one or more of these factors to improve the functioning of the heart.

3. Angiotensin-converting enzyme (ACE) inhibitors, diuretics, beta blockers, and cardiac glycosides are the four primary drug groups used to treat CHF. The combined use of ACE inhibitors, diuretics, and beta blockers has been found to decrease mortality from CHF. Cardiac glycosides do not decrease mortality, but they treat the symptoms of CHF and improve quality of life.

4. ACE inhibitors prevent the conversion of angiotensin to the active vasoconstrictor form, thereby promoting vasodilation. This decreases peripheral resistance and afterload. Angiotensin II blockers such as valsartan (Diovan), losartan (Cozaar), and candesartan (Atacand) may be used for patients who are unable to tolerate ACE inhibitors, or in some specific cases, in conjunction with an ACE inhibitor. Diuretics increase urinary output, which decreases circulating volume (preload) and peripheral resistance (afterload), reducing the workload on the failing heart.

5. Although beta blockers can decrease contractility of the heart, thereby decreasing cardiac output (which is detrimental initially in CHF), they also block the effect of the sympathetic nervous system and cause vasodilation and decreased peripheral vascular resistance (decreased peripheral resistance); this is helpful to patients with CHF. In addition, beta blockers may slow the progression of the disease by decreasing ventricular remodeling. The only beta blockers approved for use in CHF are bisoprolol (Zebeta) and sustained-release metoprolol (Lopressor), both of which selectively block beta-1 receptors, and carvedilol (Coreg), which blocks alpha-1, beta-1, and beta-2 receptors. Beta blockers are not used during acute episodes of CHF but, rather, in chronic CHF. Their use is begun, along with an ACE inhibitor, when the patient has no symptoms and a normal fluid volume. Thus, treatment with diuretics should precede treatment with beta blockers.

6. Digoxin, a cardiac glycoside, is used to manage the symptoms of CHF and to treat atrial fibrillation or flutter. It strengthens the force of contraction (positive inotropic effect), slows conduction (negative dromotropic effect), and slows heart rate (negative chronotropic effect), with a net effect of increasing cardiac output and controlling atrial rhythm.

7. Digoxin has a very long half-life; loading doses are needed to quickly achieve a therapeutic level of the drug. Digoxin undergoes little metabolism; elimination is primarily through renal excretion. Kidney disease lengthens the half-life; smaller doses may be required.

8. The most common adverse effects of digoxin are cardiotoxicity, gastrointestinal (GI) disturbances, and central nervous system (CNS) toxicity. The antidote for overdose is digoxin immune FAB. Always check the apical pulse for 1 minute before administration of digoxin. Hold the dose if the pulse is less than 60 beats/minute. Keep this drug out of the reach of children because accidental poisoning may be fatal.

9. Monitor electrolyte levels, especially potassium, during digoxin therapy. Low potassium levels increase the effect of digoxin, increasing the risk of adverse effects from digoxin. The patient with a low potassium level may have symptoms of digoxin toxicity even though the digoxin level is normal.

10. Assess digoxin blood levels when starting therapy, changing dose, or if toxicity is suspected.

KEY TERMS

Crossword Puzzle

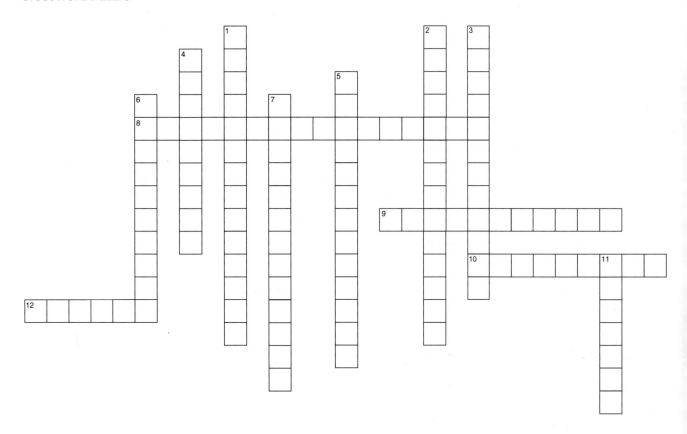

ACROSS

8. The volume of blood leaving the ventricle with contraction compared with the total amount in the ventricle before contraction
9. Pertaining to increasing or decreasing the conduction from the SA to AV node
10. Pertaining to increasing or decreasing the contractility of the heart
12. The volume of blood that leaves the ventricle with each contraction

DOWN

1. The administration of a cardiac glycoside to treat symptoms rapidly
2. A disorder in which the heart muscles enlarge
3. Pertaining to increasing or decreasing the heart rate
4. The amount of pressure the ventricle must overcome to eject blood
5. The volume of blood that leaves the left ventricle in one minute
6. The diameter of the vessel and the pressure with the vessel control peripheral
7. The force of the squeezing that the ventricle is able to achieve to eject the blood into the systemic circulation
11. The passive stretching force exerted on the ventricular muscle created by the amount of blood that has filled the heart by the end of diastole

PHYSIOLOGY AND PATHOPHYSIOLOGY: THE BODY HUMAN

Essay

1. Describe blood flow from the vena cava to the aorta.

2. What three factors influence stroke volume?

3. Compare and contrast the symptoms of right versus left heart failure.

CORE DRUG KNOWLEDGE: JUST THE FACTS

Multiple Choice

Circle the option that best answers the question or completes the statement.

1. The management of chronic heart failure includes all of the following classes of medications *except*
   a. positive inotropic agents.
   b. diuretics.
   c. angiotensin-converting enzyme inhibitors.
   d. antiarrhythmic agents.

2. The appropriate dose of digoxin is based on
   a. age.
   b. weight.
   c. lean body mass.
   d. hepatic enzyme levels.

3. Digoxin has which of the following actions on the heart?
   a. positive inotropic, positive dromotropic, negative chronotropic
   b. positive inotropic, negative dromotropic, negative chronotropic
   c. negative inotropic, positive dromotropic, positive chronotropic
   d. negative inotropic, negative dromotropic, negative chronotropic

4. Which of the following electrolyte imbalances is *not* associated with inducing digoxin toxicity?
   a. hyperkalemia
   b. hypokalemia
   c. hypomagnesemia
   d. hypercalcemia

5. Which of the following drugs may be used to treat digoxin toxicity?
   a. colestipol
   b. activated charcoal
   c. digoxin immune FAB
   d. all of the above

6. In general, the therapeutic margin for digoxin is
   a. 0.5 to 2.0 ng/mL.
   b. 0.5 to 20 ng/mL.
   c. 5 to 20 ng/mL.
   d. 0.05 to 0.2 ng/mL.

7. In addition to their inotropic effect, inamrinone and milrinone are used in the treatment of CHF because of their ability to
   a. increase conductivity through the heart.
   b. vasodilate.
   c. vasoconstrict.
   d. increase heart rate.

CORE PATIENT VARIABLES: PATIENTS, PLEASE …

Multiple Choice

Circle the option that best answers the question or completes the statement.

1. Your patient has CHF and is starting a regimen of digoxin. The patient also has a history of Graves disease and has undergone thyroidectomy and takes levothyroxine. You have assessed the patient's thyroid function test results and noted they are all within normal limits. Because of the status of the patient's thyroid disease, the dose of digoxin should be
   a. increased.
   b. decreased.
   c. unchanged.

2. Your 88-year-old patient is hospitalized for a fractured hip. The patient has a history of CHF and takes digoxin and furosemide. Before administering medications, you evaluate lab results. You note a digoxin level of 2.9 ng/mL. You should
   a. give the medication as directed.
   b. take an apical pulse and give the medication if the pulse is normal.
   c. hold the medication and contact the provider.
   d. question the patient concerning any symptoms, and give the medication unless there are cardiac abnormalities.

3. Your patient is taking digoxin 0.125 mg QD for CHF. The patient comes to the clinic today and states, "I've lost 5 pounds, I can breathe better, and my heart rate is only 70." What is your assessment of these facts?
   a. The drug is working well.
   b. The dosage should be decreased.
   c. The dosage should be increased.
   d. Use of the drug should be discontinued.

4. You are administering digoxin 0.125 mg to your patient. Before administering this drug, you should take the
   a. radial pulse 30 seconds and multiply by 2.
   b. apical pulse 15 seconds and multiply by 4.
   c. carotid pulse 1 full minute.
   d. apical pulse 1 full minute.

5. Your patient takes digoxin 0.25 mg QD with furosemide (Lasix) 40 mg QD. This morning the patient reports anorexia and nausea. The patient vomited one time yesterday. What is your best action?
   a. Contact the physician and obtain an order for a nutritional supplement.
   b. Contact the physician for an order to keep the patient NPO for 24 hours.
   c. Contact the physician for an order to obtain serum digoxin and electrolyte levels.
   d. Contact the physician for an order to obtain a potassium level.

6. Your patient is being discharged from the hospital with a prescription for digoxin. Which of the following instructions should be *omitted* from your patient teaching?
   a. how to take a pulse
   b. avoidance of OTC antihistamines
   c. keep out of the sunlight *it is not affected by light*
   d. do not stop this medication

NURSING MANAGEMENT: EVERY GOOD NURSE SHOULD …

Complete the decision tree on the next page.

Your patient was admitted at 7 AM with acute CHF. There is right- and left-sided failure. Pulse on admission is 122 beats/minute. Blood pressure is 166/110 mm Hg. Coarse rhonchi are present throughout the lungs. There is a third heart sound (S_3). Jugular veins are distended. There is +3 edema in the hands and feet.

The medication orders are:

furosemide (a loop diuretic) 20 mg IV push STAT; may repeat the dose in 2 hours if urine output is 30 cc/hour or less or if respiratory symptoms worsen
captopril (an ACE inhibitor) 25 mg PO TID
hydrochlorothiazide (a thiazide diuretic) 50 mg PO BID
digoxin 0.375 mg PO STAT as loading dose
digoxin 0.125 mg PO 6 hours after loading dose, and again 12 hours after loading dose
digoxin 0.25 mg PO daily beginning 24 hours after the loading dose

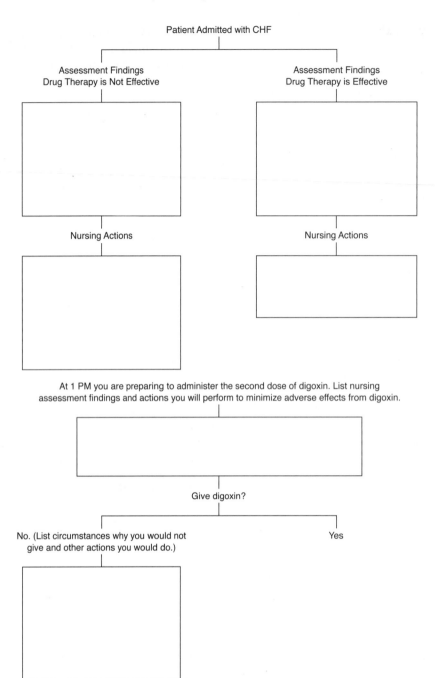

Patient Admitted with CHF

Assessment Findings
Drug Therapy is Not Effective

Assessment Findings
Drug Therapy is Effective

Nursing Actions

Nursing Actions

At 1 PM you are preparing to administer the second dose of digoxin. List nursing
assessment findings and actions you will perform to minimize adverse effects from digoxin.

Give digoxin?

No. (List circumstances why you would not
give and other actions you would do.)

Yes

The night nurse tells you in report that she has administered the STAT dose of furosemide and the STAT dose of digoxin. You will be caring for this patient today until 7 PM. At 9 AM you complete a second physical assessment to learn if the drug therapy is being effective in managing the CHF.

In the box on the left, list assessment findings that would indicate the drug therapy was not effective. In the box on the right, list assessment findings that would indicate the drug therapy was effective. Complete both sides of the decision tree (noneffective and effective).

At 1 PM you are preparing to administer the second dose of digoxin. List nursing assessment findings and actions you will perform to minimize adverse effects from digoxin.

CASE STUDY

The patient described above says to you, "Why do I have to take so many different medications? "Describe the patient education you will provide regarding the rationale for her drug regimen. (Need more help? See Chapters 27 and 28.)

CRITICAL THINKING CHALLENGE

After 24 hours of drug therapy, the patient has crackles in her lungs, 2+ edema in her hands and feet, a pulse of 96 bpm, and blood pressure of 150/96 mm Hg. She does not have a +JVD or a third heart sound now. You consult with the physician concerning these findings. What additional orders might you seek or might you expect the physician to order?

CHAPTER 30

Drugs Treating Angina

TOP TEN THINGS TO KNOW ABOUT DRUGS TREATING ANGINA

1. Three groups of drugs are used to treat angina: beta blockers, calcium channel blockers, and nitrates.
2. Beta blockers prevent the beta receptors of the heart from being stimulated; this alters cardiac function. Beta blockers slow the heart rate, depress atrioventricular (AV) conduction, decrease cardiac output, and reduce blood pressure. These effects decrease the oxygen demands of the heart, thereby decreasing angina.
3. Calcium channel blockers inhibit calcium from moving across cell membranes. This also alters cardiac function. Calcium channel blockers slow heart rate, depress impulse formation (automaticity), and slow the velocity of conduction. These effects decrease the oxygen needs of the heart. Calcium channel blockers also cause arteriolar dilation, reducing afterload so the heart does not have to work as hard.
4. Calcium channel blockers are used in chronic stable angina when the patient cannot tolerate beta blockers or nitrates or if the symptoms are not adequately controlled during the use of these therapies.
5. Nitroglycerin relaxes vascular smooth muscle and dilates both arterial and venous vessels, although more effect is on venous vessels. Venous dilation decreases preload, decreasing blood pressure. Arteriolar dilation reduces systemic vascular resistance and arterial pressure, thus reducing afterload. Myocardial oxygen consumption is decreased because of these effects. Nitroglycerin also redistributes blood flow in the heart, improving circulation to ischemic areas.
6. Nitroglycerin is used to treat acute angina (sublingually, transmucosal or translingual spray), to prevent chronic recurrent angina (topical, transdermal, translingual spray, and transmucosal or oral sustained-release), and significant hypertension (intravenously [IV]).

7. Tolerance to the vascular and antianginal effects may develop with topical administration. To minimize this, start with as small a dose as possible and remove the nitroglycerin (paste or transdermal patches) from the patient for 10 to 12 hours a day (usually overnight).
8. Nitroglycerin loses potency if exposed to light, humidity, heat, and plastic IV bags of fluid.
9. Assess the patient's blood pressure and pulse before administering nitroglycerin and throughout therapy because the drug may cause hypotension and reflex tachycardia.
10. Adjunct drug therapy used with patients who have angina include aspirin (or other antiplatelet drug such as clopidogrel or a drug from the class glycoprotein IIb/IIIa receptor antagonists), heparin, lipid-lowering agents, and morphine. These therapies do not decrease oxygen demands on the heart but slow the progression of coronary artery disease or prevent/treat complications that may arise with angina.

KEY TERMS

Matching
Match the key term with its definition.

1. _____ angina
2. _____ stable angina
3. _____ microvascular angina
4. _____ myocardial infarction
5. _____ Prinzmetal angina
6. _____ unstable angina
7. _____ variant angina

a. Cessation of oxygenation to a portion of the heart
b. Pain resulting from vasospasms in the coronary arteries
c. Pain resulting from decreased O_2 to the heart

d. Critical phase of coronary heart disease

e. Another term for Prinzmetal angina

f. Chest pain without discernible coronary blockage

g. Predictable pain that results when O_2 demand exceeds O_2 supply

PHYSIOLOGY AND PATHOPHYSIOLOGY: THE BODY HUMAN

Essay

1. What is the etiology of angina?

2. What serum coronary markers can be found in patients with unstable angina?

3. What three classes of drugs are useful in the management of angina?

4. How do antianginal drugs relieve angina?

CORE DRUG KNOWLEDGE: JUST THE FACTS

Multiple Choice
Circle the option that best answers the question or completes the statement.

1. What is the pharmacodynamics of nitrates such as nitroglycerin?

   a. decrease the contractility of the heart

   b. vasodilate vascular smooth muscle

   c. block the body's ability for an action potential

   d. thin the blood

2. Which of the following routes of administration would be appropriate for an acute angina attack?

   a. transdermal

   b. topical

   c. sustained-release tablet

   d. sublingual tablet

3. After administering nitroglycerin, the nurse should expect to see

   a. increased blood pressure and decreased pulse.

   b. increased blood pressure and increased pulse.

   c. decreased blood pressure and decreased pulse.

   d. decreased blood pressure and increased pulse.

4. What action should be taken by the nurse to safely and effectively administer IV nitroglycerin?

   a. Use pressure-sensitive tubing.

   b. Use non-PVC IV administration tubing.

   c. Use blood tubing and attachment to a D_5W main line.

   d. No special action needed.

5. How frequently can the nurse administer sublingual nitroglycerin to the patient with acute chest pain?

   a. one tablet every 5 min, to a maximum of three

   b. one tablet every 3 min, to a maximum of five

   c. one tablet every 15 min, to a maximum of three

   d. one tablet every 30 min, to a maximum of two

6. Which of the following may occur in response to sublingual nitroglycerin?

   a. hyperglycemia

   b. sedation

   c. orthostatic hypotension

   d. rash

CORE PATIENT VARIABLES: PATIENTS, PLEASE

Multiple Choice
Circle the option that best answers the question or completes the statement.

1. Your patient has been experiencing tolerance to transdermal nitroglycerin. Which of the following suggestions would be appropriate?

   a. "You should use the patch only when you have pain."

   b. "You should take the patch off when you go to bed and put a new one on in the morning."

   c. "You should stop using the patch and use only the sublingual tablet for pain."

   d. "You should change the patch every other day."

2. Which of the following patients should not use nitroglycerin for angina?
   a. Mabel, with high blood pressure
   b. Susan, with hypothyroidism
   c. Dennis, with a cerebral aneurysm
   d. Larry, with renal stenosis

3. Your patient had a myocardial infarction last night. What is the most appropriate route of administration for nitroglycerin for this patient?
   a. intravenous
   b. sublingual
   c. topical
   d. sustained-release tablets

4. Your patient has newly diagnosed angina and has been prescribed sublingual nitroglycerin as needed. Which of the following instructions would you give this patient?
   a. "Increase your fluids every day."
   b. "Be sure to sit or lie down after taking a pill in case you get dizzy."
   c. "Throw the bottle away if you get a burning sensation under your tongue."
   d. "If you have problems getting the pill out of the bottle, just put it in an envelope in your purse."

5. Your 61-year-old patient has been prescribed sublingual nitroglycerin as needed. You recognize that this patient needs additional patient teaching when the patient states
   a. "I'll place this in the pouch between my cheek and gum."
   b. "I won't drink any coffee or tea when it's in my mouth."
   c. "It might be difficult, but I'll remember not to play with it with my tongue."
   d. "After 5 minutes, I can chew the pill."

6. Your 57-year-old patient has been prescribed nitroglycerin transdermal patch. You should include which of the following in this patient's teaching?
   a. Do not apply to skin that is abraded.
   b. Wear the patch in the same area of the body for a week at a time.
   c. Change the patch daily at the same time.
   d. Wear the patch on the distal arm or leg so it can be removed quickly if needed.

NURSING MANAGEMENT: EVERY GOOD NURSE SHOULD ...

Multiple Choice
Circle the option that best answers the question or completes the statement.

1. Your patient is admitted with a diagnosis of chest pain; rule out MI. He has an order for nitroglycerin 0.3 mg SL PRN for chest pain. When he complains of chest pain, you should
   a. administer a tablet into his mouth every 3 minutes.
   b. administer three tablets under his tongue.
   c. administer a tablet under his tongue; if no relief, repeat in 5 minutes, and then again in 5 minutes.
   d. contact the physician immediately.

2. In addition to administering nitroglycerin SL for acute chest pain for the patient listed above, what other actions or assessments should you make?
   a. listen for lung sounds
   b. check pulse
   c. check pulse and blood pressure
   d. determine urinary output

3. Your patient is admitted with a history of chronic stable angina. The medication orders include 1 inch Nitrol ointment topically every 6 hours and Nitrostat tablets 0.4 mg SL PRN. The last dose of Nitrol ointment was given 2 hours ago. The patient calls you into her room complaining of chest pain. You should
   a. administer the next regularly scheduled dose of Nitrol ointment now and hold the next dose.
   b. administer an additional dose of Nitrol ointment now to her left foot.
   c. administer nothing now but repeat the Nitrol ointment when it is next due.
   d. administer a Nitrostat tablet now.

4. Your patient is being sent home with a new prescription for transdermal nitroglycerin patches. You have learned that this patient cares for her grandchildren 3 days a week. In your patient education, you should include information on
   a. measuring the correct dose of nitroglycerin.
   b. the importance of wearing the patch 24 hours a day.
   c. applying the patch at the first sign of acute chest pain.
   d. safe disposal of the used patches.

5. After being hospitalized for new onset of angina, a patient is to be sent home with a prescription for sublingual nitroglycerin tablets. They are to be used as needed at home. Patient education for this drug therapy should include to

   a. keep the tablets in the original brown bottle.

   b. keep the cap off of the bottle so the tablets can be easily accessed.

   c. continue activity, such as walking, during acute chest pain.

   d. call 911 before taking any SL nitroglycerin.

6. Which of the following should the nurse keep in mind before administering an ordered IV infusion of nitroglycerin to a hypertensive patient?

   a. The patient should be monitored in the ICU during infusion.

   b. The IV tubing provided by the manufacturer should be used.

   c. Glass bottles should be used to hold the diluted nitroglycerin.

   d. All of the above apply.

CASE STUDY

Your patient is a 40-year-old man. He has a family history of coronary artery disease (both parents died in their 50s of MI). He has insulin-controlled diabetes. He received a diagnosis of angina 3 months before being admitted to the hospital with MI. He is in stable condition now and is to be discharged with transdermal nitroglycerin, worn 14 hours a day; sublingual nitroglycerin PRN; propranolol, an oral beta blocker, twice a day; and oral low-dose aspirin daily.

Discuss the rationale for this combination drug therapy.

CRITICAL THINKING CHALLENGE

If the patient described above had asthma, in addition to his other health problems, would you expect any variation from the drug therapy prescribed above? If yes, what drugs would be added or subtracted?

CHAPTER 31

Drugs Affecting Cardiac Rhythm

TOP TEN THINGS TO KNOW ABOUT DRUGS AFFECTING CARDIAC RHYTHM

1. Contractions of the heart depend on a specialized electrical conduction system. An action potential is started in the sinoatrial (SA) node and travels through the heart, causing the atria to contract. The impulse is slowed at the atrioventricular (AV) node and then spreads through the ventricles, causing them to contract. Sodium is needed for the creation of the action potential.

2. Changes in the ionic currents (sodium, potassium, and calcium) through ion channels of the myocardial cell membrane are the main cause of cardiac arrhythmias (abnormal rhythm). These ionic changes allow arrhythmias to develop in one of three ways: through a disorder with impulse formation (the automaticity of the heart), through a disorder of the impulse conduction system, or through a combination of both.

3. Any drug used to treat an arrhythmia (or dysrhythmia) can also cause an arrhythmia.

4. Quinidine, a class IA antiarrhythmic, is used to treat atrial arrhythmias. It suppresses phase 0 of the action potential; decreases myocardial excitability, conduction velocity, and contractility; and prevents reentry phenomenon. Indirect anticholinergic effects also occur. The most common adverse effect is gastrointestinal (GI) disturbance, but serious cardiac changes and hepatic toxicity can occur. Monitor electrocardiogram (ECG), serum drug levels, liver and renal function, complete blood counts (CBC), and potassium during quinidine therapy.

5. Class IB drugs, such as lidocaine, also depress phase 0 (although not as much as class IA drugs). They also suppress automaticity. They are used primarily with ventricular arrhythmias. Lidocaine has a biphasic half-life. The half-life involved with the distribution phase is less than 10 minutes. This brevity accounts for the short duration of action when an IV bolus is given. Because of the drug's very short half-life, repeated boluses may be required to quickly achieve therapeutic level when

a continuous IV infusion is required to maintain the therapeutic effects. Lidocaine's most common adverse effects affect the cardiovascular system (arrhythmias and hypotension) and the central nervous system (dizziness/light-headedness, fatigue, and drowsiness). Excessive levels of lidocaine can produce confusion and seizures. Monitor ECG continuously during lidocaine therapy and switch to the use of another antiarrhythmic agent as soon as the patient is in stable condition.

6. Class IC drugs (flecainide and propafenone) depress phase 0 considerably, have a slight effect on repolarization, and decrease conduction significantly. Use of these drugs is usually limited to life-threatening ventricular arrhythmias because of an increased risk of mortality.

7. Class II antiarrhythmics are beta blockers, such as propranolol, although not all beta blockers are approved for use as antiarrhythmics. Propranolol depresses the cardiac action potential to control arrhythmias. Propranolol also slows heart rate and decreases cardiac output. Other uses of propranolol are for angina and hypertension.

8. Amiodarone, a class III antiarrhythmic, produces a prolonged phase 3 (repolarization). Amiodarone is used in life-threatening ventricular arrhythmias that have not responded to other drug therapies. Current research also indicates amiodarone is highly effective in treating atrial fibrillation; this is an off-label use. Amiodarone has unique pharmacokinetics and pharmacodynamics; these have an effect on dosing, therapeutic effect, adverse effects, and drug interactions. Amiodarone has three potentially fatal adverse effects: pulmonary toxicity (most common), exacerbation of the arrhythmia being treated, and liver disease (rare). Monitor patients carefully for adverse effects.

9. Class IV antiarrhythmic drugs are calcium channel blockers, such as verapamil, although not all calcium channel blockers are approved for use as antiarrythmics. Verapamil inhibits movement of calcium ions across the cardiac and arterial

muscle cell membranes. It slows conduction, depresses automaticity, depresses myocardial contractility, and dilates coronary arteries and peripheral arterioles. It is used to control ventricular rate in chronic atrial flutter or fibrillation, prophylactically (with digoxin) to treat repetitive paroxysmal supraventricular tachycardia, and to treat supraventricular tachyarrhythmias. Verapamil is also used to treat angina and hypertension. The most common adverse effect is constipation.

10. Sodium polystyrene sulfonate (Kayexalate) is a potassium-removing resin used to lower serum potassium levels to prevent serious or life-threatening arrhythmias. It is given orally or by enema. Effective lowering of potassium may take several hours; avoid use in severe hyperkalemia, where a more rapid effect is needed. Special techniques need to be used when administering via an enema.

KEY TERMS

True or False
Mark each of the following statements true or false. If the statement is false, replace the underlined word(s) with the word(s) that will make the statement true.

1. _____ Arrhythmia is the term used to describe an abnormality of cardiac rhythm.

2. _____ Absence of electrical activity is called a dysrhythmia.

3. _____ Electrical activity from the heart is captured on an electrocardiogram.

4. _____ A cycle of systole and diastole is called the cardiac cycle.

5. _____ There is an electrical gradient across the membrane of a cell called the action potential.

6. _____ Phase 0 of the action potential is called repolarization.

7. _____ Ventricular fibrillation is one of the lethal arrhythmias.

8. _____ The ability to generate an impulse spontaneously is called proarrhythmia.

9. _____ The movement of the transmembrane potential away from a positive value and toward the negative resting potential is called depolarization.

10. _____ Resting membrane potential causes repetitive cardiac stimulation, firing, and arrhythmias.

11. _____ The most common arrhythmia seen in clinical practice is atrial flutter.

12. _____ An arrhythmia produced by the use of antiarrhythmic agents is called an action potential.

13. _____ Automaticity means that the electrical impulse originated outside the SA node.

14. _____ Electrical changes that occur during an entire cycle of contraction and relaxation are called the resting membrane potential.

15. _____ Atrial fibrillation frequently converts to ventricular fibrillation.

16. _____ Atrial flutter can cause the heart to beat at 300 beats per minute.

17. _____ Another name for the transmembrane potential is the action potential.

PHYSIOLOGY AND PATHOPHYSIOLOGY: THE BODY HUMAN

Essay

1. Describe the normal electrical conduction through the heart.

2. Describe the phases of an action potential.

3. What is the purpose of the plateau phase of the action potential in cardiac muscle?

4. Differentiate between the absolute and relative refractory periods.

5. Identify the etiology of electrolyte-induced arrhythmias.

CORE DRUG KNOWLEDGE: JUST THE FACTS

Multiple Choice
Circle the option that best answers the question or completes the statement.

1. What is the purpose of antiarrhythmic drugs?
   a. to change the flow of blood through the heart
   b. to substitute for implantable cardioverter defibrillators
   c. to prevent, suppress, or treat a disturbance in cardiac rhythm
   d. to increase or decrease the contractility of the heart muscle

2. What is the prototype for class IA antiarrhythmic agents?
   a. quinidine gluconate or quinidine sulfate
   b. flecainide (Tambocor)
   c. lidocaine (Xylocaine)
   d. propranolol (Inderal)

3. What is the mechanism of action of class I antiarrhythmic agents?
   a. They block adrenergic receptors, affecting phase 4.
   b. They depress myocardial excitability, affecting phase 0.
   c. They lengthen the action potential duration, affecting phase 3.
   d. They block calcium channels, affecting phase 4 depolarization and phases 1 and 2 of repolarization.

4. Quinidine can be used in the management of
   a. atrial arrhythmias.
   b. ventricular arrhythmias.
   c. both atrial and ventricular arrhythmias.
   d. heart block only.

5. Class IB drugs, such as lidocaine (Xylocaine), are most often used in the management of
   a. atrial arrhythmias.
   b. ventricular arrhythmias.
   c. both atrial and ventricular arrhythmias.
   d. heart block only.

6. What is the prototype for class II antiarrhythmic agents?
   a. quinidine
   b. flecainide (Tambocor)
   c. lidocaine (Xylocaine)
   d. propranolol (Inderal)

7. What is the mechanism of action of class II antiarrhythmic agents?
   a. They block adrenergic receptors, affecting phase 4.
   b. They block sodium channels, affecting phase 0.
   c. They lengthen the action potential duration, affecting phase 3.
   d. They block calcium channels, affecting phase 4 depolarization and phases 1 and 2 of repolarization.

8. Amiodarone (Cordarone, Pacerone) is labeled for use only in the treatment of documented life-threatening recurrent ventricular arrhythmias because of its
   a. prohibitive cost.
   b. extremely long half-life.
   c. potential adverse effects.
   d. ability to interact with any other medication.

9. A unique feature of amiodarone (Cordarone, Pacerone) is that its mechanism of action affects
   a. electrolyte balance.
   b. acid-base balance.
   c. renal function.
   d. thyroid function.

10. What is the prototype for class IV antiarrhythmic agents?
    a. quinidine
    b. verapamil (verapamil hydrochloride, Calan, Isoptin)
    c. lidocaine (Xylocaine)
    d. amiodarone (Cordarone, Pacerone)

11. What is the mechanism of action of class II antiarrhythmic agents?

    a. They block adrenergic receptors, affecting phase 4.

    b. They block sodium channels, affecting phase 0.

    c. They lengthen the action potential duration, affecting phase 3.

    d. They block calcium channels, affecting phase 4 depolarization and phases 1 and 2 of repolarization.

12. What is the most common adverse effect to verapamil (verapamil hydrochloride, Calan, Isoptin) therapy?

    a. constipation

    b. headache

    c. diarrhea

    d. muscle aches

CORE PATIENT VARIABLES: PATIENTS, PLEASE

Multiple Choice

Circle the option that best answers the question or completes the statement.

1. Which of the following patients *should not* receive quinidine?

    a. Henry, with migraine headaches

    b. Calvin, with hypothyroidism

    c. Molly, with myasthenia gravis

    d. Leslie, with diabetes

2. Your patient comes to the clinic for a recheck of the patient's cardiac status. The patient takes quinidine. During your assessment, you note on the ECG an increased PR and QT interval, 50% widening of the QRS complex, and a short run of ventricular tachycardia. With your knowledge of this drug, what do you anticipate this patient needs?

    a. an increase in the dose of quinidine

    b. a decrease in the dose of quinidine

    c. immediate cessation of the drug

    d. immediate cessation of the drug and hospitalization

3. Your 60-year-old patient takes quinidine for arrhythmias. Which of the following electrolytes should be closely monitored while the patient is taking this medication?

    a. potassium

    b. sodium

    c. magnesium

    d. chloride

4. Your patient came to the Emergency Department and was noted to have a ventricular arrhythmia. The arrhythmia was stopped with an IV bolus of lidocaine (Xylocaine). You should prepare to

    a. administer quinidine if the arrhythmia recurs.

    b. double the initial IV dose of lidocaine if the arrhythmia recurs.

    c. hang an IV piggyback of lidocaine (Xylocaine).

    d. hang an IV piggyback of tocainide (Tonocard).

5. Which of the following patients *should not* take propranolol (Inderal) for cardiac arrhythmias?

    a. Henry, with migraine headaches

    b. Susan, with severe asthma

    c. John, with tachycardia

    d. Nancy, with hypertension

6. Your 54-year-old patient has ventricular arrhythmias despite use of multiple antiarrhythmic agents and is being prescribed amiodarone (Cordarone, Pacerone). Identification of which of the following comorbid states would preclude the use of amiodarone for this patient?

    a. hypertension

    b. myasthenia gravis

    c. Parkinson disease

    d. thyroid disease

7. Your patient is being prescribed IV amiodarone (Cordarone, Pacerone). Which body system should be *carefully* monitored during this therapy?

    a. respiratory system

    b. integumentary system

    c. GI system

    d. hematopoietic system

8. To ensure safe administration of IV amiodarone, the nurse should
   a. use nonpolyvinyl chloride administration tubing and an in-line filter.
   b. use polyvinyl chloride administration tubing, an in-line filter, and a volumetric infusion pump.
   c. use polyvinyl chloride administration tubing and a volumetric infusion pump.
   d. use nonpolyvinyl chloride administration tubing and a volumetric infusion pump.

9. Which of the following patients may receive verapamil (verapamil hydrochloride, Calan, Isoptin) therapy?
   a. Marjorie, with sick sinus syndrome
   b. Hilary, with severe CHF
   c. Kimberly, with hypertension
   d. Gina, with third-degree heart block

10. Your 67-year-old patient has begun a regimen of verapamil (verapamil hydrochloride, Calan, Isoptin) therapy. Patient teaching should include management of potential
    a. sedation.
    b. constipation.
    c. hypertension.
    d. headache.

NURSING MANAGEMENT: EVERY GOOD NURSE SHOULD ...

Multiple Choice
Circle the option that best answers the question or completes the statement.

1. A sustained-release form of quinidine is being administered to treat a patient's recurrent premature atrial contractions. Patient education regarding quinidine should include
   a. taking the drug on an empty stomach.
   b. limiting dietary intake of potassium.
   c. the need for periodic blood tests.
   d. chewing the drug thoroughly before swallowing.

2. A patient with ventricular fibrillation was treated with lidocaine, a class IB antiarrhythmic. However, the lidocaine failed to control the ventricular fibrillation. An IV infusion of amiodarone, a class III antiarrhythmic, is ordered. Nursing management in this drug therapy includes which of the following? *Mark all that apply.*
   a. helping the patient to ambulate
   b. monitoring blood pressure throughout therapy
   c. mixing the drug in polyolefin bags of 5% dextrose in water (D5W)
   d. measuring pulse oximetry regularly
   e. keeping the patient on a cardiac monitor

3. The nurse should not administer IV verapamil, a class IV antiarrhythmic and calcium channel blocker, within a few hours of administering
   a. digoxin.
   b. beta blockers.
   c. potassium.
   d. diuretics.

4. Your patient's potassium level is elevated at 5.3, and he is to receive sodium polystyrene sulfonate (Kayexalate) via an enema as treatment. What should the nurse should do? *Mark all that apply.*
   a. administer a cleansing enema first
   b. mix the drug with 100 mL sorbitol or 20% dextrose to make a suspension
   c. administer the drug using an infusion pump
   d. clamp the tube and leave it in place for at least 30 minutes after infusion
   e. monitor the patient's liver enzymes after treatment

5. Your patient is to begin a regimen of propranolol, a beta blocker, for treatment of a cardiac arrhythmia. Before administering the first dose of the drug, the nurse should assess the patient's health status and confirm that the patient does not have
   a. hypertension.
   b. angina.
   c. asthma.
   d. all of the above.

6. You are working in a coronary care unit caring for a patient who has ventricular arrhythmias after myocardial infarction. The patient is receiving lidocaine by continuous IV infusion. The dosage of lidocaine per hour has had to be increased several times to control the patient's ventricular arrhythmia. The patient is now nervous, irritable, and calling out to people not in the room. You should

   a. obtain an order for an antipsychotic drug such as haloperidol.

   b. obtain an order for a STAT lidocaine level.

   c. increase the lidocaine infusion rate per protocol.

   d. place the patient in restraints and call security.

CASE STUDY

You are caring for a patient who has recurrent paroxysmal supraventricular tachycardia. The patient also has a history of renal disease. New medication orders for this patient indicate that oral verapamil, a calcium channel blocker and class IV antiarrhythmic, is to be started.

1. What physical parameters need to be assessed before each dose of verapamil?

2. What is the impact of renal disease on verapamil therapy?

CRITICAL THINKING CHALLENGE

The patient described above returns to the clinic for a follow-up appointment 6 weeks after beginning verapamil therapy. During assessment, it is discovered that an atrial tachycardia has developed. What possible explanations related to drug therapy may explain this finding?

CHAPTER 32

Drugs Affecting Coagulation

TOP TEN THINGS TO KNOW ABOUT DRUGS AFFECTING COAGULATION

1. Anticoagulants prevent blood clots from forming. They do not break down existing clots.

2. Heparin, an anticoagulant, prevents the conversion of prothrombin to thrombin and prevents the formation of a stable clot. It is used to prevent the extension of a blood clot (particularly DVT or pulmonary embolism) and is used prophylactically in patients with short-term increased risk for thrombus formation. Heparin is administered intravenously (IV) or subcutaneously (SC) (low-molecular-weight heparin is different and given only SC). Heparin use is safe during pregnancy.

3. Monitor the active partial thromboplastin time (aPTT) to determine the patient's response to therapy; therapeutic aPTT levels are one and a half to two times the control level. The most common adverse effect is bleeding. Antidote to overdosage is protamine sulfate.

4. Warfarin, an anticoagulant, blocks vitamin K and prevents activation of prothrombin and other factors. Warfarin completes treatment of a thrombus or embolism (after heparin) and is used prophylactically for patients with a long-term risk for thrombus formation (after mitral valve replacement or chronic venous stasis). It is also used prophylactically in patients with atrial fibrillation. Warfarin is given orally. Avoid use during pregnancy because fetal warfarin syndrome will occur.

5. The maximum anticoagulant effect of warfarin takes 3 to 4 days after dosing begins, so therapy usually is begun while the patient is still receiving IV heparin. Monitor the prothrombin time (PT) or the international normalized ratio (INR) to determine the patient's response to therapy; PT should be about one and one half times the control; INR should be equal to 2 or 3. Vitamin K is the antidote. Teach patients not to greatly increase dietary vitamin K intake while taking warfarin.

6. Clopidogrel, an antiplatelet, inhibits platelet aggregation, thus prolonging the bleeding time. It is used to reduce the occurrence of atherosclerotic events (myocardial infarction, stroke, and vascular death) when aspirin is not tolerated. Adverse reactions to clopidogrel are similar to those of aspirin. The most common adverse effect is gastrointestinal (GI) distress. Severe neutropenia is possible (rare). Clopidogrel inhibits the hepatic isoenzyme P-450 2C9 and will interfere with the metabolism of other drugs metabolized through this pathway. Exact reaction cannot be predicted; observe for potential changes in drug efficacy if any of these drugs are coadministered.

7. Pentoxifylline is a hemorrheologic drug used to manage symptoms of intermittent claudication from peripheral vascular disease. Using this drug improves the patient's ability to walk for longer distances without pain. It is also used to treat acute and chronic cerebral vascular disease because it improves the psychopathologic symptoms. Pentoxifylline reduces blood viscosity and increases flexibility of the red blood cells (RBC), which decreases platelet aggregation and promotes vasodilation. Full therapeutic effects are not seen until 4 to 8 weeks of therapy. Smoking limits the effectiveness of drug therapy. Pentoxifylline's adverse effects occur primarily in the central nervous, cardiovascular, and GI systems. The effects on these systems may result from this drug's similarity to caffeine and theophylline.

8. Thrombolytic drugs break down formed blood clots. Alteplase, recombinant is indicated in the treatment of acute evolving MI and acute ischemic stroke. Therapy is most effective when initiated as soon as possible after the onset of symptoms. Intracranial bleeding (hemorrhagic stroke) must be ruled out via computed tomography (CT) scan before this agent is used to treat ischemic stroke. Alteplase, recombinant binds to the fibrin in a clot and converts the trapped plasminogen to plasmin.

Fibrinolysis, or breakdown of the clot, then occurs. Bleeding is the most frequently occurring adverse effect.

9. Antihemophilic factor (AHF) is factor VIII and is used to temporarily treat or prevent bleeding in hemophilia. It is made from pooled human sources and carries a very slight risk of hepatitis and human immunodeficiency virus (HIV) transmission. Dosage is individualized to meet patient needs. Reconstitute (without shaking) and then administer IV. Teach patient to avoid injury, not to use aspirin or ibuprofen, and carry identification of hemophilia.

10. Aminocaproic acid is a systemic hemostatic drug that stops blood loss by enhancing coagulation. It is used only in life-threatening situations. Administer with an IV pump. The most common adverse effect is GI distress. Place the patient on cardiac monitoring to detect arrhythmias. Thrombophlebitis and hypotension are also possible adverse effects.

KEY TERMS

Crossword Puzzle

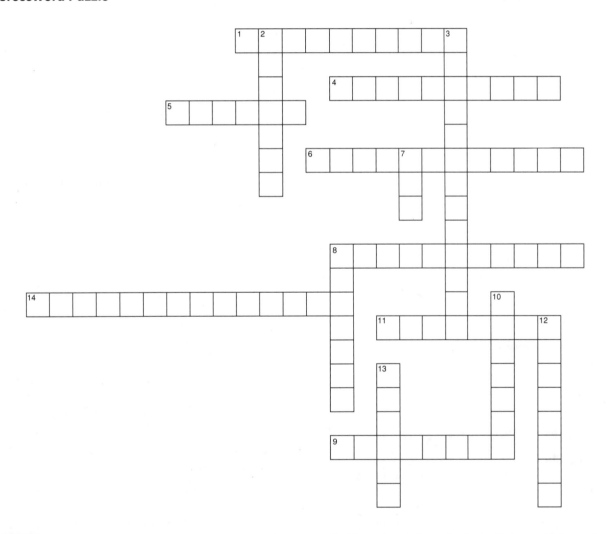

ACROSS

1. Inherited disorder of blood coagulation
4. The arrest of bleeding
5. Plasma proteins that cause blood clotting
6. Hydrolysis of fibrin
8. Transformation of solution into a gel or semi-solid mass
9. Enzyme that converts fibrinogen into fibrin
11. Thrombocyte
14. Dislodged portion of a thrombus that is floating in the bloodstream

DOWN

2. Any undissolved matter carried in a blood or lymph vessel to another location where it lodges and occludes the vessel
3. Drug that prevents clotting of blood
7. Monitoring test for anticoagulation
8. Fibrin is the end product of the clotting _____.
10. When activated, it is the substance that lyses the blood clot.
12. Attached clot in the cardiovascular (CV) system formed from constituents of blood
13. Insoluble protein product of the clotting cascade

PHYSIOLOGY AND PATHOPHYSIOLOGY: THE BODY HUMAN

Essay

1. How do anticoagulants, antiplatelet agents, hemorrheologics, and thrombolytic agents affect homeostasis?

2. What is the role of the clotting cascade?

3. What is a "factor"?

4. What is plasmin?

CORE DRUG KNOWLEDGE: JUST THE FACTS

Multiple Choice
Circle the option that best answers the question or completes the statement.

1. Anticoagulants, such as heparin, work by
   a. preventing the synthesis of factors dependent on vitamin K.
   b. lysing plasmin.
   c. inhibiting platelet synthesis.
   d. inactivating factor X.

2. The most useful test for monitoring the effectiveness of heparin is
   a. aPTT.
   b. PT.
   c. bleeding time.
   d. CBC.

3. Heparin has many potential drug–drug interactions. In general, what is the most common potential adverse effect from these interactions?
   a. bleeding
   b. headache
   c. decreased effectiveness of heparin
   d. hypertension

4. When assessing the results of heparin anticoagulation, the aPTT should be
   a. 2 to 3.
   b. 1.5 to 2 times the control.
   c. 1.4 to 1.6 times the control.
   d. 1.5 to 2.

5. Which of the following statements accurately reflects the differences between traditional heparin and low-molecular-weight heparin?
   a. Low-molecular-weight heparin has decreased bioavailability.
   b. Traditional heparin interacts less with platelets.
   c. Low-molecular-weight heparin yields a predictable dose response.
   d. Traditional heparin does not require monitoring of aPTT.

6. Anticoagulants, such as warfarin (Coumadin), work by
   a. competitively blocking vitamin K at its sites of action.
   b. lysing plasmin.
   c. inhibiting platelet synthesis.
   d. preventing conversion of fibrinogen to fibrin.

7. When assessing the results of warfarin (Coumadin) anticoagulation, the INR should be
   a. 2 to 3.
   b. 1.5 to 2 times the control.
   c. 1.4 to 1.6 times the control.
   d. 1.5 to 2.

8. Maximum effects of warfarin (Coumadin) occur within
   a. 30 minutes.
   b. 6 hours.
   c. 24 hours.
   d. 3 to 4 days.

9. Which of the following drugs is *not* classified as an antiplatelet?
   a. dipyridamole (Persantine)
   b. clopidogrel (Plavix)
   c. aspirin
   d. pentoxifylline (Trental)

10. How does clopidogrel (Plavix) work? It
    a. inhibits platelet synthesis.
    b. lyses plasmin.
    c. inhibits the binding of adenosine diphosphate (ADP) to its platelet receptor.
    d. inactivates factor X.

11. In addition to reducing the occurrence of atherosclerotic events, what other pharmacotherapeutic is appropriate for clopidogrel (Plavix)? Patients
    a. with acute coronary syndrome.
    b. undergoing percutaneous coronary intervention.
    c. undergoing coronary artery bypass graft surgery.
    d. with any of the above.

12. In the treatment of angina, dipyridamole (Persantine) works by
    a. dilating coronary arteries.
    b. inhibiting platelets.
    c. decreasing contractility of the heart.
    d. increasing oxygen consumption in the heart.

13. Glycoprotein IIb/IIIa inhibitors are frequently used after a(n)
    a. acute gastrointestinal (GI) bleed.
    b. myocardial infarction.
    c. coronary artery bypass graft (CABG).
    d. percutaneous transluminal coronary angioplasty (PTCA).

14. Which of the following drugs would be effective for intermittent claudication?
    a. heparin
    b. warfarin (Coumadin)
    c. streptokinase (Streptase)
    d. pentoxifylline (Trental)

15. Pentoxifylline (Trental) is chemically related to theophylline; therefore, adverse effects are primarily _____ in nature.
    a. central nervous system (CNS)
    b. hematologic
    c. integumentary
    d. respiratory

16. The difference between anticoagulants and thrombolytics is that
    a. anticoagulants require an unsafe dose to dissolve clots.
    b. anticoagulants dissolve clots, whereas thrombolytics prevent additional clot formation.
    c. thrombolytics dissolve clots, whereas anticoagulants prevent additional clot formation.
    d. thrombolytics decrease the risk of hemorrhage during therapy.

17. Alteplase (Activase) works by
    a. converting plasminogen to plasmin.
    b. inhibiting platelets.
    c. activating factor XIII.
    d. inhibiting fibrinogen.

18. During alteplase (Activase) infusion, the nurse should monitor (*Mark all that apply.*)
    a. arterial blood gases.
    b. vital signs.
    c. abdominal pain.
    d. changes in level of consciousness.
    e. hunger.
    f. joint pain.

19. Drotrecogin alfa, activated (Xigris) is used to
    a. prevent deep vein thrombosis.
    b. reduce mortality in critically ill patients.
    c. prevent and control excessive bleeding.
    d. treat cerebrovascular accident (CVA).

20. Antihemophilic factor (AHF) is used to
    a. prevent deep vein thrombosis.
    b. treat pulmonary emboli.
    c. prevent and control excessive bleeding.
    d. treat CVA.

21. After dilution, antihemophilic factor (AHF) should be administered within _____ hour(s).
    a. 1
    b. 24
    c. 12
    d. 3

22. Pharmacotherapeutics for hemostatic drugs include
    a. prevention of DVT.
    b. hemophilia.
    c. life-threatening bleeding disorders.
    d. disseminated intravascular coagulation (DIC).

23. The most common adverse effects of aminocaproic acid therapy affect the
    a. gastrointestinal (GI) system.
    b. cardiovascular (CV) system.
    c. genitourinary (GU) system.
    d. central nervous system (CNS).

CORE PATIENT VARIABLES: PATIENTS, PLEASE

Multiple Choice
Circle the option that best answers the question or completes the statement.

1. Which of the following patients should be closely monitored during heparin therapy?
    a. Beverly, with a history of Raynaud disease
    b. Constance, with a history of peptic ulcer disease
    c. Stanley, with a history of pancreatitis
    d. Leon, with a history of angina

2. Your patient is to receive heparin 5,000 units SC BID. To appropriately administer this medication, you should
    a. aspirate into the syringe but do not rub the area after administration.
    b. not aspirate into the syringe, but you should rub the area after administration.
    c. not aspirate into the syringe or rub the area after administration.
    d. aspirate into the syringe and rub the area after administration.

3. Your patient is receiving a continuous heparin infusion. You note bruising on the patient's arms, and the aPTT is 150 with a control of 30. You would anticipate administration of which of the following drugs?
    a. vitamin K
    b. aminocaproic acid
    c. AquaMEPHYTON
    d. protamine sulfate

4. Your patient has mitral valve prolapse and a history of pulmonary emboli, and states, "I took some kind of blood thinner, but I have not been seen for several months." Which of the following drugs do you anticipate this patient will be prescribed?
    a. heparin
    b. ticlopidine (Ticlid)
    c. warfarin (Coumadin)
    d. pentoxifylline (Trental)

5. Your patient had hip surgery today. The health care provider ordered enoxaparin (Lovenox) daily. With your knowledge of this drug, you would expect the patient's aPTT to
    a. increase.
    b. decrease.
    c. stay within the normal dosage range.

6. Your patient is taking warfarin (Coumadin) for prophylaxis for deep vein thrombosis. The patient should be scheduled for which of the following laboratory tests to monitor the effectiveness of therapy?
    a. aPTT
    b. PT
    c. INR
    d. either b or c

7. Your patient comes to the clinic for follow-up of medical problems. Current medications include clopidogrel (Plavix), phenytoin (Dilantin), cimetidine (Tagamet), and digoxin (Lanoxin). Because the patient takes clopidogrel, which of these drugs, if any, may increase this patient's risk for hemorrhage?

    a. phenytoin

    b. cimetidine

    c. digoxin

    d. all of the above

8. Your patient takes clopidogrel (Plavix) after experiencing a stroke. Patient teaching should include the need for periodic laboratory testing of (*Mark all that apply.*)

    a. complete blood count.

    b. aPTT.

    c. PT.

    d. bleeding time.

    e. platelet function.

    f. INR.

9. The patient takes pentoxifylline (Trental) for peripheral vascular disease. While you are assessing the patient's lifestyle, diet, and habits, the patient states, "I guess I should fess up–I smoke $1\frac{1}{2}$ packs of cigarettes a day." You would expect that this patient's symptoms may be

    a. increased.

    b. decreased.

    c. the same.

10. Which of the following patients should *not* receive alteplase (Activase)?

    a. Louise, 10 days postpartum

    b. Naomi, with glaucoma

    c. Carolyn, with noninsulin-dependent diabetes mellitus (NIDDM)

    d. Peter, with asthma

11. Your patient is receiving alteplase (Activase) for an acute MI. In addition to bleeding, you should monitor for

    a. sedation.

    b. muscle cramps.

    c. hypertension.

    d. arrhythmias.

12. Your patient is receiving alteplase (Activase). The patient reports abdominal pain and vomits 100 cc of dark coffee-ground emesis. The patient's blood pressure has dropped to 80/40. You should anticipate administration of which of the following drugs?

    a. protamine sulfate

    b. vitamin K

    c. aminocaproic acid (Amicar)

    d. pentoxifylline (Trental)

13. Your patient has been admitted to the emergency department with a CVA. The computed tomography (CT) scan indicates the stroke is hemorrhagic in nature. Which of the following drugs would be effective for this CVA?

    a. alteplase (Activase)

    b. urokinase (Abbokinase)

    c. streptokinase (Streptase)

    d. none of the above

14. Your patient has gone to the cardiac cath lab for a percutaneous transluminal coronary angioplasty with stent placement. Which drug class do you anticipate will be ordered for this patient?

    a. anticoagulant

    b. glycoprotein IIb/IIIa inhibitor

    c. thrombolytic

    d. hemostatic

15. Your 55-year-old patient has just started taking pentoxifylline (Trental) for intermittent claudication. Patient teaching should include:

    a. "Take on an empty stomach."

    b. "You may not see immediate results, but keep on taking the medication."

    c. "Be sure to stay out of the sunlight as much as possible."

    d. "Increase your daily intake of calcium."

16. Your patient has hemophilia and intermittently takes antihemophilic factor (AHF) at home. Patient teaching should include:

    a. "Keep the medication refrigerated until you use it."

    b. "You cannot take acetaminophen, but ibuprofen is fine."

    c. "Be sure to use sterile technique when you give yourself the subcutaneous injection."

    d. "This drug interacts with a lot of drugs, so call your doctor first."

17. Your patient has cirrhosis of the liver and is suspected of having systemic hyperfibrinolysis. What drug do you anticipate will be ordered?

    a. warfarin (Coumadin)

    b. abciximab (ReoPro)

    c. alteplase (Activase)

    d. aminocaproic acid (Amicar)

NURSING MANAGEMENT: EVERY GOOD NURSE SHOULD …

Multiple Choice
Circle the option that best answers the question or completes the statement.

1. Your patient is receiving heparin via continuous IV infusion into a peripheral vein to treat a left DVT. The patient has pneumonia and requires IV antibiotics given every 6 hours. Each antibiotic infusion requires 30 minutes. To accomplish administration of these two drug therapies, you should

    a. stop the heparin infusion every 6 hours to allow the antibiotic to be infused.

    b. piggyback the antibiotic onto the heparin line and administer both at the same time.

    c. add the antibiotic to the bag of heparin solution.

    d. use a separate IV insertion site to administer the antibiotic.

2. To prevent hematoma formation when administering subcutaneous heparin, the nurse should

    a. massage the injection site vigorously.

    b. use a 3-cc syringe.

    c. aspirate before injecting the drug.

    d. use the scapula as the preferred injection site.

3. You are caring for a 26-year-old woman who is to be discharged on warfarin, an oral anticoagulant, after a mitral valve replacement. Patient teaching regarding warfarin should include to

    a. increase dietary intake of green leafy vegetables.

    b. avoid foods high in potassium.

    c. use birth control while taking warfarin.

    d. take two doses at one time if a dose is accidentally missed.

4. Your patient has started taking clopidogrel to prevent a stroke after several mild TIAs (transient ischemic attacks). Patient education regarding clopidogrel should include which of the following? *Mark all that apply.*

    a. Take this drug with food.

    b. Blood work will be needed periodically throughout therapy.

    c. Bleeding time will be shortened.

    d. Remove throw rugs and fasten loose carpet edges in the home.

    e. Notify all health care providers that this drug has been started.

5. A patient with intermittent claudication from peripheral vascular disease in both legs begins taking pentoxifylline, a hemorrheologic drug. A follow-up telephone call is made 1 week after initiation of therapy to see if the patient has any questions or problems with the drug therapy. The patient states, "I don't feel any better. This medicine isn't working." The best response of the nurse would be

    a. "Drug therapy doesn't always work for every patient."

    b. "The drug is helping you, but you just don't realize it."

    c. "Full therapeutic effect may take 4 to 8 weeks to occur."

    d. "The drug should be stopped because it is not effective."

6. A patient is brought to the emergency room with an evolving MI and started on recombinant alteplase, a thrombolytic agent. To minimize adverse effects during this drug therapy, the nurse should

    a. assess vital signs closely throughout therapy.

    b. increase the infusion if coffee-ground emesis occurs.

    c. administer by gravity flow.

    d. give other ordered drugs by IM injection.

7. A patient with hemophilia is brought to the emergency room for uncontrolled bleeding. Antihemophyllic factor is ordered. Nursing management in this drug therapy should include which of the following? *Mark all that apply.*

   a. reconstitute the drug as soon as it is removed from the refrigerator

   b. rotate the vial of diluted drug gently to mix

   c. monitor coagulation studies during therapy

   d. administer drug by the IV route

8. Your patient had a nephrectomy 1 hour ago. Systemic hyperfibrinolysis has developed, and the patient is experiencing severe hemorrhaging. Aminocaproic acid, a hemostatic drug, has been ordered. To minimize adverse effects from this therapy, you should

   a. administer by way of an IM injection.

   b. check incision site for bleeding every 15 to 30 minutes.

   c. add the drug to other current drug infusions.

   d. obtain an electrocardiogram (ECG) at the end of therapy.

CASE STUDY

You are caring for a female patient who is 30 years old, pregnant, and has a DVT in her right leg. She is hospitalized. Her medication orders are as follows:

Heparin 35 units per kg of body weight IV push followed by 20,000 units per 24 hours per IV infusion

Additional orders read:

Bed rest
aPTT before starting heparin; repeat every 6 hours for 24 hours
Contact physician if aPTT is not in therapeutic range

1. Why is heparin used as the anticoagulant for this patient?

2. Why is some heparin ordered to be given by IV push and some heparin ordered to be given by IV infusion?

3. What is the purpose of the repeated drawing of the aPTT?

4. What is the rationale for bed rest during heparin therapy?

CRITICAL THINKING CHALLENGE

The nurse starts the heparin infusion on the patient described above and regulates it with an IV pump. The nurse checks the infusion rate hourly and assesses whether any adverse effects from the heparin have occurred. The patient tolerates the heparin infusion well. In 6 hours, her aPTT is repeated. The level is 1.25 times the control. The nurse obtains an order to increase the heparin infusion and continues to monitor the patient hourly. Three hours later, the nurse realizes that the patient has received four times the hourly rate in the last hour. The IV pump has apparently malfunctioned. The patient has no signs of bleeding, and her vital signs are stable.

What actions should the nurse take?

CHAPTER 33

Drugs Affecting Hematopoiesis

TOP TEN THINGS TO KNOW ABOUT DRUGS AFFECTING HEMATOPOIESIS

1. Hematopoietic growth factors are substances generated by the body to enhance production of blood cells. They play roles in the nonspecific and specific immune responses.
2. Deficient cell production is named by the cell involved: anemia is reduced circulating red blood cells (RBCs); neutropenia is decreased number of neutrophils; thrombocytopenia is a low platelet count; and deficient production of all cells is termed aplastic anemia.
3. Epoetin alfa functions the same as endogenous erythropoietin and stimulates the production of red blood cells. It is used in the treatment of anemia associated with chronic renal failure, use of zidovudine with human immunodeficiency virus (HIV) infection, and use of chemotherapy in cancer. It is given subcutaneously (SC). Refrigerate the drug and use aseptic technique when withdrawing it from the vial.
4. It takes as long as 8 weeks to determine the full effect of epoetin alfa. Monitor the patient's hematocrit twice a week, and adjust the dose upward after 8 weeks, if needed.
5. Filgrastim functions the same as an endogenous granulocyte colony-stimulating factor (G-CSF) and is the prototype drug for stimulating white blood cell production. Filgrastim is licensed for use in patients with cancer to increase their neutrophil count. It can be given by the intravenous (IV) or subcutaneous (SC) routes.
6. Do not discontinue treatment with filgrastim prematurely (before the expected neutrophil nadir, or lowest point, from the chemotherapy is expected). Medullary bone pain (pain within the marrow) is the only consistently observed adverse

effect that can be attributed to drug therapy; it is common and mild to moderate in severity.
7. Until the white blood cell count has risen adequately, patients receiving filgrastim are at high risk of infections. Use medical asepsis when providing care and aseptic technique when reconstituting the filgrastim. Keep the drug refrigerated but allow it to reach room temperature before administration. Teach the patient and family how to avoid infections.
8. Oprelvekin (interleukin-11) primarily alters hematopoietic activity and stimulates the production of platelets (unlike other interleukins) and functions like endogenous interleukin-11. Oprelvekin is used to prevent severe thrombocytopenia and to reduce the need for platelet transfusions after myelosuppressive chemotherapy. It is given SC. Begin oprelvekin therapy within 24 hours of the completion of chemotherapy. Continue until the postnadir platelet count is greater than or equal to 50,000 cells/mm^3, about 10 to 21 days.
9. Fluid retention with weight gain is the most common adverse effect of oprelvekin therapy. Monitor patients for signs of fluid overload. Older adults may be more likely to experience atrial arrhythmias while taking oprelvekin.
10. Reconstitute oprelvekin with the sterile water for injection (without preservative) that is provided with the medication. The protein in oprelvekin can be denatured by agitation; reconstitute by directing the spray of fluid toward the vial wall; do not aim it directly into the powdered drug. Do not shake or excessively agitate the vial; gently swirl the vial to complete dilution. Maintain aseptic technique when reconstituting and drawing up the medication.

KEY TERMS

Word Search
Write the correct answer in the space provided;
then locate the term in the word search below.

```
W   A   E   P   S   E   G   A   H   P   O   R   C   I   M   A   M   L   R   T
Y   J   N   B   W   Y   L   O   L   F   O   F   O   R   I   J   G   K   L   H
Z   C   J   E   I   N   L   C   T   R   R   D   H   N   E   D   S   S   C   R
S   E   V   R   M   O   L   P   I   B   M   E   E   G   Q   S   L   I   S   O
E   S   X   E   I   I   L   G   X   U   U   P   W   Z   D   W   I   S   E   M
T   E   B   V   E   Z   A   O   E   E   O   K   X   B   V   E   H   O   T   B
Y   T   B   Y   L   C   H   A   G   T   H   C   F   V   A   E   P   T   Y   O
C   Y   P   M   I   M   I   A   Y   I   P   Q   M   N   A   Y   O   Y   C   P
O   C   Q   Y   N   N   F   C   M   S   C   L   E   R   X   O   R   C   O   O
R   O   P   V   X   D   O   O   U   Q   E   M   A   W   Y   C   T   O   L   I
H   K   I   C   G   B   N   C   I   T   N   T   O   T   C   F   U   G   U   E
T   U   E   M   M   O   I   I   J   I   C   J   Y   D   E   Z   E   A   N   T
Y   E   D   O   C   T   R   R   Z   G   Q   H   W   C   U   L   N   H   A   I
R   L   R   Y   S   N   T   D   V   T   U   D   I   J   O   L   E   P   R   N
E   H   T   A   T   A   H   W   I   M   A   P   C   G   A   H   A   T   G   N
T   E   L   N   E   U   T   R   O   P   E   N   I   A   F   X   P   T   S   Q
S   P   H   E   M   A   T   O   P   O   I   E   S   I   S   M   M   M   O   R
A   Y   B   J   N   I   T   E   I   O   P   O   R   H   T   Y   R   E   Y   R
E   R   Y   T   H   R   O   P   O   I   E   S   I   S   V   Q   B   I   M   L
H   U   Y   L   R   E   I   F   I   D   O   M   C   I   G   O   L   O   L   B
```

1. Disorder of reduced circulating red blood cells _____

2. Deficient cell production of all types of cells_____

3. Another term for biologic modulator_____

4. Biopharmaceuticals used to alter the body's hematologic or immunologic responses_____

5. Red blood cells_____

6. Process that stimulates the production of RBCs_____

7. Major peptide hormone that stimulates production of RBCs_____

8. Most common type of leukocyte_____

9. Production of cellular components in blood_____

10. White blood cells_____

11. Mature leukocyte_____

12. Can be circulating phagocytes or can be fixed in specific tissues_____

13. Differentiate into macrophages_____

14. Decreased number of neutrophils in serum_____

15. "First line of defense" against pathogens_____

16. Process of ingesting bacteria by neutrophils_____

17. The formed element involved in blood coagulation_____

18. Low platelet count in serum_____

19. Peptide responsible for platelet production_____

PHYSIOLOGY AND PATHOPHYSIOLOGY: THE BODY HUMAN

Essay

1. What are the essential components of the immune system?

2. What are the three barrier defenses of the body against pathogens?

3. Identify the different types of leukocytes.

4. Identify the different types of lymphocytes.

CORE DRUG KNOWLEDGE: JUST THE FACTS

Multiple Choice

Circle the option that best answers the question or completes the statement.

1. A relative contraindication to the use of epoetin alfa (Epogen) is
   a. hyperthyroidism.
   b. uncontrolled hypertension.
   c. hypothyroidism.
   d. migraine headaches.

2. Which of the following types of anemia should be treated with epoetin alfa (Epogen)? *Mark all that apply.*
   a. iron or folate deficiency
   b. hemolysis
   c. gastrointestinal (GI) bleeding
   d. myelosuppressive illness

3. How frequently should the nurse schedule repeat laboratory testing for a patient with chronic renal failure who is beginning epoetin alfa (Epogen) therapy?
   a. two times a week until the target hematocrit is reached
   b. monthly until the target hematocrit is reached
   c. daily until the target hematocrit is reached
   d. weekly until the target hematocrit is reached

4. In order for epoetin alfa to be effective, the patient must have an adequate level of
   a. calcium.
   b. potassium.
   c. iron.
   d. magnesium.

5. Filgrastim (Neupogen) works to increase
   a. iron stores.
   b. red blood cells.
   c. neutrophils.
   d. platelets.

6. When administering filgrastim, the nurse should (*Mark all that apply.*)

    a. keep the drug refrigerated.

    b. shake the vial before drawing up the solution.

    c. dilute with normal saline.

    d. administer with the first cycle of chemotherapy.

    e. monitor iron stores.

7. Filgrastim (Neupogen) should be discontinued after the absolute neutrophil count remains above 1000/mm^3 for

    a. 1 week.

    b. 1 month.

    c. 3 days.

    d. 24 hours.

8. Prevention of severe thrombocytopenia may be accomplished by use of

    a. filgrastim (Neupogen).

    b. epoetin alfa (Epogen).

    c. oprelvekin (Neumega).

    d. any of the above.

9. The most common adverse effects associated with oprelvekin (Neumega) are

    a. headache and dizziness.

    b. weight gain and fluid retention.

    c. blurred vision and headache.

    d. dehydration and paresthesias.

10. Oprelvekin (Neumega) should be administered

    a. 1 month after chemotherapy is begun.

    b. 10 to 21 days postnadir.

    c. 6 to 24 hours after chemotherapy is completed.

    d. when the platelet count reaches 50,000 cells/mm^3.

CORE PATIENT VARIABLES: PATIENTS, PLEASE

Multiple Choice

Circle the option that best answers the question or completes the statement.

1. Your patient has chronic renal failure and is starting a regimen of epoetin alfa (Epogen). The patient asks, "When will you see if this works?" Your best response is

    a. 10 days.

    b. 2 to 6 weeks.

    c. 6 months.

    d. 24 hours.

2. Your patient has chronic renal failure and has been receiving epoetin alfa (Epogen) for the past 6 months. As you begin to prepare the dose for today, you note that the patient's CBC reflects a hematocrit of 40%. What is your best action?

    a. give the dose as ordered

    b. give half the dose and alert the health care provider of the CBC results

    c. hold the dose and contact the health care provider

    d. hold the dose and order a STAT CBC

3. Your patient is receiving chemotherapy and has an order for filgrastim (Neupogen). To administer this medication appropriately, you should (*Mark all that apply.*)

    a. dilute in 5% dextrose solution with albumin added.

    b. dilute in saline.

    c. shake the vial for reconstitution.

    d. administer immediately after chemotherapy.

    e. keep the medication in the patient's room.

    f. keep the medication refrigerated.

4. Which assessment finding, if identified in a patient who is receiving oprelvekin (Neumega), would require immediate follow-up by the nurse?

    a. glucose 130

    b. BP 160/100

    c. potassium level 4.0

    d. hemoglobin 13.9 %

5. Which nursing intervention should assume *priority* for the patient receiving sargramostim (Leukine) for the first time?

   a. Ice the injection site before administration.

   b. Rotate injection sites.

   c. Monitor the patient for 20 minutes after administration.

   d. Administer the medication at room temperature.

NURSING MANAGEMENT: EVERY GOOD NURSE SHOULD …

Multiple Choice
Circle the option that best answers the question or completes the statement.

1. Your patient with chronic renal failure has a hematocrit of 27, and is to start a regimen of epoetin alfa three times a week. When administering the drug, you should (*Mark all that apply.*)

   a. shake the bottle vigorously after reconstituting.

   b. refrigerate any drug remaining in the single-dose 1 mL vial to use later.

   c. administer deep into the muscle.

   d. discard any remaining drug in the single-dose 1 mL vial.

   e. coordinate twice weekly CBC.

   f. monitor the patient's blood pressure.

2. Your patient has been prescribed filgrastim, a granulocyte colony-stimulating factor (G-CSF) to prevent febrile neutropenia secondary to antineoplastic therapy for cancer. Patient education should include

   a. filgrastim use will be discontinued as soon as the neutrophil count begins to rise.

   b. filgrastim has no known adverse effects.

   c. the importance of being socially active to prevent depression.

   d. the importance of frequent handwashing to prevent infection.

3. Your patient has become anemic secondary to chemotherapy. The patient starts a regimen of epoetin alfa three times per week. You are monitoring hematocrit levels weekly. How long should you wait after initiating epoetin alfa therapy before concluding that the dose is not effective and you should seek an order for a larger dose?

   a. 2 weeks

   b. 4 weeks

   c. 8 weeks

   d. 12 weeks

4. You are to administer oprelvekin SC daily to a patient to prevent thrombocytopenia after chemotherapy. What should you do? *Mark all that apply.*

   a. plan to give the first dose of oprelvekin before giving the ordered chemotherapy dose

   b. reconstitute with sterile water for injection without preservatives

   c. keep the drug out of light

   d. administer the drug until the postnadir platelet count is $\geq$ 50,000 cells/mm^3

CASE STUDY

You are caring for a female patient who has chronic renal failure, hypertension, diabetes, and chronic heart failure (CHF). The patient goes to dialysis three times a week. The patient's blood pressure normally runs 140 to 150/80 to 90 mm Hg. Your patient's complete blood count (CBC) from today is as follows:

Patient	Normal Range
Hct 20%	Female 33%–43% Male 39%–49%
Hg 10.5 g/dL	Female 14–18 g/dL Male 11.5–15.5 g/dL
Platelets 200 × 10^3/mm^3 RBC	130–400 × 10^3/mm^3
Erythrocytes 2 × 10^5/mm^3	Female 3.5–5 × 10^5/mm^3 Male 4.3–5.9 × 10^5/mm^3
Reticulocytes 6 × 10^3/mm^3	10–75 × 10^3/mm^3
WBC 4.0 × 10^3/mm^3	3.2–9.8 × 10^3/mm^3
WBC differential	
Bands 3%	3%–5%

Patient	Normal Range
Neutrophils 56%	54%–62%
Lymphocytes 26%	25%–33%
Monocytes 3%	3%–7%
Eosinophils 1%	1%–3%
Basophils 0%	0%–0.75%

The patient is ordered epoetin alfa 100 units/kg SC three times per week.

1. Was this an appropriate order for this patient? Which lab value or values support(s) your assessment?

One week after the initiation of therapy, the patient's blood work is:

Patient	Normal Range
Hct 20%	Female 33%–43% Male 39%–49%
Hg 10.5 g/dL	Female 14–18 g/dL Male 11.5–15.5 g/dL
Platelets $200 \times 10^3/mm^3$ RBC	$130–400 \times 10^3/mm^3$
Erythrocytes $2 \times 10^5/mm^3$	Female $3.5–5 \times 10^5/mm^3$ Male $4.3–5.9 \times 10^5/mm^3$
Reticulocytes $15 \times 10^3/mm^3$	$10–75 \times 10^3/mm^3$
WBC $4.0 \times 10^3/mm^3$ WBC differential	$3.2–9.8 \times 10^3/mm^3$
Bands 3%	3%–5%
Neutrophils 56%	54%–62%
Lymphocytes 26%	25%–33%
Monocytes 3%	3%–7%
Eosinophils 1%	1%–3%
Basophils 0 %	0%–0.75%

2. Is the epoetin alfa producing a response in this patient? What lab value or values do you base your assessment upon?

3. Should you seek a change in the dose of the epoetin alfa?

CRITICAL THINKING CHALLENGE

Two weeks after the start of therapy, your patient's blood pressure is 162/94 mm Hg. The patient also reports tenderness in the back of the left calf. The patient's blood work today is:

Patient	Normal Range
Hct 26%	Female 33%–43% Male 39%–49%
Hg 14 g/dL	Female 14–18 g/dL Male 11.5–15.5 g/dL
Platelets $200 \times 10^3/mm^3$ RBC	$130–400 \times 10^3/mm^3$
Erythrocytes $3.2 \times 10^5/mm^3$	Female $3.5–5 \times 10^5/mm^3$ Male $4.3–5.9 \times 10^5/mm^3$
Reticulocytes $20 \times 10^3/mm^3$	$10–75 \times 10^3/mm^3$
WBC $4.0 \times 10^3/mm^3$ WBC differential	$3.2–9.8 \times 10^3/mm^3$
Bands 3%	3%–5%
Neutrophils 56%	54%–62%
Lymphocytes 26%	25%–33%
Monocytes 3%	3%–7%
Eosinophils 1%	1%–3%
Basophils 0%	0%–0.75%

1. What is your current assessment of these patient findings?

2. Would any additional assessment be helpful? Are any changes needed related to dialysis?

CHAPTER 34

Drugs Affecting the Immune Response

TOP TEN THINGS TO KNOW ABOUT DRUGS AFFECTING THE IMMUNE RESPONSE

1. Cytokines are chemical mediators released by leukocytes to enhance and accelerate the inflammatory responses that will destroy an invading antigen. Cytokines are generally proinflammatory, but many also have antiviral, antiproliferative, and antineoplastic properties. Cytokines are interferons and interleukins.

2. Interferon alfa-2a is a cytokine. It inhibits the growth of tumor cells, prevents their multiplication, heightens host immune response to help protect the body from tumor cells, and blocks specific viral infection by preventing viral replication.

3. Interferon alfa-2a is used to treat hairy cell leukemia, acquired immunodeficiency syndrome (AIDS)-related Kaposi sarcoma, chronic myelogenous leukemia in chronic phase Philadelphia chromosome-positive patients, and various cancers. It is given by injection. Flu-like adverse effects are common, and premedication (antipyretics, such as acetaminophen and/or antihistamines, such as diphenhydramine) is usually given.

4. Monoclonal antibodies can suppress one cell subtype or receptor site and can react with specific tumor receptor sites for diagnosis or treatment of cancer. Antitumor monoclonal antibodies include rituximab. There are also monoclonal antibodies that are used as immunosuppressants, and they are considerably different.

5. Rituximab is used to treat non-Hodgkin's lymphoma. Rituximab binds specifically to an antigen found on non-Hodgkin's lymphoma cells; no receptor is found in normal bone marrow cells. When it binds, it causes cell lysis.

6. Infusion-related effects occur in 80% of patients within 2 hours after the initiation of the first infusion. The most common infusional reactions include fever, flushing, chills, and rigors. The use of premedication (antipyretics and/or antihistamines) decreases the severity of the response.

7. Immune modulators appear to act directly on the function of T cells and B cells and either stimulate or suppress the immune response from these cells. Some drugs stimulate certain functions of the cell response but suppress other functions.

8. Cyclosporine is an immune modulator that suppresses the immune system, primarily cell-mediated immune reactions. It is used as adjunct treatment to prevent rejection after organ transplantation and to prevent graft-versus-host disease in allogeneic bone marrow or stem cell transplants. Adjunct therapy with corticosteroids is recommended.

9. There are two brands of cyclosporine, Sandimmune and Neoral, and they are different and not bioequivalent (cannot be interchanged milligram for milligram). Sandimmune formulations are available as soft gelatin capsules, an oral solution, and as an intravenous (IV) solution. Neoral formulations are available as soft gelatin capsules and an oral solution.

10. Nephrotoxicity is a fairly common and irreversible adverse effect of cyclosporine. Switch from the IV form to the oral form as soon as possible, and avoid giving the drug with food or grapefruit juice. To protect the patient from infection, use aseptic techniques and take immediate action at the first sign of infection.

KEY TERMS

Crossword Puzzle

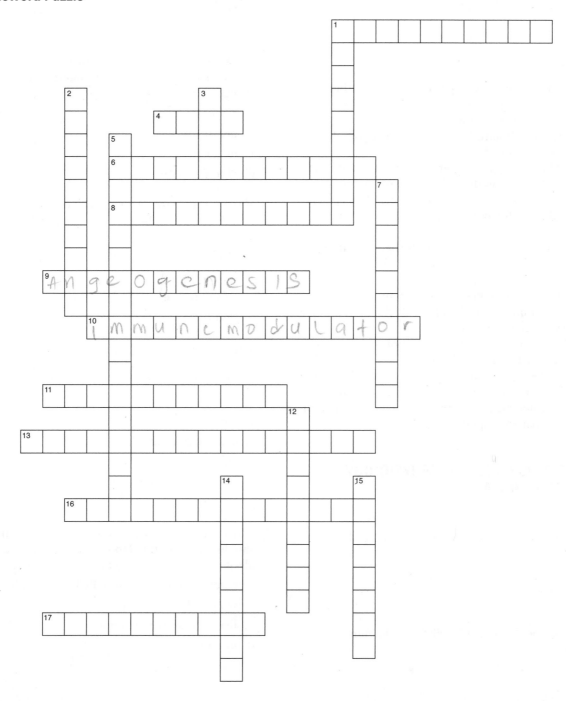

9. A n g e o g e n e s i s

10. I m m u n e m o d u l a t o r

ACROSS

1. Type of protein that destroys the antigen by altering the membrane and allowing osmotic inflow of fluid that bursts the cell

4. Abbreviation for vascular endothelial growth factor, a protein that is responsible for stimulation of new blood vessel formation

6. Chemicals secreted by active leukocytes to influence other leukocytes

8. Chemical that directly destroys a foreign cell or marks it for destruction

9. Growth of new blood vessels from pre-existing vessels

10. Group of several agents with distinctly different structures that alter T-cell or B-cell activity

11. A chemical that can cause immune system malfunction with exposure
13. Prevention of the growth of new blood vessels
16. Drug that stops growth and cellular division
17. Attraction of phagocytic cells to an area

DOWN

1. Immunologic toxins produced by white blood cells
2. Type of disease in which the body responds to specific self-antigens by producing antibodies against self-cells
3. Abbreviation for epidermal growth factor receptor. It exists on the cell surface and is activated by binding of specific ligands, including epidermal growth factor and transforming growth factor α.
5. Group of biopharmaceuticals that are naturally occurring proteins used to alter the body's immunologic responses
7. Type of antibodies that are produced by one type of immune cell and are all clones of a single parent cell
12. Compound that enhances humoral and cell-mediated immune responses
14. Synthetic retinoids
15. Type of response to destroy a foreign cell, mark it for destruction by phagocytes, and elicit an inflammatory response

PHYSIOLOGY AND PATHOPHYSIOLOGY: THE BODY HUMAN

Essay

1. Compare and contrast the types of T cells.

2. Describe the role of B cells in the immune response.

CORE DRUG KNOWLEDGE: JUST THE FACTS

Multiple Choice

Circle the option that best answers the question or completes the statement.

1. In addition to hairy cell leukemia, what other disorders may be treated with interferon alfa-2a (Roferon-A)?
   a. Kaposi sarcoma
   b. breast cancer
   c. lung cancer
   d. Hodgkin's disease

2. What is the appropriate route(s) of administration of interferon alfa-2a (Roferon-A)? *Mark all that apply.*
   a. intravenous
   b. intramuscular
   c. subcutaneous
   d. oral

3. Which of the following are the most frequent adverse effects to interferon alfa-2a therapy? *Mark all that apply.*
   a. depression
   b. confusion
   c. hypothyroidism
   d. lethargy
   e. flu-like symptoms
   f. hypotension

4. Patients receiving interferon alfa-2a (Roferon-A) should have monthly laboratory testing including all of the following *except*
   a. complete blood count (CBC).
   b. white cell differential.
   c. liver and kidney function.
   d. urinalysis.

5. Before administering rituximab (Rituxan), the nurse should check the prescriber's orders for
   a. premedications to reduce the severity of infusion reactions.
   b. postmedication to increase the efficacy of the drug.
   c. diabetic medication.
   d. frequency of vital signs.

6. To administer rituximab (Rituxin) appropriately, the nurse should (*Mark all that apply.*)
   a. mix the drug with normal saline.
   b. use glass bottles.
   c. hold administration of antihypertensive medications for 12 hours before rituximab administration.
   d. administer antihypertensive medications immediately after the rituximab infusion is completed.
   e. slow the infusion if the patient experiences an adverse effect.
   f. stop the infusion if the patient experiences an adverse effect.

7. Cyclosporine (Sandimmune, Neoral) works by suppressing
   a. T lymphocytes.
   b. B lymphocytes.
   c. cell-mediated immune reactions.
   d. phagocytosis.

8. A common yet serious adverse effect to cyclosporine (Sandimmune, Neoral) affects the _____ system.
   a. gastrointestinal
   b. genitourinary (GU)
   c. cardiovascular
   d. renal

9. Because a patient is taking interferon alfa-2a (Roferon-A), the patient should be carefully assessed for
   a. hypertension.
   b. hypoglycemia.
   c. depression.
   d. electrolyte imbalance.

10. During administration of aldesleukin (Proleukin) the nurse should constantly monitor
    a. blood pressure.
    b. level of consciousness.
    c. cardiac rhythm.
    d. heart rate.

11. Which of the following monoclonal antibodies targets the protein responsible for stimulating new blood vessel formation?
    a. Trastuzumab (Herceptin)
    b. Cetuximab (Erbitux)
    c. Bevacizumab (Avastin)
    d. Panitumumab (Vectibix)

Essay

1. List the symptoms associated with an infusion reaction to rituximab.

   Fever, flushing, chills + rigors

2. True or false: Drugs with the suffix "mab" are part of a drug class called monoclonal antibodies and can be substituted for one another with permission of the provider. Defend your answer.

   false

CORE PATIENT VARIABLES: PATIENTS, PLEASE

Multiple Choice
Circle the option that best answers the question or completes the statement.

1. Your 27-year-old patient is being treated for hairy cell leukemia with interferon alfa-2a (Roferon-A). This patient should be monitored for
   a. hypothyroidism.
   b. diabetes insipidus.
   c. constipation.
   d. GI bleeding.

2. Your patient is receiving interferon alfa-2a (Roferon-A). As you prepare to give the patient diphenhydramine, the patient asks, "Why do I need that, and why do I get this medicine in the evening?" What is your best response?

   a. "This is the way your doctor ordered it."

   b. "It is given in the evening with something to help you sleep so you will not feel the minor discomforts that the drug can cause."

   c. "It is for the possible allergic response that you might have. I just haven't had the time to give it to you sooner."

   d. "It just came up from the pharmacy."

3. Your 16-year-old patient is receiving rituximab (Rituxan) for the first time. After 1 hour of the infusion, the patient reports fever, flushing, chills, and rigors. With your knowledge of this drug, you know

   a. this is an unexpected reaction and you need to stop the drug immediately.

   b. this drug does not cause these symptoms, and the patient is just anxious.

   c. these are expected symptoms that occur with approximately 80% of patients.

   d. this is the beginning of a potentially life-threatening reaction.

4. Your patient is receiving rituximab (Rituxan). The patient also has a history of hypertension. What special considerations should be made for this patient?

   a. none

   b. Administer any antihypertensive medication just before the rituximab.

   c. Add a second type of antihypertensive medication to the patient's regimen until the rituximab therapy is complete.

   d. Do not administer the antihypertensive agent for 12 hours before rituximab administration and for 12 to 24 hours afterward.

5. Your patient is receiving abciximab (ReoPro) after a PTCA procedure. The patient states, "My friend was taking rituximab (Rituxan) for his cancer. They sure sound alike. Do I have a cancer they haven't told me about?" What is your best response?

   a. "You need to ask your doctor that question."

   b. "No, manufacturers just name the drugs any way they wish."

   c. "They are both from the same class of drugs, so the names sound alike, but the drugs are not used for the same purposes."

   d. "I've never heard of that other drug."

6. Your patient is receiving cyclosporine (Sandimmune) to prevent rejection of a heart transplant. Which of the following patient instructions is *incorrect*?

   a. "Use a glass container, not plastic, to prevent possible chemical interactions."

   b. "Mix the medication with grapefruit juice to disguise the taste."

   c. "Measure the oral solution with the dosing syringe provided, not a tablespoon."

   d. "You can mix this drug with chocolate milk."

7. Your patient had a heart transplant 6 months ago. The patient is prescribed cyclosporine (Sandimmune) and prednisone daily. The patient comes to the clinic today for laboratory tests and states, "I had a heart transplant; why are you guys so interested in my kidneys?" What is your best response?

   a. "You know how doctors are—they want to check out everything."

   b. "Cyclosporine can cause damage to your kidneys."

   c. "Prednisone can stop your kidneys from working."

   d. "I'll check—perhaps someone made a mistake."

8. Which nursing assessment should assume priority for the patient receiving rituximab (Rituxan)? Assessment of the

   a. respiratory system

   b. gastrointestinal system

   c. central nervous system

   d. integumentary system

9. The nurse should assess a patient who is receiving rituximab (Rituxin) for symptoms of infusion reaction syndrome, which include

    a. ventricular tachycardia, supraventricular tachycardia, angina, hypotension, and hypertension.

    b. profound bradycardia, pounding headache and hypotension.

    c. Cellulitis at the insertion site and fever.

    d. Increased respiratory rate, hypotension, and bradycardia.

10. A patient has been given instructions after administration of rituximab (Rituxin). Which of these responses, if made by the patient, would indicate that the patient correctly understood the instructions?

    a. "I will have a glass of wine before I go to bed tonight."

    b. "I will drink plenty of water."

    c. "I will refrain from eating dairy products for the next 24 hours."

    d. "I will take my temperature every hour for the next 12 hours."

NURSING MANAGEMENT: EVERY GOOD NURSE SHOULD …

Multiple Choice
Circle the option that best answers the question or completes the statement.

1. Your patient is to receive interferon alfa-2a to treat Kaposi sarcoma related to AIDS. Patient teaching should include

    a. how to give a subcutaneous (SC) injection.

    b. how to avoid infections.

    c. when to return for blood tests.

    d. all of the above.

    e. none of the above.

2. You are to administer the first dose of rituximab to a patient who has had a liver transplant. To minimize adverse effects from the rituximab, you should

    a. administer antipyretics after the first dose if needed.

    b. administer the drug by IV infusion using a pump.

    c. administer a high dose initially and then taper the dose.

    d. do all of the above.

    e. do none of the above.

3. Within 1 hour of starting the rituximab infusion, the patient described above has a fever of 101.4°F, is flushed, and reports feeling cold. Your best initial response is to

    a. provide warm blankets and ice chips.

    b. seek an order for acetaminophen.

    c. turn down the rate of rituximab infusion.

    d. turn off the rituximab infusion.

4. Cyclosporine, an immune modulator, has been prescribed for your patient after a bone marrow transplant. Which of these findings should concern you the most while this patient receives cyclosporine?

    a. slightly elevated serum potassium

    b. slightly low neutrophil count

    c. significantly elevated blood urea nitrogen

    d. none of the above would be a concern; they are all normal findings

5. Your patient received Sandimmune (cyclosporine) by IV just before a kidney transplant today. The dose was 5 mg/kg/day. The postoperative orders for this patient state to give 15 mg/kg/day orally beginning tomorrow. As the nurse, you should

    a. assume that this was a transcription error and administer 5 mg/kg/day orally.

    b. contact the physician for a new order.

    c. administer the 15 mg/kg/day orally as ordered.

    d. request that the pharmacist dispense Neoral instead of Sandimmune.

6. Your patient is receiving rituximab by IV infusion weekly to treat non-Hodgkin's lymphoma and is to begin taking cefamandole (second-generation cephalosporin) by IV every 6 hours for an acute urinary tract infection today. You are to administer both drugs today and will be giving the first dose of the cefamandole. You should time the administration of these two drugs in this manner:

   a. infuse both drugs at the same time by piggybacking the cefamandole into the rituximab.

   b. infuse both drugs at the same time but into two different IV insertion sites.

   c. infuse the cefamandole either 2 hours before or 2 hours after the rituximab.

   d. infuse the cefamandole and follow immediately with the rituximab.

CASE STUDY

Your patient is a 55-year-old woman who is to start taking interferon alfa-2a for treatment of hairy cell leukemia. She has poor eyesight from being a brittle type I diabetic since she was 12 years old. She lives with her husband, who has arthritis in his hands. Their daughter lives about 20 minutes away.

1. To safely administer the interferon alfa-2a, what specific information does this patient need?

2. What concerns might you have regarding this patient and her drug therapy?

CRITICAL THINKING CHALLENGE

What questions regarding the environment should you ask before discharging the patient described above to take the drug at home?

CHAPTER 35

Drugs Affecting Corticosteroid Levels

TOP TEN THINGS TO KNOW ABOUT DRUGS AFFECTING CORTICOSTEROID LEVELS

1. The two types of corticosteroids are glucocorticoids and mineralocorticoids. Mineralocorticoids influence the regulation of sodium, potassium, and water balance. Glucocorticoids, released during the stress response, have a role in the inflammatory response, the immune response, and protein, fat, and carbohydrate metabolism.

2. Prednisone (Deltasone), a glucocorticoid, is used as replacement therapy in adrenal insufficiency, anti-inflammatory therapy for various inflammatory diseases and conditions, and immunosuppressant therapy. The effects that prednisone has on the body account for its therapeutic uses but also its adverse effects.

3. Short-term treatment with prednisone may produce mild central nervous system (CNS) and gastrointestinal (GI) complaints, increased susceptibility to infections, poor wound healing, hyperglycemia, and suppression of pituitary adrenocorticotropic hormone (ACTH) release. Long-term treatment with prednisone may cause cushingoid characteristics (Cushing syndrome), osteoporosis, fluid retention, electrolyte imbalance, glucose intolerance, hyperglycemia, obesity, hirsutism, and protein wasting, among other things.

4. Systemic (metabolic) adverse effects do not usually occur with inhaled or topical glucocorticoids.

5. Sudden withdrawal of prednisone, even if used only a short time, may bring about acute adrenal insufficiency, which may be fatal. Always withdraw glucocorticoids, such as prednisone, slowly by tapering down the dose over several days or weeks.

6. The dosage of prednisone (when used as a chronic treatment), and other glucocorticoids, needs to be increased in times of stress to prevent drug-induced adrenal insufficiency.

7. Fludrocortisone has both mineralocorticoid and glucocorticoid effects but is used only for its mineralocorticoid activity as a replacement therapy in adrenocortical deficiency (Addison disease). In small doses, the mineralocorticoid effects (urinary excretion of potassium, sodium retention, and an increase in blood pressure) predominate; larger doses result in predominance of glucocorticoid effects.

8. Adverse effects of fludrocortisone usually occur if the dose is too high (edema, hypertension, chronic heart failure [CHF], cardiomegaly, hypokalemic alkalosis). Rapid withdrawal also precipitates adrenal crisis. The dosage needs to be increased in times of stress.

9. Aminoglutethimide (Cytadren) is used to treat hypercortisolism (Cushing syndrome). It does not affect the underlying pathology and is used for less than 3 months. Orthostatic and persistent hypotension may occur. Monitor blood pressure carefully.

10. Patients receiving corticosteroids or their antagonists should carry a Medic Alert card or wear a bracelet to alert medical personnel of special needs related to drug therapy in the event of emergency.

KEY TERMS

Fill in the Blanks
Read each statement carefully and, using the chapter's key terms, write the correct answer in the space provided.

1. Water and electrolyte balance of the body is mediated by _____ hormones.

2. Chronic adrenocortical insufficiency is also known as _____.

3. In secondary _____ _____, the deficiency of cortisol secretion is secondary to insufficient secretion of ACTH by the anterior pituitary.

4. A congenital abnormality, _____, results in excess ACTH.

5. _____ exerts a major influence on regulating potassium, sodium, and water balance.

6. A disorder caused by excessive secretion of aldosterone is called _____.

7. The _____ hormones are potent anti-inflammatory agents.

8. Symptoms of a(n) _____ include severe hypotension, hyponatremia, dehydration, hyperkalemia, and hyperthermia

9. _____ is a disorder resulting from increased adrenocortical secretion of cortisol.

10. _____ sensitizes the arterioles to norepinephrine for vasopressor effects and allows epinephrine and glucagon to activate gluconeogenesis and glycogenolysis.

11. Drugs that suppress adrenal cortical function are called _____.

PHYSIOLOGY AND PATHOPHYSIOLOGY: THE BODY HUMAN

Essay

1. What are the catecholamines secreted by the adrenal medulla?

2. What hormones are secreted by the adrenal cortex?

3. What are the major effects of glucocorticoid steroids on the body?

4. List the metabolic effects of the glucocorticoids on the body.

5. What is the long-term effect of exogenous glucocorticoid therapy?

6. What is the major mineralocorticoid produced by the adrenal gland?

7. What are the major glucocorticoids produced by the adrenal gland?

CORE DRUG KNOWLEDGE: JUST THE FACTS

Multiple Choice
Circle the option that best answers the question or completes the statement.

1. Which of the following is *not* a primary use of prednisone (Deltasone)?
   a. replacement therapy for adrenal insufficiency
   b. maintenance of water and electrolyte balance
   c. anti-inflammatory therapy
   d. immunosuppressant effects

2. What is the most dangerous complication of prednisone (Deltasone) therapy?
   a. GI ulceration
   b. hyperglycemia
   c. immune system compromise
   d. vertigo

3. Which of the following body systems is *unaffected* by the potential complications of long-term prednisone (Deltasone) therapy?

   a. respiratory
   b. gastrointestinal
   c. integumentary
   d. every system of the body

4. Which of the following statements regarding drug–drug interaction with prednisone (Deltasone) therapy is correct?

   a. There are only a few drug–drug interactions, and they are minor.
   b. There are only a few drug–drug interactions, but many are serious.
   c. There are many drug–drug interactions, and many are serious.
   d. There are many drug–drug interactions; some are serious, and many are life threatening.

5. Alternate-day dosing of prednisone (Deltasone) may decrease

   a. potential drug–drug interactions.
   b. some adverse effects.
   c. sodium loss.
   d. GI distress.

6. Patients taking corticosteroids for a long period of time need to

   a. have the drug dosages tapered when use of the drug is discontinued.
   b. increase their intake of potassium-rich foods.
   c. take "drug holidays" at least once a week.
   d. take dietary supplements to counteract their weight loss.

7. Which of the following adverse effects is associated with the use of fludrocortisone (Florinef)?

   a. hypotension
   b. dehydration
   c. chronic heart failure (CHF)
   d. sedation

8. Patients taking fludrocortisone (Florinef) need to limit their intake of

   a. potassium.
   b. sodium.
   c. magnesium.
   d. chloride.

9. Patients taking fludrocortisone (Florinef) need to increase their intake of

   a. potassium.
   b. sodium.
   c. magnesium.
   d. chloride.

10. Which of the following drugs would be useful in the treatment of hypercortisolism?

    a. fludrocortisone (Florinef)
    b. methylprednisolone (Solu-Medrol)
    c. aminoglutethimide (Cytadren)
    d. spironolactone (Aldactone)

11. During aminoglutethimide (Cytadren) therapy, the nurse should closely monitor

    a. temperature.
    b. blood pressure.
    c. respiratory rate.
    d. pulse.

12. Which of the following baseline lab tests should be completed before initiating amino-glutethimide (Cytadren) therapy?

    a. CBC and arterial blood gas
    b. iron stores and glucose tolerance
    c. thyroid function and CBC
    d. urinalysis and thyroid function

13. The nurse should assess patients transitioning from systemic prednisone to an inhaled corticosteroid for symptoms of corticoid withdrawal syndrome, which include

    a. malaise, myalgia, nausea, headache, and low-grade fever.
    b. nausea, vomiting, and diarrhea.
    c. tachycardia and hypertension.
    d. hyperactivity, subnormal temperature, and myalgia.

CORE PATIENT VARIABLES: PATIENTS, PLEASE …

Multiple Choice
Circle the option that best answers the question or completes the statement.

1. Your 41-year-old patient had a renal transplant today. The patient has been prescribed prednisone (Deltasone). Which of the following nursing actions is *most* important for this patient?

   a. monitor for constipation

   b. take vital signs at least once a day

   c. assess for CNS depression

   d. monitor for signs of infection

2. Your 6-year-old patient has severe asthma. The patient's mom states, "I always feel so much better when my child takes prednisone (Deltasone). Why can't my child just stay on it?" Which of the following is your best response?

   a. "The cost of prednisone therapy is just too high."

   b. "Long-term therapy could result in short stature for your child."

   c. "Your child would come home crying because the adverse effects make the face puffy."

   d. "It would quit working if you gave it for a long time."

3. Your 50-year-old patient is receiving long-term prednisone (Deltasone) therapy. Which of the following diet restrictions should this patient follow?

   a. limit carbonated beverages

   b. increase potassium intake

   c. increase sodium intake

   d. decrease protein intake

4. Your patient takes prednisone (Deltasone) for chronic obstructive pulmonary disease (COPD). This patient should have frequent follow-up clinic visits to assess for

   a. CHF and headaches.

   b. hyperglycemia and osteoporosis.

   c. weight loss and hypoglycemia.

   d. dermatitis and headaches.

5. Your patient has adrenal insufficiency and is starting a regimen of a daily dose of prednisone (Deltasone). Which of the following instructions is appropriate?

   a. Take your medication at bedtime.

   b. Take one pill 6 times a day.

   c. Take your medication whenever you remember it.

   d. Take your medication in the early morning.

6. Your patient takes prednisone (Deltasone) daily for adrenal insufficiency. The patient is admitted to the hospital after a serious motor vehicle accident with multiple fractures and blunt head trauma. During hospitalization, this patient's prednisone dose may need to

   a. increase.

   b. decrease.

   c. stay the same.

7. Your patient started taking fludrocortisone (Florinef) 3 months ago. In comparison with the patient's baseline physical assessment, you would expect the blood pressure to have

   a. increased.

   b. decreased.

   c. stayed the same.

8. Your patient takes fludrocortisone (Florinef) for replacement therapy. The patient calls the clinic and states, "I am getting occasional headaches. What type of analgesia can I take?" Which of the following would be best for this patient?

   a. meperidine

   b. aspirin

   c. acetaminophen

   d. any of the above

9. Your patient is taking fludrocortisone (Florinef) and reports a 25-pound weight gain. You should assess for

   a. sodium intake.

   b. magnesium intake.

   c. cigarette smoking.

   d. increased exercise regimen.

10. Your patient has newly diagnosed hypercortisolism and is starting to take aminoglutethimide (Cytadren). Patient teaching should include which of the following instructions?

    a. Take only three meals per day to decrease GI distress.

    b. Assess sedation before driving a vehicle.

    c. This drug will not interfere with your attempts to become pregnant.

    d. Take a "drug holiday" at lease once a week.

NURSING MANAGEMENT: EVERY GOOD NURSE SHOULD …

Multiple Choice

Circle the option that best answers the question or completes the statement.

1. Your patient is receiving oral prednisone after a kidney transplant. To minimize adverse effects of the prednisone, you should

    a. administer the drug on an empty stomach.

    b. administer the drug with milk or food.

    c. decrease the dose in times of physical stress.

    d. decrease the dose if proton pump inhibitors are prescribed.

2. Your patient receives prednisone because of adrenal insufficiency. He is to take one dose every day. To most closely mimic the normal physiologic action of glucocorticoids, you should instruct your patient to take the drug

    a. early in the morning.

    b. late in the evening.

    c. in the middle of the day.

    d. at any time of day.

3. You are caring for a patient who receives fludrocortisone (Florinef), a mineralocorticoid, for Addison disease. You would evaluate the drug therapy as being effective if

    a. hypertension develops.

    b. hypokalemia occurs.

    c. weight increases.

    d. all of the above occur.

    e. none of the above occurs.

4. Your patient is to begin therapy with fludrocortisone (Florinef) for Addison disease. Teaching about fludrocortisone drug therapy should include which of the following?

    a. decrease potassium intake

    b. increase sodium intake

    c. stop drug therapy during periods of illness

    d. wear or carry a Medic Alert bracelet or card

5. Your patient is to begin aminoglutethimide (Cytadren) therapy for Cushing syndrome. You should monitor which of the following while this patient receives aminoglutethimide?

    a. thyroid function

    b. blood pressure

    c. adrenal insufficiency

    d. all of the above

    e. none of the above

CASE STUDY

You are caring for a patient who is 65 years old and has chronic asthma. The patient receives a limited income from a Social Security pension. The patient is given a prescription for beclomethasone, an inhaled glucocorticoid. The drug is administered through a metered-dose inhaler. One puff twice a day is the dose.

1. Why was a glucocorticoid ordered for this patient? *bronchio spasm dilation tx of choice for asthma*

2. What teaching is indicated for the beclomethasone therapy? (Need help? See Chapter 48.)

CRITICAL THINKING CHALLENGE

The patient described above receives inhaled beclomethasone for 2 years and then starts a regimen of oral prednisone. After 1 year of the oral prednisone therapy, the patient is brought to the emergency room with severe hypotension. The lab work shows the patient's sodium levels are low and potassium levels are elevated. The patient appears somewhat dehydrated and has a temperature of 100.6°F, although the white count is not elevated. The patient has lost 10 pounds since the previous year.

1. What is your assessment of these findings?

2. What explanations might account for the presence of these findings?

CHAPTER 36

Drugs That Are Cell Cycle–Specific

TOP TEN THINGS TO KNOW ABOUT DRUGS THAT ARE CELL CYCLE–SPECIFIC

1. Chemotherapeutic drugs interfere either with the synthesis of DNA, RNA, or proteins or with the appropriate functioning of the preformed molecule; in response, a proportion of cells die. Chemotherapy works on the principle of first-order kinetics: the number of tumor cells killed by an antineoplastic drug is proportional to the dose used. The proportion of cells killed after chemotherapy administration is a constant percentage of the total number of malignant cells present, not a specific number of cells. Because only a portion of the cells die, multiple doses of chemotherapy must be given. Cell cycle–specific drugs are toxic to the cell at a particular phase of the cell cycle and cause no significant harm during the other phases.

2. The major toxicities of antineoplastic drugs are seen on rapidly dividing cells, such as the bone marrow, gastrointestinal (GI) mucosa, hair follicles, and gonadal cells. Avoid use during pregnancy. Precautions must be used in the handling and disposal of all chemotherapy drugs.

3. 5-Fluorouracil (5-FU), an antimetabolite, works in the S phase of cell division and interferes with the synthesis of DNA and RNA by acting as a false antimetabolite, causing thiamine deficiency (thiamine is needed for DNA and RNA cell division and growth). 5-FU, like other anti-metabolites, is most effective against tumors with a high growth fraction. It is used to treat various solid tumors, especially malignant GI tumors.

4. Myelosuppression (anemia, leukopenia, and thrombocytopenia) is the dose-limiting adverse effect of 5-FU. Monitor WBC closely at nadir. Other serious adverse effects are GI ulceration and hemorrhage (can be fatal) and cardiotoxicity (during the first 72 hours of the initial treatment cycle).

5. Vincristine, a vinca alkaloid, works in the M (mitotic) phase of cell division by preventing cell division in the metaphase stage of mitosis. It is used in treating acute lymphoblastic leukemia and some other cancers. Dose-limiting adverse effects are neurologic (motor, sensory, and autonomic neuropathy). Neurotoxicity appears weeks or months after drug administration and lasts a long time. The severity of neurotoxicity is related to the cumulative dose. Vincristine is given only intravenously (IV). It is a vesicant. Use extravasation precautions when administering this drug.

6. Etoposide, a podophyllotoxin, works in the G_2 and S phases of the cell cycle, preventing cells from entering mitosis and prophase by inhibiting DNA synthesis. Etoposide is used in combination therapy for refractory testicular tumors, small-cell lung cancer, and some other cancers. Myelosuppression (granulocytopenia) is etoposide's dose-limiting adverse effect. Monitor white blood cell (WBC) count closely at nadir. Etoposide may be given by mouth (PO) or IV. It causes nausea and vomiting when given PO; it is an irritant when given IV. If administered too rapidly by IV, hypersensitivity or anaphylactic-like reactions can occur. If this occurs, stop the infusion and give IV fluids, corticosteroids, antihistamines, and volume expanders as ordered.

7. Paclitaxel (a taxane) inhibits the normal dynamic reorganization of the microtubular network during interphase and mitosis. Paclitaxel also prevents transition from the G_0 and G_1 phases into the S phase by blocking cellular response to protein growth factors. Paclitaxel is used in treating ovarian and breast cancers. Myelosuppression is a dose-limiting adverse effect of paclitaxel. Significant neurotoxicity can also occur.

8. Hypersensitivity reactions occur in about 10% of patients who receive paclitaxel during the first 10 minutes of the infusion. Premedicate with corticosteroids (Decadron), diphenhydramine (Benadryl), and H_2 antagonist (Cimetidine) to prevent severe reactions.

9. Topotecan HCl, a semisynthetic derivative of camptothecin, inhibits the enzyme needed for

maintaining DNA structure during replication, transcription, and translation of genetic materials (S phase). This inhibition leads to breakage of DNA strands and cell death. Topotecan is used to treat patients with metastatic ovarian cancer after the failure of initial or subsequent chemotherapy. It is also effective in treating small-cell lung cancer. The dose-limiting toxicity of topotecan is myelosuppression, especially neutropenia. Assess the adequacy of bone marrow reserve before starting therapy and reassess WBC at nadir. Hematopoietic growth factors may be needed.

10. Hydroxyurea, a miscellaneous antineoplastic agent, is used in managing hematologic cancers. It is an inhibitor of the enzyme ribonucleotide reductase, causing inhibition of DNA, without inhibiting RNA or protein synthesis. It is S-phase specific and may hold other cells in the G_1 phase of the cell cycle. Myelosuppression (especially leukopenia) is the major toxicity and is dose related.

KEY TERMS

Crossword Puzzle

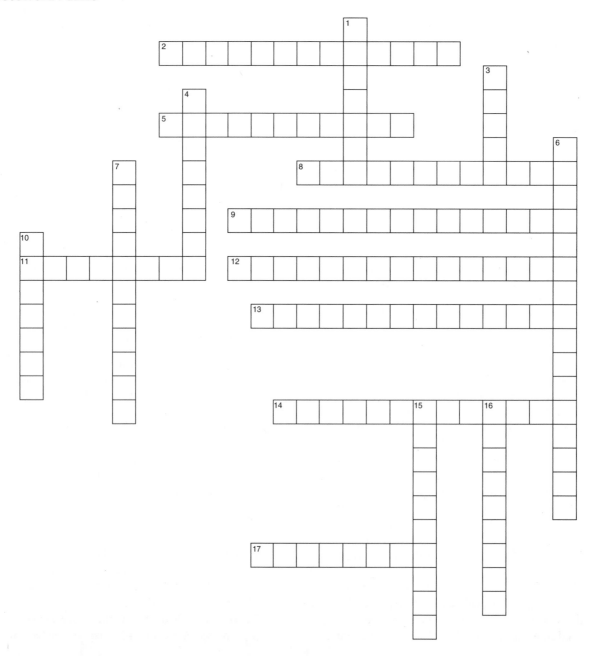

ACROSS

2. Type of therapy given after induction therapy has achieved a complete remission
5. This therapy involves the use of adjuvant chemotherapeutic drugs during the preoperative or perioperative periods
8. Term that describes the use of cytotoxic agents to destroy cancer cells
9. Ability of the body to react to radiation treatment after it is completed
11. Any agent causing irritation
12. After complete remission is achieved, the same agents used for induction therapy are given at higher doses
13. Fraction of the cell population that is in any phase of the cell cycle
14. Chemotherapeutic drugs that are most effective during a particular phase of the cycle are known as cell _____
17. This therapy is administered after radiation or surgery to destroy residual tumor cells

DOWN

1. This therapy is given to a patient whose symptoms have recurred or whose treatment by another regimen has failed
3. Time at which the maximum cytotoxic effect is exerted on the bone marrow
4. Extremely acidic drugs that may cause significant and undesired tissue damage
6. Drugs that act independently of a specific cell cycle are called cell _____
7. This therapy involves using single or combination, low-dose cytotoxic drugs on a long-term basis
10. Process of reproduction of cells, resulting in the formation of two daughter cells
15. This therapy is done to control symptoms, provide comfort, and improve the patient's quality of life if a cure is not achievable
16. This term commonly describes treatment of hematologic concerns

PHYSIOLOGY AND PATHOPHYSIOLOGY: THE BODY HUMAN

Matching
Match the following phases of the reproductive cell cycle.

1. _____ mitotic spindles constructed and RNA synthesized
2. _____ waiting for reproductive stimulus
3. _____ cell division

4. _____ DNA and RNA assembled
5. _____ resting phase

a. G_0
b. G_1
c. S
d. G_2
e. M

ESSAY

1. What are the four phases of mitosis?

2. What is cytokinesis?

3. Describe generation time.

4. What differentiates the cancer cell from the normal cell?

5. Define first-order kinetics.

CORE DRUG KNOWLEDGE: JUST THE FACTS

Multiple Choice
Circle the option that best answers the question or completes the statement.

1. Antimetabolites such as 5-fluorouracil (5-FU) inhibit tumor growth by
   a. interfering with the metaphase of mitosis.
   b. inhibiting DNA synthesis in the S and G_2 phases.
   c. inhibiting the normal dynamic reorganization of the microtubular network during interphase and mitosis.
   d. inducing thiamine deficiency, which deprives the cells of DNA and RNA.

2. Which of the following would necessitate close monitoring of a patient receiving 5-FU therapy?
   a. poor nutritional status
   b. depressed bone marrow function
   c. concurrent serious infection
   d. all of the above

3. 5-FU therapy is particularly effective in the treatment of
   a. central nervous system (CNS) lesions.
   b. malignant gastrointestinal (GI) tumors.
   c. lymphoma.
   d. leukemia.

4. Which of the following adverse effects would necessitate cessation of therapy with 5-FU?
   a. WBC >3,500
   b. constipation
   c. stomatitis
   d. hypertension

5. Which of the following chemotherapeutic agents is most useful in the treatment of lymphoblastic leukemia?
   a. floxuridine (FUDR)
   b. etoposide (VePesid)
   c. vincristine (Oncovin)
   d. docetaxel (Taxotere)

6. Patients receiving vincristine (Oncovin) should be closely monitored for
   a. fever spike.
   b. extravasation.
   c. diarrhea.
   d. hypertension.

7. Which of the following interventions is necessary to assure safe administration of vincristine (Oncovin)? *Mark all that apply.*
   a. protect from light
   b. keep at room temperature
   c. monitor for extravasation
   d. monitor CBC at least once per month

8. Administration of etoposide (VePesid) should be
   a. IVP within 3 minutes.
   b. IVPB over 30 to 60 minutes.
   c. IVP over 10 minutes.
   d. IVPB over 1 to 2 hours.

9. An adverse effect associated with etoposide (VePesid) therapy is
   a. bronchospasm and cough.
   b. CNS depression and tachycardia.
   c. increased intraocular pressure and visual disturbances.
   d. radiation recall and alopecia.

10. Paclitaxel (Taxol) therapy has been very successful in patients with
    a. brain and ovarian cancer.
    b. ovarian and breast cancer.
    c. GI and ovarian cancer.
    d. brain and pancreatic cancer.

11. Patients receiving paclitaxel (Taxol) may experience which of the following adverse effects?
    a. hypersensitivity reaction
    b. neurotoxicity
    c. myelosuppression
    d. all of the above

12. A unique adverse effect associated with docetaxel (Taxotere) therapy is
    a. fluid retention syndrome.
    b. increased appetite.
    c. increased thickness of hair.
    d. decreased intraocular pressure.

13. Topotecan HCl (Hycamtin) works by
    a. inhibiting the activity of an enzyme involved in gene transcription and DNA replication.
    b. inhibiting DNA synthesis in the S and G2 phases.
    c. inhibiting the normal dynamic reorganization of the microtubular network during interphase and mitosis.
    d. inducing thiamine deficiency, which deprives the cells of DNA and RNA.

14. Which of the following statements concerning drug–drug interactions of topotecan HCl (Hycamtin) is accurate?

    a. There are no known drug–drug interactions.

    b. There are a few drug–drug interactions, but they are minor.

    c. There are a few drug–drug interactions, and they are serious.

    d. There are many drug–drug interactions, and they are serious.

15. Hydroxyurea (Hydrea) is administered

    a. via IV push.

    b. via IV piggyback.

    c. by subcutaneous injection.

    d. orally.

16. Which of the following instructions should be included for the patient receiving hydroxyurea (Hydrea)?

    a. "You need to stay out of the sun as much as possible."

    b. "You should drink plenty of fluids to prevent problems with your kidneys."

    c. "You should eat lots of green leafy vegetables."

    d. "Be sure to check your blood glucose every day."

ESSAY

1. List the lab tests that should be monitored in patients receiving chemotherapeutic drugs.

2. Generate a list of major teaching points for patients receiving chemotherapeutic drugs.

Matching

Match the following drugs with their Black Box warnings. Match all that apply.

1. _____ 5-FU

2. _____ Vincristine

3. _____ Etoposide

4. _____ Paclitaxel

5. _____ Topotecan

6. _____ Hydroxyurea

    a. Carcinogenic

    b. Myelosuppression

    c. Extravasation

    d. Anaphylaxis

    e. Neutropenia

    f. Severe toxicities

    g. Cutaneous vasculit toxicities

    h. Hospitalization for initial administration

    i. Fatal with intrathecal administration

    j. Mutagenic

CORE PATIENT VARIABLES: PATIENTS, PLEASE

Multiple Choice

Circle the option that best answers the question or completes the statement.

1. Your patient is prescribed 5-fluorouracil (5-FU) drug therapy. Which of the following adverse effects would limit the use of this drug therapy?

    a. hepatotoxicity

    b. neurotoxicity

    c. myelosuppression

    d. pulmonary toxicity

2. Before initiating 5-FU therapy, which of the following should be documented?

    a. pulmonary function results

    b. condition of skin, nails, and hair

    c. visual acuity

    d. blood pressure

3. Your patient is receiving 5-FU therapy. She is scheduled to receive her third cycle. Before initiating this infusion, you should evaluate this patient's

   a. WBC and differential count.

   b. urinalysis.

   c. BUN and creatinine.

   d. hepatic enzymes.

4. Your patient is prescribed vincristine (Oncovin) therapy. The patient experiences a loss of deep tendon reflexes and weakness. The patient also reports constipation. You suspect

   a. hepatotoxicity.

   b. neurotoxicity.

   c. pulmonary toxicity.

   d. cardiotoxicity.

5. During an infusion of etoposide (VePesid), your patient experiences facial flushing, bronchospasm, and tachycardia. This might be attributable to

   a. pulmonary toxicity.

   b. infusing medication over too long a time period.

   c. infusing medication over too short a time period.

   d. cardiotoxicity.

6. Your patient is receiving combination therapy with paclitaxel (Taxol) and cisplatin (Platenol). Which of the drugs should be administered first?

   a. paclitaxel

   b. cisplatin

   c. It does not matter.

   d. They should never be used in combination.

7. Which of the following interventions are necessary when your patient receives paclitaxel (Taxol)?

   a. Shield medication from light.

   b. Assess vital signs frequently during the first 15 minutes of infusion.

   c. Monitor urine output for discoloration.

   d. Assess the patient's level of consciousness during first the 15 minutes of infusion.

8. To minimize the potential for fluid retention syndrome with docetaxel (Taxotere) therapy, which of the following premedications may be administered?

   a. corticosteroids

   b. histamine antagonists

   c. diuretics

   d. all of the above

9. Your patient is receiving topotecan HCl (Hycamtin). The patient asks, "How many times do I need to get this drug?" What is your best response?

   a. "This is the only time."

   b. "You will need only five doses."

   c. "You will need one dose for 5 consecutive days and need to repeat that series three more times."

   d. "You need to get it one time every 21 days for four courses."

10. Your patient is receiving hydroxyurea (Hydrea) for leukemia. Which of the following should be closely monitored with this patient?

    a. hepatic function

    b. pulmonary function

    c. CBC

    d. ECG

11. Your patient calls the clinic and states, "I do not seem to be able to keep any food down." What is your best response?

    a. "That is normal. You will get your appetite back again."

    b. "Not to worry—try to swallow protein shakes."

    c. "Stop your medication immediately."

    d. "Has it been more than 24 hours?"

12. Your patient is receiving chemotherapeutic drugs for breast cancer. She asks, "What does that word 'nadir' mean?" You would respond that it is the

    a. length of time it takes for the drug to clear your body.

    b. length of time before your hair starts to fall out.

    c. period that the drug can cause the most damage to your white cells.

    d. period that the drug works the hardest.

NURSING MANAGEMENT: EVERY GOOD NURSE SHOULD …

Multiple Choice
Circle the option that best answers the question or completes the statement.

1. You are caring for a patient who is receiving 5-FU for stomach cancer and who has developed mouth sores. What teaching is appropriate regarding treatment of these mouth sores?
   a. Drink hot tea with honey and lemon.
   b. Rinse the mouth after every meal with a commercial mouthwash.
   c. Eat more gelatin and pudding.
   d. Use aspirin to control the discomfort.

2. Because your patient is receiving the initial round of chemotherapy with 5-FU, the nurse must carefully assess the_____ system for the first 72 hours.
   a. respiratory
   b. cardiovascular
   c. renal
   d. gastrointestinal

3. Your patient is to begin receiving vincristine as treatment for lymphoblastic leukemia. Which of the following would be most important for you to emphasize in patient education?
   a. brush hair vigorously
   b. eat a bland, low-residue diet
   c. report immediately if heart rate seems slow
   d. report immediately if IV site is burning or looks red

4. The patient decscribed above receives several doses of vincristine. This time, while checking the IV site during drug infusion, the nurse notices some swelling at the insertion site. An appropriate nursing action would be to
   a. turn off the infusion.
   b. administer isotonic sodium thiosulfate.
   c. apply iced compresses.
   d. do all of the above.
   e. do none of the above.

5. To minimize the risk of a hypersensitivity reaction to etoposide, a podophyllotoxin, the nurse should
   a. administer the drug by IV push.
   b. administer the drug slowly over at least 30 to 60 minutes.
   c. make sure the patient has a call light handy.
   d. make sure the patient's family stays with the patient.

6. You are caring for a woman who is to receive paclitaxel for treatment of breast cancer because other treatment has not been effective. She is concerned that she will lose her hair and asks whether this is likely with paclitaxel treatment. The best response of the nurse would be:
   a. "No. Hair loss does not occur with paclitaxel."
   b. "Yes. Hair loss may occur and may be severe."
   c. "Yes. Hair loss may occur, but it is usually mild and unnoticeable."
   d. "You shouldn't worry about possible hair loss; other adverse effects are more important."

7. Your patient is to receive hydroxyurea and then radiation for treatment of acute blastic leukemia. To minimize adverse effects from the drug therapy, the nurse should
   a. monitor the CBC before and during therapy.
   b. begin drug therapy 1 week before radiation therapy.
   c. monitor for elevated BUN and creatinine levels.
   d. do all of the above.
   e. do none of the above.

8. Which of the following should the nurse do to prevent accidental personal exposure to hazardous drugs such as antineoplastics? *Mark all that apply.*
   a. Use caution when purging IV lines with an antineoplastic.
   b. Discard syringes that held antineoplastics in the trash can at the patient's bedside.
   c. Use a sterile gauze pad around the IV tubing when disconnecting it from the angiocath after drug administration.
   d. Wash your hands during drug preparation if you are eating while preparing the drug.
   e. Use goggles or a face shield if splashing of the drug is possible

CASE STUDY

Your patient has colorectal cancer. He is to receive 5-FU 450 mg/m^2 IV on days 1 through 5, and day 28 of drug therapy, then weekly thereafter. In addition, he is to receive levamisole 50 mg PO every 8 hours for days 1 through 3 of therapy, then every 2 weeks for 1 year.

1. Why is this patient receiving these two drug therapies? (Hint: Need help? See Chapter 37.)

2. Discuss the monitoring that should be done while the patient receives these drug therapies.

CRITICAL THINKING CHALLENGE

Your patient described above complains, "I'm having diarrhea. It is all black."

1. What is your assessment of these findings?

2. What actions should you take when your patient reports these findings to you?

CHAPTER 37

Drugs That Are Cell Cycle–Nonspecific

TOP TEN THINGS TO KNOW ABOUT DRUGS THAT ARE CELL CYCLE–NONSPECIFIC

1. Cell cycle–nonspecific drugs kill cells regardless of their phase in the cell cycle. This nonspecificity is why these drugs are considered more toxic than cell cycle–specific drugs. Like cell cycle–specific drugs, they should be avoided during pregnancy.

2. Cyclophosphamide is an alkylating agent that is derived from nitrogen mustard. When the liver metabolizes cyclophosphamide, it becomes a cytotoxic agent. The active metabolite has broad-spectrum antitumor effects. Cyclophosphamide is used in the treatment of hematologic cancers and solid tumors. It is also part of the regimen used in stem cell transplantation.

3. The dose-limiting adverse effect of cyclophosphamide is leukopenia. Long-term lower dose therapy can cause secondary cancers later in the patient's life; adolescent patients are at highest risk. High-dose therapy can cause hemorrhagic cystitis; to prevent this, give the uroprotectant drug mesna and hydrate the patient well before, during, and after therapy.

4. Carmustine, a nitrosourea drug, is used in the palliative therapy of several disorders. It works by alkylating DNA and RNA and thus blocking synthesis and repair. Adverse effects of carmustine include nausea and vomiting, delayed bone marrow suppression (thrombocytopenia and leukopenia 6 weeks after drug administration), and pulmonary toxicity (associated with prolonged therapy and higher cumulative doses). To minimize adverse effects, give antiemetics within 2 hours of treatment, monitor WBC and pulmonary function, and prevent infection.

5. Doxorubicin, an antitumor antibiotic, has wide clinical activity, particularly against hematologic cancers and solid tumors. Doxorubicin blocks the synthesis of RNA and DNA. Doxorubicin also binds to nucleic acids, causing destruction and prolonged tissue damage.

6. Adverse effects of doxorubicin are acute (nausea, vomiting, bone marrow suppression, mucositis, alopecia, and other cutaneous reactions), chronic (cardiotoxicity, the dose-limiting toxicity; cumulative dose influences cardiotoxicity; children and older adults are more susceptible), and local (extravasation injury and radiation recall). To minimize adverse effects, give cardioprotective drugs, such as dexrazoxane, with treatment and prevent extravasation (good IV technique, use large veins, monitor closely during infusion).

7. Tamoxifen, an antiestrogen, is used as first-line therapy to treat advanced breast cancer (that is estrogen-receptor positive) in both premenopausal and postmenopausal women. It is the only drug approved to prevent breast cancer in high-risk women. It competes with estrogen for binding sites in tissues and thus deprives estrogen-sensitive tumors of estrogen.

8. Most patients do not have adverse effects from short-term use of tamoxifen. The infrequently occurring adverse effects of tamoxifen are related to loss of estrogen's effects (hot flashes, vaginal bleeding or discharge, menstrual irregularities, fluid retention). Possible serious effects are liver abnormalities, which may be fatal, and endometrial cancer (with long-term use). Increased bone and tumor pain (disease flare) are signs of positive tumor response.

9. Combination chemotherapy uses two or more drugs against a tumor. Combination therapy maximizes cell kill, has a broader range of kill, increases duration of remission, and minimizes emergence of cancer cells resistant to chemotherapy. Dosage of each drug can be kept to a minimum, thus decreasing serious toxicities from each drug.

10. Targeted cancer therapies, the newest cancer drugs, block the growth and spread of cancer. Many of these therapies focus on proteins that are involved in the signaling process. By blocking the signals that tell cancer cells to grow and divide uncontrollably, the growth and division of cancer

cells are stopped. The advantages in comparison with current treatment are that these therapies are more effective, are less harmful to normal cells, and have fewer adverse effects. Most are under development, but the approved ones include "small-molecule" drugs, which block specific enzymes and growth factor receptors (GFRs) involved in cancer cell growth, and "apoptosis-inducing" drugs, which cause cancer cells to undergo apoptosis (cell death) by interfering with the proteins involved in the process. Monoclonal antibodies (see Chapter 34) can be considered to be targeted therapies because they interfere with the growth of cancer cells.

KEY TERMS

Fill in the Blank
Read each statement carefully and, using the chapter's key terms, write the correct answer in the space provided.

1. Drugs that mimic the actions of radiation therapy on cells are named _____.

2. The _____ and _____ are a diverse group of drugs that are beneficial in treating neoplasms that originate from tissues whose growth is hormonally mediated.

3. To limit the potential toxicities of chemotherapeutic drugs, _____ may be used.

4. Cytoxan, a type of drug, has a broad spectrum of _____ antitumor activity.

5. _____ are a subcategory of the alkylating drugs, which are highly lipid soluble.

6. *Streptomyces* bacteria broths are the etiology of most _____.

7. A positive tumor response to drug therapy may be indicated by a local _____.

8. Antineoplastic drugs that are not limited to a specific phase in the cell's life cycle are called _____.

9. _____ are microscopic spherical vesicles that encapsulate the drug molecules.

10. _____ occurs within 24 hours of receiving chemotherapy.

11. Vomiting 5 days after chemotherapy is referred to as _____.

12. The _____ is the number of cells that make up the tumor.

13. Drugs that have a high potential for causing severe nausea and vomiting are called _____.

CORE DRUG KNOWLEDGE: JUST THE FACTS

Multiple Choice
Circle the option that best answers the question or completes the statement.

1. Pharmacotherapeutics for cyclophosphamide (Cytoxan) include all of the following *except*
   a. uterine cancer.
   b. hematologic cancers.
   c. stem cell transplantation.
   d. pancreatic cancer.

2. In addition to hematopoietic abnormalities, adverse effects associated with high-dose cyclophosphamide (Cytoxan) therapy include
   a. sterile hemorrhagic cystitis and diabetes insipidus.
   b. nephrotoxicity and diabetes insipidus.
   c. ototoxicity and CNS sedation.
   d. syndrome of inappropriate antidiuretic hormone (SIADH) and hemorrhagic cystitis.

3. Patients receiving cyclophosphamide (Cytoxan) should be informed for the potential development of
   a. secondary malignancies.
   b. excessive hair growth.
   c. gray-colored skin.
   d. gout.

4. Patients receiving PO cyclophosphamide (Cytoxan) should be advised to
   a. limit fluids to 4 glasses per day.
   b. increase consumption of green leafy vegetables.
   c. increase fluid consumption to 10 to 12 glasses per day.
   d. decrease intake of sodium.

5. Cisplatin (Cisplatinum) is well known for its ability to cause
   a. hair loss.
   b. nausea and vomiting.
   c. hyperkalemia.
   d. sedation.

6. Pharmacotherapeutics for carmustine (BCNU) include
   a. uterine cancer.
   b. brain tumors.
   c. pancreatic cancer.
   d. breast cancer.

7. Adverse effects from carmustine (BCNU) affect the
   a. cardiac and respiratory systems.
   b. CNS and cardiac systems.
   c. hematopoietic and respiratory systems.
   d. hematopoietic system.

8. Patients receiving doxorubicin (Adriamycin) should be monitored frequently for
   a. CNS depression.
   b. respiratory depression.
   c. thrombophlebitis.
   d. extravasation.

9. The major limiting factor of doxorubicin (Adriamycin) therapy is
   a. hepatotoxicity.
   b. nephrotoxicity.
   c. neurotoxicity.
   d. cardiotoxicity.

10. First-line therapy for advanced breast cancer in postmenopausal women is
    a. bleomycin (Blenoxane).
    b. tamoxifen (Nolvadex).
    c. streptozocin (Zanosar).
    d. cisplatin (Platinol).

11. In the treatment of breast cancer, tamoxifen (Nolvadex) works by
    a. increasing estrogen reception at receptor sites.
    b. decreasing androgen reception at receptor sites.
    c. inhibiting DNA synthesis in tumor cells.
    d. depriving estrogen-sensitive tumors of estrogen.

12. Which of the following statements concerning adverse effects of tamoxifen (Nolvadex) therapy is correct?
    a. There are many adverse effects, and most are very significant.
    b. There are few adverse effects, but all are very significant.
    c. There are few adverse effects, and they are modest.
    d. There are many adverse effects, and most are life threatening.

13. Although each cell cycle–nonspecific drug has different dose-limiting factors, they all have a potential common adverse effect that requires frequent monitoring of
    a. CBC.
    b. liver enzymes.
    c. pulmonary function tests.
    d. renal function.

Matching
Match the following drugs with its appropriate Black Box warning. Match all that apply.

1. _____ cisplatin
2. _____ doxorubicin
3. _____ tamoxifen
4. _____ carmustine

a. Nausea and vomiting
b. Myelosuppression
c. Tissue necrosis with extravasation
d. Pulmonary toxicity
e. Thromboembolic events
f. Delayed bone marrow suppression
g. Cardiotoxicity
h. Ototoxicity

i. Secondary leukemia

j. Overwhelming infection

k. Anaphylaxis

l. Nephrotoxicity

m. Cancer

CORE PATIENT VARIABLES: PATIENTS, PLEASE

Multiple Choice

Circle the option that best answers the question or completes the statement.

1. Your 27-year-old patient is prescribed cyclophosphamide (Cytoxan). The patient states, "What type of reaction will I probably have to this drug?" Which of the following is the best response?

   a. "Your hair will probably fall out, almost right away."

   b. "You will probably experience nausea and vomiting."

   c. "This drug causes severe constipation."

   d. "Probably none."

2. Your patient is receiving cyclophosphamide (Cytoxan). The patient complains of dizziness, nasal stuffiness, and rhinorrhea. What is your best action?

   a. stop the infusion immediately

   b. give diphenhydramine (Benadryl) IVP

   c. slow the infusion rate

   d. a and b

3. Your patient is to receive cyclophosphamide (Cytoxan). To administer this drug safely, you should

   a. prehydrate the patient orally and intravenously with at least 1 to 2 L of normal saline solution with potassium and magnesium additives.

   b. keep the patient NPO until the solution is infused.

   c. prehydrate the patient with tap water.

   d. decrease fluid ingestion 24 hours before administration of cyclophosphamide.

4. Which of the following patients has an increased risk for adverse effects if given carmustine (BCNU) therapy? Patients with

   a. cardiovascular disorders.

   b. pulmonary disorders.

   c. integumentary disorders.

   d. CNS disorders.

5. Your patient is receiving carmustine (BCNU). The patient complains of an intense burning sensation at the IV site. What should you do?

   a. increase the rate of infusion and bring an ice compress

   b. increase the rate of infusion and bring a warm compress

   c. decrease the rate of infusion and bring a warm compress

   d. decrease the rate of infusion and bring an ice compress

6. Your patient had chemotherapy and radiation therapy 6 months ago. Today, he comes to the clinic with complaints of blisters, swelling, and skin loss at the site of the cancer. After reviewing the patient's chart, you note that the patient received doxorubicin (Adriamycin). With your knowledge of this drug, you suspect the patient is experiencing

   a. a delayed hypersensitivity.

   b. chemotherapy extravasation.

   c. radiation recall.

   d. a routine sunburn.

7. Your 66-year-old patient is receiving doxorubicin (Adriamycin) therapy. To minimize the potential for cardiotoxicity, the patient has been prescribed dexrazoxane (Zinecard). You should administer dexrazoxane

   a. 3 hours after completion of doxorubicin infusion.

   b. 24 hours before initiation of doxorubicin infusion.

   c. 30 minutes before initiation of doxorubicin infusion.

   d. 1 hour after completion of doxorubicin infusion.

8. Which of the following instructions should be given to your patient concerning doxorubicin (Adriamycin) therapy?

    a. "You may feel very sleepy after therapy."

    b. "This drug may turn your urine a reddish color."

    c. "Many patients have intractable hiccups after therapy."

    d. "Some patients may experience a floating sensation during therapy."

9. Your patient comes to the clinic for a follow-up visit after carmustine (BCNU) therapy 3 weeks ago. The patient states he feels "OK" but now feels better knowing that his CBC is not abnormal. Which of the following statements is most appropriate?

    a. "We need to continue to check your lab values because this drug can cause bone marrow suppression weeks after administration."

    b. "You can see your regular doctor in 6 months now."

    c. "You are one of the lucky ones, but it's best to get rechecked in a few months."

    d. "This drug doesn't usually affect the results of your blood count."

NURSING MANAGEMENT: EVERY GOOD NURSE SHOULD …

Multiple Choice
Circle the option that best answers the question or completes the statement.

1. You are caring for a patient who has small-cell lung cancer and is receiving cyclophosphamide, an alkylating agent, as treatment. To minimize adverse effects from the cyclophosphamide, you should

    a. administer diuretics to increase urinary output.

    b. prehydrate with 1 to 2 L of normal saline with potassium and magnesium.

    c. administer an aminoglycoside antibiotic.

    d. limit dietary potassium and magnesium.

2. Your 15-year-old female patient is to receive long-term cyclophosphamide therapy to treat her chronic leukemia. Which of the following should be included in her teaching? *Mark all that apply.*

    a. Amenorrhea may occur.

    b. Nausea, vomiting, and anorexia are possible.

    c. A secondary malignancy is possible later in life.

    d. Daily fluid intake of 1 to 2 L is necessary while taking the drug.

3. Your patient is an 8-year-old child who is receiving doxorubicin to treat leukemia. To minimize adverse effects, you should

    a. use a small, peripheral vein to administer doxorubicin.

    b. offer aspirin to relieve discomforts from drug administration.

    c. monitor for rales and dyspnea.

    d. monitor for reddish-colored urine.

4. Your patient has right breast cancer. She is receiving tamoxifen and reports bone pain and pain in her right breast. Your most appropriate action is to

    a. hold the next dose of tamoxifen.

    b. decrease the next dose of tamoxifen.

    c. administer the next dose of tamoxifen as ordered.

    d. contact the physician immediately.

5. Your patient is receiving carmustine, a nitrosourea, as treatment for a brain tumor. He returns in 6 weeks for a second treatment. Before administering the next dose, you should check the patient's

    a. weight.

    b. blood pressure.

    c. platelets.

    d. BUN.

6. You are to administer IV doxorubicin. Before starting the infusion, you should

    a. verify patency of the IV site.

    b. apply ice to the arm.

    c. apply a tourniquet above the IV insertion site.

    d. massage the vein.

CASE STUDY

You are caring for a patient who has received a diagnosis of ovarian cancer. She is to receive the following chemotherapy:

Doxorubicin 60 mg/m^2 IV every 21 days
Cyclophosphamide 300 mg/m^2 IV on day 1 every 4 weeks

1. What is the rationale for two different antineoplastic drugs being ordered?

2. Describe the adverse effects this patient is most likely to experience while taking these two drugs.

CRITICAL THINKING CHALLENGE

Your patient receives the first doses of doxorubicin and cyclophosphamide and is discharged. When she returns to restart the drug cycle, she has diagnostic tests done before the next doses of doxorubicin and cyclophosphamide. The findings include:

BUN	20
Creatinine	1.2
Platelets	101,000
WBC	4,200
SGOT	33
SGPT	33
ECG	normal sinus rhythm

1. What is your evaluation of the combined chemotherapy to this date?

2. Should you administer the next doses of cyclophosphamide and doxorubicin?

CHAPTER 38

Principles of Antimicrobial Therapy

TOP TEN THINGS TO KNOW ABOUT THE PRINCIPLES OF ANTIMICROBIAL THERAPY

1. Antimicrobial drugs are classified by their susceptible organism or by their mechanism of action.
2. Antimicrobials work in six ways. They inhibit bacterial cell wall synthesis, protein synthesis, nucleic acid synthesis, metabolic pathways, and viral enzymes. Lastly, they disrupt cell membrane permeability.
3. Selective toxicity is the ability of a drug to suppress or kill an infecting microbe without harming the patient's cells.
4. Microbes develop resistance to antimicrobial therapy because of the production of drug-inactivating enzymes, changes in receptor structure, changes in drug permeation and transport, development of alternative metabolic pathways, emergence of drug-resistant microbes, and antimicrobial usage that facilitates the development of resistance.
5. Resistance is more likely to occur from the use of broad-spectrum drugs. Resistance is facilitated if the drug dose is too low, the time between doses is too long, therapy stops too soon, or the drug is used prophylactically.
6. Four important antibiotic-resistant microbes are methicillin-resistant *Staphylococcus aureus* (MRSA), penicillin-resistant *Streptococcus pneumoniae*, vancomycin-resistant enterococci (VRE), and multiple drug–resistant *Mycobacterium tuberculosis*.
7. Drug selection to treat an infection is based on identification of the pathogen, drug susceptibility, drug spectrum, drug dose, duration of therapy, site of infection, and patient assessment.
8. Gram staining and culturing determine the organism, whereas a sensitivity test determines which antimicrobials are effective in killing the organism. Culture and sensitivity tests should be done before administration of any antimicrobial drug.
9. Empiric therapy or broad-spectrum drugs may be used before an organism has been identified.

Combination drug therapy is often used initially for severe infections or for mixed infections. There are advantages and disadvantages to combination therapy.
10. The patient's response to drug therapy (positive and negative) should be assessed carefully. For drug therapy that may cause serious adverse effects, monitor serum drug levels, peak and trough levels, and other relevant laboratory values. Individualize monitoring based on the patient, the drug therapy, and the infecting microbe.

KEY TERMS

True or False
Mark each of the following statements true or false. If the statement is false, replace the underlined word(s) with the word(s) that will make the statement true.

1. _____ Classifications of <u>antimicrobial drugs</u> include antibacterial drugs, antiviral drugs, antifungal drugs, antiprotozoal drugs, and anthelminthic drugs.

2. _____ Antibacterial drugs that actually kill bacteria are called <u>bacteriostatic</u>.

3. _____ Antibiotics that exhibit a <u>bacteriocidal</u> effect inhibit bacterial growth despite undetectable drug levels. *Postantibiotic*

4. _____ An infection that occurs in the hospital environment is called <u>nosocomial</u>.

5. _____ The ability to suppress or kill an infecting microbe without injury to the host is known as <u>spontaneous mutation</u>. *Selective mutation*

6. _____ A <u>sensitivity</u> indicates whether the pathogen is gram positive or gram negative. *Gram staining*

7. _____ The range of microbes against which a drug is active is its <u>culture</u>. *Spectrum*

8. _F_ Organisms that are capable of producing disease are called <u>microbes</u>.

9. _F_ Prescribing antibiotic treatment before the pathogen has been definitively identified is called <u>rational therapy</u>.

10. _T_ Another term for antimicrobials is <u>anti-infective</u>.

11. _F_ A <u>pathogen</u> is a unicellular or small multicellular organism. *Microbe*

12. _F_ The <u>sensitivity</u> determines the identity of the microbe, and the culture determines which antimicrobial agent will be therapeutic.

13. _T_ A <u>superinfection</u> is one that occurs during the course of treatment for a primary infection.

CORE DRUG KNOWLEDGE: JUST THE FACTS

Essay

1. How are antimicrobials classified?

   According to susceptibility + mechanism of the org.

2. List the classifications of antimicrobial drugs by susceptible organism.

   Antibiotic
   Antivirus
   Antiprotozoa
   Antifungi

3. List the mechanism of action of the major antimicrobial classifications.

   destroy cell membrane
   inhibit protein synthesis
   destroy nucleus

4. List the most common antibiotic-resistant microbes in the United States.

   Streptococci methicillin Resistant
   Penicillin, staphylococci
   Vancomycin Resist. en
   Multiple drug resistant tuberculosis

5. List general considerations for selecting antimicrobial therapy.

   narrow spectrum
   dose / duration
   Identify microbe, site of
   infection, Pt assessment

6. List the Centers for Disease Control and Prevention's objectives to decrease antimicrobial resistance that the nurse has a primary responsibility to perform.

   Use aseptic technique in all procedure

7. List the factors that contribute to the development of nosocomial infections.

   A prevalent of host
   pathogen
   medium of transmission

CORE PATIENT VARIABLES: PATIENTS, PLEASE

Essay

1. What important health status assessments should be made before antimicrobial therapy?

   check immune
   Allergy,
   hypersensitivity

2. Why are infants and the elderly more vulnerable to antimicrobial toxicity?

   immunity immature infant
   low immunity for elderly
   dysfunction of liver / kidney

3. Identify key elements of patient education for patients receiving antimicrobial therapy.

   complete dose, take p regular
   dose, interval

4. Identify the most important nursing action to limit the occurrence of nosocomial infections.

   wash hand

5. What is the purpose of obtaining peak and trough levels of certain antibiotics? When should they be obtained?

   peak - 30 - 1hr p last dose
   trough 30 - 1hr bp next dose

CHAPTER 39

Antibiotics Affecting the Bacterial Cell Wall

TOP TEN THINGS TO KNOW ABOUT ANTIBIOTICS AFFECTING THE BACTERIAL CELL WALL

1. Drugs that affect the bacterial cell wall penetrate the cell wall and bind to molecular targets on the cytoplasmic membrane in the cell. They then disrupt the strength of the cell wall. This permits the high oncotic pressure inside the cell to draw fluid into the cell. Fluid is drawn in until the cell bursts. The patient's immune system cleans up the debris and fights any remaining infection.

2. Beta-lactam antibiotics are so called because their chemical structure contains a beta-lactam ring, which is required for antibacterial action. Penicillins, cephalosporins, monobactams, carbapenems, and beta-lactamase inhibitors are all considered beta-lactam antibiotics.

3. Penicillins were the first antibiotics used clinically. They are classified as narrow spectrum, broad spectrum, or extended spectrum; they may also be penicillinase resistant. Penicillin G aqueous, the prototype penicillin, is a narrow-spectrum, bactericidal drug that is effective against mostly gram-positive organisms. It is most commonly given intravenously (IV). The most serious adverse effect is allergic reactions. Most common adverse effects are gastrointestinal (GI). For optimum effectiveness, administer doses around the clock. Assess patients carefully, especially during the first dose, for allergic reactions.

4. Patients allergic to one penicillin should be considered allergic to all penicillins. Carbapenems also have a beta-lactam ring structure and may create a cross-sensitivity in patients allergic to a penicillin. Monobactam antibiotics have a significantly different chemical structure from other beta-lactams and are safe to give to penicillin-allergic patients.

5. Resistance to beta-lactams may occur because of the bacteria's ability to produce beta-lactamase.

Clavulanic acid, tazobactam, and sulbactam are beta-lactamase inhibitors that are combined with penicillins to eradicate the microbe despite its ability to produce beta-lactamase.

6. Imipenem, meropenem, and ertapenem are the carbapenems approved for use in the United States. They are very broad-spectrum antibiotics with activity against gram-positive cocci, gram-negative cocci, and bacilli, and they are the most effective beta-lactam antibiotics for use against anaerobes.

7. Cephalosporins are similar to penicillins in structure and activity. Penicillin-allergic patients have an increased risk of being allergic to cephalosporins. Four generations of cephalosporins have been introduced, each with a different spectrum of activity. Cephalosporins are the most commonly prescribed antibiotics; this is leading to cephalosporin-resistant bacteria.

8. Cefazolin, the prototype cephalosporin, is a first generation drug. Most frequent adverse effects are hypersensitivity and GI; nephrotoxicity is possible and is more likely if the patient is also receiving aminoglycoside antibiotics. Acute alcohol intolerance (disulfiram-like reaction) may occur as an interaction of cefazolin and alcohol.

9. Vancomycin, a tricyclic glycopeptide antibiotic, is the only drug in its class. In addition to altering the bacterial cell wall, it inhibits the synthesis of RNA. Because of serious toxicity, vancomycin is used only in serious infections when other antibiotics have failed. Vancomycin-resistant enterococci (VRE) is becoming a common problem.

10. Vancomycin has adverse effects of nephrotoxicity, ototoxicity, and significant histamine release (resulting in anaphylactoid reactions and "red man" or "red neck" syndrome). Administer drug slowly IV (at least over 60 minutes), and avoid extravasation. Monitor peak and trough levels and hepatic and renal function. Assess for change in balance and hearing loss.

KEY TERMS

Matching
Match the key term with its definition.

1. ___A___ bacterial cell envelope
2. ___d___ beta-lactam
3. ___f___ beta-lactamases
4. ___e___ cephalosporinases
5. ___B___ penicillinases
6. ___C___ penicillin-binding proteins

a. Composed of a thick cell wall and cytoplasmic membrane
b. Enzymes that inactivate penicillin
c. Located inside the bacterial cell wall
d. Active chemical structure of many antibiotics
e. Enzymes that inactivate cephalosporins
f. Enzymes that disrupt the beta-lactam ring

CORE DRUG KNOWLEDGE: JUST THE FACTS

Multiple Choice
Circle the option that best answers the question or completes the statement.

1. Which of the following classes of antibiotics is *most* likely to induce an allergic reaction?
   a. aminoglycosides
   b. macrolides
   c. penicillins
   d. cephalosporins

2. Generally speaking, penicillin G is *ineffective* in the management of
   a. most gram-negative bacteria infections.
   b. gram-positive anaerobic infections.
   c. gram-positive spirochete infections.
   d. endocarditis prophylaxis.

3. Which of the following routes is *inappropriate* for administration of penicillin?
   a. oral
   b. subcutaneous
   c. intramuscular
   d. intravenous

4. Before the administration of penicillin, it is important to
   a. check the CBC results.
   b. determine if any previous reactions to antibiotics have occurred.
   c. ask the patient to void.
   d. check the patient's pregnancy status.

5. Penicillin has a cross sensitivity to which of the following drug classes?
   a. aminoglycosides
   b. cephalosporins
   c. erythromycins
   d. tetracyclines

6. In contrast to narrow-spectrum penicillins, aminopenicillins such as amoxicillin (Amoxil) have increased effectiveness against
   a. gram-negative bacteria infections.
   b. gram-positive anaerobic infections.
   c. gram-positive spirochete infections.
   d. endocarditis prophylaxis.

7. Extended-spectrum penicillins are extremely effective against
   a. gonorrhea.
   b. *Streptococcus.*
   c. *Pseudomonas.*
   d. *Staphylococcus.*

8. Beta-lactamase inhibitors are given in conjunction with penicillin to
   a. change the protein binding sites.
   b. increase the spectrum of activity.
   c. target the enzyme that may decrease the efficacy of penicillin.
   d. decrease the potential for adverse effects.

9. A benefit of aztreonam (Azactam) therapy is that it
   a. has increased spectrum of activity.
   b. may be used in penicillin-allergic patients.
   c. has decreased potential for adverse effects.
   d. has decreased potential for drug–drug interactions.

10. What is the difference between imipenem (Primaxin) and meropenem (Merrem)?

    a. Meropenem has a narrow spectrum of activity, and imipenem does not.

    b. Imipenem has a narrow spectrum of activity, and meropenem does not.

    c. Meropenem is easily inactivated and must be administered with cilastatin.

    d. Imipenem is easily inactivated and must be administered with cilastatin.

11. What is the major difference between the different "generations" of cephalosporin agents?

    a. pharmacodynamics

    b. spectrum of activity

    c. emergence of drug resistance

    d. ability to induce allergic responses

12. Generally speaking, cephalosporin antibiotics should be taken for

    a. 7 to 10 days.

    b. 2 to 3 days.

    c. 1 to 5 days.

    d. 10 to 21 days.

13. Hypersensitivity to cephalosporins frequently presents with

    a. shortness of breath.

    b. hives.

    c. nausea and vomiting.

    d. maculopapular rash.

14. Vancomycin is used in the management of

    a. sexually transmitted diseases.

    b. urinary tract infection.

    c. serious systemic bacterial infections.

    d. cellulitis.

15. The most serious adverse effects to vancomycin are

    a. sinus tachycardia and hypotension.

    b. ototoxicity and nephrotoxicity.

    c. hepatotoxicity and neurotoxicity.

    d. histamine release and phlebitis.

CORE PATIENT VARIABLES: PATIENTS, PLEASE

Multiple Choice

Circle the option that best answers the question or completes the statement.

1. Your patient is prescribed penicillin V for a dental infection. Which of the following instructions would you give?

    a. "Take the medication with food for best results."

    b. "Although it is ordered 4 times a day, you can double the dose and take it twice a day."

    c. "You can take it every other day if you experience GI distress."

    d. "Take the medication 1 hour before or 2 hours after a meal.

2. Your 86-year-old patient has pneumonia and is prescribed penicillin. She has a history of renal insufficiency. Which of the following lab tests should be done before initiating therapy?

    a. pulmonary function tests

    b. BUN and creatinine

    c. ALT and AST

    d. urinalysis

3. Your patient is hospitalized with bacteremia. He is prescribed IV penicillin G and gentamicin. How would you administer these drugs?

    a. Wait at least 2 hours between administration of these drugs.

    b. Wait 30 minutes between administration of these drugs.

    c. Administer each drug on an alternate day.

    d. Administer the first drug, flush the tubing, then administer the second drug.

4. Your patient comes to the clinic and receives a diagnosis of infection. When asked about allergies, the patient stated, "I have an allergy to penicillin, but I can take ampicillin." With your knowledge about these drugs, you know that

    a. this is a possibility because they are two different types of penicillins.

    b. the patient should not take any form of drug with "cillin" in its name if he has an allergy to penicillin.

    c. as long as they are not taken together, it is alright for your patient to take either drug.

    d. you should substitute another type of antibiotic.

5. Your patient has just received an injection of IM procaine penicillin. Within 30 seconds, the patient becomes confused and agitated and runs from the exam room. You suspect

   a. the patient has been taking some type of illicit drugs.

   b. an allergy to penicillin.

   c. a toxic response of penicillin.

   d. a procaine reaction.

6. Your patient has an order for IV cefazolin (Kefzol). As you take the medication out of the refrigerator, you note that the solution was reconstituted yesterday. You should

   a. allow the solution to warm for 15 minutes, then administer.

   b. give the infusion now.

   c. call the pharmacy and have a replacement sent.

   d. warm the solution in the microwave, then administer.

7. Your patient has been receiving IV cefazolin for the past 24 hours, and the next dose is now due. You note that the culture and sensitivity test results indicate the infection is resistant to cephalosporins. You should

   a. hang the cefazolin, and write a note in the progress notes.

   b. hang the cefazolin.

   c. hold the cefazolin, contact the health care provider, and get an order for a new antibiotic.

   d. hold the cefazolin and tell the next shift to discuss the test results with the physician when he or she makes rounds in the evening.

8. Your patient is receiving IV vancomycin. To minimize adverse effects, the health care provider has ordered peak-and-trough blood levels. When is the optimal time for you to obtain the peak blood level?

   a. 30 minutes before the next infusion

   b. 20 minutes after the onset of the infusion

   c. 1 hour before the next infusion

   d. 1 hour after the completion of the infusion

9. Your patient is scheduled to receive IV vancomycin. To safely administer this medication, you should infuse it

   a. over 20 minutes.

   b. over 60 minutes.

   c. over 2 to 3 hours.

   d. within 10 minutes.

10. Your patient with a GI infection is prescribed vancomycin by mouth. The patient states, "My friend had this drug, but she got it in her veins. Isn't that a better way to get it?" What is your response?

   a. "Since your problem is in your GI system, giving the drug this way will have a localized action on the infection."

   b. "Why don't you ask the doctor that question."

   c. "I'm sure your friend received a different drug."

   d. "I have no idea."

NURSING MANAGEMENT: EVERY GOOD NURSE SHOULD …

Multiple Choice

Circle the option that best answers the question or completes the statement.

1. To maximize the therapeutic effect of penicillin G, you should administer

   a. the drug with milk.

   b. the doses only during normal waking hours.

   c. IV forms directly from the refrigerator.

   d. the drug for at least 2 days after the patient feels better.

2. Your patient is to be discharged on cefazolin, a cephalosporin. The nurse should teach the patient to avoid which of the following while taking this drug?

   a. wine

   b. potassium chloride elixirs (such as Kay Ciel)

   c. cough medicine

   d. all of the above

   e. none of the above

3. Your patient is receiving vancomycin as treatment for endocarditis. To minimize adverse effects from the drug therapy, the nurse should administer the drug by

   a. IV push.

   b. slow IV infusion.

   c. subcutaneous injection.

   d. the oral route.

4. You are to administer the first IV dose of penicillin G to treat a patient's pneumonia. To minimize adverse effects, you should
   a. determine if a sputum culture and sensitivity has been obtained.
   b. ask her if she has any drug allergies.
   c. monitor her closely during drug administration.
   d. do all of the above.
   e. do none of the above.

5. You are to administer procaine penicillin to a patient in the outpatient department who has syphilis. To maximize therapeutic effects and minimize adverse effects, you should
   a. administer the drug into the deltoid muscle.
   b. keep the drug in the refrigerator until the time of administration.
   c. locate anatomic landmarks to determine the injection site.
   d. do all of the above.
   e. do none of the above.

6. Your patient has a mixed infection and is receiving cefazolin, a cephalosporin, and gentamicin, an aminoglycoside antibiotic. To minimize adverse effects, the nurse should most closely monitor which lab value?
   a. hematocrit
   b. aPTT
   c. BUN
   d. cefazolin blood levels

7. You are caring for an 80-year-old patient who has a respiratory infection caused by vancomycin-resistant enterococci (VRE). The patient also has chronic renal failure. The patient has been prescribed daptomycin to treat the infection. You would expect to administer to this patient
   a. the standard adult dose.
   b. more than the standard adult dose.
   c. less than the standard adult dose. *It is used to treat VRE*
   d. a different drug because daptomycin is not effective against VRE.

CASE STUDY

One of your patients is 70 years old and receiving vancomycin 1 g IV every 6 hours for osteomyelitis. This morning, while going to the bathroom, the patient fell but was not injured. As you help the patient back to bed, she laughs a little and says to you, "I don't know what came over me. I'm acting like I'm tipsy." Later, you hear the patient say to the housekeeper, "There must be crickets in this room. I keep hearing little noises." The housekeeper checks the room carefully and assures the patient that there are no crickets in the room.

1. What assessment do you make from these incidents?

2. Is there any additional data you would like to help confirm your assessment?

CRITICAL THINKING CHALLENGE

After your assessment of the patient described above, you obtain an order and have a peak-and-trough level drawn around the next scheduled dose of vancomycin. The trough is drawn immediately before the dose, and the peak is drawn 1 hour after the infusion is complete. You also have the patient's BUN and creatinine levels checked. The results are:

Vancomycin	Patient	Normal	Toxic
Trough	22 µg/mL	5.0–10.0 µg/mL	>20 µg/mL
Peak	86 µg/mL	30–40 µg/mL	>80–100 µg/mL
BUN	20 mg/dL	8–18 mg/dL	
Creatinine	1.2 mg/dL	0.6–1.2 mg/dL	

1. What is your assessment of these lab findings?

2. What action would you take based on your assessment?

CHAPTER 40

Antibiotics Affecting Protein Synthesis

TOP TEN THINGS TO KNOW ABOUT ANTIBIOTICS AFFECTING PROTEIN SYNTHESIS

1. Drugs that affect protein synthesis in the bacteria may be either bactericidal or bacteriostatic. These drugs are usually reserved for serious infections.

2. Gentamicin, an aminoglycoside, is reserved for serious infections because of the severe adverse effects of nephrotoxicity, ototoxicity, and neurotoxicity. Monitor drug peak and trough levels to dose appropriately and prevent adverse effects. Neonates (younger than 1 month) and adults older than 65 years have an increased risk for ototoxicity and nephrotoxicity. Many bacteria can resist all aminoglycosides from entering their cells; to overcome this, gentamicin often is given with other antibiotics (such as penicillin) to increase their effectiveness or alter the cell wall, allowing the gentamicin to enter.

3. Clindamycin, a lincosamide, is used to treat serious to life-threatening infections. It works by entering the bacterial cell, binding to bacterial ribosomes, suppressing protein synthesis, and causing cell death. Most common adverse effects are gastrointestinal (GI); serious adverse effects are pseudomembranous colitis and blood abnormalities.

4. Erythromycin, a macrolide, inhibits RNA-dependent protein synthesis at the chain elongation step. This either prevents the cell from dividing or causes cell death. It is the drug of choice for penicillin-allergic patients. Absorption is diminished by food, dairy products, and antacids. The drug frequently causes GI distress even if given intravenously (IV). IV infusions are very irritating to the veins, so administer very slowly.

5. Telithromycin (Ketek) is the first drug in a new class of antibiotics called ketolides. It is approved for community-acquired pneumonia. Telithromycin is contraindicated for patients with myasthenia gravis, patients with a history of hepatitis or other hepatic dysfunction,

patients receiving drugs that affect the QT interval, and patients with disorders that are considered prodysrhythmic such as uncorrected hypokalemia or hypomagnesia, and clinically important bradycardia. Telithromycin may cause hepatic dysfunction including acute hepatic failure, severe liver injury, fulminant hepatitis, and hepatic necrosis.

6. Linezolid, an oxazolidinone, was developed to treat methicillin-resistant *Staphylococcus aureus* (MRSA) infections; it is also used to treat vancomycin-resistant enterococci (VRE) infections. Approval may be required from the infectious disease department or committee before the drug is administered to a patient. Linezolid blocks the early stages of protein synthesis, unlike other antibiotics; this may prevent the development of resistance and cross resistance. Linezolid also is a monoamine oxidase (MAO) inhibitor. Drug–food interactions can be serious; avoid foods with tyramine, caffeine, and alcohol. Most common adverse effects are GI.

7. Quinupristin/dalfopristin are the only streptogramins and are marketed as a combination drug. Quinupristin/dalfopristin is used to treat life-threatening VRE infections ("superbugs"). Approval may be required from the infectious disease department or committee before the drug is administered to a patient. Quinupristin/dalfopristin irreversibly blocks ribosome functioning, thus inhibiting protein synthesis. Quinupristin/dalfopristin is a potent inhibitor of P-450, so many drug interactions are possible. Administer by IV infusion, preferably through a central line. Flush lines with 5% dextrose and water only.

8. Tetracycline, one of the tetracyclines, retards bacterial growth by inhibiting protein synthesis and preventing cell division and replication. It is used to treat a variety of serious infections (e.g., Rocky Mountain spotted fever) when penicillin cannot be used, and to treat acne vulgaris, and chlamydia. Overuse is leading to resistance.

Dairy products and antacids interfere with the absorption of tetracycline. Adverse effects of tetracycline include GI (most common), photosensitivity (advise patients to stay out of direct sunlight), and mottling and discoloration of developing teeth (avoid use during pregnancy and in children younger than 8 years).

9. Tigecycline (Tygacil), the first drug in a new class of drugs called glycylcycline antibiotics, is indicated for the management of complicated skin and skin structure infections and complicated intra-abdominal infections. Tigecycline is structurally similar to tetracyclines, so it has many of the same contraindications and adverse effects.

10. Chloramphenicol has a broad range of activity but is reserved for serious infections where other antibiotics have been ineffective. Chloramphenicol inhibits protein synthesis in both bacterial and human cells. Life-threatening adverse effects include "gray baby" syndrome (newborns have progressive blue-gray skin and vasomotor collapse), blood dyscrasias, and reversible or nonreversible bone marrow depression (dose related or nondose related). Serious adverse effects are optic neuritis (blindness) and peripheral neuritis. Monitor drug levels.

KEY TERMS

Matching
Match the key term with its definition.

1. ___F___ azotemia
2. ___D___ cylindruria
3. ___H___ hyposthenuria
4. ___B___ nephrotoxicity
5. ___I___ ototoxicity
6. ___C___ peak and trough
7. ___J___ proteinuria
8. ___A___ pyuria
9. ___E___ xeroderma
10. ___G___ xerophthalmia

a. Pus in the urine
b. Adverse effect affecting the kidneys
c. Determines if drug levels remain therapeutic
d. Casts in the urine
e. Dryness of the skin

f. Excessive urea levels in the blood
g. Dryness of the conjunctiva
h. Loss of the ability to concentrate urine
i. Adverse effect affecting hearing
j. Protein in the urine

CORE DRUG KNOWLEDGE: JUST THE FACTS

Multiple Choice
Circle the option that best answers the question or completes the statement.

1. Patients with aminoglycoside therapy should be monitored for
   a. cardiotoxicity and nephrotoxicity.
   b. ototoxicity and nephrotoxicity.
   c. peripheral neuropathy and cardiotoxicity.
   d. hepatotoxicity and ototoxicity.

2. What is the correct time to obtain a trough level of gentamicin?
   a. 30 minutes after IM administration
   b. 60 minutes after IV administration
   c. 2 hours before the next dose
   d. 30 minutes before the next dose

3. Which of the following statements concerning drug–drug interactions with gentamicin is correct? There are
   a. many interactions, and most are very significant.
   b. many interactions, and most are insignificant.
   c. very few interactions, and most are significant.
   d. very few interactions, and most are insignificant.

4. The appropriate route of administration for neomycin is
   a. oral.
   b. subcutaneous.
   c. intramuscular.
   d. intravenous.

   Its too toxic to be administered parenteral
   not used for ampicic

5. Clindamycin is reserved for the management of
   a. severe systemic gram-positive bacteria.
   b. severe systemic gram-negative bacteria.
   c. infections by bacteria with known sensitivity.
   d. anaerobes only.

6. Although clindamycin is reserved for serious infections, topical clindamycin is useful in the treatment of
   a. hives.
   b. Stevens-Johnson syndrome.
   c. acne vulgaris.
   d. pruritus.

7. Clindamycin is associated with the development of
   a. hearing loss.
   b. pseudomembranous colitis.
   c. azotemia.
   d. migraine headaches.

8. The antibiotic class of choice for penicillin-allergic patients is
   a. cephalosporins.
   b. macrolides.
   c. fluoroquinolones.
   d. aminoglycosides.

9. The most common adverse effects of erythromycin affect the _____ system.
   a. central nervous
   b. respiratory
   c. hematopoietic
   d. GI

10. A benefit of clarithromycin therapy is
    a. twice-a-day dosing.
    b. that it is less expensive than erythromycin.
    c. alternate-day dosing.
    d. all of the above.

11. Linezolid (Zyvox) is indicated for use in the management of
    a. pseudomembranous colitis.
    b. bacterial meningitis.
    c. methicillin-resistant *Staphylococcus aureus*.
    d. all of the above.

12. The pharmacokinetics of linezolid (Zyvox) is unusual in that
    a. the oral formulation has a duration twice as long as the IV formulation.
    b. the oral formulation has 100% bioavailability.
    c. the IV formulation has 98% bioavailability.
    d. the IV onset is longer than the PO onset.

13. The most common adverse effects associated with the use of linezolid (Zyvox) include
    a. pseudomembranous colitis.
    b. rebound hypertension.
    c. diarrhea, headache, nausea, and vomiting.
    d. constipation.

14. Quinupristin/dalfopristin (Synercid) is indicated for the management of
    a. brain abscesses.
    b. pseudomembranous colitis.
    c. trichomoniasis.
    d. vancomycin-resistant enterococci.

15. Potential serious adverse effects to quinupristin/dalfopristin (Synercid) include all of the following *except*
    a. pseudomembranous colitis.
    b. superinfection.
    c. nephrotoxicity.
    d. hepatotoxicity.

16. During quinupristin/dalfopristin (Synercid) therapy, the nurse should arrange for which of the following lab tests?
    a. hepatic function and bilirubin
    b. complete blood count (CBC) and renal function
    c. hepatic and renal function
    d. hepatic function and CBC

17. To maximize the absorption of tetracycline, the patient should avoid concurrent administration of
    a. antacids.
    b. fluids.
    c. corticosteroids.
    d. all of the above.

18. Chloramphenicol is the drug of choice in the treatment of
    a. methicillin-resistant *Staphylococcus aureus*.
    b. serious systemic fungal infections.
    c. brain abscesses.
    d. urinary tract infections.

19. A serious adverse effect associated with chloramphenicol therapy in newborn infants is
    a. gray baby syndrome.
    b. red neck syndrome.
    c. pseudomembranous colitis.
    d. hypotension.

20. In an adult, a common serious adverse effect associated with chloramphenicol therapy is
    a. hepatic insufficiency.
    b. diverticulitis.
    c. central nervous system (CNS) depression.
    d. aplastic anemia.

CORE PATIENT VARIABLES: PATIENTS, PLEASE

Multiple Choice
Circle the option that best answers the question or completes the statement.

1. Your patient is receiving IV gentamicin (Garamycin) therapy. After the blood technician draws a specimen, the patient asks, "Why are they taking so much blood?" Which of the following is the best response?
    a. "They want to be sure that this is the right drug for you."
    b. "It is important to keep gentamicin levels within a certain range to avoid adverse effects."
    c. "The lab frequently makes mistakes and has to redraw the specimen."
    d. "They are really only taking a little bit each time."

2. Your patient has been receiving IV gentamicin (Garamycin) for the past 2 days. The patient is scheduled for surgery today. To ensure the patient's safety, you should
    a. be sure to tape a note to the front of the chart documenting the administration of gentamicin.
    b. refrain from giving any benzodiazepine as a preoperative medication.
    c. refrain from giving any anticholinergic before surgery.
    d. ask the anesthesiologist for an increased dose of premedication.

3. Your patient is to start PO clindamycin. To maximize the therapeutic effects of the drug, you should administer the first dose
    a. on an empty stomach.
    b. with a high-fat meal.
    c. with small, frequent meals.
    d. with grapefruit juice.

4. Your patient is using clindamycin lotion on her skin. The patient reports that her skin is extremely dry. You would suggest
    a. hydration.
    b. moisturizing cream.
    c. hydration and moisturizing cream.
    d. soaking in a bathtub.

5. Your patient is hospitalized with a serious infection and is receiving IV clindamycin. This patient should be monitored for which of the following symptoms?
    a. rash
    b. facial rigidity
    c. respiratory depression
    d. blood-tinged diarrhea

6. Your 55-year-old patient has had type 1 diabetes since the age of 12 years and experiences diabetic gastroparesis. Which of the following drugs may be helpful in this disorder?
    a. cefixime
    b. neomycin
    c. erythromycin
    d. lincomycin

7. Your patient has asthma and takes theophylline. The patient has an acute exacerbation of bronchitis and is prescribed erythromycin. This patient should be monitored for
    a. treatment failure of erythromycin.
    b. treatment failure of theophylline.
    c. toxicity of erythromycin.
    d. all of the above.

8. Your patient has an order for IV erythromycin. To safely administer this medication, you should

   a. dilute with sterile water and administer refrigerated solutions within 8 hours.

   b. dilute with normal saline and administer nonrefrigerated solutions within 24 hours.

   c. dilute with sterile water and administer refrigerated solutions within 24 hours.

   d. dilute with normal saline and administer nonrefrigerated solutions within 8 hours.

9. During linezolid (Zyvox) therapy, the nurse should assist the patient to choose a diet that limits the intake of

   a. potassium.

   b. sugar.

   c. salt.

   d. tyramine.

10. Your patient is receiving linezolid (Zyvox) therapy. Despite the attempts by the staff to educate the patient regarding needed dietary restrictions, the patient insists on having food brought in by the family. You should monitor this patient's

    a. weight.

    b. lung sounds.

    c. blood pressure.

    d. intake and output.

11. Your patient is scheduled to receive IV quinupristin/dalfopristin (Synercid). To safely administer this medication, you should flush the line with

    a. D₅W.

    b. saline.

    c. heparin.

    d. saline or heparin.

12. The optimal infusion time for IV quinupristin/dalfopristin (Synercid) is

    a. 20 minutes.

    b. 1 hour.   Hundates vein

    c. 10 minutes.

    d. 1 minute.

13. Your female patient has received a diagnosis of acne vulgaris and is prescribed tetracycline. What assessment should be done before initiating therapy?

    a. pregnancy status

    b. blood pressure

    c. skin turgor

    d. temperature

14. Your 16-year-old pregnant patient comes to the prenatal clinic crying and states her boyfriend has chlamydia. His doctor gave him a prescription for doxycycline for both himself and the patient. Which of the following statements would be most appropriate?

    a. "Take the medication. Let's gets this resolved before it causes you any discomfort."

    b. "You can take the medication, but be sure you take your prenatal vitamins at least 2 hours after the doxycycline."

    c. "It's best you do not take this medication because it may cause problems with the baby's teeth and bones."

    d. "I would advise against it, but you can do what you wish."

15. Your patient has recently completed a 10-day course of chemotherapy. The patient now has bacterial meningitis and is prescribed chloramphenicol. This patient should be closely monitored for

    a. bone marrow suppression.

    b. renal toxicity.

    c. ototoxicity.

    d. superinfection.

16. Which of these assessment findings, if identified in a patient who has been prescribed telithromycin, should the nurse report to the prescriber prior to administration of the drug? Current use of

    a. antihistamines

    b. antiarrhythmic drugs

    c. beta-blocking agents

    d. aminoglycoside antibiotics

NURSING MANAGEMENT: EVERY GOOD NURSE SHOULD …

Multiple Choice
Circle the option that best answers the question or completes the statement.

1. Your 65-year-old patient is receiving gentamicin, an aminoglycoside, for peritonitis. To minimize adverse effects, what should you do? *Mark all that apply.*

   a. monitor intake and output closely

   b. assess for tinnitus

   c. assess for loss of balance

   d. monitor BUN and creatinine levels

2. You are administering IV erythromycin, a macrolide, to your patient to treat bacterial endocarditis. The patient reports burning during the infusion. Your most appropriate initial action is to

   a. document that the patient is allergic to erythromycin.

   b. apply a warm compress to the vein.

   c. slow the rate of the infusion.

   d. remove the IV from the patient.

3. Your patient is receiving clindamycin for treatment of pelvic inflammatory disease. She begins to have diarrhea, with loose stools five or six times a day. You should

   a. obtain an order for an antidiarrheal.

   b. obtain an order for laboratory examination of the stool specimen.

   c. obtain an order for a high-roughage diet.

   d. do all of the above.

   e. do none of the above.

4. You are caring for a patient who is to be discharged on a regimen of tetracycline as treatment for a chlamydia infection. She has a 2-year-old child at home. Patient education should emphasize which of the following? *Mark all that apply.*

   a. Take the drug with milk.

   b. Stop taking the drug when symptoms are gone.

   c. Exposure to sunlight will increase effectiveness of this drug.

   d. Keep this drug secured and out of reach of children.

5. Your patient is receiving chloramphenicol for meningitis. For which of the following adverse effects should you withhold administration of the drug and contact the physician?

   a. excessive bruising

   b. elevation of hepatic enzymes

   c. fatigue

   d. all of the above

   e. none of the above

6. You are to administer a dose of quinupristin/dalfopristin to a patient who has a severe VRE infection. The patient is NPO and has a peripherally inserted central catheter (PICC) line in the left arm. This patient also receives diazepam for seizures. What are the appropriate nursing actions? *Mark all that apply.*

   a. administer the quinupristin/dalfopristin orally

   b. flush the PICC line before and after the drug is given with D_5W solution

   c. flush the PICC line after the drug is given with heparin flush solution

   d. avoid administering the diazepam while the patient is taking quinupristin/dalfopristin

   e. notify the physician that you cannot safely administer this drug

7. Which of the following foods should a patient who is receiving linezolid avoid?

   a. bleu cheese

   b. strawberries

   c. graham crackers

   d. carrots

8. Your patient has community-acquired pneumonia caused by multidrug-resistant *Streptococcus pneumoniae*. Telithromycin (Ketek), the new ketolide antibiotic, is prescribed. The patient questions why he must take a "new fancy drug" that is not available as a generic and will likely cost more. What should patient education about this drug therapy include? *Mark all that apply.*

   a. This drug will kill the organism that is making him sick; other medications will not work because the organism is resistant to their effects.

   b. This drug needs to be taken only once a day.

   c. This drug needs to be taken only for 5 to 10 days.

   d. This drug quickly reaches a therapeutic concentration in the respiratory tract.

CASE STUDY

You are caring for a patient who has type 1 diabetes and diminished renal function. The patient was admitted to the hospital after developing osteomyelitis after a cut on his foot failed to heal. The results of a culture and sensitivity of the foot reveal that the infecting organism is resistant to many antibiotics. It is susceptible to gentamicin, and the patient begins a regimen of this drug. The order reads: Start gentamicin 60 mg q8h. Peak and trough level after third dose. Pharmacist to follow and adjust dose based on lab work.

1. Consider this patient's core patient variables. What core patient variables place the patient at additional risk for adverse effects from the gentamicin?

2. Why are peak and trough levels ordered? When should you collect them? Are there any special concerns with collecting peak and trough samples?

CRITICAL THINKING CHALLENGE

You are the nurse administering the first two doses of gentamicin to the patient described above with osteomylitis. You know that a peak and trough are ordered around the next dose.

1. What implications does this have on your administration of gentamicin?

2. In addition to administering the drug therapy and monitoring for its effectiveness and adverse effects, are there any other actions you think are appropriate when caring for this patient?

CHAPTER 41

Drugs That Are Miscellaneous Antibiotics

TOP TEN THINGS TO KNOW ABOUT DRUGS THAT ARE MISCELLANEOUS ANTIBIOTICS

1. Miscellaneous antibiotics have a mechanism of action other than disrupting the cell wall or protein synthesis of bacteria. Miscellaneous antibiotics include the fluoroquinolones, rifampin, metronidazole, daptomycin, and polymyxin B.

2. Naldixic acid, a quinolone antibiotic, is actually the first generation of fluoroquinolone drugs. Fluoroquinolones are so named because a fluorine atom was added to the quinolone structure. Naldixic acid is used only for the treatment of uncomplicated urinary tract infections.

3. There are four generations of fluoroquinolone drugs; however, the fourth generation fluoroquinolones are not available in the United States. Like cephalosporins, each generation has a different spectrum of activity.

4. Ciprofloxacin, a second generation drug, works by inhibiting DNA gyrase, an enzyme needed for bacterial DNA replication. It is most effective against aerobic gram-negative organisms. It has previously been used extensively for serious gram-negative infections, but some types of bacteria have developed resistance to ciprofloxacin. Ciprofloxacin is generally also active against aerobic gram-positive organisms, but resistance has been noted in *Staphylococcus aureus* and *Pneumococcus* species. For this reason, ciprofloxacin should be used cautiously in skin infections.

5. Ciprofloxacin has a prolonged postantibiotic effect. This means that organisms will not resume growing for 2 to 6 hours after exposure to the drug, even when the drug blood level is too low to be detected.

6. The most common adverse effects of cipro-floxacin are gastrointestinal (GI). Arthropathy (joint disease) is possible and is the most serious adverse effect. Children younger than 18 years have a higher risk for the development of arthropathy.

7. Give ciprofloxacin through a large vein and infuse slowly over 60 minutes to reduce the risk of venous irritation. If the patient has GI adverse effects from oral ciprofloxacin, small, frequent meals should be given.

8. Polymyxin B is an older antibiotic used to treat most gram-negative bacteria. Polymyxin B is administered by topical, ophthalmic, and otic routes, and is frequently mixed with other drugs.

9. Daptomycin is the only drug in a new class of antibiotics called cyclic lipopeptides. Daptomycin is used to manage serious infections that have not responded to other types of antibiotics, including complicated skin and skin structure infections (including from methicillin-resistant *Staphylococcus aureus* [MRSA]), infections from gram-positive bacteria that are resistant to vancomycin and linezolid, and bacterial endocarditis.

10. Daptomycin works by binding to the bacterial membrane and interfering with the integrity of the cell wall. This disruption causes a rapid depolarization of the membrane potential that leads to inhibition of protein, DNA, and RNA synthesis and, eventually, bacterial cell death. Daptomycin also has a postantibiotic effect that lasts approximately 6 hours. Daptomycin can retain potency against antibiotic-resistant gram-positive bacteria; no mechanism of resistance to daptomycin has been identified. Daptomycin's most common adverse effects are GI.

KEY TERMS

Fill in the Blanks

Read each statement carefully and, using the chapter's key terms, write the correct answer in the space provided.

1. _____ differ from first generation drugs by the addition of a fluorine atom to the quinolone structure.

2. Uncomplicated UTIs may be treated with a first generation drug known as _Naldixic_

3. The most significant adverse effect to the use of ciprofloxacin is _Arthropathy_

4. A class of drugs with a unique mechanism of action is_Daptomycin, cyclic lipopetide_

CORE DRUG KNOWLEDGE: JUST THE FACTS

Multiple Choice
Circle the option that best answers the question or completes the statement.

1. How do fluoroquinolone antibiotics work? They
   a. interrupt cell wall synthesis.
   b. inhibit DNA replication.
   c. block the action of folic acid.
   d. interrupt protein synthesis.

2. Ciprofloxacin (Cipro) is available in all of the following dosage forms *except*
   a. oral.
   b. parenteral.
   c. topical.
   d. inhalation.

3. Fluoroquinolones such as ciprofloxacin (Cipro) are *ineffective* in the management of
   a. gram-negative organisms.
   b. aerobic gram-positive organisms.
   c. anaerobic organisms.
   d. sexually transmitted diseases.

4. The most common adverse effects to ciprofloxacin (Cipro) therapy affect the _____ system.
   a. GI
   b. central nervous
   c. hematopoietic
   d. respiratory

5. Unlike ciprofloxacin (Cipro), nalidixic acid (NegGram) is approved for the management of
   a. genitourinary infections only.
   b. anaerobic infections.
   c. meningitis.
   d. acne only.

6. Levofloxacin (Levaquin) should be administered
   a. once daily.
   b. every other day.
   c. four times a day.
   d. twice a day.

7. When administered for systemic circulation, polymyxin B may induce
   a. cardiotoxicity.
   b. immunotoxicity.
   c. hepatotoxicity.
   d. nephrotoxicity.

8. Daptomycin (Cubicin) works by
   a. displacing protein binding sites.
   b. inhibiting protein synthesis.
   c. binding to the bacterial membrane and interfering with the integrity of the cell wall.
   d. inhibiting cross-banding of the bacterial cell wall.

CORE PATIENT VARIABLES: PATIENTS, PLEASE

Multiple Choice
Circle the option that best answers the question or completes the statement.

1. Your patient brought her 5-year-old son to the clinic today. He has an eye infection and was prescribed ophthalmic ciprofloxacin (Cipro). Your patient asks, "My pediatrician says that this drug is not OK for kids. Why did this doctor order it?" What is your best response?
   a. "Just because one doctor does not want to use it doesn't mean all of them feel the same way."
   b. "This is something you should ask the doctor."
   c. "Your pediatrician is right. Oral preparations of this drug should not be given to children, but the topical drops are approved." _Arthropathy_
   d. "No, I think you are wrong."

2. Your 25-year-old female patient has been prescribed ciprofloxacin (Cipro) for a respiratory infection. Patient teaching should include which of the following instructions?

    a. If taking birth control pills, use a backup method while taking the drug.

    b. Do not use any bronchodilator inhalers while taking this drug.

    c. Wear high-top shoes to avoid tendon rupture.

    d. Stop the medication as soon as you feel better.

3. Your patient has just been prescribed ciprofloxacin (Cipro) for a skin infection. After reviewing his medical record, you note that he has a history of gastroesophageal reflux disease (GERD). Patient teaching for this patient should include which of the following instructions?

    a. "Do not take any medication for your stomach while taking this drug."

    b. "Take any antacids at least 1 hour before or 2 hours after the Cipro."

    c. "Be sure to take the Cipro at the same time you take your vitamins."

    d. "Take Cipro with a full glass of cranberry juice."

4. Your patient has an order for IV ciprofloxacin (Cipro). To administer this medication safely, you should

    a. dilute in 5 mL NS and infuse IV push over 1 to 2 minutes.

    b. dilute in 10 mL sterile water and infuse IV push in 30 seconds.

    c. infuse IV piggyback over 15 to 20 minutes.

    d. infuse IV piggyback over 1 hour.

5. Your female patient has just completed a 7-day course of ciprofloxacin (Cipro). The patient calls the clinic today and reports having a thick white vaginal discharge. You suspect a

    a. hypersensitivity reaction.

    b. toxic reaction.

    c. superinfection.

    d. sexually transmitted disease.

6. Your patient has an order for IV daptomycin (Cubicin). To administer this drug safely, you should administer with a

    a. dextrose solution.

    b. dextrose/normal saline solution.

    c. bacteriostatic water solution.

    d. normal saline or lactated Ringer's solution.

7. Your patient receiving IV daptomycin (Cubicin) states, "My muscles hurt all over, and I started to have diarrhea today." Which of the following statements is most appropriate?

    a. "I'll be sure to write that in my nursing notes."

    b. "I will let your doctor know right away."

    c. "Those are expected effects from the drug."

    d. "Perhaps you have caught some kind of bug."

NURSING MANAGEMENT: EVERY GOOD NURSE SHOULD …

Multiple Choice
Circle the option that best answers the question or completes the statement.

1. To minimize adverse effects from ciprofloxacin, the nurse should teach the patient to

    a. use a sunscreen.

    b. limit fluid intake.

    c. take a double dose if one is missed.

    d. eat three large meals.

2. You are caring for a patient who takes theophylline for chronic obstructive pulmonary disease (COPD). The patient now has peritonitis and is prescribed ciprofloxacin. To minimize adverse effects, you should

    a. encourage aerobic exercise.

    b. monitor for tachycardia and insomnia.

    c. place the patient's bed in front of a sunny window.

    d. administer the theophylline in the morning and the ciprofloxacin in the evening.

3. A patient who has been taking oral ciprofloxacin at home to treat pneumonia from *Klebsiella pneumoniae* calls the advice hotline for her HMO. The patient tells you, the advice nurse, "I must be allergic to this drug because I have terrible nausea and abdominal pain since I started it." You should advise the patient to

    a. stop taking the drug because she is allergic to it.

    b. crush the drug and mix in a small amount of yogurt.

    c. take the drug after meals.

    d. eat small, frequent meals, but continue the drug.

CASE STUDY

A female patient age 27 years was seen in the outpatient center and received a diagnosis of severe urinary tract infection. A prescription for ciprofloxacin 500 mg twice a day was written. Describe the patient education that this patient needs for ciprofloxacin.

Take full course
Take small frequent meals for GI upset

CRITICAL THINKING CHALLENGE

Three days later, the patient described above returns to the outpatient center reporting that the symptoms have not improved much. The patient tells you that she has taken the drug twice a day for the last 3 days, as prescribed. The lab report from 3 days ago indicates that the bacteria are susceptible to ciprofloxacin.

What other questions might you ask to determine why this patient is still having symptoms of a urinary tract infection?

Is she taking it c̄ any acid containing food or drug?

CHAPTER 42

Drugs Treating Urinary Tract Infections

TOP TEN THINGS TO KNOW ABOUT DRUGS TREATING URINARY TRACT INFECTIONS

1. Sulfamethoxazole-trimethoprim is a combination of a sulfonamide and another antibiotic. The name is abbreviated as SMZ-TMP. Some sources list it as trimethoprim-sulfamethoxazole or TMP-SMZ.
2. SMZ-TMP interferes with the synthesis of folic acid (folate) needed for biosynthesis of RNA, DNA, and proteins. This prevents the formation of new bacteria, so SMZ-TMP is bacteriostatic. Avoid giving this drug to patients with folate deficiency disorders.
3. SMZ-TMP is used to treat a variety of organisms and illnesses, including urinary tract infections (UTI), respiratory infections (such as *Pneumocystis carinii* pneumonia [PCP] seen in HIV and AIDS), gastrointestinal (GI) infections, and sexually transmitted diseases.
4. Immunocompromised patients are more likely to have adverse effects from SMZ-TMP.
5. Nausea, vomiting, and diarrhea are the most common adverse effects of SMZ-TMP. Serious adverse effects are crystalluria (resulting in renal damage), allergic reactions (such as urticaria, pruritus, photosensitivity, and Stevens-Johnson syndrome), and hematologic effects (such as anemia and agranulocytosis).
6. To minimize adverse effects from SMZ-TMP, give with food, and increase fluid intake to at least 1.5 L/day, unless contraindicated by the physical condition of the patient.
7. Other antibiotic classes are also used to manage UTI. These include aminoglycocides, cephalosporins, fluoroquinolones, penicillins, tetracyclines, and the miscellaneous antibiotic fosfomycin.
8. Urinary tract antiseptics work by a local action in the urinary tract. They do not achieve high serum levels and so have few systemic effects. There is no prototype.
9. Urinary tract antiseptics include methenamine (avoid giving to patients with upper UTI or indwelling urinary catheters because these don't allow sufficient time for drug to work), nitrofurantoin, and the quinolone antibiotic nalidixic acid.
10. Phenazopyridine is a urinary analgesic. It does not have antibacterial activity, but it relieves pain, burning, frequency, and urgency caused by irritation of the urinary tract from the UTI. Phenazopyridine will make the urine look orange or red.

KEY TERMS

Anagrams
Using the definitions, unscramble each of the sets of letters to form a word. Write your response in the spaces provided.

1. A recurrent UTI caused by a different organism from the initial infection

N R O E I N T F C E

r e i n f e c t i o n

2. Infection of the bladder

S T C I Y T S I

c y s t i t i s

3. Another term for acute urethral syndrome

S U I R T E I T R H

u r e t h r i t i s

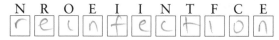

4. Infection of the kidneys

S P I Y T E I L R O H N P E

P y e l o n e p h r i t i s

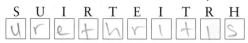

5. A recurrent UTI caused by the same organism from the initial infection

E R S E A P L

r e l a p s e

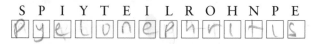

Give c food increase fluid

6. Symptoms of a UTI after the initial infection resolved

| T | R | N | E | E | C | R | U | R |

R e c u r r e n t

7. Infection caused by microbes invading the prostate

| S | P | I | R | T | O | I | S | T | T | A |

P r o s t a t i t i s

8. Potential adverse effect to the use of sulfonamides

| A | C | I | R | R | Y | U | S | L | T | L | A |

C r y s t a l i u r e a

9. First-line drugs in the management of UTI

| S | S | E | U | D | L | I | F | M | O | A | N |

S u l f o n a m i d e s

10. Necessary for the biosynthesis of RNA, DNA and proteins

| A | B | A | P |

P A B A

PHYSIOLOGY AND PATHOPHYSIOLOGY: THE BODY HUMAN

Essay

1. Name the components of the urinary system.

Kidney, urethers, bladder urethra

2. Identify the host defenses that protect an individual from a UTI. *mucin*

3. Why are women more prone to UTIs than men?

Ascention of bacteria through outside through the urethra. short proximity

CORE DRUG KNOWLEDGE: JUST THE FACTS

Multiple Choice

Circle the option that best answers the question or completes the statement.

1. Pharmacotherapeutics of SMZ-TMP include all of the following *except*
   a. *Pneumocystis carinii* pneumonia.
   b. Legionnaire's disease.
   c. histoplasmosis.
   d. urinary tract infections.

2. Sulfonamides work by
   a. inhibiting protein synthesis.
   b. interfering with folic acid synthesis.
   c. disrupting cell wall matrix.
   d. inhibiting replication of DNA.

3. During therapy with sulfamethoxazole-trimethoprim (SMZ-TMP), the patient should be advised to
   a. avoid sunlight.
   b. avoid cranberry juice or foods that acidify urine.
   c. increase fluid intake.
   d. do all of the above.

4. A potential adverse effect associated with the administration of sulfamethoxazole-trimethoprim (SMZ-TMP) is
   a. crystalluria.
   b. chronic heart failure.
   c. iron deficiency anemia.
   d. migraine headache.

5. A potential adverse effect to the infant who receives sulfamethoxazole-trimethoprim (SMZ-TMP) from breast-feeding is
   a. kernicterus.
   b. hepatitis.
   c. pancreatitis.
   d. aplastic anemia.

6. A benefit of fosfomycin (Monurol) therapy is
   a. one-time-a-day dosing.
   b. 3-day duration of therapy.
   c. one-time-only dosing.
   d. one-time-a-week dosing.

7. Which of the following statements concerning urinary tract antiseptics is accurate?

   a. They reach low systemic levels.

   b. They have many adverse effects because of their toxicity.

   c. They have many drug–drug interactions.

   d. They are the drug of choice for acute UTI.

8. Nitrofurantoin (Macrodantin) is associated with adverse effects in the

   a. CNS.

   b. cardiovascular system.

   c. pulmonary system.

   d. urinary system.

9. Treatment with which of the following drugs will result in bright orange-red urine?

   a. phenazopyridine (Pyridium)

   b. sulfisoxazole (Novosoxazole)

   c. nitrofurantoin (Macrodantin)

   d. spectinomycin

10. Although phenazopyridine (Pyridium) is frequently used in the management of UTI, it

    a. has more adverse effects than benefits.

    b. has no antibacterial activity.

    c. is more frequently used in the management of viral illness.

    d. is not FDA approved.

CORE PATIENT VARIABLES: PATIENTS, PLEASE

Multiple Choice
Circle the option that best answers the question or completes the statement.

1. Your 66-year-old patient is a homeless alcoholic who comes to the clinic with a report of dysuria and hematuria. The patient receives a diagnosis of pyelonephritis and is prescribed a course of SMZ-TMP. Because of this patient's health status history, which of the following lab tests would be appropriate before initiating therapy?

   a. renal function and arterial blood gas

   b. folate level and complete blood count (CBC)

   c. hepatic enzymes and folate level

   d. arterial blood gas and hepatic enzymes

2. To maximize the effects of SMZ-TMP, a patient should be advised to take the medication

   a. on an empty stomach.

   b. with a glass of cranberry juice.

   c. with a high-fat meal.

   d. at bedtime.

3. Your patient is taking sulfamethoxazole-trimethoprim (SMZ-TMP) for PCP prophylaxis. What instructions should be given to this patient?

   a. Limit your intake of water.

   b. Drink at least four glasses of cranberry juice per day.

   c. Increase your fluids to at least 1 liter per day.

   d. Increase your intake of dairy products.

4. Patients receiving long-term therapy with sulfamethoxazole-trimethoprim (SMZ-TMP) should have periodic laboratory testing, including

   a. uric acid levels and liver function.

   b. pulmonary function tests and CBC.

   c. ophthalmic exams and renal function tests.

   d. CBC, liver function, and renal function tests.

5. Your patient is taking sulfamethoxazole-trimethoprim (SMZ-TMP) for PCP prophylaxis. Jeffrey comes to the clinic today with a report of fatigue, sore throat, and easy bruising. What do you suspect may be the problem?

   a. viral pharyngitis

   b. anemia

   c. strep throat

   d. mononucleosis

6. Your patient has been prescribed fosfomycin (Monurol) for an acute UTI. Patient education should include instructions to

   a. drink the medication immediately after dissolving the powder.

   b. crush the capsules and mix in applesauce.

   c. inhale from the metered-dose inhaler as needed.

   d. let the dissolved powder sit for 1 hour before consuming.

7. Your 81-year-old patient has a urinary tract infection. This patient has an indwelling catheter. Which of the following medications would be *inappropriate* for the treatment of this patient's UTI?

    a. sulfamethoxazole-trimethoprim (SMZ-TMP)

    b. sulfisoxazole (Novosoxazole)

    c. methenamine (Hiprex)

    d. nitrofurantoin (Furadantin)

8. Your patient has pyelonephritis. The patient reports a constant burning sensation in the lower abdomen and frank pain with voiding. Which of the following drugs would be helpful in alleviating the discomfort this patient is experiencing?

    a. phenazopyridine (Pyridium)

    b. nitrofurantoin (Macrodantin)

    c. methenamine (Hiprex)

    d. sulfasalazine (Azulfidine)

NURSING MANAGEMENT: EVERY GOOD NURSE SHOULD …

Multiple Choice
Circle the option that best answers the question or completes the statement.

1. Your patient is being given a prescription for sulfamethoxazole-trimethoprim to treat a urinary tract infection. Teaching should emphasize which of the following?

    a. Take the drug with food if GI upset occurs.

    b. Drink at least 1,500 mL per day.

    c. Use sunscreen and protective clothing outside.

    d. all of the above

    e. none of the above

2. Your patient is 70 years old, uroseptic, and begins a regimen of IV sulfamethoxazole-trimethoprim. To minimize the risk of adverse effects, you should closely monitor the patient's

    a. CBC.

    b. fasting blood glucose/sugar (FBG or FBS).

    c. daily weight.

    d. distance vision.

3. You are following up on a patient with AIDS who has received SMZ-TMP therapy for several months to prevent *Pneumocystis carinii* infections. As part of ongoing assessment and evaluation of therapy when the patient returns for follow-up appointments, you should

    a. determine intake and output levels.

    b. assess for urine pH below 5.5.

    c. assess urine for crystals.

    d. do all of the above.

    e. do none of the above.

4. You are to administer SMZ-TMP via IV infusion to a patient with a severe urinary tract infection. To minimize adverse effects, you should

    a. administer as an IV bolus.

    b. refrigerate diluted solutions before administration.

    c. avoid flushing IV lines used to administer SMZ-TMP.

    d. do all of the above

    e. do none of the above

5. Which of these statements, if made by a patient who has been prescribed SMZ-TMP, would indicate a need for further teaching?

    a. "I will limit my sun exposure."

    b. "I will not breast-feed my daughter while I am taking this drug."

    c. "I will limit drinking alcohol to just on the weekends when someone else can drive me home."

    d. " I will increase the amount of water I drink."

CASE STUDY

Your patient is to start a regimen of oral SMZ-TMP for a urinary tract infection. As the nurse about to administer the first dose, you ask if he is allergic to sulfa drugs used as antibiotics. The patient states, "No, the only drug I'm allergic to is that blood pressure drug hydrochlorothiazide." You administer the drug as ordered. The next day the patient states, "You know, I must be allergic to the soap used to wash these sheets. I'm really itchy." On examination, you see reddened areas, some of them raised, over his chest and back.

What is your assessment?

He is reacting to SMZ-TMP

CRITICAL THINKING CHALLENGE

What piece of data did you overlook that contributed to this patient's rash and itchiness?

cross allergic reactions SMZ-TMP and Hydrochlorothiazide

CHAPTER 43

Drugs Treating Mycobacterial Infections

TOP TEN THINGS TO KNOW ABOUT DRUGS TREATING MYCOBACTERIAL INFECTIONS

1. Drug therapy to treat tuberculosis (TB) frequently includes three or four drugs because multidrug-resistant TB has developed. Unless the organism is resistant to isoniazid (INH), isoniazid is always included in the treatment for TB.
2. Isoniazid can be used as prophylaxis or as treatment of TB. INH is bactericidal or bacteriostatic; it works by disrupting the synthesis of the tuberculin bacterial cell wall. Isoniazid also may inhibit plasma monoamine oxidase (MAO) inhibitor.
3. Common adverse effects of isoniazid include hepatitis and peripheral neuropathy.
4. To minimize the adverse effect of hepatitis, avoid giving INH to patients who already have hepatitis or who have a history of INH-induced hepatitis; monitor liver enzymes carefully; and teach patients to avoid alcohol.
5. To minimize and prevent peripheral neuropathy, give vitamin B$_6$ (pyridoxine) and complete routine eye examinations. To prevent drug–food interactions, avoid excessive tyramine-rich food and histamine-rich food.
6. Other first-line drugs used to treat TB are rifampin, ethambutol, pyrazinamide (PZA), and streptomycin. Rifampin inhibits bacterial and mycobacterial RNA synthesis. Ethambutol appears to work by inhibiting RNA synthesis; it is effective only against bacilli that are actively dividing. Pyrazinamide's mechanism of action is unknown; it is most effective in the initial stages of treatment.
7. Second-line drugs to treat TB are cycloserine, ethionamide, para-aminosalicylic acid, and fluorquinolone or aminoglycoside antibiotics. Second-line drugs for TB are always given concurrently with first-line drugs. The main adverse effects from other TB drugs include optic neuritis (ethambutol), hepatotoxicities (all), arthralgias (all), gastrointestinal disturbances (all), photosensitivity (pyrazinamide), nephrotoxicity, and ototoxicity (aminoglycoside antibiotics).
8. Rifampin is also used to treat leprosy. Adverse effects are similar to those of INH, especially hepatic injury. Rifampin also discolors body fluids (urine, saliva, tears, sputum) and can permanently stain soft contact lenses. Rifampin has many drug interactions because it is a potent inducer of the P-450 hepatic enzyme system.
9. Patients with TB may also have HIV or AIDS. Determine other drug therapies because many HIV and AIDS drugs are contraindicated with rifampin use.
10. Teach patients about the risk of multidrug-resistant TB and the importance of completing the entire course of drug therapy to treat TB.

KEY TERMS

True or False

Mark each of the following statements true or false. If the statement is false, replace the underlined word(s) with the word(s) that will make the statement true.

1. ____T____ Mycobacteria are slow-growing microbes that cause disease in humans.

2. ____F____ *Mycobacterium leprae* is spread by in-halation of spores into the lungs.

3. ____F____ The combination of the primary lung lesion and lymph node granulomas is referred to as leprosy. *Ghon complex*

4. ____F____ Multiple-drug therapy is used for patients with a positive skin test but a negative chest x-ray. *Chemoprophylaxis*

5. ____T____ Hansen disease and leprosy are the same disease.

6. __F__ _Mycobacterium leprae_ frequently causes disease in patients who are HIV positive.

7. __F__ _Mycobacterium avium_ complex is a disease that mainly affects the skin. _leprosy_

8. __F__ High fevers, chills, diarrhea, and weight loss are symptoms of _leprosy_.

9. __F__ _M. avium_ causes leprosy.

CORE DRUG KNOWLEDGE: JUST THE FACTS

Multiple Choice
Circle the option that best answers the question or completes the statement.

1. Isoniazid is the drug of choice in the management of
   a. Hansen disease.
   b. _Mycobacterium avium_ complex.
   c. tuberculosis.
   d. a and c.

2. Isoniazid (INH) works by
   a. inhibiting protein synthesis.
   b. inhibiting synthesis of the bacterial cell wall.
   c. disrupting the change of RNA to DNA.
   d. interfering with folic acid synthesis.

3. The most common adverse effects associated with the use of INH are
   a. renal failure and increased seizure activity.
   b. CNS depression and peripheral neuropathy.
   c. memory impairment and renal failure.
   d. hepatitis and peripheral neuropathy.

4. Which of the following statements concerning INH is correct?
   a. INH has very few drug–drug interactions, but the few are very significant.
   b. INH has very few drug–drug interactions, and they are very insignificant.
   c. INH has many drug–drug interactions, and most are very significant.
   d. INH has many drug–drug interactions, but they are very insignificant.

5. To minimize the potential for peripheral neuropathy, INH may be given in combination with
   a. rifampin (Rifadin).
   b. pyridoxine (vitamin B_6).
   c. spectinomycin.
   d. ethambutol (Myambutol).

6. A serious adverse effect associated with the administration of ethambutol (Myambutol) is
   a. optic neuritis.
   b. hepatitis.
   c. pancreatitis.
   d. CNS depression.

7. Pyrazinamide (PZA) therapy may exacerbate
   a. chronic heart failure.
   b. diabetes.
   c. gout.
   d. asthma.

8. Rifampin (Rifadin) works by
   a. inhibiting protein synthesis.
   b. inhibiting synthesis of the bacterial cell wall.
   c. disrupting RNA synthesis.
   d. interfering with folic acid synthesis.

9. Like INH, rifampin (Rifadin) may cause injury to the
   a. kidneys.
   b. liver.
   c. heart.
   d. lungs.

10. Which of the following statements concerning drug–drug interactions with rifampin (Rifadin) is accurate?
    a. Rifampin has very few drug–drug interactions, but the few are lethal.
    b. Rifampin has very few drug–drug interactions, and they are very insignificant.
    c. Rifampin has many drug–drug interactions, and most are very significant.
    d. Rifampin has many drug–drug interactions, but they are very insignificant.

11. Which of the following drugs would be *inappropriate* for use in the treatment of leprosy?

    a. dapsone (Avlosulfan)

    b. clofazimine (Lamprene)

    c. spectinomycin

    d. rifapentine (Priftin)

12. The most serious adverse effect from dapsone (Avlosulfan) therapy affects the _____ system.

    a. hematopoietic

    b. cardiovascular

    c. respiratory

    d. integumentary

CORE PATIENT VARIABLES: PATIENTS, PLEASE

Multiple Choice

Circle the option that best answers the question or completes the statement.

1. Your 51-year-old patient has recently been exposed to TB. The patient had a negative TB skin test 6 months ago; however, the current test is positive. Which of the following interventions should be done while this patient receives INH prophylaxis?

    a. baseline CBC and repeat CBC every 6 months

    b. baseline renal function tests and repeat test every 3 months

    c. baseline hepatic function test and repeat test every month

    d. baseline pyridoxine level and repeat test every 6 months

2. A patient receiving INH for TB prophylaxis reports anorexia, malaise, fatigue, jaundice, and nausea. The nurse should recognize these symptoms as indicative of

    a. hepatitis.

    b. peripheral neuropathy.

    c. tyramine reaction.

    d. anemia.

3. Your patient has been taking triple antimicrobial therapy for active TB for the past 3 months. The patient comes to the clinic today and states, "My soft contact lenses have turned red." Which of the following medications may have caused this problem?

    a. INH

    b. rifampin (Rifadin)

    c. ethambutol (Myambutol)

    d. spectinomycin

4. Your patient has been diagnosed with active TB. This patient has multiple medical problems including HIV, steroid-dependent asthma, and type 2 diabetes. Which of the following drugs, given concurrently with the patient's previously prescribed medications, would be the most problematic?

    a. spectinomycin

    b. ethambutol (Myambutol)

    c. pyrazinamide (PZA)

    d. rifampin (Rifadin)

5. Your 33-year-old patient is taking multidrug therapy for TB. The patient has a history of hepatic dysfunction. Which combination of drugs would be contraindicated for this patient?

    a. INH and rifampin

    b. INH and ethambutol

    c. rifampin and spectinomycin

    d. ethambutol and PZA

6. Your 32-year-old patient is taking triple antimicrobial therapy for TB. The patient takes isoniazid (INH), rifampin (Rifadin), and ethambutol (Myambutol). In addition to serial liver function tests, which of the following should be done for this patient?

    a. chest x-ray

    b. ophthalmology exam

    c. ECG

    d. HbA$_{1C}$

7. Your patient is to receive IV rifampin (Rifadin). To safely administer this medication, you should

    a. premedicate the patient with IV diazepam (Valium).

    b. administer IVP over 30 seconds.

    c. infuse IVPB over 3 hours.

    d. administer IVP over 2 to 3 minutes.

NURSING MANAGEMENT: EVERY GOOD NURSE SHOULD …

MULTIPLE CHOICE

Circle the option that best answers the question or completes the statement.

1. You are caring for a patient who has active TB. He is prescribed isoniazid, rifampin, and ethambutol. He protests at taking so many medicines. Your best action would be to

   a. rotate the drugs, offering one each day.

   b. administer only the isoniazid and mark the others as "refused."

   c. force him to take all three drugs.

   d. explain the rationale for triple-drug therapy.

2. Patient education about INH should include limiting the intake of which of the following?

   a. avocados

   b. chocolate

   c. tuna fish

   d. all of the above

   e. none of the above

3. To minimize adverse effects from isoniazid, the nurse should monitor

   a. AST and ALT levels.

   b. creatinine clearance.

   c. BUN.

   d. vital capacity.

4. You work in a large city as a nurse in the health department. Because the incidence rate of TB is very high in the city, with multidrug resistance becoming more of a problem, the deputy director of the health department has issued a directive that the health department will actively work with patients to confirm their adherence with prescribed drug therapy. Thus, you would expect to do which of the following for the patients you visit who have active TB and have been prescribed drug therapy?

   a. Instruct the caregiver to encourage the patient to take the medication.

   b. Tell the patient that as long as one of the drugs prescribed is taken he or she will be cured.

   c. Give each patient the medication and watch him or her swallow it.

   d. Ask the patient if he or she is taking the medicine.

CASE STUDY

You are caring for a patient who is 38 years old and homeless. The patient is an alcoholic and has TB. He comes to the clinic that provides health care for the homeless every day to get his medication (INH, rifampin, ethambutol, and pyrazinamide).

1. For which adverse effects is the patient most at risk?

2. What will you do to minimize these adverse effects?

CRITICAL THINKING CHALLENGE

To help keep the patient described above from drinking alcohol, the doctor has also prescribed disulfiram (Antabuse). When the patient returns to the clinic the next time, you notice that his mood is very changeable. When the patient first comes into the clinic, he acts very angry with you and the other staff members, but after a short while, the patient is cracking jokes and talking nonstop. The patient says to you, "I hope you won't punish me for being so abrupt. It is just the way I am these days."

1. What may have brought this on?

2. What action should you take?

CHAPTER 44

Drugs Treating Fungal Infections

TOP TEN THINGS TO KNOW ABOUT DRUGS TREATING FUNGAL INFECTIONS

1. Fungal infections range from mildly annoying to life-threatening infections.
2. Fungal infections are systemic or superficial. Systemic infections can cause serious medical problems, especially in patients who are immunocompromised. They are classified as those that are opportunistic and those that occur in the general population. Superficial mycoses can be dermatophytic (skin related) or mucous membrane related; the most common of these infections are tinea and candidiasis.
3. Fungi can be separated into two groups—yeasts and molds. The yeasts are single-celled organisms, approximately the size of a red blood cell, that reproduce by a budding process. The buds separate from the parent cell and mature into identical daughter cells. Molds produce long, hollow, branching filaments called hyphae.
4. Amphotericin B, a polyene antifungal, is fungicidal or fungistatic, and works by binding to membrane sterols in fungal cell membranes, resulting in increased cell permeability, cell leakage, and death. Damage to host cells can also occur. Amphotericin B is used in treating progressive and potentially fatal systemic infections caused by severe adverse effects.
5. Adverse effects of amphotericin B include nephrotoxicity (in more than 80% of patients), infusion-related reactions, electrolyte abnormalities, anemia, leukopenia, thrombocytopenia, and others.
6. Administer other drugs as ordered before infusion to decrease adverse effects, administer a test dose before a full dose (central line preferred), use an in-line filter and IV pump, keep the patient well hydrated, and monitor electrolytes, complete blood count (CBC), and renal and hepatic function throughout therapy. Educate patients regarding the likelihood of a transfusion reaction and other adverse effects.
7. Nystatin, an antifungal related to amphotericin B, is not used for systemic infections. It is used to treat topical, vaginal, and oral fungal infections. Oral suspension of nystatin should be swished through the mouth and then swallowed or spit out, as directed by the prescriber. Oral troches should be dissolved in the mouth.
8. Fluconazole, an azole antifungal, is used to treat esophageal, oropharyngeal, and vulvovaginal candidiasis, and systemic fungal infections. It may be used prophylactically in immunocompromised patients with a CD4+ T-cell counts of less than 200. Fluconazole works by altering the fungal cell membrane, resulting in increased cellular permeability and leakage of cell contents.
9. Most common adverse effects of fluconazole are gastrointestinal (GI), headache, and dizziness. Mild elevations in liver enzymes may occur, which usually return to pretreatment levels after drug therapy is over. The patient should be encouraged to avoid alcohol.
10. Some of the azole antifungal agents are administered by intravenous infusion; others are given orally; and others are only available for topical administration. Many of the topical agents can be purchased over-the-counter without a prescription.

PHYSIOLOGY AND PATHOPHYSIOLOGY: THE BODY HUMAN

Essay

1. How do yeasts reproduce?

2. What are hyphae?

3. In the human host, where would you find an infection with a dermatophyte?

4. How is a systemic mycosis different from a dermatophyte?

KEY TERMS

Matching
Match the following key terms with their correct definitions.

1. _____ *Candida*

2. _____ cryptococcosis

3. _____ dermatophytes

4. _____ dimorphic fungi

5. _____ tinea

a. Capable of growing as yeasts at one temperature and as molds at another

b. Mold-like fungi

c. Yeast-like fungus that is almost always present as part of the normal population of organisms in the mouth, skin, intestinal tract, and vagina

d. Common name for dermatophytic infections

e. Most serious of the fungal infections in immunocompromised patients

CORE DRUG KNOWLEDGE: JUST THE FACTS

Multiple Choice
Circle the option that best answers the question or completes the statement.

1. Amphotericin B (Fungizone) is used in the care of patients with
   a. tinea.
   b. onychomycosis.
   c. a serious systemic mycotic disease.
   d. a serious systemic viral disease.

2. What is the mechanism of action of amphotericin B (Fungizone)?
   a. alters fungal cell membrane permeability
   b. inhibits protein synthesis
   c. disrupts fungal mitotic spindle structure
   d. interrupts DNA synthesis

3. Which of the following laboratory tests should be done before and throughout amphotericin B (Fungizone) therapy?
   a. CBC
   b. electrolytes
   c. renal function
   d. all of the above

4. Amphotericin B (Fungizone) is thought to have a suppressive effect on erythropoietin production. This may result in
   a. renal toxicity.
   b. hepatic toxicity.
   c. anemia.
   d. seizure activity.

5. Nystatin (Mycostatin), an antifungal drug nearly identical to amphotericin B (Fungizone), is indicated for the treatment of
   a. severe systemic mycoses.
   b. oral, cutaneous, mucocutaneous, or vaginal candidiasis.
   c. severe systemic viruses.
   d. HIV.

6. Flucytosine (5-FC) should be administered cautiously to patients receiving other medications that are known to induce
   a. hepatotoxicity.
   b. nephrotoxicity.
   c. hematologic toxicity.
   d. all of the above.

7. Which of the following drugs is used as primary fungal prophylaxis in immunocompromised patients?
   a. fluconazole (Diflucan)
   b. ketoconazole (Nizoral)
   c. butenafine (Mentax)
   d. amphotericin B (Fungizone)

8. The most common adverse effects to fluconazole (Diflucan) therapy affect the _____ system.

    a. cardiovascular

    b. gastrointestinal

    c. reproductive

    d. endocrine

CORE PATIENT VARIABLES: PATIENTS, PLEASE

Multiple Choice
Circle the option that best answers the question or completes the statement.

1. Your patient is receiving IV amphotericin B (Fungizone). Which of the following electrolyte imbalances may be induced by this therapy?

    a. hypokalemia

    b. hyponatremia

    c. hyperkalemia

    d. hypernatremia

2. Patients receiving IV amphotericin B have the greatest risk for the development of

    a. blurred vision.

    b. arachnoiditis.

    c. nephrotoxicity.

    d. hypertension.

3. Before initiation of amphotericin B (Fungizone) therapy, what patient teaching should you do?

    a. "This infusion may make you feel tired. I'll leave the side rails down."

    b. "Many patients have a reaction to this medication. I will premedicate you to diminish this possible response."

    c. "This medication may cause a minor tingling at the IV site. Let me know if that occurs."

    d. "This infusion will last for about 30 minutes. I'll be back then to take it down."

4. Your female patient is being treated with griseofulvin (Grisactin) for a fungal infection in her toenails. The nurse explains that the patient may need to take the medication for 6 to 12 months. Which of the following instructions should also be given to this patient?

    a. "Keep this medication out of the light."

    b. "Take this medication with a fatty meal."

    c. "If you take birth control pills, use another method of contraception."

    d. "Stop taking the medication 1 week each month."

5. Your patient is receiving IV fluconazole (Diflucan). What is the appropriate rate of infusion for this medication?

    a. 200 mg over 20 minutes

    b. 200 mg per hour

    c. 200 mg over 3 to 4 hours

    d. 200 mg IV push over 2 minutes

6. Your patient has HIV and is being prescribed fluconazole (Diflucan) for fungal prophylaxis. Your patient also has type 2 diabetes and takes glimepiride (Amaryl). Because of this combination of drugs, you should monitor this patient's

    a. blood pressure.

    b. blood glucose.

    c. kidney function.

    d. T-cell count.

NURSING MANAGEMENT: EVERY GOOD NURSE SHOULD …

Multiple Choice
Circle the option that best answers the question or completes the statement.

1. You are to administer the first dose of amphotericin B for a systemic fungal infection. Before beginning the infusion, you should

    a. administer a test dose.

    b. assess vital signs.

    c. administer an antipyretic, such as ibuprofen.

    d. do all of the above.

    e. do none of the above.

2. During the infusion of amphotericin B, your patient experiences wheezing, nausea, and a drop in blood pressure. You should
   a. increase the rate of infusion.
   b. change the IV site to a peripheral line with a smaller vein.
   c. slow the IV rate.
   d. do all of the above.
   e. do none of the above.

3. Your patient is receiving fluconazole prophylaxis against histoplasmosis because of low CD4 and T-cell counts. The patient experiences diarrhea while taking fluconazole. You should
   a. discontinue use of the fluconazole.
   b. seek an order for an antidiarrheal.
   c. obtain stool cultures.
   d. do all of the above.
   e. do none of the above.

4. You are caring for a patient who has been treated with several antibiotics for a surgical infection after repair of a fractured hip. The patient now has oral candidiasis and is to receive nystatin suspension. To increase the effectiveness of the drug, you should
   a. shake the suspension and apply to the surgical wound.
   b. mix the suspension in water and have the patient drink it.
   c. have the patient swish the suspension in her mouth before swallowing it.
   d. avoid shaking, draw up in a syringe, and administer to the back of the patient's throat.

5. Which of the following instructions should the nurse give to the patient receiving posaconazole (Noxafil)? *Mark all that apply.*
   a. "Take this medication on an empty stomach."
   b. "Be sure to limit your exposure to the sun."
   c. "Use the spoon that comes with the medication to take the appropriate amount."
   d. "Shake the medication before pouring into the spoon."
   e. "Swallow the capsule whole. Do not open or crush it."
   f. "Take the medication with food or a nutritional supplement."

CASE STUDY

Your patient has a history of chronic heart failure and takes digoxin, hydrochlorothiazide, and captopril for this. The patient recently was treated with prednisone, an oral steroid, for a severe asthmatic attack. Unfortunately, now the patient has experienced a serious *Aspergillus* infection. The organism is resistant to the usually effective antimicrobials, except for amphotericin B. There are orders to begin amphotericin B therapy.

1. Consider the patient-related variables. Are there any that place this patient at increased risk of adverse effects from the amphotericin? If yes, what are they?

2. What can you do to minimize possible adverse effects?

CRITICAL THINKING CHALLENGE

1. What factors do you think contributed to this patient having a serious *Aspergillus* infection?

2. Should you administer the amphotericin B?

CHAPTER 45

Drugs Treating Viral Infections

TOP TEN THINGS TO KNOW ABOUT DRUGS TREATING VIRAL INFECTIONS

1. Viruses are responsible for many infectious disorders, ranging from the common cold to life-threatening meningitis.
2. Few antiviral drugs have been developed because viruses have no metabolic enzymes of their own, so they can replicate only within a living host cell by using the metabolic processes of the host. Because most antiviral drugs target the metabolic processes used to replicate, the drug may also do substantial harm to the host.
3. Antiviral drugs have a narrow spectrum of activity, and each drug's clinical application is limited to a particular viral disorder
4. Acyclovir, an antiviral drug, competes for a position in the DNA chain of the herpes virus and then terminates DNA synthesis. Uninfected cells allow for minimum uptake of acyclovir. It is used to treat herpes simplex (cold sores, genital sores), herpes zoster (shingles), Epstein-Barr virus, and cytomegalovirus (CMV). It has no effect on HIV.
5. Use acyclovir during periods of active lesions. Teach patient to wear gloves and wash hands when applying topically to prevent spread of infection. The drug is generally well tolerated, but nephrotoxicity from crystallization may occur. Encourage the patient to drink fluids.
6. Ganciclovir (Cytovene) is the drug of choice to prevent or treat CMV infection in immunocompromised patients, such as patients with HIV or transplant recipients. Other drugs used to treat CMV infection include cidofovir (Vistide), foscarnet (Foscavir), and valganciclovir (Valcyte).
7. Antiviral drugs are also available as topical or ophthalmic drugs. Docosanol (Abreva) is an OTC topical drug used to treat herpes simplex, and penciclovir (Denavir) is a prescription topical antiviral drug for herpes labialis. Trifluridine (Viroptic) and vidarabine (Vira-A) are both prescription ophthalmologic drugs.

Topical antiviral agents need multiple applications throughout the patient's waking hours.
8. There are several antiviral preparations used prophylactically to treat the symptoms of, or to decrease the duration of, influenza. These are amantadine, rimantadine, oseltamivir, and zanamivir. Oseltamivir is the drug of choice for avian (H5N1) flu.
9. Interferon alfa and beta are used in the management of viral hepatitis. Peginterferon combined with oral ribavirin is the treatment of choice for HCV. Other drugs to manage viral hepatitis include adefovir dipivoxil (Hepsera), entecavir (Baraclude), lamivudine (Epivir HBV), and telbivudine (Tyzeka). Lamivudine is also approved for treatment of HIV; however, the dose to treat HIV is much higher than the dose used to to viral hepatitis.
10. Respiratory syncytial virus (RSV) is treated with several different types of drugs. Palivizumab (Synagis) is a humanized monoclonal antibody to RSV that is administered monthly during the RSV season. Ribavirin (Virazole) is administered as an inhaled drug for RSV and as an oral drug (Rebetol) for the treatment of hepatitis C.

KEY TERMS

Matching
Match the key term with its definition.

1. _____ cytomegalovirus

2. _____ herpes simplex virus

3. _____ herpes zoster

4. _____ phosphorylation

5. _____ respiratory syncytial virus

a. Process needed to produce the activity of acyclovir

b. Common respiratory virus that affects children

c. Type of herpes that is life threatening

d. Virus that is spread by direct contact with fluid from active lesions

e. Infection caused by the virus that also causes chickenpox

PHYSIOLOGY AND PATHOPHYSIOLOGY: THE BODY HUMAN

Essay

1. What are the five steps of viral reproduction?

2. List the different types of hepatitis found in North America and how they are transmitted.

3. How do the transmissions of herpes simplex and herpes zoster differ?

CORE DRUG KNOWLEDGE: JUST THE FACTS

Multiple Choice
Circle the option that best answers the question or completes the statement.

1. Which of the following viruses is unaffected by acyclovir (Zovirax)?
   a. herpes
   b. human immunodeficiency virus (HIV)
   c. cytomegalovirus (CMV)
   d. Epstein-Barr

2. What is the mechanism of action of acyclovir (Zovirax)?
   a. inhibition of viral cell wall
   b. disruption of protein synthesis
   c. termination of DNA synthesis
   d. increased permeability of viral cell wall

3. Patients receiving IV acyclovir (Zovirax) should be monitored for
   a. hepatotoxicity.
   b. anemia.
   c. neurotoxicity.
   d. nephrotoxicity.

4. Which of the following antiviral agents are effective for the treatment of cytomegalovirus (CMV)?
   a. cidofovir (Vistide) and penciclovir (Denavir)
   b. famciclovir (Famvir) and ganciclovir (Cytovene)
   c. ganciclovir (Cytovene) and valganciclovir (Valcyte)
   d. cidofovir (Vistide) and valacyclovir (Valtrex)

5. Amantadine (Symmetrel) may be useful in the treatment of influenza A and
   a. acetaminophen toxicity.
   b. diverticulitis.
   c. HIV disease.
   d. Parkinson disease.

6. Oseltamivir phosphate (Tamiflu) and zanamivir (Relenza) are used in the management of
   a. cytomegalovirus.
   b. herpes simplex.
   c. herpes zoster.
   d. influenza.

7. Which of the interferons is FDA approved for the treatment of both hepatitis B and C?
   a. interferon alfa-2b (Intron-A)
   b. interferon alfa-2a (Roferon-A)
   c. interferon alfa-2b (PRG-Intron)
   d. interferon alfa-2a and ribavirin (Rebetron)

8. Ribavirin (Virazole), palivizumab (Synagis), and RSV-IG (RespGam) are used to treat or prevent
   a. herpes simplex and zoster.
   b. cytomegalovirus.
   c. hepatitis B.
   d. respiratory syncytial virus

CORE PATIENT VARIABLES: PATIENTS, PLEASE

Multiple Choice

Circle the option that best answers the question or completes the statement.

1. Your patient is receiving IV acyclovir (Zovirax). This patient has additional medical problems, including migraine headaches, HIV, diabetes mellitus, and drug addiction. Which of the patient's medical problems requires cautious use of acyclovir?
   a. diabetes mellitus
   b. HIV
   c. migraine headaches
   d. drug addiction

2. Your patient is receiving IV acyclovir (Zovirax). To safely administer this drug, you should administer it
   a. over 20 minutes and keep the patient NPO.
   b. over 20 minutes and keep the patient well hydrated.
   c. over 60 minutes and keep the patient NPO.
   d. over 60 minutes and keep the patient well hydrated.

3. Your 60-year-old patient calls the clinic and states, "I don't need to get my flu shot today. I am going to use that new Tamiflu." Which of the following is your best response?
   a. "You might be able to do that, but the doctor needs to check your medical history first."
   b. "I'll cancel your appointment. Thank you for calling."
   c. "The drug is not approved for use in people your age."
   d. "You should have both."

4. Your neighbor comes over and states that she can feel a "herpes cold sore" coming. She asks, "Do you have anything I can take for it?" Your best response is
   a. "I'll see if I have any antibiotics."
   b. "I have some leftover penciclovir (Denavir). I'll get it for you."
   c. "There is a great OTC med called docosanol (Abreva) that you can get at the drugstore."
   d. "I have some ganciclovir (Cytovene). Maybe that will help."

5. Your patient has the flu and is prescribed zanamivir (Relenza). Patient teaching should include how to
   a. use a metered-dose inhaler.
   b. use a Diskhaler.
   c. give a SC injection.
   d. give an IM injection.

NURSING MANAGEMENT: EVERY GOOD NURSE SHOULD …

Multiple Choice

Circle the option that best answers the question or completes the statement.

1. A patient being treated for genital herpes with acyclovir calls the patient information hotline at the HMO and speaks to the nurse. The patient states, "These herpes lesions are now red and warm. Is this okay? Should I do something about it?" What advice should the nurse give?
   a. Take aspirin and continue with the acyclovir.
   b. Stop taking the acyclovir.
   c. Come in to the health center to be examined.
   d. Take a warm bath.

2. You are caring for an immunocompromised patient with CMV retinitis. The health care provider has ordered IV ganciclovir (Cytovene) to be administered. Which of the following lab tests need to be evaluated prior to administration? *Mark all that apply.*
   a. renal function tests
   b. liver function tests
   c. complete blood count
   d. electrolytes

3. Your patient has been prescribed lamivudine (Epivir HBV) for chronic hepatitis B. Which of the following lab tests is **most important** for the nurse to assess prior to administration of this drug?
   a. HIV status
   b. complete blood count
   c. renal function
   d. platelet count

4. The nurse should assess a patient who is prescribed telbivudine (Tyzeka) for chronic HBV for a history of
   a. fatigue, malaise.
   b. myopathy.
   c. jaundice.
   d. easy bruising.

CASE STUDY

You are a dialysis nurse in an acute care hospital. You are assigned to dialyze a 45-year-old male with acute renal failure. While you are setting up your equipment, the patient tells you that he was diagnosed with infectious endocarditis after using IV drugs for many years. His kidneys abruptly failed after he left the hospital against medical advice "to get my fix." The patient states, "I don't have any organs left that aren't diseased. I even have hepatitis C."

1. Do you have a legal responsibility to care for this patient?

2. What type of immunization will protect you from hepatitis C?

3. What steps should you take to protect yourself from getting hepatitis C?

CRITICAL THINKING CHALLENGE

You are working in an outpatient clinic. Your patient has just been diagnosed with genital herpes and prescribed valacyclovir (Valtrex). The patient states, "I'm getting married in a month. Do I need to break my engagement? Will this medication cure me?" What will you include in your patient teaching?

CHAPTER 46

Drugs Treating HIV Infection and AIDS

TOP TEN THINGS TO KNOW ABOUT DRUGS TREATING HIV INFECTION AND AIDS

1. HIV infection and AIDS are chronic diseases that historically have had a poor prognosis, but their prognosis has significantly improved since the establishment of HAART therapy. HIV infection and the effectiveness of drug therapy are monitored by CD4 cell counts and HIV RNA counts (viral load).

2. Pharmacotherapy may be used for patients with or without symptoms. There are benefits and risks of treatment. Exact protocols and treatment strategies for HIV and AIDS are evolving constantly as new drugs are being developed and more is learned about these infections. These drugs are used in combinations to decrease the emergence of viral resistance. Resistance can develop in all types of anti-HIV agents even when the therapeutic regimen is followed, but occurs most frequently when it is not.

3. Pharmacotherapy for HIV and AIDS is complex and requires lifestyle changes and accommodations by the patient. The timing of doses is very important. Some of the drugs need to be taken on an empty stomach and some with food. With the advent of combination drug therapy, the number of pills/capsules taken daily has decreased; however, some patients continue to need multiple medications throughout the day. All anti-HIV drugs have adverse effects that may decrease the quality of the patient's life. Drug therapy can be very expensive. These factors make it difficult for a patient to comply with drug therapy effectively.

4. Zidovudine (AZT) is a nucleoside reverse transcriptase inhibitor (NRTI) used to treat HIV infection; it was the first FDA-approved drug for treating HIV. It works by incorporating itself into the DNA of the virus. This stops the building process and prevents the creation of a new virus. It is one of the few antiretroviral drugs used to reduce the risk of perinatal transmission of HIV. Patients should eat a high-carbohydrate, moderate-protein, and low-fat diet because fatty meals decrease absorption.

5. Common adverse effects of zidovudine are gastrointestinal (GI) intolerance, headache, rash, and fever. Black Box warnings for zidovudine include: hematologic toxicities, symptomatic myopathy (including cardiomyopathy), lactic acidosis, and severe hepatomegaly. Monitor the patient carefully and assess blood work for adverse effects and response to therapy.

6. Nonnucleoside reverse transcriptase inhibitors (NNRTIs) such as efavirenz (Sustiva) also inhibit HIV reverse transcriptase. NNRTIs are not incorporated into the viral DNA. They inhibit a specific site on the enzyme reverse transcriptase that is required to carry out the process of DNA synthesis. This results in the inability to convert viral RNA into DNA. It is always used in combination with other classes of anti-HIV drugs. The most common adverse effects of efavirenz are CNS in nature. Symptoms such as dizziness, impaired concentration, insomnia, abnormal dreams, and hallucinations occur with approximately 50% of patients; however, these symtoms tend to spontaneously resolve within a month. Rarely, life-threatening skin reactions such as erythema multiforme, Stevens-Johnson syndrome, or toxic epidermal necrolysis may occur. Efavirenz interacts with drugs that are metabolized by P-450 CYP3A4.

7. Saquinavir mesylate, a protease inhibitor (PI), is responsible for packaging infected polyproteins so that the new virus carries the disease. Protease inhibitors block this step so that the new virus is noninfectious. Protease inhibitors also block reverse transcriptase (decrease viral replication) and inhibit replication of HIV in the macrophages (major reservoirs of HIV). It is used in combination therapy with reverse transcriptase inhibitors. Combination therapy enhances suppression of viral replication and limits the development of resistance. Therapeutic adherence for every dose is crucial to prevent increases in viral load and drug resistance.

8. The bioavailability of saquinavir is increased with high-fat, high-protein meals. It has many drug–drug interactions; always check for compatibility. Common adverse effects are GI and central nervous system (CNS). Saquinavir, like other PIs, causes abnormal fat deposits at the base of the posterior neck ("buffalo hump") and the abdominal area ("protease paunch") and changes in the handling of fats, resulting in hyperlipidemia (substantial increases in triglycerides or cholesterol). Hyperglycemia and insulin resistance are other adverse effects.

9. Entry inhibitors or fusion inhibitors are a new class of drugs that inhibit the HIV virus from binding to, fusing with, and entering the human cell. Enfuvirtide, the prototype, is approved for managing HIV infection in patients who have experienced treatment failure with drugs from each existing class of antiretrovirals or who have been unable to tolerate previous antiretroviral regimens. It is given as a subcutaneous injection; injection site reactions occur in almost all patients receiving enfuvirtide. Teach patients to rotate injection sites and use aseptic technique. Enfuvirtide is associated with the development of bacterial pneumonia. This drug is extremely expensive.

10. Patients with HIV infections are at high risk for opportunistic infections. Some of these infections occur so commonly that drug therapy for prophylaxis is routinely prescribed. Prophylaxis therapy is often used for *Pneumocystis carinii* pneumonia (sulfamethoxazole-trimethoprim), tuberculosis (isoniazid), and *Toxoplasma gondii* (sulfamethoxazole-trimethoprim), *Mycobacterium avium* complex (azithromycin or clarithromycin), varicella-zoster virus (acyclovir, valacyclovir, or famciclovir). Vaccines that are usually administered to prevent infection are *Streptococcus pneumoniae*, hepatitis B, hepatitis A, and influenza.

KEY TERMS

True or False
Mark each of the following statements true or false. If the statement is false, replace the underlined word(s) with the word(s) that will make the statement true.

1. _____ A provirus is the virus before it exits the cell.

2. _____ The polymerase chain reaction test and viral load test detect antibodies produced in response to HIV infection.

3. _____ Viral load indicates the current immunologic status of the patient.

4. _____ In HIV disease, the virus has an affinity for attaching to plasma cells.

5. _____ Rapid HIV testing results are available in approximately 30 minutes.

6. _____ CD4 cell counts are reported as copies per milliliter.

7. _____ The newest class of antiretroviral drugs is protease inhibitors.

8. _____ After a patient has a positive ELISA test, a viral load is completed.

9. _____ The most potent class of antiretroviral drugs are the nonnucleoside reverse transcriptase inhibitors.

10. _____ Current protocols for the management of HIV and AIDS are called viral loads.

11. _____ Two classes of drugs that affect the same enzyme in two different ways are the nucleoside reverse transcriptase inhibitors and the nonnucleoside reverse transcriptase inhibitors.

PHYSIOLOGY AND PATHOPHYSIOLOGY: THE BODY HUMAN

Essay

1. What are the potential benefits of delayed antiretroviral therapy?

2. What are the potential risks of delayed antiretroviral therapy?

3. Why is monotherapy contraindicated for the treatment of HIV disease and AIDS?

4. In addition to the enzyme immunoassay (EIA) or Western blot (WB) tests, what other laboratory tests are available for diagnosing HIV?

CORE DRUG KNOWLEDGE: JUST THE FACTS

Multiple Choice

Circle the option that best answers the question or completes the statement.

1. What is the difference in the mechanism of action between nucleoside reverse transcriptase inhibitors (NRTIs) and nonnucleoside reverse transcriptase inhibitors (NNRTIs)?
   a. The mechanism of action occurs in a different site within the virus.
   b. NRTI drugs inhibit replication by binding to reverse transcriptase, and NNRTI drugs cause chain termination by incorporation into the viral DNA.
   c. NRTI drugs cause chain termination by incorporation into the viral DNA, and NNRTI drugs inhibit the end production of the virus before being expelled from the CD4+ T cell.
   d. NRTI drugs cause chain termination by incorporation into the viral DNA, and NNRTI drugs inhibit replication by binding to reverse transcriptase.

2. To decrease the potential for maternal transmission of HIV to the fetus, which of the following drugs should be administered to the woman during pregnancy?
   a. zidovudine (Retrovir)
   b. stavudine (Zerit)
   c. delavirdine (Rescriptor)
   d. ritonavir (Norvir)

3. Zidovudine (Retrovir) therapy has many adverse reactions. In which of the following body systems do the most serious effects occur?
   a. CNS
   b. respiratory
   c. endocrine
   d. hematologic

4. To increase the bioavailability of protease inhibitors such as saquinavir (Invirase, Fortovase), the medication should be administered
   a. 1 hour before meals.
   b. 2 hours after meals.
   c. with a high-fat meal.
   d. with a low-fat meal.

5. Which of the following statements concerning drug–drug interactions with saquinavir (Invirase, Fortovase) is correct?
   a. There are multiple interactions, and many may produce subtherapeutic levels of saquinavir.
   b. There are multiple interactions, and many may produce toxic levels of saquinavir.
   c. There are multiple interactions, and some may produce subtherapeutic levels of saquinavir, whereas others may produce toxic levels of saquinavir.
   d. There are very few interactions, and they are all insignificant.

6. A rare but very serious adverse effect that may occur with efavirenz therapy is
   a. cardiac arrhythmias.
   b. pulmonary edema.
   c. pulmonary emboli.
   d. Stevens-Johnson syndrome.

7. Patients receiving antiretroviral therapy should have serial laboratory tests done. These include
   a. CBC.
   b. renal and hepatic function.
   c. T-cell count and viral load.
   d. all of the above.

8. The drug of choice for prophylaxis of *Pneumocystis carinii* pneumonia is
   a. atovaquone (Mepron).
   b. sulfamethoxazole-trimethoprim (Bactrim, Septra).
   c. pentamidine (NebuPent).
   d. pyrimethamine (Daraprim).

9. The drugs of choice for *Mycobacterium avium* complex (MAC) prophylaxis include
   a. dapsone (Avlosulfon).
   b. azithromycin or clarithromycin (Biaxin).
   c. pyrimethamine (Daraprim).
   d. sulfamethoxazole-trimethoprim (Bactrim, Septra).

10. Enfuvirtide (Fuzeon) is approved for use in patients who
    a. are allergic to other antiretroviral drugs.
    b. experienced treatment failure with other antiretroviral drugs.
    c. have newly diagnosed HIV.
    d. have a viral load greater than 5,000.

11. Enfuvirtide (Fuzeon) is administered by
    a. pills or troches.
    b. intramuscular injection.
    c. subcutaneous injection.
    d. intravenous infusion.

12. Darunavir (Prezista), like many other antiretroviral drugs, is administered in combination with ritonavir. Why?
    a. Ritonavir decreases the potential for severe adverse effects.
    b. Ritonavir is a different class of antiretroviral drug.
    c. Ritonavir increases the bioavailability of darunavir.
    d. Ritonavir buffers the stomach and allows darunavir to be absorbed.

MATCHING

Match the following antiretroviral drugs with their appropriate Black Box warning. Match all that apply. *

1. _____ Lactic acidosis
2. _____ Stevens-Johnson syndrome
3. _____ Pancreatitis
4. _____ Hematologic toxicity
5. _____ Pregnancy
6. _____ Hypersensitivity reactions
7. _____ Hepatotoxicity
8. _____ Drug–drug interactions
9. _____ Myopathy
10. _____ Intracranial hemorrhage
11. _____ HBV exacerbation

----

* Other antiretroviral drugs may also have these symptoms as potential adverse effects; however, they are not listed as Black Box warnings.

a. abacavir
b. amprenavir
c. didanosine
d. emtricitavine
e. lamivudine
f. nevirapine
g. ritonavir
h. stavudine
i. tenofovir
j. tipranavir
k. zidovudine

CORE PATIENT VARIABLES: PATIENTS, PLEASE

Multiple Choice
Circle the option that best answers the question or completes the statement.

1. Your patient has AIDS. The patient is currently taking zidovudine (Retrovir), efavirenz (Sustiva), and saquinavir (Invirase). The patient has received a diagnosis of CMV retinitis, and ganciclovir (Cytovene) has been prescribed. Because of this combination of drugs, which of the following lab tests should be closely monitored?
   a. intraocular pressure
   b. CBC
   c. hepatic enzymes
   d. renal enzymes

2. Your patient is taking zidovudine (Retrovir). What diet education should be done with this patient?
   a. high carbohydrate, moderate protein, low fat
   b. low carbohydrate, high protein, low fat
   c. moderate carbohydrate, moderate protein, high fat
   d. low carbohydrate, low protein, high fat

3. Your patient is receiving zidovudine, efavirenz, and fosamprenavir for the past year? In addition to a viral load and T-cell count, which of the following lab tests is *most important* to assess?
   a. complete blood count
   b. electrolytes
   c. renal status
   d. hepatic enzymes

4. Your patient is taking saquinavir for HIV disease. The patient has tuberculosis. Which of the following drugs would be contraindicated for use with this patient?

    a. isoniazid (INH)

    b. ethambutol (Myambutol)

    c. spectinomycin

    d. rifampin (Rifadin)

5. Your 30-year-old patient is taking ritonavir (Norvir) oral capsules. It is important to include which of the following statements in patient teaching for this patient?

    a. Shield the medication from light.

    b. Refrigerate the medication.

    c. Keep the medication in a warm cabinet.

    d. Keep the medication in a damp place, such as the bathroom.

6. Your patient is taking triple antiretroviral therapy for HIV disease. The patient comes to the clinic for a routine checkup. Lab results include a CD4+ T-cell count of 455 and an undetectable viral load. The patient states, "Shouldn't I be taking more medications to keep me from getting other diseases?" Which of the following would be the best response?

    a. "You probably should, but this is an HMO."

    b. "Yes, but then you run the risk of inducing more adverse effects."

    c. "You might develop drug resistance if we add any more drugs."

    d. "At this point, your immune system is capable of providing that protection."

7. Your patient has been receiving highly active antiretroviral therapy (HAART) for 5 years that includes a protease inhibitor. In addition to monitoring T-cell and viral load counts, you should monitor for

    a. increased blood sugar.

    b. frequent headaches.

    c. abnormal fat distribution.

    d. constipation.

8. The teaching plan for a patient who is taking enfuvirtide (Fuzeon) should include instructions for

    a. reconstituting the drug.

    b. subcutaneous administration.

    c. safe discard of used syringes.

    d. all of the above.

9. Which of the following patients would require additional assessment prior to administering darunavir (Prezista)?

    a. Diane, with a history of an anxiety disorder

    b. Carol, who is pregnant

    c. Lindsey, with a history of type 2 diabetes

    d. Anna, with a history of asthma

NURSING MANAGEMENT: EVERY GOOD NURSE SHOULD …

Multiple Choice
Circle the option that best answers the question or completes the statement.

1. To maximize the effectiveness of zidovudine, the nurse should

    a. administer the drug with meals.

    b. administer the drug one time a day.

    c. instruct the patient to avoid fatty foods.

    d. do all of the above.

    e. do none of the above.

2. To maximize the therapeutic effects of saquinavir, the nurse should

    a. administer the drug 30 minutes after meals.

    b. skip administering a dose if the patient reports mild nausea.

    c. instruct the patient to avoid fatty foods.

    d. do all of the above.

    e. do none of the above.

3. When a patient taking abacavir has a rash, fever, nausea, and body aches, which action should the nurse take?

    a. Obtain an order for Tylenol and calamine lotion.

    b. Do not administer the drug and contact the physician.

    c. Administer the medication with food or juice.

    d. Nothing, these are signs of a viral illness.

4. Your patient has HIV infection and recently received a diagnosis of oral infection (candidiasis). In addition to treating the candidiasis, which of the following drugs would you expect to administer?

   a. isoniazid

   b. rifampin

   c. amphotericin B

   d. sulfamethoxazole-trimethoprim

5. Patient education for a patient receiving zidovudine and saquinavir to treat HIV infection should include

   a. these drugs should not be taken at the exact same time.

   b. GI upset may occur; the effects may resolve after 3 to 4 weeks of therapy.

   c. drug resistance can develop if doses are skipped or drugs are taken intermittently.

   d. all of the above.

   e. none of the above.

6. To help a patient be adherent with HIV drug therapy, what should the nurse do? *Mark all that apply.*

   a. Recommend that the drugs be taken at a time of a routine activity (such as brushing the teeth or eating a meal).

   b. Help the patient plan a daily schedule to take the drugs.

   c. Provide oral and written instructions about taking the drugs.

   d. Provide specific instructions of when the drugs should be taken with regard to meals.

7. You are providing teaching for a patient who will be receiving enfuvirtide at home. What information should be included? *Mark all that apply.*

   a. Powdered enfuvirtide may be stored at room temperature.

   b. After being reconstituted, enfuvirtide should be refrigerated in the vial.

   c. Inject the drug intramuscularly into the vastus lateralus.

   d. Two sizes of syringes are packed with the enfuvirtide; use the 3-mL one for reconstituion and the 1-mL one for administration

8. Your hospitalized patient has been taking tipranavir (Aptivus), zidovudine (Retrovir), ritonavir (Norvir), and efavirenz (Sustiva) for the past year. Which of the following assessments should take priority?

   a. lung sounds

   b. intake and output

   c. skin integrity

   d. level of consciousness

CASE STUDY

Your patient is a 21-year-old woman. She has a history of IV drug abuse and alcohol abuse. She states she hasn't used drugs or alcohol in the 6 months since she received a diagnosis of HIV. She is being treated with saquinavir and zidovudine. She was admitted to the hospital this time with *Pneumocystis carinii* pneumonia and was treated successfully with sulfamethoxazole-trimethoprim (SMZ-TMP) IV. She will be going home with a regimen of oral SMZ-TMP. In report, you learn that she frequently refuses her medications, and the nurses need to go in three or four times to get her to take everything. The nurse giving report says, "I don't know why we bother. When she leaves the hospital, she'll be noncompliant and then will be right back in here. What else can you expect?"

Consider the core drug knowledge and this patient's core patient variables. What teaching do you think might be needed?

CRITICAL THINKING CHALLENGE

1. What additional questions do you think you should ask this patient to more fully assess her?

2. How might this knowledge alter your teaching plan or teaching strategies?

CHAPTER 47

Drugs Treating Parasitic Infections

TOP TEN THINGS TO KNOW ABOUT DRUGS TREATING PARASITIC INFECTIONS

1. Parasites include protozoa, helminths, and arthropods. Pharmacologic intervention for parasites must be specific not only to the type of parasite, but also to the stage of its life cycle.

2. Chloroquine is used to treat malaria. It is also used in rheumatoid arthritis and discoid lupus. It is taken up inside the infected erythrocyte and interrupts the synthesis of RNA and DNA. In treating rheumatoid arthritis, it antagonizes histamine and serotonin, inhibiting prostaglandin synthesis; this creates an anti-inflammatory effect.

3. Common adverse effects of chloroquine are hypotension, electrocardiogram (ECG) changes, nausea, vomiting, diarrhea, and abdominal pain. Give this drug on the same day of the week if given on a weekly basis. Have patients take the drug with food to minimize gastrointestinal (GI) problems. Encourage patients to change positions slowly to minimize symptoms of hypotension.

4. Metronidazole, a synthetic antibacterial and antiprotozoal drug, is used to treat various organisms causing infection. It works by entering anaerobic bacteria and inhibiting DNA synthesis, causing bacterial cell death. Avoid use during pregnancy (at least through the first trimester) and in alcoholics (disulfiram-like reaction can occur). Common adverse effects are GI and central nervous system (CNS).

5. Give oral (PO) metronidazole with food to minimize GI effects; give intravenous (IV) metronidazole slowly over 1 hour. Monitor for thrombophlebitis and secondary infections. Educate patients that sex partners need to be treated simultaneously for trichomonal infections.

6. Pentamidine is used to prevent or treat *Pneumocystis carinii* pneumonia (PCP). Its action is unclear, but it appears to interfere with nucleotide, phospholipid, and protein synthesis of the parasite. Pentamidine is given through aerosolization for prophylaxis and IV for treatment of PCP.

7. Sudden, severe effects may develop after a single dose of pentamidine. Cough and bronchospasm, and sudden severe hypotension are the most frequent adverse effects. Other adverse effects are thrombocytopenia, leukopenia, anemia, arrhythmias, tachycardia, acute hypoglycemia (especially in diabetics), pancreatitis, and elevated liver enzymes (especially in patients with pre-existing hepatic disease).

8. Keep the patient in bed while administering pentamidine, monitor blood pressure carefully throughout therapy, give a bronchodilator before inhaled pentamidine, protect the IV solution from light, and use respiratory precautions.

9. Mebendazole is an oral, broad-spectrum, synthetic antihelminthic that treats a variety of worms, especially nematodes. It acts by damaging the cells of the helminth but not the host. Common adverse effects are transient GI, CNS, and fever during expulsion of worms. Potential serious adverse effects are blood abnormalities and hepatotoxicity. Avoid use during pregnancy (teratogenic and embryo toxic). Monitor blood counts and liver function test results if the therapy is long term. Instruct the patient to chew the drug or crush it and mix with food.

10. Permethrin, an antiectoparasitic drug, is used to treat scabies and pediculosis. It is applied topically, where it is absorbed through the exoskeleton of parasites. Permethrin disrupts the parasite's nerve cell membrane, resulting in paralysis and death. Avoid use in abraded skin to prevent systemic absorption into the patient. Teach patients how to apply and how to prevent reinfection.

KEY TERMS
Crossword Puzzle

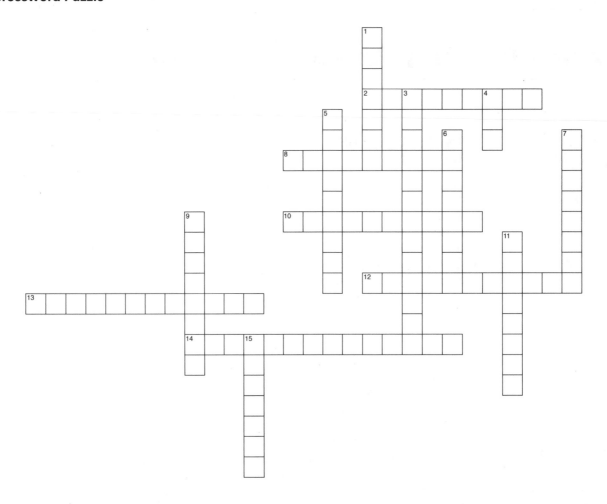

ACROSS

2. Vectors of disease such as mites
8. Flukes
10. Infection with a protozoan parasite that causes diarrhea, dyspepsia, and occasionally malabsorption
12. Sexually active organism that produces active amebiasis
13. Disease caused by infection with a species of protozoa of the genus *Trichomonas* or related genera
14. Type of parasite that infects external body surfaces

DOWN

1. Disease spread by the bite of an infected mosquito
3. Disease caused by the protozoan parasite
4. Abbreviation for type of pneumonia that affects many people with AIDS
5. Disease caused by the microorganism *Entamoeba histolytica*
6. Worms

7. Roundworm
9. Organism that lives on or in another and draws its nourishment therefrom
11. Unicellular organism
15. Tapeworm

CORE DRUG KNOWLEDGE: JUST THE FACTS

Multiple Choice

Circle the option that best answers the question or completes the statement.

1. In addition to the treatment of malaria, which of the following is a pharmacotherapy of chloroquine (Aralen)?

    a. scabies

    b. lice

    c. rheumatoid arthritis

    d. *Pneumocystis carinii* pneumonia

2. Which of the following body systems can be affected by chloroquine therapy?

   a. genitourinary

   b. endocrine

   c. hematologic

   d. sensory

3. Which of the following procedures should be done before initiating chloroquine therapy?

   a. pulmonary function test

   b. coronary stress test

   c. breast examination

   d. ophthalmologic examination

4. Which of the following is *not* a disorder treatable with metronidazole (Flagyl)?

   a. Crohn disease

   b. trichomonas

   c. amebiasis

   d. *Pneumocystis carinii* pneumonia

5. Metronidazole (Flagyl) is contraindicated for which of the following patients?

   a. Nancy, with alcoholism

   b. Beth, with anemia

   c. Tom, with prostatic hypertrophy

   d. Nelson, with bipolar disease

6. For patients with an allergy to sulfa drugs, the drug of choice for *Pneumocystis carinii* pneumonia (PCP) prophylaxis is

   a. cotrimoxazole (Bactrim, Septra).

   b. pentamidine (NebuPent).

   c. atovaquone (Mepron).

   d. any of the above.

7. Which of the following is an approved route of administration for pentamidine?

   a. inhalation

   b. oral

   c. intravenous

   d. a and c

   e. a and b

8. Which of the following interventions for the administration of pentamidine is *incorrect*?

   a. Shield IV pentamidine from light.

   b. Administer pentamidine within 24 hours of preparation.

   c. Administer bronchodilator before pentamidine by inhalation.

   d. Dilute IV pentamidine with normal saline.

9. Mebendazole (Vermox) is administered by which of the following routes?

   a. subcutaneous

   b. intravenous

   c. oral

   d. all of the above

10. Which of the following drugs would be useful in the treatment of flukes and tapeworms?

    a. mebendazole (Vermox)

    b. praziquantel (Biltricide)

    c. thiabendazole (Mintezol)

    d. niclosamide (Niclocide)

11. Permethrin (Elimite) should be applied to

    a. clean, dry hair.

    b. dry hair.

    c. clean, damp hair.

    d. wet hair.

12. Which of the following statements is correct concerning crotamiton (Eurax) use?

    a. A second application should be done in 1 week.

    b. Only one application is necessary.

    c. A second application is needed in 24 hours.

    d. If symptoms remain, a second application can be done in 3 days.

CORE PATIENT VARIABLES: PATIENTS, PLEASE

Multiple Choice

Circle the option that best answers the question or completes the statement.

1. Your 66-year-old patient has recently returned from a trip and has malaria. Which of the following disorders would contraindicate the use of chloroquine (Aralen)?

   a. hypertension

   b. retinopathy

   c. peptic ulcer disease

   d. Crohn disease

2. Your patient has just returned from a vacation in a malaria-endemic country. The patient took chloroquine (Aralen) 2 weeks before leaving and once a week during the vacation. The patient is symptom-free and asks, "Can I stop this medication now?" Which of the following is the best response?

   a. "You can stop the medication because you have no symptoms."

   b. "Take the medication 1 more week, then you can stop."

   c. "Take the remainder of the medication at bedtime tonight."

   d. "No, you need to continue the medication for an additional 4 weeks."

3. Your patient is taking chloroquine (Aralen) for malaria. Which of the following instructions should be given to this patient?

   a. "Be sure to keep this medication out of the reach of your children."

   b. "Take the medication on the same day each week."

   c. "The medication can make you dizzy; be sure to change positions slowly."

   d. all of the above

4. Your patient is taking metronidazole (Flagyl) for trichomoniasis. The patient asks you what type of adverse effects may occur. Which of the following groups of symptoms is correct?

   a. xerostomia, dysgeusia, nausea, and vomiting

   b. chest pain, nausea, and vomiting

   c. constipation, dysgeusia, and vomiting

   d. urinary frequency, xerostomia, and vomiting

5. Your 52-year-old patient has multiple medical problems, including a history of chronic heart failure (CHF) for which the patient takes digoxin (Lanoxin) and furosemide (Lasix). The patient also has a history of deep vein thrombosis and takes warfarin (Coumadin). The patient has *Helicobacter pylori* and is prescribed metronidazole (Flagyl) for 3 weeks. In light of this patient's history, what interventions should be done during the metronidazole therapy?

   a. monitor for disulfiram reaction

   b. perform an exercise stress test before initiation of therapy

   c. monitor for signs of bleeding

   d. monitor for pancreatitis

6. Your female patient calls the clinic concerned that her urine has discolored. She states she is being treated for trichomoniasis and is taking metronidazole (Flagyl). Which of the following statements is most appropriate?

   a. "Trichomoniasis is a sexually transmitted disease; maybe you have another type as well."

   b. "Perhaps you have a urinary tract infection."

   c. "I would stop the medication immediately and come to the clinic."

   d. "This is a common occurrence with this medication, but it is harmless."

7. Your patient is to receive IV pentamidine (NebuPent). Which nursing intervention should be taken with this patient immediately after the infusion?

   a. take the blood pressure

   b. take a blood glucose

   c. order a nebulizer treatment

   d. give a saline laxative

8. Your patient has HIV disease and seizures. The patient is prescribed carbamazepine (Tegretol) for seizures and receives pentamidine (NebuPent) by inhalation every month. The patient should be advised to call the health care provider if which of the following symptoms occur?

   a. increased urine output

   b. spontaneously resolved abdominal pain

   c. sore throat, easy bruising, or bleeding

   d. cough

9. Your 21-year-old patient has vaginal trichomonas and is prescribed metronidazole (Flagyl) 2 grams to be taken one time. Before administration of metronidazole, which of the following laboratory tests should be completed?

   a. complete blood count

   b. pregnancy test

   c. liver function tests

   d. kidney function tests

10. Your patient has brought her 4-year-old child to the clinic because of rectal itching. The child is found to have pinworms. Which of the following instructions should be given to this patient?

   a. "Keep your child away from the other children in the family until the child is no longer contagious."

   b. "It's best to treat all members of the family at the same time because pinworms are so contagious."

   c. "This is not an easy disease to acquire, so you do not have to worry about it."

   d. "Give this medication to your child on an empty stomach."

NURSING MANAGEMENT: EVERY GOOD NURSE SHOULD …

Multiple Choice
Circle the option that best answers the question or completes the statement.

1. A patient is seen in the clinic where you work and is given a prescription for chloroquine because she will be traveling out of the country to a region known to have malaria. Teaching regarding chloroquine therapy should include instructions to

   a. begin drug therapy 2 weeks before the planned travel schedule.

   b. discontinue drug therapy when leaving the malarial area.

   c. take the drug every day at the same time.

   d. take the drug on an empty stomach.

2. Patients taking metronidazole for a giardiasis infection should be taught to avoid which of the following?

   a. milk

   b. over-the-counter (OTC) liquid cold medicines

   c. OTC antipyretics

   d. rice

3. Your patient is a 22-year-old woman who is being treated for a *Trichomonas* infection with metronidazole. You should ask the patient

   a. whether she has a current sexual partner.

   b. whether she could be pregnant.

   c. whether she is taking anticoagulants.

   d. all of the above.

   e. none of the above.

4. Because your patient is receiving IV metronidazole, the patient should be carefully assessed for

   a. cardiac arrhythmias.

   b. peripheral edema.

   c. blood-tinged diarrhea.

   d. decreased urine production.

5. You are caring for a patient who has a current PCP infection. The patient is to receive IV pentamidine. To minimize adverse effects from the drug, you should

   a. mix the drug in a saline solution.

   b. monitor temperature every hour during infusion.

   c. administer IM morphine before infusion.

   d. do all of the above.

   e. do none of the above.

6. Which nursing measure should assume priority prior to administration of trimetrexate (NeuTrexin) for your immunocompromised patient with PCP pneumonia?

   a. schedule CBC test twice weekly

   b. verify the order for leucovorin has been written

   c. assess lung sounds

   d. perform urine dip to assess for hematuria

7. Your patient has traveler's diarrhea and has been prescribed nitazoxanide (Alinia). What pertinent medical information should you obtain from the patient before completing your patient education? A history of

   a. diabetes mellitus

   b. chronic heart failure

   c. cardiac arrhythmias

   d. gastrointestinal esophageal reflux disease (GERD)

8. Patient teaching regarding the use of mebendazole to treat a pinworm infection should include which of the following?

   a. Chew the tablets.

   b. Take with milk.

   c. All family members should be treated.

   d. all of the above

   e. none of the above

CASE STUDY

A patient is admitted from the emergency room to the hospital's medical floor with a diagnosis of PCP. He also has diabetes and AIDS. The patient's vital signs are temperature, 101.5°F; heart rate, 92; respirations, 32; and blood pressure, 138/80. The patient has a nonproductive cough and is short of breath. The physician writes an order for this patient to receive pentamidine 250 mg IV per day for 14 days. By the time the pentamidine arrives from the pharmacy, it is 10:30 PM. The nurse hangs the drug.

1. What parameters should the nurse monitor while administering the pentamidine?

2. What other actions should the nurse perform to minimize adverse effects?

CRITICAL THINKING CHALLENGE

The patient's infusion of pentamidine goes well, and the evening nurse reports off duty to the night nurse at 11:30 PM. When the night nurse gets in to this patient's room on his rounds at 12:30 AM, he finds the patient ashen, diaphoretic, and hard to arouse.

Consider the core drug knowledge and the core patient variables. What assessment might you make of this patient's current status?

CHAPTER 48

Drugs Affecting the Upper Respiratory System

TOP TEN THINGS TO KNOW ABOUT DRUGS AFFECTING THE UPPER RESPIRATORY SYSTEM

1. The most common conditions affecting the upper respiratory system initiate an inflammatory response.
2. Antitussives are used to suppress the cough reflex, when chronic nonproductive coughing accompanies a disorder of the respiratory tract. Dextromethorphan, an antitussive, is often used in over-the-counter (OTC) products. Dextromethorphan has few adverse effects, although interaction with other central nervous system (CNS) depressants may exacerbate sedation. Avoid giving to patients who depend on their cough reflex to keep their airway clear (such as those with asthma or emphysema).
3. Decongestants decrease nasal congestion from inflammation secondary to upper respiratory infections. Pseudoephedrine, a decongestant, achieves nasal decongestion by mimicking the sympathetic nervous system, causing vasoconstriction. The shrinkage reduces membrane size and allows for sinus drainage and improved air flow.
4. Adverse effects from pseudoephedrine are related to other sympathetic receptors being stimulated. The primary adverse effects are from sympathetic stimulation of the CNS and cardiovascular systems (e.g., anxiety, insomnia, tachycardia, and elevated blood pressure [BP]). Use caution in patients with conditions that may be adversely affected by these stimulation effects.
5. Antihistamines are used to treat symptoms associated with allergies. Histamine is released during the inflammatory response to an antigen invasion. Antihistamines block the H_1 receptor sites, preventing histamine action. Antihistamines restore normal air flow through the upper respiratory system. Many antihistamines are available over the counter.
6. Fexofenadine, an antihistamine, is used to relieve symptoms associated with seasonal and perennial allergic rhinitis, and some other conditions. It is most effective when given before symptoms occur.
7. Fexofenadine also has some anticholinergic effects and antipruritic effects. However, as a second-generation antihistamine, it causes fewer anticholinergic effects than do first-generation drugs such as diphenhydramine (Benadryl).
8. Expectorants decrease the viscosity of secretions so they can be more easily coughed up and improve air flow. As the cough becomes productive, less coughing is stimulated. They are available in many OTC preparations.
9. Guaifenesin, an expectorant, is used as symptomatic relief of respiratory conditions, such as colds, acute bronchitis, and influenza that have a dry, nonproductive cough. Available OTC, it is often combined with decongestants and antihistamines.
10. Assess the cause of the cough before using guaifenesin. A chronic cough from smoking will not be alleviated by guaifenesin. Long-term use should be avoided because it may mask a more serious condition. Teach patients to consult with a physician if cough doesn't go away after a week's use of guaifenesin. Most oral solutions contain alcohol. Assess patients for alcohol abuse or the use of disulfiram (Antabuse; treatment for alcoholism).

KEY TERMS

True or False
Mark each of the following statements true or false. If the statement is false, replace the underlined word(s) with the word(s) that will make the statement true.

1. _____ Drugs that block the cough reflex are called <u>antihistamines</u>.

2. _____ <u>Dopamine</u> is a chemical released during the inflammatory process.

3. _____ Drugs that block the effects of histamine are called <u>antihistamines</u>.

4. _____ <u>Antitussives</u> are drugs that decrease the overproduction of respiratory secretions.

5. _____ The <u>sinuses</u> are in constant motion, moving the mucus and any trapped substance toward the throat.

6. _____ <u>Bronchodilators</u> increase a productive cough to clear the airways.

7. _____ <u>Influenza</u> is a viral infection that starts in the upper respiratory tract.

8. _____ <u>Laryngitis</u> is an inflammation or infection of the throat.

9. _____ Sinusitis occurs when the epithelial lining of the <u>oral</u> cavities becomes inflamed.

10. _____ <u>Influenza</u> is an infection caused by any of several strains of myxoviruses.

11. _____ Inflammation of the nose is known as <u>rhinitis</u>.

12. _____ An inflammation of the voice box is called <u>pharyngitis</u>.

13. _____ <u>Rebound congestion</u> occurs when the drug effect wears off and the body compensates by vasodilating the same nasal arterioles that the drug constricted.

PHYSIOLOGY AND PATHOPHYSIOLOGY: THE BODY HUMAN

Essay

1. Identify the components of the upper respiratory system.

2. What is the purpose of goblet cells in the epithelial lining of the respiratory tract?

3. How are entrapped particles in the respiratory tract expelled from the body?

4. What are two mechanisms, stimulated by the CNS, that are initiated to clear airways?

CORE DRUG KNOWLEDGE: JUST THE FACTS

Multiple Choice

Circle the option that best answers the question or completes the statement.

1. Dextromethorphan (Benylin) works by
   a. inhibition of the cough center in the medulla.
   b. inhibition of respiratory tract secretions.
   c. stimulation of opiate receptors.
   d. bronchodilation.

2. Which of the following statements concerning the adverse effects of dextromethorphan (Benylin) is correct?
   a. There are many adverse effects, but few are serious.
   b. There are many adverse effects, and many are serious.
   c. There are a few minor adverse effects.
   d. There are only a few adverse effects, but all of them are serious.

3. Pseudoephedrine (Sudafed) works by
   a. mimicking the action of the parasympathetic nervous system.
   b. mimicking the action of the sympathetic nervous system.
   c. blocking the action of the parasympathetic nervous system.
   d. blocking the action of the sympathetic nervous system.

4. Pseudoephedrine (Sudafed) is indicated for the treatment of which of the following?
   a. viral upper respiratory infection
   b. asthma
   c. bronchitis
   d. cerebral palsy

5. Which of the following adverse effects may occur during pseudoephedrine (Sudafed) therapy?
   a. urinary retention
   b. bradycardia
   c. tachycardia
   d. hunger

6. How does oxymetazoline (Afrin) differ from pseudoephedrine (Sudafed)?
   a. route and decreased incidence of adverse effects
   b. contraindications and increased dosing frequency
   c. route and increased adverse effects
   d. contraindications and decreased dosing frequency

7. Which of the following nasal sprays is a steroidal anti-inflammatory drug?
   a. oxymetazoline (Afrin)
   b. phenylephrine (Neo-Synephrine)
   c. ephedrine (Kondon's Nasal)
   d. dexamethasone sodium phosphate (Turbinaire)

8. Antihistamines, such as fexofenadine (Allegra), are the treatment of choice for
   a. viral upper respiratory infections.
   b. allergic rhinitis.
   c. influenza.
   d. asthma.

9. Fexofenadine (Allegra), a second-generation antihistamine, differs from first-generation antihistamines such as diphenhydramine (Benadryl) by
   a. increased adverse effect profile.
   b. decreased sedation.
   c. decreased incidence of allergy.
   d. increased anticholinergic effects.

10. An expectorant drug, such as guaifenesin (Robitussin), is used to relieve
    a. a dry, hacking cough.
    b. nasal congestion.
    c. chest congestion.
    d. sinus congestion.

11. Which of the following statements concerning drug–drug interactions of guaifenesin (Robitussin) is accurate?
    a. There are no known drug–drug interactions.
    b. There are a few drug–drug interactions, but they are minor.
    c. There are a few drug–drug interactions, and they are serious.
    d. There are many drug–drug interactions, and they are serious.

12. Cromolyn sodium (NasalCrom) works by
    a. vasoconstriction of nasal vessels.
    b. depressing the medulla.
    c. preventing the breakdown of mast cells.
    d. antagonizing the effects of histamine.

CORE PATIENT VARIABLES: PATIENTS, PLEASE

Multiple Choice
Circle the option that best answers the question or completes the statement.

1. Your patient has a viral upper respiratory infection, and dextromethorphan (Benylin) is prescribed every 4 hours. You note that the patient is taking fluoxetine, a selective serotonin reuptake inhibitor (SSRI). You would advise this patient to
   a. refuse to take the dextromethorphan at all.
   b. take the dextromethorphan every other day.
   c. skip the 6 PM dose and double the bedtime dose.
   d. call if symptoms such as fever, nausea, or hallucinations occur.

2. For the hospitalized patient, a priority nursing diagnosis for the patient receiving hydrocodone bitartrate is
   a. risk for ineffective airway clearance.
   b. risk for ineffective gas exchange.
   c. risk for injury.
   d. risk for constipation.

3. Which of the following patients should refrain from pseudoephedrine (Sudafed) therapy?
   a. Maria, with constipation
   b. Janice, with headaches
   c. Tyler, with severe hypertension
   d. James, with depression

4. Which of the following statements would be appropriate for patient teaching regarding pseudoephedrine (Sudafed) therapy?
   a. "You can take this medication for 30 days."
   b. "This medication does not have any major drug interactions."
   c. "This medication can make you really drowsy."
   d. "In addition to this medication, you should use a humidifier and drink at least 10 glasses of water a day."

5. Which of the following patients should refrain from fexofenadine (Allegra) therapy?
   a. Marilyn, who is breast-feeding
   b. Heather, who has Parkinson disease
   c. Evelyn, who has peripheral venous stasis
   d. Charlene, who has diabetes mellitus

6. Your 5-year-old patient has allergic rhinitis. Which of the following drugs would be best for this?
   a. cetirizine (Zyrtec)
   b. fexofenadine (Allegra)
   c. desloratadine (Clarinex)
   d. diphenhydramine (Benadryl)

7. Your 46-year-old patient calls the clinic to speak with the advice nurse. The patient reports having a cough for the past 4 weeks and says she has been self-treating with guaifenesin (Robitussin) from the local drug store. The patient states, "This is barely helping me. I need something else." Which of the following statements is most appropriate?
   a. "This medication will work better if you stop smoking."
   b. "Have you been drinking lots of water with this medication?"
   c. "Because your cough has been with you for so long, it's best if you come to the clinic for a checkup."
   d. "As long as you do not have a fever, I would just double the dose."

8. Patient teaching for the patient receiving dextromethorphan (Benylin) should include
   a. "Do not drive until you see how this drug affects you."
   b. "Do not eat or drink any dairy products with this drug."
   c. "Take the drug only at bedtime."
   d. "Do not take this drug within 2 hours of your vitamin tablets."

9. Patient teaching for the patient receiving pseudoephedrine (Sudafed) should include
   a. "Do not take this drug for more than 30 days."
   b. "Do not take any other OTC medications without asking your doctor or pharmacist."
   c. "Be sure to drink milk at least once a day to decrease the GI effects."
   d. "This drug may make you very tired."

10. Patient teaching for the patient taking fexofenadine (Allegra) should include
    a. "Limit your intake of water while you are taking this drug."
    b. "You should not take this drug for more than 3 days."
    c. "This drug may give you insomnia."
    d. "Try sugarless gum or candy if your mouth is dry."

NURSING MANAGEMENT: EVERY GOOD NURSE SHOULD …

Multiple Choice

Circle the option that best answers the question or completes the statement.

1. A patient is seen in the outpatient center for a chronic cough and receives a prescription for dextromethorphan, an antitussive. Which of the following should the nurse include in patient education?

   a. Do not drive until the effects of the drug on you are known.

   b. Do not drink alcohol while taking this drug.

   c. Keep this medicine out of the reach of children.

   d. all of the above

   e. none of the above

2. What recommendations would you give a patient to maximize the therapeutic effect of pseudoephedrine, a nasal decongestant?

   a. Eat a diet high in fiber.

   b. Drink plenty of liquids.

   c. Avoid taking hot, steamy showers.

   d. Do not take for more than 14 days.

3. You are the nurse working a telephone hot line to answer questions about health problems. A patient calls and tells you he has been taking fexofenadine, an antihistamine, for seasonal allergies. The drug is effective, but the patient reports having an upset stomach after taking it and wonders if he must stop taking the drug. What advice should you give?

   a. Stop taking the drug immediately.

   b. Take half of the prescribed dosage.

   c. Take the drug with food.

   d. Take another antihistamine in addition to the fexofenadine.

4. Your next call, as the telephone advice nurse, is from a patient who reports having a chronic nonproductive cough. The patient states: "Would it be better to take Robitussin or Benylin for my cough? I have both at home." Which of the following questions would you include in your assessment to give him the best answer?

   a. Do you have chronic asthma or emphysema?

   b. Do you smoke?

   c. What other medications do you take?

   d. all of the above

   e. none of the above

5. You are caring for a 14 year-old patient who came to the clinic with her mother. Privately, the mother tells you that she is concerned that her child might be smoking because she is constantly asking her to buy Robitussin (dextromethorphan) for a cough. With your knowledge of this drug, what further information would you need from the mother?

   a. "Can you smell cigarette smoke when she comes home?"

   b. "Have you noticed any unusual or agitated behavior?"

   c. "Does anyone in your family smoke?"

   d. "Has she been recently ill or running a temperature?"

CASE STUDY

Your patient is 72 years old and has been prescribed fexofenadine, an antihistamine, to treat his seasonal allergies. To minimize adverse effects and provide appropriate patient education, what questions about lifestyle, diet, habits, and environment would you want to ask?

CRITICAL THINKING CHALLENGE

The patient described above has been taking fexofenadine for about 2 months and does not have adverse effects from the drug. At this time, the patient's wife calls the outpatient department and speaks to the nurse. She is very concerned about her husband. She says, "He was working in the garden and got a rash from some weeds. He took some medicine for the rash and itching, and now I can't get him to stay awake."

1. What medicine do you think this patient took for his rash and itching?

2. What leads you to this belief?

CHAPTER 49

Drugs Affecting the Lower Respiratory System

TOP TEN THINGS TO KNOW ABOUT DRUGS AFFECTING THE LOWER RESPIRATORY SYSTEM

1. Acetylcysteine is a mucolytic used to break up thick, tenacious sputum in patients whose physical conditions make it difficult to cough up these secretions (e.g., chronic obstructive pulmonary disease [COPD], cystic fibrosis, pneumonia, tuberculosis [TB]). It is most frequently given by nebulizer, usually in an acute care setting. It is a fast-acting drug with onset of action within 1 minute. Main adverse effects are respiratory (bronchospasm, bronchoconstriction, chest tightness, burning in upper airway, rhinorrhea). Acetylcysteine is the antidote for severe acetaminophen overdosage.

2. Albuterol is a relatively selective beta-2 agonist used as a bronchodilator for patients with COPD and asthma. It may be given orally or inhaled by way of a metered-dose inhaler or nebulizer. Bronchodilation occurs quickly (in 15 minutes or less) after inhalation. Because of this, inhaled albuterol is considered a "rescue drug" when there is an acute attack of bronchoconstriction. It is the drug patients should use first when they begin to experience symptoms. There are also long-acting beta-2 agonist drugs. Long-acting beta-2 agonists have been associated with a higher risk for asthma-related deaths. Teach the patient that long-acting drugs are not appropriate for acute symptoms because the onset of action is too slow.

3. Although albuterol is relatively selective for beta-2 receptors, some stimulation of beta-1 receptors occurs. Adverse effects are related to these sympathomimetic effects, such as tachycardia, anxiety, and tremor. Oral doses are more likely to cause systemic adverse effects.

4. Ipratropium is an anticholinergic that decreases the formation of cyclic guanosine monophosphate (cGMP), creating relaxation of the smooth muscle in the bronchial tree. It is used as maintenance treatment for bronchospasm from chronic asthma, bronchitis, emphysema, or COPD. It is given by inhalation or intranasal spray.

5. Ipratropium is taken daily to decrease the frequency and severity of future asthma attacks. It will not provide "rescue relief" for an attack in progress. Patient education is important to achieve the full therapeutic effect.

6. Theophylline, a xanthine, has a direct effect on the smooth muscle of the respiratory tract and produces bronchodilation. It is used to treat or prevent bronchial asthma and bronchospasms in COPD. It is given orally. Aminophylline, a very similar drug that is water soluble, is given IV when acute symptoms occur.

7. Adverse effects of theophylline are gastrointestinal (nausea, vomiting, diarrhea), central nervous system stimulation (headache, insomnia, irritability), and possibly cardiovascular (hypotension, arrhythmias). Adverse effects most frequently occur when serum levels are elevated above the therapeutic range, although they may occur with therapeutic levels. Monitor serum levels throughout therapy.

8. Cromolyn sodium is a mast cell stabilizer that is used in prophylaxis for mild to moderate asthma. It prevents the mast cell from rupturing and spilling its contents (degranulation) after it has contact with an antigen. Thus, it has anti-inflammatory effects. It is administered by inhalation or intranasal spray. Cromolyn sodium must be taken daily as prophylaxis; it is not effective during an acute asthmatic attack. However, it may be used before exercise to prevent exercise-induced bronchospasm.

9. Zafirlukast blocks the receptors for leukotrienes, which are potent bronchoconstrictors. This is how zafirlukast improves the wheezing, coughing, and dyspneic symptoms of asthma. Zafirlukast is used in the treatment of chronic

asthma; it does not relieve the symptoms of an acute asthmatic attack. It is given orally. Food impairs the absorption of zafirlukast; give 1 hour before or 2 hours after eating.

10. Glucocorticoid steroids are the most effective anti-inflammatory drugs used in the management of respiratory disorders. They may be given orally, parenterally, or by inhalation. Inhaled glucocorticoids need to be used daily for their peak effect to occur. IV doses may be used in acute respiratory flare-ups, in combination with a xanthine or a beta-2 agonist. Inhaled glucocorticoids do not have the systemic adverse effects that occur with oral and parenteral forms. The adverse effects from inhaled steroids are localized in the respiratory tract (sore throat, hoarseness, cough).

KEY TERMS

Matching
Match the key term with its definition.

1. ___c___ bronchodilators
2. ___e___ bronchospasm
3. ___i___ chemoreceptors
4. ___f___ CAL
5. ___d___ COPD
6. ___h___ mucolytics
7. ___a___ perfusion
8. ___g___ respiration
9. ___b___ statis asthmaticus
10. ___j___ ventilation

a. Delivery of blood to the alveoli
b. A life-threatening bronchospasm
c. Drugs that open the airways in the lungs
d. Umbrella term for a group of respiratory disorders
e. Muscle spasm that occurs in the airways
f. Current name for COPD
g. Exchange of gases at the alveolar level
h. Drugs that break down mucus in the airways
i. Neuroreceptors sensitive to CO_2 and acid levels
j. The act of breathing

PHYSIOLOGY AND PATHOPHYSIOLOGY: THE BODY HUMAN

Essay

1. Identify the components of the lower respiratory system.

2. When assessing a patient, the nurse determines vital signs including blood pressure, pulse, temperature, and respirations. Is the term "respiration" accurate? Why or why not?

3. What is the action of the vagus nerve in the respiratory system?

4. In the respiratory system, what response is expected when stimulation of the sympathetic nervous system occurs?

CORE DRUG KNOWLEDGE: JUST THE FACTS

Multiple Choice
Circle the option that best answers the question or completes the statement.

1. The action of acetylcysteine (Mucomyst) is to
   a. dilate the bronchioles.
   b. decrease inflammation in the bronchioles.
   c. break down mucoproteins in the airways that block airflow.
   d. stop the breakdown of the mast cell.

2. Acetylcysteine (Mucomyst) is the drug of choice in the treatment of

   a. viral upper respiratory diseases.

   b. cystic fibrosis.

   c. allergic rhinitis.

   d. sinusitis.

3. In addition to action on the respiratory system, acetylcysteine (Mucomyst) is used in the management of

   a. acetaminophen overdose.

   b. migraine headaches.

   c. nephrotoxicity.

   d. pancreatitis.

4. The action of albuterol (Proventil) is to

   a. dilate the bronchioles.

   b. decrease inflammation in the bronchioles.

   c. break down mucoproteins in the airways that block airflow.

   d. stop the breakdown of the mast cell.

5. When albuterol (Proventil) is administered by inhalation, relief of symptoms should occur within

   a. 30 seconds.

   b. 1 hour.

   c. 30 minutes.

   d. 5 minutes.

6. Adverse effects associated with the use of albuterol (Proventil) include

   a. bradycardia and sedation.

   b. tachycardia and palpitations.

   c. constipation and bradycardia.

   d. sedation and constipation.

7. Ipratropium bromide (Atrovent) works by

   a. stimulating the action of the sympathetic nervous system.

   b. blocking the action of the sympathetic nervous system.

   c. stimulating the action of the parasympathetic nervous system.

   d. blocking the action of the parasympathetic nervous system.

8. Adverse effects of inhaled ipratropium bromide (Atrovent) include

   a. paradoxic acute bronchospasm.

   b. bronchodilation.

   c. tachycardia.

   d. headache.

9. In general, ipratropium bromide (Atrovent) should be used

   a. every 2 hours as needed.

   b. 3 to 4 times a day.

   c. once a day.

   d. not more than twice a day.

10. Theophylline (Theo-Dur) works by

    a. stimulating the sympathetic nervous system.

    b. blocking the rupture of a mast cell.

    c. directly affecting the smooth muscle of the respiratory tract.

    d. blocking the action of the parasympathetic nervous system.

11. The optimal therapeutic range for theophylline (Theo-Dur) is

    a. 10 to 20 mcg/mL.

    b. 30 to 35 mcg/mL.

    c. 2 to 5 mcg/mL.

    d. 20 to 25 mcg/mL.

12. Which of the following statements concerning theophylline (Theo-Dur) therapy is correct?

    a. There are very few drug–drug interactions with theophylline.

    b. Although there are many drug–drug interactions with theophylline, they are minor and require no special intervention.

    c. There are many drug–drug interactions with theophylline that may require dosage changes.

    d. CNS adverse effects rarely occur with theophylline.

13. Patients taking theophylline (Theo-Dur) should avoid large amounts of

    a. milk.

    b. charcoal-broiled beef.

    c. chicken.

    d. green leafy vegetables.

14. Flunisolide (Aerobid) works by
    a. inhibiting the production of leukotrienes and prostaglandins.
    b. decreasing the activity of the inflammatory cells.
    c. enhancing the responsiveness of beta receptors in airway smooth muscle.
    d. all of the above.

15. Flunisolide (Aerobid) should be given cautiously to patients with
    a. diabetes mellitus.
    b. hypotension.
    c. active infection of the respiratory system.
    d. hypothyroidism.

16. Which of the following statements concerning flunisolide (Aerobid) therapy is correct?
    a. There are very few drug–drug interactions with flunisolide.
    b. Although there are many drug–drug interactions with flunisolide, they are minor and require no special intervention.
    c. There are many drug–drug interactions with flunisolide that may require dosage changes.
    d. CNS adverse effects rarely occur with flunisolide.

17. Cromolyn sodium (Intal) works by
    a. blocking the action of the sympathetic nervous system.
    b. blocking the action of the parasympathetic nervous system.
    c. bronchodilation.
    d. preventing the release of chemicals that stimulate the inflammatory process.

18. Cromolyn sodium (Intal) is contraindicated for patients
    a. with hepatotoxicity.
    b. having an acute asthma attack.
    c. with nephrotoxicity.
    d. with chronic asthma.

19. Which of the following statements concerning cromolyn sodium (Intal) therapy is correct?
    a. There are no drug–drug interactions with cromolyn.
    b. Although there are many drug–drug interactions with cromolyn, they are minor and require no special intervention.
    c. There are many drug–drug interactions with cromolyn that may require dosage changes.
    d. CNS adverse effects rarely occur with cromolyn.

20. Zafirlukast (Accolate) works by
    a. blocking the rupture of a mast cell.
    b. blocking leukotriene receptor sites.
    c. blocking the action of the sympathetic nervous system.
    d. blocking the action of the parasympathetic nervous system.

21. Serious adverse effects to zafirlukast (Accolate) therapy include
    a. CNS obtundation.
    b. kidney failure.
    c. hepatic failure.
    d. respiratory depression.

22. Zafirlukast should not be given to children younger than
    a. 18 years.
    b. 5 years.
    c. 12 years.
    d. 10 years.

23. Which of the following drugs is indicated for treatment of an acute asthma attack?
    a. flunisolide (Aerobid)
    b. zafirlukast (Accolate)
    c. ipratropium bromide (Atrovent)
    d. albuterol (Proventil)

24. The most serious adverse effect associated with omalizumab (Xolair) is
    a. neoplasm.
    b. cardiac toxicity.
    c. neurotoxicity.
    d. respiratory depression.

CORE PATIENT VARIABLES: PATIENTS, PLEASE

Multiple Choice

Circle the option that best answers the question or completes the statement.

1. Your 7-year-old patient has cystic fibrosis and is receiving acetylcysteine therapy. Before the therapy, you should anticipate the need for
   a. flunisolide (Aerobid).
   b. zafirlukast (Accolate).
   c. ipratropium bromide (Atrovent).
   d. albuterol (Proventil).

2. Which of the following patients should be closely monitored when using IV acetylcysteine (Mucomyst)?
   a. Susan, with a history of asthma
   b. Sean, with a history of chronic hepatitis C
   c. Nancy, with a history of hypothyroidism
   d. Ben, with a history of hypertension

3. Your 16-year-old patient received a diagnosis of asthma at the age of 11 years. The patient uses an albuterol (Proventil) inhaler. The patient comes to the clinic today and states, "This inhaler is worthless. I have to use it every 2 hours." With your knowledge of this drug, you suspect the patient may be
   a. noncompliant.
   b. experiencing rebound bronchoconstriction.
   c. experiencing addiction.
   d. smoking.

4. Your 27-year-old patient comes to the clinic for renewal of a prescription for albuterol (Proventil). She states that the drug works well, but she can feel her heart race, cannot sleep, and feels "wired" all the time. Which of the following core patient variables is important to assess at this time?
   a. health status
   b. culture
   c. lifespan and gender
   d. diet, lifestyle, and habits

5. Your 21-year-old patient has asthma and takes albuterol (Proventil) as needed. The patient is seen at the clinic today, and the health care provider adds ipratropium bromide (Atrovent) to the asthma regimen. It is important for you to teach this patient to use this inhaler
   a. only when the albuterol is not helping.
   b. only when the patient feels bad.
   c. twice a day, regardless of how the patient feels.
   d. twice a day, if the patient feels tightness in the chest.

6. Your 22-year-old patient has asthma and an order for ipratropium bromide (Atrovent). Before administration, you should assess for allergies to
   a. eggs.
   b. milk.
   c. pasta.
   d. legumes.

7. Your 42-year-old patient has asthma and takes oral theophylline. The patient states, "I hate those pills. I'm up all night and nervous." Which of the following interventions would be most helpful to this patient?
   a. Administer the medication every other day.
   b. Contact the health care provider for an order for an inhaled steroid.
   c. Give the theophylline with milk.
   d. Break the pill in half and give each half 2 hours apart.

8. Despite a long history of asthma, your patient continues to smoke a pack of cigarettes per day. During theophylline therapy, you would expect to administer
   a. a higher dose of theophylline.
   b. a lower dose of theophylline.
   c. a dose that would be the same as that for a nonsmoker.

9. Patient teaching for patients receiving inhaled steroids should include:
   a. "Rinse your mouth after use to avoid adverse effects."
   b. "Drink a glass of milk immediately after using your inhaler."
   c. "Use your inhaler when you have tightness in your chest."
   d. "Drink lots of water during the day."

10. Your patient has exercise-induced asthma and the health care provider has just prescribed cromolyn sodium (Intal). Patient education should include instructions to

    a. use the inhaler at the first sign of an acute attack.

    b. use the inhaler only on days that the patient expects symptoms.

    c. use the inhaler 15 to 20 minutes before participating in exercise.

    d. use the inhaler 4 times a day, regardless of how the patient feels.

11. Your patient has severe persistent asthma that is not controlled by inhaled steroids. Which of the following should be documented before initiation of omalizumab (Xolair) therapy?

    a. adequate iron stores

    b. normal renal and hepatic function

    c. negative skin test for TB

    d. positive skin test for perennial allergens

12. Your patient has asthma and uses albuterol (Proventil), ipratropium bromide (Atrovent), and beclomethasone dipropionate (Beclovent) inhalers. The patient comes to the clinic for a routine checkup and states, "I can never remember which of these I should take first." Which of the following statements is most appropriate in response?

    a. "It really does not matter; just be sure to take them all 4 times a day."

    b. "Use the albuterol first. That will help the other two disperse further into your lungs."

    c. "Take the ipratropium first and then rinse your mouth. The other two can follow."

    d. "Use the beclomethasone first and then rinse your mouth. Take the ipratropium second and the albuterol last."

NURSING MANAGEMENT: EVERY GOOD NURSE SHOULD …

Multiple Choice

Circle the option that best answers the question or completes the statement.

1. You are the nurse providing a nebulizer treatment of acetylcysteine for a patient with bilateral lower lobe pneumonia. Which of the following should you remember while administering drug therapy and caring for the patient?

    a. Keep diluted acetylcysteine at room temperature.

    b. The patient should avoid coughing after drug therapy.

    c. Nebulization of the drug initially produces a sweet smell.

    d. A sticky residue may form on the patient's face from therapy.

2. A patient has been started on an IV drip of aminophylline, a xanthine bronchodilator, for an acute COPD exacerbation. Which of the following should be included in the nursing care of this patient while he receives IV aminophylline?

    a. Assess breath sounds every 2 to 4 hours.

    b. Assess for insomnia, tachycardia, and irritability.

    c. Inform him that he will have blood drawn regularly while taking the drug.

    d. all of the above

    e. none of the above

3. A patient with asthma has been prescribed zafirlukast (a mast cell stabilizer), beclomethasone (a glucocorticoid steroid) metered-dose inhaler, and albuterol (a beta-2 agonist) metered-dose inhaler. The patient says, "Why do I need three medications, including two inhalers? Can't I just take one pill?" Patient education should include

    a. the drugs work in different ways to provide better, more complete treatment.

    b. the zafirlukast and the beclomethasone work to prevent asthmatic attacks, and the albuterol works to provide quick relief of asthmatic attacks.

    c. giving beclomethasone and albuterol by inhalers helps to reduce their adverse effects.

    d. all of the above.

    e. none of the above.

4. A female patient has been prescribed cromolyn sodium as part of the treatment for her asthma. She has a history of irregular menstrual periods and lactose intolerance. What teaching does this patient need regarding the cromolyn sodium?

   a. Contact the provider if nausea, bloating, or abdominal cramps occur while taking this drug.

   b. Use the inhaler when an asthmatic attack occurs.

   c. Use the inhaler by first inhaling deeply and then triggering the inhaler to release a dose.

   d. all of the above

   e. none of the above

5. Your patient begins a regimen of oral theophylline. In your patient education, you'll need to tell this patient that he needs to avoid, or limit, the intake of which of these favorite foods and beverages?

   a. lemon meringue pie (eats once every 4 or 5 months)

   b. fettuccine alfredo (eats once every 6 weeks to 2 months)

   c. iced tea (drinks daily)

   d. Sprite soda (drinks daily)

   e. Cheerios cereal (eats 5 or 6 days in a row every 3 months)

6. A patient returns for a checkup after beginning a regimen of zafirlukast for asthma. Which of these findings would alarm you, the nurse, the most?

   a. absence of wheezing

   b. mild headache

   c. whites of the eyes are yellowed

   d. upset stomach

CASE STUDY

An asthmatic patient with a history of smoking one half pack of cigarettes a day is seen in the outpatient department and given a prescription for theophylline, a bronchodilator, to help control his asthma. The patient's serum theophylline level after 1 week on the drug is checked, and it is 15 mcg/mL, which is within the therapeutic range. The patient is told to continue taking this dose but to stop smoking. The patient returns to the clinic for a visit 6 weeks after starting the theophylline regimen. The serum theophylline level is now 25 mcg/mL, which is above the therapeutic range. The patient says to you, "I gave up smoking like they told me, but, boy, now I feel rotten. I have a headache all the time, and I can't sleep. I thought giving up smoking would make me feel better, not worse."

1. What explanations may account for this patient's complaints?

2. What actions might be necessary to correct these complaints?

CRITICAL THINKING CHALLENGE

The patient described above is stabilized on theophylline. Nine months later, he is hospitalized for pneumonia and ordered 400 mg ciprofloxacin IV every 12 hours as treatment. The patient continues to receive the same dose of theophylline. On the third day of treatment with the ciprofloxacin, the nurse caring for this patient notes that he is very irritable, compared with his mood previously. The patient also is experiencing diarrhea and some nausea.

1. What do you think might be causing these problems?

2. What lab work is needed to confirm your assessment?

CHAPTER **50**

Drugs Affecting the Upper Gastrointestinal Tract

TOP TEN THINGS TO KNOW ABOUT DRUGS AFFECTING THE UPPER GASTROINTESTINAL TRACT

1. Peptic ulcers are caused by the bacteria *Helicobacter pylori*, not by smoking, caffeine use, or stress. To eradicate *H. pylori*, a combination of antibiotics is used, in combination with a proton pump inhibitor, or possibly with an H$_2$ receptor antagonist.

2. Omeprazole is a proton pump inhibitor used in the treatment of duodenal ulcers associated with *H. pylori*, and for the treatment of heartburn and other symptoms of gastroesophageal reflux disease (GERD). Omeprazole suppresses the last phase of gastric acid production. In the elderly, the action of PPIs (raising the pH) decreases the absorption of calcium, thus there is an increased risk for fractures, especially of the hip. Teach the patient to take omeprazole before meals, for the entire time prescribed, and not to crush or chew the medicine.

3. Ranitidine, an H$_2$ receptor antagonist, blocks histamine action at the parietal cells in the stomach, thus inhibiting all phases of gastric acid secretion. Ranitidine inhibits both daytime and nocturnal basal gastric acid secretions, as well as gastric acid secretion stimulated by food, betazole, and pentagastrin. It is used in treating the symptoms of active duodenal ulcers, benign gastric ulcers, GERD, pathologic hypersecretory conditions, endoscopically diagnosed erosive esophagitis, and as maintenance therapy to promote healing of erosive esophagitis. Ranitidine is available in prescription and over-the-counter (OTC) formulas.

4. Ranitidine is generally well tolerated. Administer intravenous ranitidine therapy slowly to prevent hypotension and cardiac arrhythmias. Teach the patient to take the drug orally exactly as directed for the entire course of therapy; symptoms disappear before the ulcer will totally heal.

5. Antacids are base salts that increase gastric pH. They relieve symptoms of hyperacidity, GERD, and the pain caused by duodenal ulcers. All antacids are closely related and used in various combinations. Aluminum hydroxide with magnesium hydroxide, like other antacids, interacts with many other drugs and may affect their pharmacokinetics and therapeutic effect. Give such agents 2 hours after other drugs to prevent interactions. Assess patients for the use of OTC antacids.

6. Aluminum antacids cause constipation, and magnesium antacids cause diarrhea. The combination of the two usually has no effect. Avoid using aluminum hydroxide with magnesium hydroxide (or other magnesium antacids) in patients with chronic renal failure; magnesium toxicity may occur. Aluminum carbonate is used in chronic renal failure because it binds with phosphorus and reduces hyperphosphatemia.

7. Gastrointestinal (GI) stimulants, such as metoclopramide, apparently increase the effect of acetylcholine in the GI tract, increasing peristalsis and gastric emptying, without stimulating gastric, pancreatic, or gallbladder secretions. Metoclopramide also is a dopamine receptor antagonist that produces antiemetic effects. It is used to treat diabetic gastroparesis and symptoms of GERD and to prevent nausea and vomiting after surgery and during chemotherapy. Serious adverse effects, related to the dopamine-blocking effects, are not common but include depression, extrapyramidal symptoms, Parkinson-like symptoms, and tardive dyskinesia.

8. Digestive enzymes such as pancrelipase are a replacement for the body's intrinsic enzymes when the body produces too little (e.g., cystic fibrosis, chronic pancreatitis, after pancreatectomy). Administer pancrelipase with meals.

9. Orlistat inhibits the digestive enzyme lipase; this decreases the absorption of digested fat. Orlistat is used in the management of obesity in addition to

a weight-loss diet. GI adverse effects are common. Teach the patient to take orlistat with every meal that has fat in it; no dose should be taken if a meal is skipped or if it has no fat in it.

10. Ondansetron is a selective serotonin receptor antagonist (5-HT$_3$ receptor antagonist). It blocks stimulation of special serotonin receptors in the chemoreceptor trigger zone (CTZ), preventing nausea and vomiting. Ondansetron is used to prevent the nausea and vomiting associated with chemotherapy and after surgery when nausea and vomiting must be avoided. Ondansetron should be administered before chemotherapy or induction into anesthesia.

KEY TERMS

Crossword Puzzle

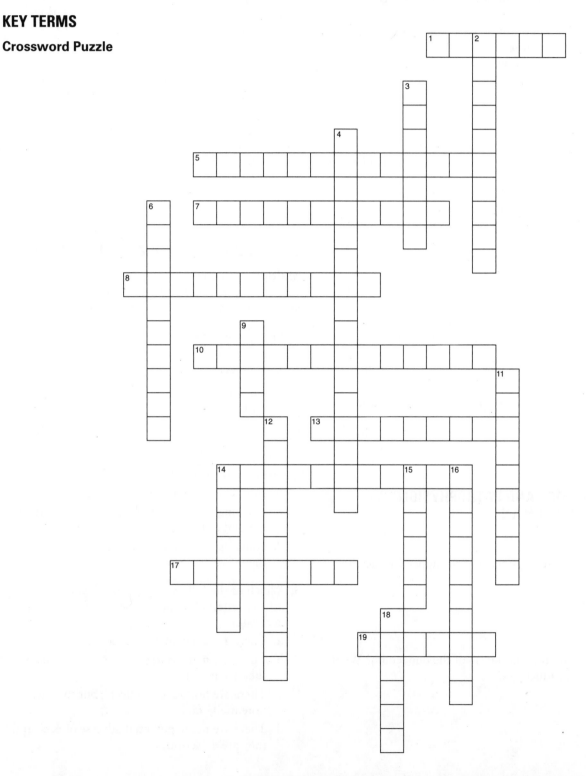

ACROSS

1. Type of ulcer that erodes of all layers of the wall of the stomach or duodenum
5. Stomach acid washes through esophagus into the mouth
7. Drugs that inhibit vomiting
8. Waves of alternate circular contraction and relaxation of the intestine by which the contents are propelled onward
10. Stimulation of this trigger zone of the brain results in vomiting
13. Difficulty swallowing
14. Vomiting of blood
17. Part of the small intestine
19. Dark tarry stools

DOWN

2. Drug that increases the effect of acetylcholine on the GI system
3. Drugs that stimulate vomiting
4. Responsible for the breakdown of food
6. Sudden appearance of a slightly sour or salty fluid in the mouth
9. Characterized by heartburn, regurgitation, dysphagia, and waterbrash
11. Burning sensation that rises from the stomach, up the chest towards the neck
12. Located in the medulla of the brain
14. Bacterial organism found in 90% of patients with ulcers
15. Type of ulcer that occurs with critically ill patients
16. Drugs that increase the transit time of gastric contents
18. Upward movement of gastric juices into the esophagus

PHYSIOLOGY AND PATHOPHYSIOLOGY: THE BODY HUMAN

Essay

1. Name the components of the upper GI tract.

2. What are the four layers of the duodenum? What are their functions?

3. Name the cells in the stomach responsible for the production of "gastric juice."

4. What part of the autonomic nervous system (ANS) stimulates the production of gastric secretions?

5. Name the pancreatic enzymes. What are their functions?

CORE DRUG KNOWLEDGE: JUST THE FACTS

Multiple Choice

Circle the option that best answers the question or completes the statement.

1. Omeprazole (Prilosec) is used in the management of
   a. diarrhea.
   b. constipation.
   c. GERD.
   d. nausea.

2. Omeprazole (Prilosec) works by
   a. neutralizing gastric acid.
   b. suppressing the $H^+/K^+ATPase$ enzyme system.
   c. blocking histamine at the H_2 receptor site of parietal cells.
   d. adhering to the ulcer lesions and protecting them from stomach acids.

3. Which of the following statements concerning adverse effects to omeprazole (Prilosec) therapy is accurate?
   a. There are a few minor adverse effects.
   b. There are many potential adverse effects, but they are minor.
   c. There are few adverse effects, but they are potentially fatal.
   d. There are many potential adverse effects, and they are all serious.

4. Sucralfate (Carafate) works by
   a. neutralizing gastric acid.
   b. suppressing the H^+/K^+ ATPase enzyme system.
   c. blocking histamine at the H_2 receptor site of parietal cells.
   d. adhering to the ulcer lesions and protecting them from stomach acids.

5. Ranitidine (Zantac) is used in the management of
   a. nausea and vomiting.
   b. diarrhea.
   c. peptic and duodenal ulcers.
   d. constipation.

6. Ranitidine (Zantac) works by
   a. neutralizing gastric acid.
   b. suppressing the H^+/K^+ ATPase enzyme system.
   c. blocking histamine at the H_2 receptor site of parietal cells.
   d. adhering to the ulcer lesions and protecting them from stomach acids.

7. Which of the following statements concerning potential adverse effects of ranitidine (Zantac) therapy is accurate?
   a. There are few potential adverse effects, and they are minor.
   b. There are few potential adverse effects, but they are all serious.
   c. There are many potential adverse effects, and they are all minor.
   d. There are many potential adverse effects, and some of them are serious.

8. Which of the following statements concerning potential drug–drug interactions during ranitidine (Zantac) therapy is accurate?
   a. There are a few potential drug–drug interactions that are not significant.
   b. There are many potential drug–drug interactions, but they are not significant.
   c. There are a few potential drug–drug interactions, and they are very significant.
   d. There are many potential drug–drug interactions, and many are very significant.

9. Misoprostol (Cytotec) is used to
   a. prevent gastric ulcer disease.
   b. treat gastric ulcer disease.
   c. prevent GERD.
   d. treat GERD.

10. Which of the following drugs is classified as an antacid?
    a. ranitidine (Zantac)
    b. misoprostol (Cytotec)
    c. sucralfate (Carafate)
    d. aluminum hydroxide

11. Which of the following adverse effects may occur with the use of aluminum-based antacids?
    a. diarrhea
    b. constipation
    c. anemia
    d. peptic ulceration

12. When taken after meals, aluminum- and magnesium-based antacids should be effective for approximately
    a. 30 to 60 minutes.
    b. 3 hours.
    c. 6 hours.
    d. 24 hours.

13. What is a major difference between aluminum hydroxide and sodium bicarbonate?
    a. There is no difference.
    b. Aluminum hydroxide may be systemically absorbed, resulting in metabolic alkalosis.
    c. Sodium bicarbonate may be systemically absorbed, resulting in metabolic alkalosis.
    d. Sodium bicarbonate has less acid rebound than does aluminum hydroxide.

14. Metoclopramide (Reglan) is effective in the treatment of
    a. peptic ulcers.
    b. duodenal ulcers.
    c. diabetic gastroparesis.
    d. diarrhea.

15. Which of the following statements concerning potential drug–drug interactions of metoclopramide (Reglan) is accurate?

    a. There are only a few potential drug–drug interactions.

    b. There are many drug–drug interactions because of its ability to disrupt the metabolism of many drugs.

    c. There are many drug–drug interactions because of its ability to disrupt the absorption of many drugs.

    d. There are many drug–drug interactions because of its ability to disrupt the excretion of many drugs.

16. During metoclopramide (Reglan) therapy, elderly females have an increased risk for

    a. fatigue.

    b. tardive dyskinesia.

    c. mental depression.

    d. restlessness.

17. Which of the following drugs would be an effective replacement for digestive enzymes?

    a. pancrelipase (Pancrease, Viokase)

    b. sucralfate (Carafate)

    c. ranititine (Zantac)

    d. metoclopramide (Reglan)

18. Contraindications to the administration of pancrelipase (Pancrease, Viokase) include an allergy to

    a. sulfa.

    b. dairy products.

    c. pork.

    d. seafood.

19. Orlistat (Xenical) is used in the management of

    a. diabetes.

    b. pancreatic insufficiency.

    c. peptic ulcer disease.

    d. morbid obesity.

20. Adverse effects to orlistat (Xenical) therapy usually affect the _____ system.

    a. CNS

    b. GI

    c. cardiovascular

    d. respiratory

21. Ondansetron (Zofran) is used to prevent

    a. morbid obesity.

    b. peptic ulcer disease.

    c. GERD.

    d. nausea and vomiting.

22. Which of the following statements concerning the potential adverse effects of ondansetron (Zofran) is accurate?

    a. There are only a few potential adverse effects, and they are all serious.

    b. There are many potential adverse effects, and a few are serious.

    c. There are only a few potential adverse effects, and they are minor.

    d. There are many potential adverse effects, and they are minor.

CORE PATIENT VARIABLES: PATIENTS, PLEASE

Multiple Choice

Circle the option that best answers the question or completes the statement.

1. Your 55-year-old patient comes to the clinic today for renewal of a prescription for omeprazole (Prilosec). The patient states, "This drug really works for me. I'm concerned about what will happen when I reach the time limit for taking it. What will they do for me then?" What is your best response?

    a. "That's a question you need to ask the nurse practitioner."

    b. "You will have to go back to using antacids as needed."

    c. "You can take a combination of antacids and sucralfate (Carafate)."

    d. "Because your condition is chronic, you should be able to stay on this medication indefinitely."

2. Your patient has a duodenal ulcer and takes sucralfate (Carafate). The patient states, "I still have gastric discomfort. Can I take an antacid as well?" The most appropriate response would be:

   a. "Sure, that's no problem."

   b. "You can take the antacid, but you will probably have a real problem with constipation."

   c. "You can take the antacid, but it's important to take it at least 30 minutes after the sucralfate."

   d. "No, that would be two drugs that are increasing the pH, and that would be dangerous."

3. Your patient has a hip fracture and is scheduled for surgery in the morning. You note an order for ranitidine (Zantac) but are unable to find a history of GERD or ulcers. This medication is being given to prevent

   a. stress ulcers.

   c. constipation.

   b. diarrhea.

   d. vomiting.

4. Your patient has GERD and takes ranitidine (Zantac). The patient states, "I still have gastric discomfort. Can I take an antacid as well?" Which of the following responses is correct?

   a. "No, that would be two drugs that are decreasing the pH and that would be dangerous."

   b. "You can take the antacid, but you will probably have a real problem with diarrhea."

   c. "Sure, that's no problem."

   d. "You can take the antacid, but it's important to take it at least 2 hours after the ranitidine."

5. Which of the following drugs would be an *absolute* contraindication for your patient's peptic ulcer during pregnancy?

   a. aluminum hydroxide

   b. misoprostol (Cytotec)

   c. cimetidine (Tagamet)

   d. magnesium hydroxide

6. A patient calls the clinic and states, "My 14-year-old son had an upset stomach after eating spicy food. I gave him an antacid. How soon will it work?" What answer would you give? Within

   a. 5 minutes

   b. 3 hours

   c. 1 hour

   d. 6 hours

7. Your 50-year-old patient has chronic renal failure and remembers being told something about reading the labels on antacids but cannot remember what it was. What would you tell this patient?

   a. "Do not take an antacid that is aluminum based."

   b. "Do not take an antacid that is magnesium based."

   c. "Do not take an antacid."

   d. "Take whatever type of antacid is available."

8. Which of the following patients should refrain from metoclopramide (Reglan) therapy?

   a. Jason, with hypertension

   b. Billy, with GERD

   c. Alex, with seizure disorder

   d. Bob, with asthma

9. Your patient is taking metoclopramide (Reglan) for diabetic gastroparesis. Which of the following instructions for this patient is correct?

   a. "Take the medication 1 hour after eating."

   b. "Take the medication at bedtime."

   c. "Take the medication 30 minutes before meals."

   d. "Take the medication 2 hours before meals."

10. Your patient is receiving chemotherapy for breast cancer. To minimize the adverse effects of chemotherapy, you should administer metoclopramide (Reglan)

    a. IV 30 minutes before chemotherapy.

    b. IM at bedtime.

    c. PO before each meal.

    d. IV 30 minutes after chemotherapy.

11. Your 12-year-old patient is receiving IV metoclopramide (Reglan). You note involuntary movements of the limbs, facial grimacing, and rhythmic protrusion of the tongue. You suspect the patient is experiencing

    a. parkinsonism.

    b. tardive dyskinesia.

    c. overdose.

    d. extrapyramidal effects.

12. Your patient is hospitalized for acute pancreatitis. At home, the patient takes pancrelipase. The patient states, "I'm worried that I'm not getting my pancrelipase. Do you know why?" What is your best response?

    a. "I'm not sure, but I will ask the doctor."

    b. "Pancrelipase should not be given until after your acute pancreatitis has subsided."

    c. "I'll get an order for it right away."

    d. "I'm sure the doctor knows what he is doing."

13. Your patient takes pancrelipase. The patient also takes albuterol for asthma. What instructions should you give to this patient?

    a. "Do not use your albuterol inhaler within 30 minutes of taking pancrelipase."

    b. "Be careful not to inhale the pancrelipase because it may trigger an asthma attack."

    c. "Use your inhaler just before taking pancrelipase."

    d. all of the above

14. Your patient has type 2 diabetes caused by morbid obesity. The patient has been prescribed orlistat (Xenical). After 6 weeks, the patient has lost 15 pounds. You anticipate that the patient's diabetic medication dose may need to be

    a. increased.

    b. decreased.

    c. left alone.

15. Patient education for patients receiving orlistat (Xenical) needs to include instructions to

    a. take your vitamins 1 hour before or 4 hours after a meal.

    b. take your vitamins with meals.

    c. increase intake of fats.

    d. increase intake of cholesterol-rich foods.

16. Your patient has breast cancer and is receiving radiation therapy. The patient has an order for ondansetron (Zofran). In this situation, how should ondansetron be administered?

    a. IV 30 minutes before the procedure

    b. PO 15 minutes before the procedure

    c. IV 1 to 2 hours before the procedure

    d. PO 1 to 2 hours before the procedure

NURSING MANAGEMENT: EVERY GOOD NURSE SHOULD ...

Multiple Choice

Circle the option that best answers the question or completes the statement.

1. A patient is to start taking liquid aluminum hydroxide with magnesium hydroxide to treat recurrent esophageal reflux. To maximize the therapeutic effect of the drug therapy, the nurse should teach the patient to

    a. shake the bottle well before measuring the dose.

    b. administer 1 hour before meals.

    c. mix the drug with water before administering.

    d. do all of the above.

    e. do none of the above.

2. A patient with GERD is to receive 30 mL of aluminum hydroxide with magnesium hydroxide orally every 4 hours while awake and ranitidine, an H_2 receptor antagonist, 800 mg orally twice a day. To maximize therapeutic or minimize adverse effects, the nurse should

    a. stagger doses of the two drugs so they are given 2 hours apart.

    b. give the ranitidine immediately before meals and the aluminum hydroxide with magnesium hydroxide immediately after meals.

    c. crush the ranitidine and mix with the aluminum hydroxide with magnesium hydroxide.

    d. do all of the above.

    e. do none of the above.

3. Your patient had abdominal surgery 2 days ago. He is now experiencing nausea and vomiting every time he eats. He begins taking metoclopramide 10 mg orally 3x/day. For effective nursing management of this drug therapy, you should

    a. administer the metoclopramide 30 minutes before each meal.

    b. monitor the patient for depression while he is taking this drug.

    c. caution the patient that the drug may cause drowsiness or fatigue.

    d. do all of the above.

    e. do none of the above.

4. A 1½-year-old child receives a diagnosis of cystic fibrosis and is to begin taking pancrelipase. What teaching would be important for this child's parents?

   a. The drug should be administered on an empty stomach.

   b. They should avoid inhaling the powdered drug.

   c. Steatorrhea stools are an adverse effect of the drug.

   d. The drug should be taken once a day.

5. Your patient has a gastric ulcer and is to begin a combined drug therapy of amoxicillin, metronidazole, and omeprazole, a proton pump inhibitor. The patient is known to be allergic to salicylates. The patient says, "Are all these medicines really necessary? I never heard of taking antibiotics for an ulcer. I thought you took Maalox." As his nurse, your best response to him is:

   a. "Infections of the stomach frequently occur secondary to gastric ulcers; all three drugs are needed to treat the infection."

   b. "The antibiotics are to prevent an infection; the omeprazole is to treat the gastric ulcer."

   c. "*H. pylori* organisms are normally responsible for gastric ulcers; the antibiotics will eradicate the organisms. The omeprazole decreases gastric acid, relieving pain and helping to eradicate the *H. pylori* organisms."

   d. "*H. pylori* organisms can multiply after a gastric ulcer is formed. The antibiotics prevent infection from *H. pylori*. The omeprazole decreases pain from the gastric ulcer."

6. You are caring for a 66-year-old patient who has been hospitalized for a GI bleed. The patient is being discharged home with a prescription for omeprazole (Prilosec). Which of the following should be included in your patient teaching?

   a. "You will need to return to the clinic daily for a complete blood count until it returns to normal."

   b. "You should supplement your diet with calcium citrate."

   c. "You should increase your intake of milk."

   d. "Be sure to take an antacid at the same time every day if you are still experiencing abdominal discomfort."

7. When performing a nursing assessment, which of these observations would be the most significant finding of a patient who is taking omeprazole (Prilosec)?

   a. decreased bowel sounds

   b. subnormal temperature

   c. low blood pressure

   d. crackles in the lungs

8. Your patient has been prescribed orlistat to assist in weight loss. You know from taking a diet history that this patient often skips breakfast, but has a snack, usually from the vending machine at work, at 4 PM. Currently, about 40% of the patient's daily calories come from fat. Which of the following would you include in your teaching?

   a. Take the orlistat in the morning, at noon, and at dinnertime.

   b. Divide your fat intake evenly among the meals you eat.

   c. Keep the same amount of fat in your diet as you have now.

   d. This medication reduces your need for exercise.

9. Your patient is to receive IV ondansetron to prevent nausea and vomiting from chemotherapy. To maximize the therapeutic effect from the ondansetron, you should

   a. give the drug 30 minutes before the start of chemotherapy.

   b. administer the drug quickly via IV push.

   c. avoid redosing after chemotherapy.

   d. do all of the above.

   e. do none of the above.

CASE STUDY

A patient with a pathologic hypersecretory condition has begun taking ranitidine, an H₂ receptor antagonist. He also smokes one pack of cigarettes per day and drinks two gin and tonics every night before dinner.

What teaching would be appropriate and relevant to the ranitidine drug therapy?

CRITICAL THINKING CHALLENGE

The patient described above returns to the clinic for follow-up in 3 weeks and appears to be doing well. The patient continues taking the ranitidine for another 3 weeks. When the patient returns to the clinic this time, he reports confusion, headaches, and dizziness.

1. What questions should you ask to help determine the cause of these adverse effects?

2. Are there any lab tests that would assist you to fully assess this patient and determine the cause of these problems?

CHAPTER 51

Drugs Affecting the Lower Gastrointestinal Tract

TOP TEN THINGS TO KNOW ABOUT DRUGS AFFECTING THE LOWER GASTROINTESTINAL TRACT

1. Simethicone, an antiflatulent, changes the surface tension of gas bubbles so they can be passed more easily. It is not systemically absorbed. Administer after meals. Tablets should be chewed well.

2. Diphenoxylate HCl with atropine sulfate, an antidiarrheal, acts on the smooth muscle of the intestine to slow intestinal motility, prolong transit time, and promote reabsorption of fluid. Diphenoxylate HCl is similar to a narcotic in structure; the dose is not high enough to provide pain relief. Atropine, an anticholinergic, is added to discourage deliberate abuse. Locally acting antidiarrheals, such as kaolin, pectin, and bismuth salicylate, are sold over the counter. They are commonly used, but their efficacy is not well established.

3. Laxatives are used to treat constipation. They are for short-term use. Laxatives are classified as: saline, hyperosmotics, stimulants, and bulk-forming. Laxatives are contraindicated in patients who have severe abdominal pain that has not been diagnosed, are nauseated and vomiting, or have a bowel obstruction.

4. Magnesium hydroxide is a saline laxative. It attracts and retains water in the large intestine, resulting in an increase in peristalsis and a bowel movement. Repeated use may cause fluid and electrolyte imbalance. It is also used as an antacid. Avoid use in patients with renal failure because the patient may experience significant hypermagnesemia.

5. Lactulose, a hyperosmolar laxative, pulls water into the colon like magnesium sulfate. In the colon, it is metabolized into acids and carbon dioxide. The acids also pull ammonia into the stool; thus, lactulose is used to decrease the elevated blood ammonia levels found in hepatic coma and hepatic encephalopathy.

6. Stimulant laxatives include bisacodyl, cascara sagrada, senna, and castor oil. These drugs have a direct stimulatory effect on the intestinal mucosa or nerve plexus and increase peristalsis. Stimulant laxatives are the most frequently abused type of laxative. Chronic use may induce loss of normal bowel function and laxative dependency.

7. Bulk laxatives, such as psyllium, polycarbophil, and methylcellulose increase the bulk of the fecal material, stimulating peristalsis and evacuation. They are considered the safest type of laxative because they mimic the natural process of fecal elimination.

8. Lubricants and stool softeners alter the characteristic of the stool and allow for easier passage, but they are not laxatives. Mineral oil is a lubricant that coats the walls of the intestine and the fecal matter to ease passage of the stool. Stool softeners, such as docusate, promote the movement of water into the stool to keep the stool soft and promote easier passage. Stool softeners are used to prevent constipation, not treat it.

9. Alosetron is used in the treatment of women with diarrhea-predominant irritable bowel syndrome (IBS-D). Its use is restricted to those with severe symptoms that have not responded to other therapies. Alosetron blocks the 5-HT$_3$ receptor, resulting in decreased visceral sensation, abdominal discomfort and pain. It requires a signed patient-physician agreement because the potential adverse effect of constipation can be serious, with potentially life-threatening complications. Teach the patient to increase his or her fluid intake to at least 2,000 mL/day. Encourage the patient to read the medication guide that accompanies every refill of the drug. Other drugs used to treat IBS include antispasmotics, antidiarrheals, laxatives, and tricyclic antidepressants (depending on the type of IBS). For constipation-predominant IBS (IBS-C), lubiprostone (Amitiza), a selective chloride channel activator may be prescribed.

Tegaserod has historically been prescribed for IBS-C; however, its use is severely restricted because of its ability to induce cardiovascular events such as MI, stroke, and worsening of angina. It is approved for use in patients for whom no other treatment options are viable under a special program similar to alosetron.

10. Mesalamine is the drug of choice for inflammatory bowel disease (IBD). The action of mesalamine is unclear; however, it is thought to inhibit the cyclooxygenase and lipoxygenase pathways, thereby decreasing the production of prostaglandins, leukotrienes, and hydroxyeicosa-tetraenoic acids. It is contraindicated for patients with a hypersensitivity to sulfites, salicylates, or those with active peptic ulcer disease.

KEY TERMS

Word Search

```
F  I  D  E  F  G  L  N  O  I  T  A  P  I  T  S  N  O  C  D
L  K  H  T  F  V  Q  X  U  R  H  S  J  F  S  J  L  J  I  L
A  S  L  P  G  E  D  G  K  Q  H  Q  C  B  R  H  S  A  K  A
T  D  H  Y  N  X  C  C  Z  U  O  U  V  L  F  I  R  B  X  U
U  E  C  C  J  Y  P  A  W  N  P  I  E  Y  T  R  D  O  X  U
S  L  H  I  B  M  X  P  L  R  M  R  M  I  H  B  Q  U  G  H
C  X  N  P  W  Z  T  D  F  I  S  H  L  E  T  D  L  S  A  V
Y  M  Z  Q  S  S  F  E  K  E  M  O  A  Y  A  R  Z  X  Q  J
T  U  D  Y  I  W  O  Q  P  V  C  P  G  S  J  L  E  C  S  O
B  L  Q  G  O  Z  X  L  T  E  P  E  A  R  H  K  U  O  F  L
D  O  B  K  E  B  Y  N  V  E  N  R  L  C  R  N  W  X  L  G
X  W  T  C  A  H  D  I  R  D  C  Y  T  B  T  G  Y  F  B  P
Y  D  L  B  D  K  T  I  M  O  Y  B  S  Z  A  I  U  Y  C  X
T  M  F  C  S  A  S  Y  T  Y  I  Z  L  M  H  T  O  C  J  S
G  D  S  J  R  T  W  S  L  F  P  W  O  K  C  L  I  N  U  Q
P  B  N  E  A  C  L  F  M  W  F  H  T  G  B  D  G  R  Q  H
I  I  C  L  X  J  Q  Z  F  I  K  A  F  Q  X  Z  K  E  R  A
N  L  S  R  F  N  L  L  H  J  A  Z  T  C  M  X  S  B  I  I
U  I  L  X  N  Q  U  N  Y  R  O  T  A  M  M  A  L  F  N  I
S  D  F  L  M  X  T  M  E  S  A  E  S  I  D  N  H  O  R  C
```

Using the definitions provided, determine the key terms and locate them in the word search.

1. Wave-like muscular contraction of the intestine

2. Abbreviation for irritable bowel syndrome

3. Abbreviation for inflammatory bowel disease

4. Infrequent or incomplete passage of stool

5. Frequent, watery stools

6. Inability to pass hardened mass of feces

7. By-product of digestion that may be painful

8. Inflammatory disease characterized by inflammation extending into the deeper layers of the intestinal wall

9. Inflammatory disease of the large intestine

10. General term that includes both ulcerative colitis and Crohn disease.

11. Inflammatory disease of the large intestine in which ulcers form in the mucosa of the colon or rectum

PHYSIOLOGY AND PATHOPHYSIOLOGY: THE BODY HUMAN

Essay

1. The large intestine consists of:

2. What are the four components of the colon?

3. The defecation reflex causes:

4. In a healthy person, fecal material consists of:

5. Bacteria in the colon produce which important vitamins?

CORE DRUG KNOWLEDGE: JUST THE FACTS

Multiple Choice
Circle the option that best answers the question or completes the statement.

1. Which of the following drugs is used to decrease gas production?
   a. magnesium hydroxide
   b. simethicone (Mylicon)
   c. diphenoxylate HCl (Lomotil)
   d. docusate (Colace)

2. Which of these statements concerning the adverse effects of simethicone (Mylicon) is accurate?
   a. There are no potential adverse effects to its use.
   b. There are a few potential adverse effects, but they are minor.
   c. There are many potential adverse effects, but they are minor.
   d. There are a few potential adverse effects, and they are serious.

3. Which of the following drugs are used in the treatment of diarrhea? *Mark all that apply.*
   a. magnesium hydroxide (Milk of Magnesia)
   b. loperamide (Imodium)
   c. kaolin
   d. diphenoxylate HCl (Lomotil)

4. Diphenoxylate (Lomotil) works by
   a. decreasing the absorption of fats and carbohydrates.
   b. increasing the water absorption from the bowel.
   c. slowing intestinal motility and prolonging intestinal transit time.
   d. decreasing water absorption from the bowel.

5. Administration of diphenoxylate (Lomotil) to a patient with diarrhea caused by bacteria may result in
   a. impaction.
   b. prolongation of symptoms.
   c. headache.
   d. no known interaction.

6. Magnesium hydroxide (Milk of Magnesia) works by
   a. increasing the bulk of fecal material.
   b. stimulating peristalsis of the bowel.
   c. softening the stool for easy passage.
   d. retaining water in the intestinal lumen to increase pressure.

7. Potential adverse effects of long-term magnesium hydroxide (Milk of Magnesia) therapy include
   a. headaches.
   b. sedation.
   c. electrolyte imbalance.
   d. peptic ulcer.

8. Which of the following laxatives may also be used in the treatment of hepatic coma?
   a. magnesium hydroxide (Milk of Magnesia)
   b. polyethylene glycol-electrolyte solution
   c. lactulose (Cephulac)
   d. bisacodyl (Dulcolax)

9. What adverse effect is associated with long-term use of lubricant laxatives?
   a. headache
   b. hypertension
   c. decreased absorption of fat-soluble vitamins
   d. decreased absorption of fat and cholesterol

10. Alosetron (Lotronex) is used for patients with irritable bowel syndrome (IBS) who have (*Mark all that apply.*)
    a. not experienced response to other modalities
    b. any degree of intermittent constipation
    c. frequent bowel urgency
    d. decreased absorption of fat and cholesterol
    e. fecal incontinence

11. What common adverse effect is associated with alosetron (Lotronex)?

    a. headache

    b. hypertension

    c. constipation

    d. diarrhea

12. 5-ASA preparations such as mesalamine (Asacol) should not be given to patients with a history of allergy to

    a. sulfa.

    b. aspirin.

    c. penicillin.

    d. all of the above.

13. Infliximab (Remicade) is used primarily for

    a. diarrhea-predominant IBS.

    b. constipation-predominant IBS.

    c. ulcerative colitis.

    d. Crohn disease.

CORE PATIENT VARIABLES: PATIENTS, PLEASE

Multiple Choice

Circle the option that best answers the question or completes the statement.

1. Your patient is prescribed simethicone (Mylicon) as needed for flatus. Patient teaching should include instructions to

    a. smash the tablet and place it in food.

    b. chew the tablet thoroughly.

    c. take the medication only at bedtime.

    d. allow the suspension to separate before taking.

2. Your patient has diarrhea and is taking diphenoxylate (Lomotil). The patient also has a seizure disorder and is prescribed phenobarbital. You should monitor this patient for

    a. increased sedation.

    b. profound nausea.

    c. abdominal discomfort.

    d. headache.

3. Which of the following patients would have a high risk for atropine toxicity when taking diphenoxylate (Lomotil)?

    a. Lisa, with a history of migraine headache

    b. Susan, with Down syndrome

    c. Allison, with ulcerative colitis

    d. Francine, with peptic ulcer disease

4. Your 35-year-old patient is hospitalized for diarrhea and dehydration and prescribed diphenoxylate (Lomotil). After reviewing the patient's medical history, you note the patient has been taking Nardil, a monoamine oxidase inhibitor. You should monitor this patient for

    a. tachycardia.

    b. hypertension.

    c. fever.

    d. blood dyscrasias.

5. Your patient has frequent constipation and takes magnesium hydroxide (Milk of Magnesia). In addition, the patient takes theophylline (Theo-Dur), beclomethasone (Beclovent), and phenytoin (Dilantin). This patient should be monitored for

    a. exacerbation of asthma symptoms.

    b. theophylline toxicity.

    c. seizure activity.

    d. diarrhea.

6. Which of the following patients should refrain from using psyllium, a bulk-forming laxative, for constipation?

    a. Julie, with a mental health disorder

    b. Adam, with asthma

    c. Tom, with benign prostatic hypertrophy

    d. Dixie, with chronic heart failure

7. Your patient states, "I have constipation all the time. What type of laxative should I take?"

    a. bulk-forming

    b. saline

    c. stimulant

    d. lubricant

8. Your 17-year-old patient has irritable bowel syndrome (IBS). Which of the following drugs would you anticipate administering to this patient?

   a. simethicone (Mylicon)

   b. magnesium hydroxide (Milk of Magnesia)

   c. dicyclomine (Bentyl)

   d. kaolin

9. Your patient has severe IBS and is prescribed alosetron (Lotronex). Before administering the drug, you should assess the most recent

   a. complete blood count.

   b. electrolyte balance.

   c. liver function test.

   d. cholesterol level.

10. Your patient with IBS states, "I am so miserable. When will I know if this drug works?" What is your best response?

    a. 1 to 3 hours

    b. 4 to 6 weeks

    c. 5 days

    d. 1 week

NURSING MANAGEMENT: EVERY GOOD NURSE SHOULD …

Multiple Choice
Circle the option that best answers the question or completes the statement.

1. Which of the following should be included in patient education for simethicone, an antiflatulent?

   a. Chew tablets before swallowing.

   b. Administer before meals or 2 hours after meals.

   c. Increase dietary intake of cabbage, cucumbers, and onions.

   d. Decreased belching is expected.

2. Your patient is a 10-year-old child being treated with diphenoxylate HCl with atropine sulfate for severe diarrhea. At the beginning of your shift, you, the nurse, perform a physical assessment of this patient. You note the following findings: temperature, 100°F orally; pulse, 110 bpm; respirations, 24/minute. Suprapubic distention is noted, with tenderness to palpation. No urine output for 8 hours is recorded. Stools have decreased in frequency but still are loose. The patient is due for another dose of diphenoxylate HCl with atropine sulfate. How should you act based on these findings?

   a. Administer another dose of diphenoxylate HCl with atropine sulfate.

   b. Administer another dose of diphenoxylate HCl with atropine sulfate, acetaminophen (Tylenol), and extra fluids.

   c. Hold the next dose of diphenoxylate HCl with atropine sulfate and place an indwelling catheter in the patient to drain her bladder.

   d. Hold the next dose of diphenoxylate HCl with atropine sulfate and contact the doctor.

3. You are caring for a patient with chronic renal failure who reports being extremely constipated. You, the nurse, believe that more than one dose of a laxative may be necessary to correct the constipation. Which of the following laxatives would not be appropriate for this patient?

   a. senna (Senokot)

   b. lactulose (Cephulac)

   c. magnesium sulfate (Milk of Magnesia)

   d. bisacodyl (Dulcolax)

4. You are caring for a 75-year-old patient who reports frequent constipation. The patient asks if he should take magnesium sulfate every day to prevent constipation. The best nursing response would be

   a. "Yes, this will help you be regular in bowel patterns."

   b. "Yes, the extra magnesium will correct any dietary deficiencies."

   c. "No, magnesium sulfate is not intended for long-term use."

   d. "No, magnesium sulfate has only antacid effects."

5. Your patient has been ordered polyethylene glycol-electrolyte solution, also known as PEG-ES (GoLYTELY), before an x-ray of the lower GI tract. Teaching related to this drug therapy should include that PEG-ES will

a. prevent constipation after the x-ray.

b. induce diarrhea within 4 hours.

c. stop diarrhea within 4 hours.

d. reduce blood ammonia levels.

CASE STUDY

You are caring for a 65-year-old patient admitted to the hospital for a bleeding gastric ulcer. While hospitalized, the patient had a myocardial infarction. The patient is currently on bed rest; consuming a low-fat, bland diet; and has medication orders for docusate (Colace) daily.

What patient-related variables are relevant to the order for docusate? Why?

CRITICAL THINKING CHALLENGE

Why are patients who have had myocardial infarctions ordered docusate routinely?

CHAPTER 52

Drugs Affecting Blood Glucose Levels

TOP TEN THINGS TO KNOW ABOUT DRUGS AFFECTING BLOOD GLUCOSE LEVELS

1. All insulins manage hyperglycemia by promoting cellular glucose uptake and metabolism. Insulins vary by onset, peak, and duration of action. The standard source of insulin is now recombinant DNA, also referred to as human. Insulins are used in type 1 diabetes and sometimes in type 2 diabetes. Excessive exogenous insulin produces hypoglycemia. and insufficient exogenous insulin produces hyperglycemia. Patient teaching about insulin should include how to administer accurately, diet modifications, exercise, testing for blood glucose, storage of insulin, and disposal of used needles and syringes.

2. Regular insulin is rapid acting and short lasting. It may be used alone or in combination regimens with longer-acting insulins. All insulins are given subcutaneously (rotate injection sites serially within an anatomic location), but regular insulin may also be given intravenously. Regular insulin is used when sliding scale insulin is ordered; it can be administered via an implantable insulin pump. Aspart (NovoLog), lispro (Humalog), and glulisine (Apidra) are all rapid-acting insulins. They have a faster onset, an earlier peak, and a shorter duration of action than regular insulin. They are taken just before a meal because of their rapid onset. All can be used in implantable insulin pumps and, if the order specifies them by name, in sliding scale situations. They may be used in regimens with longer-acting insulins; however, they should not be combined with these insulins when being administered via an external insulin infusion pump. Both aspart (Novolog Mix 70/30) and lispro (Humalog Mix 75/25 or Humalog Mix 50/50) are also available in combination with protamine. This allows an immediate onset of action and an additional action that prolongs its duration; thus, in this combination they are classified as intermediate-acting insulins. *To avoid confusion, the drugs should be referred to by their generic names, not their trade names.* Exubera is the only insulin that is not given parenterally; it is inhaled. Its onset, peak, and duration are similar to rapid-acting insulins. It is contraindicated for patients with respiratory disorders such as asthma or for patients who have been smokers in the past 6 months. In 2007, the manufacturer voluntarily ceased production of Exubera in the United States because of poor sales.

3. NPH is an intermediate-acting insulin. It is cloudy in appearance because it is a suspension; roll the vial to mix carefully before withdrawing into the syringe. NPH is not used for sliding scale insulin or implantable insulin pumps. Compared with regular insulin, it has a longer time to onset and peak and a longer duration of action.

4. Insulin glargine (Lantus) and insulin detemir (Levemir) are long-acting insulins. They have several unique properties. They are clear (unlike NPH), with an onset of action and duration of action longer than those of regular insulin. They do not have a peak effect but create a relatively constant glucose-lowering effect (flat effect). They cannot be mixed with other insulins or solutions.

5. Glyburide is an oral, sulfonylurea antidiabetic drug. Used in type 2 diabetes, it stimulates insulin release and reduces glucagon levels. Glyburide also reduces the glucose output from the liver by decreasing liver glycogenolysis (breakdown of glycogen stored in liver into glucose) and gluconeogenesis (formation of glycogen from fatty acids and proteins, rather than from carbohydrates). Glyburide also increases insulin sensitivity at cellular sites. It should not be used in a patient allergic to sulfa drugs. Hypoglycemia is the most common adverse effect of sulfonylurea drugs such as glyburide, although it is usually milder than hypoglycemia associated with insulins.

6. Metformin is an oral antidiabetic used in type 2 diabetes. It is considered an "insulin sensitizer" drug. It suppresses hepatic glucose production, enhances insulin sensitivity in the muscle, and promotes glucose uptake. It requires some pancreatic insulin to work. In addition, metformin lowers triglyceride levels, total and low-density

lipoprotein (LDL) cholesterol levels, and promotes weight loss.

7. Rosiglitazone and pioglitazone are oral antidiabetics used in type 2 diabetes. Like metformin, they are considered "insulin sensitizers." However, they do not lower triglyceride levels or total or LDL cholesterol levels, and they do not promote weight loss. They lower the blood glucose levels by improving the cellular response to insulin (makes insulin have more effect on cell). They are prescribed for monotherapy or in combination with a sulfonylurea, metformin, or insulin when adequate glycemic control is not achieved.

8. Acarbose and miglitol are also oral antidiabetic drugs used in patients with type 2 diabetes and mild to moderate hyperglycemia who are at risk for hypoglycemia or lactic acidosis. They delay the digestion of carbohydrates, resulting in a smaller postprandial rise of blood glucose. Use oral glucose tablets if hypoglycemia occurs, because cane sugar found in candy and orange juice will not be absorbed because of the drug's action.

9. Exenatide (Byetta) and pramlintide (Symlin) are parenteral antidiabetic drugs used for both type 1 and type 2 diabetes. Exenatide is a synthetic incretin mimetic. By mimicking the actions of incretin hormones, it decreases blood glucose levels, helping them to return to normal. Pramlintide is a synthetic analogue of human amylin, a naturally occurring neuroendocrine hormone that contributes to glucose control during the postprandial period. In addition to their ability to decrease blood glucose levels, both drugs also inhibit glucagon secretion, slow gastric emptying time, and promote satiety with resultant weight loss.

10. Glucagon, a naturally occurring substance, is given as a drug therapy to restore consciousness in extreme hypoglycemia. It stimulates glycogenolysis in the peripheral tissues.

KEY TERMS

Crossword Puzzle

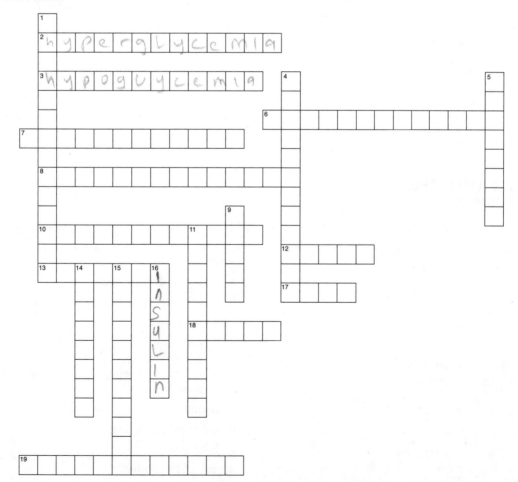

ACROSS

2. Breakdown of subcutaneous fat
3. Additional dose of insulin to correct any elevations in blood glucose
6. Elevated serum glucose level
7. Severe complication of type 1 diabetes mellitus
8. Breakdown of glycogen stored in liver into glucose
10. Another term for correctional insulin
12. Patients with this type of diabetes are insulin dependent
13. Rebound phenomenon of reactive hypoglycemia
17. Phenomena of early morning hyperglycemia
18. Patients with this type of diabetes are not insulin dependent
19. Low serum glucose

DOWN

1. Formation of glycogen from fatty acids and proteins, rather than from carbohydrates
4. Type of lab test to assess long-term glucose control
5. The insulin secretion stimulated in response to meals
9. Continuous secretion of insulin that maintains glucose homeostasis
11. Abbreviation for hyperosmolar hyperglycemic nonketotic syndrome
14. Type of diabetes caused by relative or absolute deficiency of insulin
15. Type of diabetes that occurs during pregnancy
16. Hormone that promotes glucose utilization, protein synthesis, and the formation and storage of neutral lipids

PHYSIOLOGY AND PATHOPHYSIOLOGY: THE BODY HUMAN

Essay

1. Which two hormones have the most influence on the regulation of blood glucose?

2. Identify the cells in the islets of Langerhans and the hormones they produce.

3. What are the functions of insulin?

4. What is the single most important factor influencing the rate of insulin synthesis and release?

5. Other than insulin, what other factors influence blood glucose levels?

CORE DRUG KNOWLEDGE: JUST THE FACTS

Multiple Choice
Circle the option that best answers the question or completes the statement.

1. The onset of NPH is approximately
   a. 30 to 60 minutes.
   b. 1 to 1.5 hours.
   c. 1 to 2.5 hours.
   d. 4 to 8 hours.

2. Regular insulin is effective for approximately
   a. 3 to 4 hours.
   b. 8 to 12 hours.
   c. 24 hours.
   d. more than 36 hours.

3. The peak effect of long-acting insulin glargine (Lantus) occurs approximately _____ after administration?
   a. It has no defined peak
   b. 7 to 15 hours
   c. 4 to 12 hours
   d. 2 to 4 hours

4. Which of the following types of insulin can be given intravenously?
   a. regular
   b. intermediate-acting
   c. long-acting
   d. any of the above

5. To decrease the potential for lipodystrophy, the patient should
   a. monitor glucose levels.
   b. dip urine for ketones daily.
   c. rotate injection sites.
   d. trim toenails evenly.

6. Ingestion of alcohol with insulin therapy may result in
   a. hyperglycemia.
   b. hypoglycemia.
   c. both a and b.
   d. neither a nor b.

7. Which of the following insulin preparations may be used in an insulin pump delivery system? Mark all that apply.
   a. NPH
   b. aspart
   c. regular
   d. detemir

8. Maximal effects of glyburide (DiaBeta) occur within
   a. 40 to 60 minutes.
   b. 10 to 25 minutes.
   c. 2 hours.
   d. 3 to 4 hours.

9. Sulfonylurea drugs are contraindicated for use in patients with an allergy to
   a. insulin.
   b. sulfonamides.
   c. aminoglycosides.
   d. penicillin.

10. Which of the following drugs should be used for type 2 diabetes during pregnancy?
    a. glyburide (DiaBeta)
    b. glucagon
    c. insulin
    d. rosiglitazone (Avandia)
    Oral agents are contra-indicated in pregnancy

11. Which of the following statements is correct concerning repaglinide (Prandin)?
    a. It is unsuitable for use in elderly patients.
    b. It is contraindicated for patients with renal insufficiency.
    c. It has an extremely long half-life and duration of action.
    d. It can be omitted when the patient skips a meal.

12. The effects of metformin (Glucophage) include
    a. suppression of hepatic glucose production.
    b. lowering of triglyceride levels.
    c. enhancement of insulin sensitivity.
    d. all of the above.

13. Metformin (Glucophage) should be administered
    a. with morning and evening meals.
    b. 1 hour before meals.
    c. 2 hours after meals.
    d. at bedtime.

14. Which of the following adverse effects is *specific* to metformin (Glucophage) therapy?
    a. hypoglycemia
    b. GI distress
    c. lactic acidosis
    d. diarrhea

15. Acarbose (Precose) works by
    a. sensitizing insulin receptors.
    b. decreasing carbohydrate absorption from the small intestine.
    c. increasing insulin secretion from the pancreas.
    d. decreasing hepatic production of glucose.

16. Acarbose (Precose) is contraindicated for use in patients with
    a. diverticulitis.
    b. hepatic insufficiency.
    c. anemia.
    d. chronic obstructive pulmonary disease (COPD).

17. Thiazolidinedione antiglycemics such as rosiglitazone (Avandia) work by
    a. enhancing insulin production.
    b. sensitizing insulin receptors.
    c. decreasing hepatic production of glucose.
    d. inhibiting carbohydrate absorption from the small intestine.

18. Rosiglitazone (Avandia) may be given concurrently with
    a. metformin (Glucophage).
    b. glyburide (DiaBeta).
    c. acarbose (Precose).
    d. all of the above.

19. The duration of action of glucagon is approximately
    a. 24 hours.
    b. 5 to 10 minutes.
    c. 1 to 2 hours.
    d. 6 to 12 hours.

20. Glucagon is administered via the _____ route. *Mark all that apply.*
    a. subcutaneous
    b. intramuscular
    c. intravenous
    d. oral

21. Sitagliptin (Januvia) lowers blood glucose by
    a. Protecting the endogenous incretin hormones and enhancing their actions
    b. Blocking gluconeogenesis
    c. Increasing the sensitivity of insulin receptors
    d. Blocking the uptake of carbohydrates from the intestine

22. In addition to lowering blood glucose, pramlintide (Symlin) also
    a. increases gastric emptying time.
    b. causes weight gain.
    c. promotes satiety.
    d. increases the secretion of glucagon.

Matching
Match the type of insulin with its correct duration of action.

1. ___C___ isophane (NPH)
2. ___b___ regular (Humulin R)
3. ___A___ lispro (Humalog)
4. ___d___ insulin glargine (Lantus)
5. ___c___ insulin lispro protamine (Humalog Mix 50/50)
6. ___A___ insulin aspart (NovoLog)
7. ___A___ insulin glulisine (Apidra)
8. ___d___ insulin detemir (Levemir)
9. ___C___ insulin aspart protamine (Novolog Mix 70/30)

a. Rapid acting
b. Short acting
c. Intermediate acting
d. Long acting

Matching
Match the oral agent with its appropriate class.

1. ___b___ metformin (Glucophage)
2. _____ rosiglitazone (Avandia)
3. _____ nateglinide (Starlix)
4. _____ glipizide (Glucotrol)
5. _____ tolbutamide (Orinase)
6. _____ pioglitazone (Actos)
7. _____ glyburide (DiaBeta)
8. _____ repaglinide (Prandin)
9. _____ acarbose (Precose)
10. _____ miglitol (Glyset)

a. Sulfonylurea
b. Biguanide
c. Alpha-glucosidase inhibitor
d. Thiazolidinedione
e. Meglitinide

CORE PATIENT VARIABLES: PATIENTS, PLEASE

Multiple Choice
Circle the option that best answers the question or completes the statement.

1. Your 38-year-old patient has type 1 diabetes and takes regular insulin. The patient is hospitalized for pneumonia. As you enter the patient's room, you note that the patient is trembling and tachycardic. The patient reports having a headache and feeling nervous. You suspect that this patient is experiencing
   a. hyperglycemia.
   b. hypoglycemia.
   c. hyperosmolar hyperglycemic states.
   d. none of the above.

2. Your patient has type 1 diabetes. The patient's regimen is changing to include lispro (Humalog) insulin. What instructions should be given to this patient regarding the administration of this medication? Administer the medication
   a. 1 hour before meals.
   b. 1 hour after meals.
   c. 10 to 15 minutes before a meal.
   d. only at bedtime.

3. Your 22-year-old patient with diabetes takes NPH insulin twice a day. NPH was administered to your patient at 7:30 AM. At what time is this patient *most* likely to experience a hypoglycemic episode?
   a. 8:30 to 9:00 AM
   b. 9:30 to 11:30 AM
   c. 11:30 AM to 7:30 PM
   d. 10:30 AM to 12:00 noon

4. Your patient has newly diagnosed type 1 diabetes. The patient is prescribed a combination of regular and intermediate-acting insulin. When preparing this combination, this patient should be taught to draw up which medication first?
   a. regular insulin
   b. intermediate-acting insulin
   c. it does not matter

5. Your 43-year-old patient has type 2 diabetes. The patient has taken glyburide (DiaBeta) but experiences hypoglycemia frequently. Which of the following drugs would be helpful in treating this patient's diabetes?
   a. metformin (Glucophage)
   b. regular insulin
   c. repaglinide (Prandin)
   d. tolbutamide (Tolinase)

6. Your patient takes metformin (Glucophage) for diabetes. Which of the following interventions would be necessary throughout therapy?
   a. serial CBC
   b. electrocardiogram (ECG)
   c. periodic hepatic and renal function studies
   d. arterial blood gas

7. Your patient is hospitalized for complications of a tubal ligation. She has a history of type 2 diabetes and takes acarbose (Precose). The patient is experiencing a hypoglycemic episode. Which of the following interventions would be appropriate?
   a. orange juice
   b. hard candy
   c. milk and crackers
   d. oral glucose tablet

8. Your patient has been hospitalized for brittle type 1 diabetes. Upon entering the patient's room, you find the patient unconscious, with a glucometer reading of 32. Which of the following drugs would be most appropriate to treat this?
   a. IV glucose
   b. glucagon IM
   c. diazoxide
   d. dissolved glucose tablets

9. A patient's daughter calls and tells you her mother had an insulin reaction and was found unconscious. The daughter states she gave her mother a glucagon injection 20 minutes ago, and she woke up but is still groggy and does not make sense. Which of the following instructions would you give?
   a. "Let her wake up on her own, then give her something to eat."
   b. "Place a couple of hard candies in her mouth."
   c. "Just let her sleep. She needs the rest."
   d. "Give her another injection and call the paramedics."

10. Your patient's mother reports that she has administered glucagon to her child five times in the past month. The nurse should obtain additional information regarding *(Mark all that apply)*

    a. current medications
    b. smoking or recreational drug use
    c. routine diet
    d. daily insulin use
    e. latest glycosylated hemoglobin result
    f. recent stress

11. Which of these statements, if made by a patient who takes insulin detemir would indicate a need for further teaching?

    a. "I will give myself a shot in a different place every day."
    b. "I will save money by putting both detemir and aspart in the same syringe."
    c. "I will not put it in my insulin pump."
    d. "I will check my glucose daily."

12. Your 66-year old female patient has type 2 diabetes that has not been well controlled with metformin. Today the health care provider prescribes pioglitazone (Actos). Which of the following should be included in your patient teaching?

    a. aseptic technique for subcutaneous administration
    b. separate administration of these two medications by at least 12 hours
    c. fall-proofing her home
    d. checking her blood glucose at least 4 times a day

13. When taking a history from a patient who has just been prescribed exenatide (Byetta), which of the following questions would be most important for the nurse to ask?

    a. "How long have you had diabetes?"
    b. "Do you take any other medications?"
    c. "Are you afraid of needles?"
    d. "Do you have any allergies to foods?"

14. Which of these statements, if made by a patient who is prescribed both insulin and pramlintide (Symlin), would indicate a need for further teaching?

    a. "I will wash my hands before I give myself a shot."
    b. "I will keep a supply of glucose tablets in my car."
    c. "I will combine both drugs in the same syringe."
    d. "I will stop driving my car if I feel weak or dizzy."

NURSING MANAGEMENT: EVERY GOOD NURSE SHOULD …

Decision Tree
Use this information to complete the decision tree.

Your patient has type 1 diabetes and is hospitalized for cellulitis of the left foot. His medication orders include the following:

NPH insulin 20 units SC Q AM before breakfast. Sliding scale with regular insulin SC, before meals and at bedtime:
If blood glucose is 70 to 160, give zero units.
If blood glucose is 161 to 200, give 2 units.
If blood glucose is 201 to 240, give 4 units.
If blood glucose is 241 to 280, give 6 units.
If blood glucose is 281 to 310, give 8 units.
If blood glucose is <70 or >310, contact physician.

7:30 AM blood glucose 190
Give NPH and ☐ units regular insulin

11:30 AM blood glucose 255
Give ☐ units regular insulin

2 PM patient complains of
nervousness, sweating
Recheck blood glucose
Glucose is 69

Your assessment:

Your action:

Recheck blood glucose
in ☐ minutes

Glucose now 138
Patient no longer
complains of nervousness

Your assessment:

Your action:

11:30 AM blood glucose 45, patient
confused, very hard to arouse

Your assessment:

Your action:

Blood glucose 118 at 12 noon

Your assessment:

Your action:

2 PM patient has fruity breath
Hard to arouse
Recheck blood glucose; glucose is 600

Your assessment:

Your action:

Recheck blood glucose in ☐ minutes

Blood glucose is 450; patients more alert

Your assessment:

Your action:

Recheck blood glucose in ☐ minutes;
if stable, repeat at next scheduled time

CASE STUDY

Your patient is a 60-year-old African American who
is 30 pounds over ideal body weight. The patient has
type 2 diabetes. The medical history shows an allergy
to penicillin and sulfa drugs. This patient is to start
taking metformin (Glucophage), an oral antidiabetic.

1. Why was this patient not prescribed insulin?

2. Why was this patient not started on a regimen of
   a sulfonylurea, such as glyburide?

3. What teaching is necessary for this patient?

CRITICAL THINKING CHALLENGE

The patient described above takes metformin for
1 year. The blood glucose levels have been stabilized
at 120 mg/dL. At this time, the patient cuts his right
foot, experiences an infection, and is hospitalized.
The blood glucose level now is 297 mg/dL.

   Would you expect to see any changes made in this
patient's drug therapy to control his diabetes? Why
or why not?

CHAPTER 53

Drugs Affecting Pituitary, Thyroid, Parathyroid, and Hypothalamic Function

TOP TEN THINGS TO KNOW ABOUT DRUGS AFFECTING PITUITARY, THYROID, PARATHYROID, AND HYPOTHALAMIC FUNCTION

1. Drugs given to treat disorders of the pituitary, thyroid, or parathyroid glands either supply additional hormone because the gland does not produce enough or prevent the release of additional hormone because the gland produces too much.

2. Somatropin is a recombinant-DNA formulation of growth hormone. It is used as long-term replacement therapy for children who have a growth failure because of inadequate endogenous growth hormone secretion and for those with short stature caused by Turner syndrome.

3. Desmopressin is a synthetic analogue of the naturally occurring antidiuretic hormone (ADH), also known as the hormone vasopressin. It is used to treat diabetes insipidus (a problem of excessive water loss caused by partial or total deficiency in the production or secretion of ADH). Like the naturally occurring vasopressin, ADH desmopressin interacts with V1 and V2 receptors. Stimulation of V1 receptors creates vasoconstriction. Unlike naturally occurring vasopressin, desmopressin has very few pressor effects. The stimulation of V2 receptors, found on renal tubule cells, has an antidiuretic and hemostatic response. The antidiuretic effects are from increasing the renal collecting tubules' permeability to water and resorption of water. The antidiuretic effect of desmopressin is longer acting than that from natural occurring ADH/vasopressin.

4. Patients taking desmopressin, especially young children and older adults, are at risk for water intoxication if they drink excessive fluids. Caution patients to drink only enough to quench their thirst.

5. Levothyroxine, a synthetic T_4, is used as replacement in hypothyroidism. It produces the same effects as endogenous thyroid, such as increased metabolic effects, elevating pulse and blood pressure. Treatment is usually lifelong.

6. Adverse effects of levothyroxine are usually signs of hyperthyroidism (hypertension, tachycardia, hyperreflexia, anxiety, increased sweating). If signs of hypothyroidism occur, the dose is insufficient and should be increased.

7. Methimazole is an antithyroid compound used to treat hyperthyroidism; it reduces the amount of functional thyroid tissue. Methimazole inhibits the synthesis of thyroid hormones (T_4 and T_3), so new T_3 and T_4 are not produced. Methimazole is used for palliative treatment of hyperthyroidism, as adjunct in preparation for surgery (thyroidectomy) or radioactive iodine therapy, or to manage thyrotoxic crises. Minor adverse effects such as gastrointestinal (GI) disturbance and dizziness are common. Teach the patient to eat small frequent meals or divide the daily dosage into two or three doses to minimize GI disturbances and to use safety precautions to prevent injury or accidents.

8. Low doses of iodine are needed for the formation of thyroid hormone. High doses inhibit thyroid function. Strong iodide solutions are used for preoperative suppression of the thyroid or in acute thyrotoxicosis. Radioactive iodine is used to diagnose an overactive thyroid and to destroy thyroid tissue in severe Graves disease.

9. Calcitonin, salmon is a synthesized form of naturally occurring calcitonin. It has a role in the regulation of calcium and bone metabolism. It increases the renal loss of phosphate, calcium, and sodium. It is used to prevent bone resorption in Paget disease and postmenopausal osteoporosis and in the early treatment of hypercalcemic emergencies (SC or IM only). Because of potential systemic

allergic reactions, skin testing is often done before initiation of therapy.

10. Calcitriol is a fat-soluble vitamin that increases GI absorption of calcium and increases serum calcium. It is used in the management of hypocalcemia, especially in patients receiving chronic renal dialysis. Common adverse effects are GI and central nervous system (CNS) in nature. If serum calcium levels increase too much, cardiac arrhythmias may occur. Monitor serum calcium levels.

KEY TERMS

Matching Exercise
Match the key term with its definition.

1. _____ acromegaly

2. _____ bone resorption

3. _____ cretinism

4. _____ diabetes insipidus

5. _____ gigantism

6. _____ Graves disease

7. _____ hyperthyroidism

8. _____ effector hormones

9. _____ hypothyroidism

10. _____ myxedema coma

11. _____ osmolarity

12. _____ Paget disease

13. _____ thyrotoxicosis

14. _____ thyroid crisis

15. _____ SIADH

a. The concentration of osmotically active particles in solution

b. Caused from excessive antidiuretic hormone (ADH)

c. Caused from a deficiency in antidiuretic hormone (ADH)

d. Hormones that produce an effect when stimulated

e. An abnormality of the thyroid gland in which secretion of thyroid hormone is increased

f. Diminished production of thyroid hormone, leading to clinical manifestations of thyroid insufficiency

g. Characterized by retardation of both physical and mental development

h. A disorder marked by progressive enlargement of peripheral parts of the body

i. A life-threatening condition manifested by coma, hypothermia, bradycardia, hypoglycemia, and hypoventilation

j. A condition of abnormal size or overgrowth of the entire body or of any of its parts

k. A generalized skeletal disease, frequently familial, in which bone resorption and formation are both increased, leading to thickening and softening of bones

l. Another term for hyperthyroidism

m. A type of hyperthyroidism thought to be an autoimmune disorder

n. Loss or destruction of bone tissue

o. Another term for thyrotoxicosis

PHYSIOLOGY AND PATHOPHYSIOLOGY: THE BODY HUMAN

Essay

1. What is the master gland of the body?

2. What are the regulatory functions of the hypothalamus?

3. What are the releasing factors that have controlling effects on the anterior lobe of the pituitary?

4. What are the hormones released by the anterior pituitary?

5. What are the hormones released by the posterior pituitary?

6. Optimal production of thyroid hormones depends on what element in the body?

7. Why is thyroxine (T_4) thought to be the more important thyroid hormone?

8. What body processes are influenced by the thyroid hormones?

9. What hormone has the most influence on serum calcium in the body?

10. What body processes are influenced by calcium?

CORE DRUG KNOWLEDGE: JUST THE FACTS

Multiple Choice
Circle the option that best answers the question or completes the statement.

1. Somatropin (Humatrope) is used in the management of_____hormone deficiency.
   a. parathyroid
   b. growth
   c. thyroid
   d. pituitary

2. Serious adverse effects that may occur with the use of somatropin (Humatrope) include
   a. renal failure.
   b. hepatic failure.
   c. leukemia.
   d. pancreatitis.

3. Because of its potential adverse effects, children receiving somatropin (Humatrope) should have which of the following done before the start of therapy?
   a. electrocardiogram (ECG)
   b. pulmonary function tests
   c. urinalysis (UA)
   d. hip x-rays

4. Patients receiving somatropin (Humatrope) should be monitored for which of the following disorders?
   a. hypertension
   b. hyperthyroidism
   c. hypothyroidism
   d. hypotension

5. Which of the following medications would be contraindicated for the management of growth hormone hypersecretion?
   a. somatropin (Humatrope)
   b. octreotide acetate (Sandostatin)
   c. bromocriptine mesylate (Parlodel)
   d. all of the above

6. Desmopressin (DDAVP) is used in the management of
   a. diabetes insipidus.
   b. diabetes mellitus.
   c. hyperthyroidism.
   d. hypothyroidism.

7. Desmopressin (DDAVP) can be administered by
   a. oral tablets.
   b. intranasal inhalation.
   c. IV or SC.
   d. all of the above.

8. Which of the following drugs is used in the management of hypothyroidism?

   a. somatropin (Humatrope)

   b. levothyroxine (Synthroid)

   c. propylthiouracil (PTU)

   d. calcitriol (Rocaltrol)

9. Maximal effect of levothyroxine (Synthroid) occurs in

   a. 6 to 7 weeks.

   b. 24 to 48 hours.

   c. 6 to 8 hours.

   d. 1 to 3 weeks.

10. Which of the following adverse effects may occur with levothyroxine (Synthroid) therapy?

    a. tachycardia

    b. bradycardia

    c. hypotension

    d. constipation

11. During pregnancy, the dose of levothyroxine (Synthroid) may need to be

    a. discontinued.

    b. increased.

    c. decreased.

    d. kept the same.

12. Which of the following drugs is used in the management of hyperthyroidism?

    a. somatropin (Humatrope)

    b. levothyroxine (Synthroid)

    c. methimazole (MMI)

    d. calcitriol (Rocaltrol)

13. The time it takes methimazole (MMI) to induce lower T_4 levels to normal is

    a. 1 to 2 days.

    b. 24 hours.

    c. 3 to 6 minutes.

    d. 5 to 6 weeks.

14. Common adverse effects of methimazole (MMI) include

    a. headache.

    b. nausea and vomiting.

    c. diarrhea.

    d. rash.

15. In addition to methimazole (MMI), what other drugs may be useful in the management of hyperthyroidism?

    a. levothyroxine (Synthroid)

    b. I-131

    c. calcitriol (Rocaltrol)

    d. liothyronine (Cytomel)

16. I-131 is a pregnancy category _____ drug.

    a. A

    b. B

    c. D

    d. X

17. Calcitonin, salmon (Miacalcin) is used in the management of

    a. Paget disease.

    b. Graves disease.

    c. acromegaly.

    d. cretinism.

18. To optimize the benefit of bisphosphonate therapy, the patient should take the medication with

    a. 6 to 8 ounces of water 30 minutes before ingesting other medication, food, or beverages.

    b. 6 to 8 ounces of juice 30 minutes after ingesting other medication, food, or beverages.

    c. 6 to 8 ounces of water at bedtime.

    d. food at the breakfast meal.

19. Calcitriol (Rocaltrol) is used in the management of

    a. hypercalcemia.

    b. hypocalcemia.

    c. hyperthyroidism.

    d. hypothyroidism.

20. Adverse effects to calcitriol include

    a. hypertonicity and diarrhea.

    b. blood dyscrasias.

    c. rash, diarrhea, and bone pain.

    d. weakness, headache, and dry mouth.

CORE PATIENT VARIABLES: PATIENTS, PLEASE

Multiple Choice

Circle the option that best answers the question or completes the statement.

1. Your 7-year-old patient is taking somatropin (Humatrope) for growth deficiency. Throughout therapy, this patient should be monitored for
   a. cancer.
   b. hyperthyroidism.
   c. CNS depression.
   d. hyperglycemia.

2. You are giving instructions for somatropin (Humatrope) therapy to the patient's mother. Which of the following statements is *inappropriate*?
   a. "Be sure to wash your hands thoroughly before giving the injection."
   b. "Jennifer may develop a limp, but that is expected so don't worry about it."
   c. "If Jennifer complains of muscle discomfort, you may give her acetaminophen."
   d. "Call us immediately if you notice Jennifer drinking a lot of fluids and going to the bathroom more frequently."

3. Your 7-year-old patient is receiving somatropin (Humatrope) therapy. Which of the following lab values should be obtained periodically?
   a. CBC and liver function
   b. glucose and thyroid function
   c. hepatic and kidney function
   d. CBC and glucose

4. Your patient is being treated for diabetes insipidus with desmopressin (DDAVP). As you enter the patient's room, you note that the patient is confused, drowsy, listless, and reports having a headache. Which of the following conditions would you suspect is the problem?
   a. water intoxication
   b. dehydration
   c. desmopressin allergy
   d. CHF

5. Which of the following patients has the highest risk for adverse effects from desmopressin (DDAVP) therapy?
   a. Kenneth, with a history of hepatitis
   b. Julie, with a history of asthma
   c. Carmen, with a history of myocardial infarction
   d. Henry, with a history of bipolar disease

6. Your 45-year-old patient takes desmopressin (DDAVP). Which of the following laboratory tests should be done to evaluate the effectiveness of therapy?
   a. BUN and creatinine
   b. CBC
   c. chest x-ray
   d. urine specific gravity

7. Your 24-year-old patient has hypothyroidism and is prescribed levothyroxine (Synthroid). Which of the following situations would contraindicate the use of this drug?
   a. pregnancy
   b. asthma
   c. osteoporosis
   d. breast-feeding

8. Your 55-year-old patient takes levothyroxine (Synthroid) for hypothyroidism and warfarin (Coumadin) for deep vein thrombosis prophylaxis. What is the possible interaction between these drugs?
   a. There is no interaction between these drugs.
   b. There is an increased risk for bleeding.
   c. There is a increased risk for cardiovascular effects from levothyroxine.
   d. The warfarin dose may need to be increased to anticoagulate the blood.

9. Your 45-year-old patient has primary hypothyroidism and is taking levothyroxine (Synthroid). The patient asks, "Just how long do I need to take this medication?" You would respond:

   a. "Generally, people with hypothyroidism need to take their medication for the rest of their life."

   b. "You should really ask the nurse practitioner that question."

   c. "Just until your thyroid function tests are in the normal range again."

   d. "Usually, they try to taper you off the drug after a year."

10. Which of the following instructions should be given to your patient who is beginning methimazole (MMI) therapy?

    a. "Take small frequent meals to minimize GI distress."

    b. "Decrease your fluid intake."

    c. "Drink dairy products to decrease hunger."

    d. "Take the drug every 12 hours."

11. Your 45-year-old patient has hyperthyroidism and has been taking methimazole (MMI) for the past 8 months. As you assess her health status, you note that this patient is also taking warfarin (Coumadin). With this drug combination, you should monitor for

    a. a decreased anticoagulation effect.

    b. an increased anticoagulation effect.

    c. nothing; there is no interaction between these drugs.

12. Your patient has hyperthyroidism and takes methimazole (MMI). She called today and states, "I think I'm pregnant—at least my home pregnancy kit is positive." What instructions should you give this patient?

    a. "Stop taking the drug immediately."

    b. "You really will need to increase your dose now that you are pregnant."

    c. "Can you come in to be seen today?"

    d. "You can continue your medication. There is no problem with pregnancy and taking this drug."

13. Your patient has been taking methimazole (MMI) for the past year. What laboratory tests should be done?

    a. thyroid and parathyroid function tests

    b. CBC and thyroid function

    c. renal and parathyroid function tests

    d. ECG and thyroid and hepatic function tests

14. Your patient has drug-induced hypercalcemia. Which of the following lab tests should be done before initiating calcitonin, salmon (Calcimar)? Calcium and

    a. CBC

    b. renal function tests

    c. hormone status

    d. thyroid function tests

15. Your patient has Paget disease and takes SC calcitonin, salmon (Calcimar). Patient education should include:

    a. "You may experience increased transient bone pain."

    b. "You can change to the intranasal form in the future."

    c. "You can put ice packs on if you experience bone pain."

    d. "This drug may give you constipation."

16. Your 54-year-old patient has osteoporosis. Which of the following drugs would you anticipate using for this patient?

    a. alendronate (Fosamax)

    b. bromocriptine (Parlodel)

    c. calcitriol (Rocaltrol)

    d. levothyroxine (Synthroid)

17. Your patient who receives dialysis takes calcitriol (Rocaltrol). Patient teaching for this patient should include to refrain from taking antacids with a(n)

    a. aluminum base.

    b. calcium base.

    c. magnesium base.

    d. sodium bicarbonate base.

NURSING MANAGEMENT: EVERY GOOD NURSE SHOULD …

Multiple Choice
Circle the option that best answers the question or completes the statement.

1. An 8-year-old child has started taking somatropin, a growth hormone, because of deficient intrinsic growth factor. Patient teaching necessary for the child and parents includes
   a. how to administer an SC injection.
   b. proper storage of the drug is in a sunny location.
   c. adverse effects such as limping are not serious problems.
   d. all of the above.
   e. none of the above.

2. Your patient had a thyroidectomy yesterday because of hyperthyroidism. The patient begins a regimen of levothyroxine (Synthroid) as thyroid hormone replacement. You should monitor the patient for
   a. bradycardia.
   b. hypertension.
   c. intolerance to heat or cold.
   d. all of the above.
   e. none of the above.

3. A patient receiving methimazole for hyperthyroidism calls the advice nurse helpline at an HMO. The patient reports having a great deal of nausea and abdominal pain. The nurse should advise the patient to
   a. take the methimazole on an empty stomach.
   b. eat small, frequent meals.
   c. take the total daily dose of methimazole all at one time in the evening after dinner.
   d. stop taking the methimazole at once.

4. Your patient has chronic renal failure, receives dialysis, and is taking calcitriol, an antihypocalcemic drug. Lab values relevant to drug therapy for which the nurse should monitor include
   a. potassium.
   b. calcium.
   c. BUN.
   d. SGOT.
   e. all of the above.

5. You, the nurse, are to administer the first dose of calcitonin, salmon, and an antihypercalcemic drug to a patient with acute severe hypercalcemia. The drug is to be given IM. Before giving the first dose, you should
   a. administer calcium.
   b. administer vitamin D.
   c. perform a skin test with calcitonin, salmon.
   d. assess for bone deformities.

CASE STUDY

Your patient has been determined to be hyperthyroid and is to start taking methimazole, an antithyroid drug, before having a thyroidectomy. The medical history also shows that the patient has a history of a mitral valve replacement 5 years ago and takes 2.5 mg of warfarin daily for this.

The patient says, "Why can't I just have the surgery. I hate to take medicine!"

What teaching should you give?

CRITICAL THINKING CHALLENGE

The patient described above complains, "I'm having a terrible time with my gums bleeding when I brush my teeth. And I'm bruising so easily too."

1. What could be a possible cause of these problems?

2. What lab value should be evaluated?

3. Why should this patient have frequent lab testing?

CHAPTER 54

Drugs Affecting Men's Health and Sexuality

TOP TEN THINGS TO KNOW ABOUT DRUGS AFFECTING MEN'S HEALTH AND SEXUALITY

1. Testosterone is the primary male sex hormone. Adequate levels of sex hormones are needed to develop the sexual and reproductive organs, create and maintain the secondary sexual characteristics, and induce and stop the growth spurt of adolescence. Testosterone also causes retention of sodium, potassium, and phosphorus and decreased urinary excretion of calcium.

2. Testosterone is used as a replacement therapy for males with low or absent endogenous testosterone. In postmenopausal women, testosterone may be used in advanced, inoperable metastatic breast cancer.

3. The most adverse effects of testosterone are related to high doses of the drug. The most common male adverse effects are gynecomastia, excessive frequency and duration of penile erections, decreased ejaculatory volumes, and oligospermia (low sperm counts). Females will experience masculinization if they receive testosterone.

4. Other adverse effects of testosterone are related to the actions of testosterone on fluid and electrolytes. They include hypernatremia, hypercalcemia, hyperchloremia, hyperkalemia, hyperphosphatemia, fluid overload, edema, and hypercholesterolemia.

5. Sildenafil is used in the treatment of erectile dysfunction. It is administered orally, usually 1 hour before sexual activity. Sildenafil is effective only with accompanying sexual stimulation. Sildenafil promotes vasodilation and increases blood flow to the penis; this helps to achieve and maintain an erection. Sildenafil should not be used if nitrates are also used. Adverse effects are usually mild and transient.

6. Sildenafil, sold under the trade name of Revatio, is used as treatment for pulmonary arterial hypertension. It can be given to women for this use. When given for pulmonary hypertension,

sildenafil is dosed differently; it is administered three times a day, with or without food—also can

7. Finasteride is used to treat benign prostatic hyperplasia (BPH) and male pattern baldness; the dose for male hair loss is much smaller than that for BPH. Two separate trade names are used to differentiate these preparations.

8. Finasteride prevents testosterone from being converted to dihydrotestosterone (DHT; the hormone responsible for prostate growth). This decreases the circulating DHT levels and also boosts testosterone levels. These changes improve BPH-related symptoms, increase maximum urinary flow rates, and decrease prostate size.

9. With male pattern hair loss, DHT is found in increased amounts in the scalp. Finasteride decreases scalp and serum DHT concentrations in these men.

10. Topical minoxidil is used to treat male pattern baldness. It can also be used in women with diffuse hair loss or thinning in the frontal parietal areas. The exact cause of action is unknown. At least 4 months of twice-daily applications are needed for hair growth. Therapy will be effective in more than half of patients but must be continued to maintain the new hair.

KEY TERMS

True or False
Mark each of the following statements true or false. If the statement is false, replace the underlined word(s) with the word(s) that will make the statement true.

1. ____ <u>Luteinizing hormones</u> are naturally occurring or synthetic steroidal compounds that produce the masculinization and tissue building properties of testosterone.

2. ____ During puberty, the pituitary gland secretes large volumes of <u>FSH and LH.</u>

3. ____ <u>Benign prostatic hypertrophy</u> is the inability to achieve or maintain an erection in at least every three of four attempts at intercourse.

4. ____ Prostatic enlargement that is not caused by cancer is called <u>erectile dysfunction.</u>

5. ____ <u>Male pattern baldness</u> is also known as androgenetic alopecia.

PHYSIOLOGY AND PATHOPHYSIOLOGY: THE BODY HUMAN

Essay

1. What is the primary male sex hormone(s)?

2. In addition to maintaining male secondary sexual characteristics, what effect does testosterone have on the body?

3. How does the body achieve an erection?

CORE DRUG KNOWLEDGE: JUST THE FACTS

Multiple Choice

Circle the option that best answers the question or completes the statement.

1. Which of the following disorders *in women* may be treated with testosterone?
   a. delayed puberty
   b. breast cancer
   c. hair loss
   d. decreased libido

2. Testosterone may be contraindicated for use in patients with a history of cardiovascular disorders because of the potential for
   a. arrhythmias.
   b. tachycardia.
   c. bradycardia.
   d. chronic heart failure (CHF).

3. Adverse effects of testosterone therapy in females include
   a. breast enlargement.
   b. loss of voice.
   c. menstrual irregularities.
   d. hair loss.

4. Patients using testosterone (Testoderm TTS) should replace the patch
   a. weekly.
   b. daily.
   c. monthly.
   d. every other day.

5. In contrast to patients using testosterone (Testaderm TTS), patients using Androderm transdermal patches should replace the patch
   a. weekly.
   b. daily.
   c. monthly.
   d. every other day.

6. Appropriate pharmacotherapy with anabolic steroids includes all of the following *except*
   a. improvement of athletic performance.
   b. controlling metastatic breast cancer in women.
   c. hereditary angioedema.
   d. specific anemias.

7. Adverse effects of anabolic steroids include damage to the
   a. heart.
   b. kidneys.
   c. liver.
   d. eyes.

8. Erectile dysfunction is currently treated with
   a. testosterone.
   b. minoxidil (Rogaine).
   c. finasteride (Proscar).
   d. sildenafil (Viagra).

9. Sildenafil (Viagra) is contraindicated for patients taking
   a. calcium channel blocking drugs.
   b. diuretics.
   c. antibiotics.
   d. nitrates.

10. Benign prostatic hypertrophy is currently treated with
    a. testosterone.
    b. minoxidil (Rogaine).
    c. finasteride (Proscar).
    d. sildenafil (Viagra).

11. In addition to BPH, finasteride may be used in the treatment of
    a. erectile dysfunction.
    b. adrenal suppression.
    c. migraine headache.
    d. male pattern baldness.

12. Minoxidil (Rogaine) should be applied to
    a. wet hair and scalp after shampooing.
    b. wet hair and scalp two times a day.
    c. dry hair and scalp after shampooing and drying.
    d. dry hair and scalp two times a day.

CORE PATIENT VARIABLES: PATIENTS, PLEASE

Multiple Choice

Circle the option that best answers the question or completes the statement.

1. Your 12-year-old patient takes testosterone because of delayed puberty. This patient should be monitored for which of the following adverse effects?
   a. altered bone maturation
   b. excessive hair growth
   c. testicular atrophy
   d. tachycardia

2. Your 14-year-old patient is taking testosterone. Patient education should include the potential for
   a. headaches.
   b. impotence.
   c. gynecomastia.
   d. testicular hypoplasia.

3. Appropriate follow-up care for prepubescent boys receiving testosterone treatment includes
   a. weekly testosterone levels.
   b. radiographs every 6 months.
   c. monthly CBC and creatinine levels.
   d. daily testosterone levels for the first 2 weeks.

4. Your 42-year-old patient is receiving testosterone for adrenal insufficiency. Which of the following lab tests should be monitored during therapy?
   a. cholesterol, liver function tests, and a CBC
   b. chest x-ray, CBC, and urinalysis
   c. cholesterol and urinalysis
   d. liver function and chest x-ray

5. Your patient has newly diagnosed erectile dysfunction. He is starting to take sildenafil (Viagra). Appropriate patient teaching should include instructions to take the medication
   a. 6 to 10 hours before sexual activity.
   b. with a high-fat meal to increase its absorption.
   c. approximately 1 hour before sexual activity.
   d. 3 to 4 hours before sexual activity.

6. Your patient presented to the clinic with a request for sildenafil (Viagra). While taking his medical history, you note that he has a history of hypertension, diabetes mellitus, and depression. In his social history, you note that he is a pack-a-day smoker. What advice would you give this patient?
   a. "This drug must be used cautiously with you due to your medical history and current smoking status."
   b. "This drug is contraindicated for you, but if you use it only weekly, you should be OK."
   c. "You can use this drug without any problems."
   d. "You can use this drug, but be sure not to take any other medications for at least 2 hours before you take it."

7. Your 42-year-old male patient states, "I have been taking sildenafil (Viagra) for awhile. It always worked before, but now it is not always effective." Which of the following core patient variables would you assess?

    a. health status

    b. life span and gender

    c. lifestyle, diet, and habits

    d. environment

8. Your female patient comes to the clinic for advice about her hair loss. She states that her husband takes finasteride (Propecia) and his hair growth is "great." She wants to know if she may also have a prescription for finasteride. What is your best response?

    a. "Why don't you try some of your husband's pills to see if it works for you."

    b. "That should be no problem."

    c. "Finasteride is actually contraindicated for women because it causes birth defects."

    d. "I can get you a few samples to try."

9. Your male patient is taking finasteride (Proscar) for BPH. He reports erectile dysfunction, decreased libido, and decreased volume of ejaculate. With your knowledge of this drug, what would you tell this patient?

    a. "If I were you, I would stop this drug today."

    b. "These are expected adverse effects to the drug. Sometimes they go away on their own."

    c. "These are expected adverse effects to the drug. You have to choose if you want to be able to urinate or have sexual activity."

    d. "Sounds like you have an allergy to the drug."

10. Your patient has male pattern baldness and is starting minoxidil (Rogaine) therapy. He asks, "Just when will I see a difference in my hair?" What is your best response?

    a. 1 week

    b. 1 month

    c. 4 months

    d. 6 months

NURSING MANAGEMENT: EVERY GOOD NURSE SHOULD …

Multiple Choice

Circle the option that best answers the question or completes the statement.

1. You are caring for an 11-year-old boy who has hypogonadism. He is to start taking testosterone (short acting) as replacement therapy. You should do which of the following to minimize adverse effects from the drug therapy?

    a. Administer the drug intravenously.

    b. Verify that x-rays are taken every 6 months.

    c. Assess BUN and creatinine levels regularly.

    d. all of the above

    e. none of the above

2. Your patient is a 28-year-old man who is starting a regimen of Testoderm TTS, a transdermal system of testosterone administration, for treatment of his secondary hypogonadotropic hypogonadism. Which of the following should you include in teaching for this patient?

    a. Apply the patch to skin that is dry.

    b. Replace the patch every 2 hours.

    c. Apply the patch to skin on the arm, back, or upper buttocks.

    d. Secure the patch to the skin using an Ace wrap.

3. Your patient is a 58-year-old man who is to begin taking sildenafil for erection dysfunction. He has a family history of cardiovascular disease and is being treated for elevated blood cholesterol levels with lovastatin. He takes no other medications. Patient education for this patient should include:

    a. sexual stimulation is needed for sildenafil to be effective.

    b. take the drug about 1 hour before sexual intercourse.

    c. if symptoms of chest pain, shortness of breath, or nausea occur during intercourse, stop sexual activity.

    d. all of the above.

    e. none of the above.

4. Your patient is a 73-year-old man who lives with his 30-year-old daughter. This patient has BPH and is to begin taking finasteride, an androgen inhibitor. He has trouble swallowing pills. His daughter tells you that she frequently crushes medication for him to help him swallow it. To minimize adverse effects, you should

   a. insist the patient swallow the pills whole.

   b. show the patient how to insert the pill through the urethra.

   c. instruct the daughter not to handle or to get any crushed or broken drug on her skin.

   d. teach the daughter to administer the drug just before her father urinates.

5. A male patient is in the clinic for a routine visit. During that time, he tells the nurse of his plan to buy minoxidil to treat his thinning hair line. He says, "I'll give it a try for a little while and see if it helps." Patient education regarding this drug therapy should include that

   a. this drug is available only by prescription.

   b. fine, soft colorless hair may grow first.

   c. this drug may increase your blood pressure.

   d. hair growth should be seen within 2 weeks.

6. Your 68-year-old female patient is given a prescription for sildenafil to treat

   a. sexual dysfunction

   b. hormone imbalance

   c. pulmonary hypertension

   d. adrenal insufficiency

CASE STUDY

You are caring for a male patient who has had diabetes for 35 years and has coronary artery disease, which is asymptomatic at this time. He is to begin a regimen of testosterone topical patches because it was found that his endogenous testosterone levels are greatly below normal levels.

What lab values should be monitored when this patient returns for a follow-up visit 6 weeks after starting drug therapy?

CRITICAL THINKING CHALLENGE

When the patient described above returns for a second follow-up visit 12 weeks after starting drug therapy, he reports being short of breath and that his wedding ring is tight. On examination, you auscultate rales and crackles in his lungs and you see that he has +2 edema in his hands and feet.

What is a possible cause of these symptoms?

CHAPTER 55

Drugs Affecting Women's Health and Sexuality

TOP TEN THINGS TO KNOW ABOUT DRUGS AFFECTING WOMEN'S HEALTH AND SEXUALITY

1. Estrogens and progestin are the primary female sex hormones. Adequate levels of sex hormones are needed to develop the sexual and reproductive organs, create and maintain the secondary sexual characteristics, induce and stop the growth spurt of adolescence, create a normal menstrual cycle, and achieve and maintain a pregnancy.

2. Endogenous estrogen also affects the cardiovascular system (positively and negatively depending on dose, route, and whether the woman is menopausal), increases bone density, and maintains the tone and elasticity of the urogenital structures. Other actions of estrogen include increased fluid retention, protein anabolism, and conservation of calcium and phosphorus.

3. Conjugated estrogen is used as hormone replacement therapy (HRT) when endogenous levels of estrogen are low or absent, as treatment of abnormal uterine bleeding, and as treatment for moderate to severe vasomotor response (hot flashes) during menopause (treated with as small a dose as possible for as short a time as possible—not lifelong therapy—because of the increased risk of cardiovascular complications). In males, it is used as palliative therapy in prostatic and breast cancers.

4. Estrogen replacement therapy (ERT) in combination with progestin in postmenopausal women increases the risk of stroke; coronary heart disease; breast cancer (and when detected, it is at a more advanced stage); ovarian cancer, and dementia or mild cognitive impairment. Estrogen use alone increases the risk for endometrium cancer but does not increase the risk of coronary heart disease or breast cancer. When estrogen is used to treat menopausal symptoms, the adverse effects may be minimized by using a topical form, instead of an oral, systemic form.

5. Adverse effects of estrogen are related to estrogen's effects on the body and may be dose related. Common adverse effects include menstrual changes (breakthrough bleeding, changes in menstrual flow, dysmenorrhea, premenstrual-like syndrome), nausea, headache, bloating, photosensitivity, and breast tenderness.

6. Progestins are composed of progesterone and its derivatives. They regulate, through stimulation or inhibition, the secretion of pituitary gonadotropins, thus regulating development of ovarian follicle. Progestins also inhibit spontaneous uterine contractions.

7. Progestins are used to treat amenorrhea and dysfunctional uterine bleeding. Progestins are given with estrogen as HRT; the combination helps prevent endometrial cancer but increases the risk of breast cancer and other problems (see above).

8. Oral contraceptives are combinations of estrogen and progestins. Formulations with high doses of estrogen may cause serious adverse effects (thromboembolism, stroke, myocardial infarction). Therefore, the lowest effective dose of estrogen should be used. Other forms of contraceptives include a transdermal system, a vaginal ring, subdermal implants, and intrauterine implants.

9. Alendronate inhibits normal and abnormal bone resorption. It is used to treat and prevent osteoporosis in postmenopausal women and to treat Paget disease.

10. Gastrointestinal (GI) complaints are common adverse effects from alendronate. Very specific administration techniques help to minimize or prevent these problems. Teach the patient to take alendronate at least 30 minutes before eating, drinking any beverage other than plain water, or taking any other medication. The patient should also not lie down after taking alendronate.

KEY TERMS

True or False

Mark each of the following statements true or false. If the statement is false, replace the underlined word(s) with the word(s) that will make the statement true.

1. _____ The female body produces six different <u>progestins</u>.

2. _____ <u>Estrogen</u> is the primary endogenous progestational substance.

3. _____ Estrogen, which is secreted by the hypothalamus and then perfused throughout the anterior pituitary, stimulates the release of <u>gonadotropin-releasing hormone</u> and <u>progestins</u>.

4. _____ The ending of monthly menstrual cycles is known as <u>menopause</u>.

5. _____ <u>Paget disease</u>, characterized by low bone mineral density, is a loss in bone mass sufficient to compromise normal function.

6. _____ During the <u>proliferative phase</u>, the follicle is transformed into the corpus luteum, which secretes much progesterone and estrogen.

7. _____ During the <u>secretory phase</u>, estrogen increases the vascularity of the uterine lining, preparing it for implantation of a fertilized egg.

8. _____ The female sex <u>hormones</u> are responsible for the production of female sexual characteristics.

9. _____ <u>Osteoporosis</u> is an idiopathic bone disease characterized by chronic focal areas of bone destruction.

PHYSIOLOGY AND PATHOPHYSIOLOGY: THE BODY HUMAN

Essay

1. What is the primary female sex hormone(s)?

2. Which of the estrogen hormones is the most potent?

3. In addition to maintaining female secondary sexual characteristics, what effect does estrogen have on the body?

4. Describe the hormonal control of the menstrual cycle.

CORE DRUG KNOWLEDGE: JUST THE FACTS

Multiple Choice

Circle the option that best answers the question or completes the statement.

1. Which of the following disorders is an *inappropriate* use of conjugated estrogen?
   a. HRT in female hypogonadism
   b. prophylaxis of cardiovascular disease
   c. primary ovarian failure
   d. abnormal uterine bleeding

2. Conjugated estrogen should be used cautiously in patients with (*Mark all that apply.*)
   a. incomplete bone growth.
   b. epilepsy
   c. hypertension
   d. hypothyroidism
   e. cardiac dysfunction
   f. migraine headache

3. Conjugated estrogens may be given safely to patients with
   a. non–estrogen-dependent neoplastic diseases.
   b. undiagnosed abnormal genital bleeding.
   c. active thrombophlebitis or thromboembolic disorders.
   d. history of cerebrovascular accident (CVA).

4. Postmenopausal women receiving hormone replacement therapy with estrogen and progestin should be advised of an increased risk for (*Mark all that apply.*)
   a. hyperthyroidism
   b. coronary heart disease
   c. breast cancer
   d. renal failure
   e. dementia
   f. CVA.

5. Common adverse effects to the use of conjugated estrogens include all of the following *except*
   a. breakthrough bleeding.
   b. shortness of breath.
   c. nausea and vomiting.
   d. bloating and abdominal cramps.

6. Pharmacotherapeutics for progesterone include (*Mark all that apply.*)
   a. dysfunctional uterine bleeding
   b. estrogen-dependent tumors
   c. hormone replacement therapy
   d. contraception
   e. gynecomastia
   f. amenorrhea

7. Patients with a history of _____ should be closely monitored while taking progesterone (Gesterol).
   a. hypotension
   b. blood dyscrasias
   c. asthma
   d. diabetes mellitus

8. When given to postmenopausal women, progesterone in combination with estrogen increases the risk for _____ cancer. *Mark all that apply.*
   a. breast
   b. uterine
   c. ovarian
   d. lung
   e. bone
   f. brain

9. Which of the following drugs are used in the treatment of ovulatory failure?
   a. clomiphene (Clomid)
   b. conjugated estrogens
   c. progestins
   d. all of the above

10. Danazol (Danocrine) is used in the management of
   a. primary ovarian failure.
   b. endometriosis.
   c. birth control.
   d. amenorrhea.

11. Megestrol acetate (Megace), a progestin-like progesterone, is used in the treatment of
   a. AIDS.
   b. CVA.
   c. pregnancy complications.
   d. COPD.

12. What is the route of administration for Norplant?
   a. subdermal
   b. subcutaneous
   c. intrathecal
   d. intramuscular

13. Mifepristone (Mifeprex) is used to
   a. stop conception.
   b. treat ovarian failure.
   c. abort an early pregnancy.
   d. treat adrenal insufficiency.

14. To be optimally effective, emergency contraceptive medication should be taken

    a. 6 hours after intercourse, then daily for 3 days.

    b. within 24 hours of intercourse, then 12 hours later.

    c. within 24 hours of intercourse, then 24 hours later.

    d. 72 hours after the event.

15. Transdermal hormone contraceptive patches should be placed on the (*Mark all that apply.*)

    a. abdomen

    b. breast

    c. upper outer arm

    d. buttocks

    e. lower arm

    f. leg

16. Alendronate (Fosamax) from used in the management of

    a. unwanted pregnancy.

    b. primary ovarian failure.

    c. hair loss.

    d. osteoporosis.

17. Common adverse effects from alendronate (Fosamax) occur in the _____ system.

    a. CNS

    b. cardiovascular

    c. GI

    d. integumentary

Essay

1. Compare and contrast the three types of combination oral contraceptives.

2. Develop a list of potential serious adverse effects associated with oral contraceptives.

3. Develop a list of common adverse effects associated with oral contraceptives.

CORE PATIENT VARIABLES: PATIENTS, PLEASE

Multiple Choice

Circle the option that best answers the question or completes the statement.

1. Your 54-year-old patient came to the clinic because of a lack of menstruation in the past 12 months. Laboratory tests confirm this patient is postmenopausal. The patient states she is confused about the use of estrogen after menopause. Which of the following facts is correct about estrogen use after menopause?

    a. There is a decreased risk for breast cancer in women with a family history of breast cancer.

    b. There is an increased risk for cardiac events in women without a history of coronary heart disease.

    c. Postmenopausal women on estrogen have an decrease in bone density.

    d. It decreases the risk for uterine cancer.

2. Your 62-year-old patient has been prescribed both estrogen and progestin for her postmenopausal symptoms. The patient states, "My friends all just take estrogen. Why do I have to take both pills?" Your best response would be:

    a. "This is the regimen that your health care provider prefers."

    b. "Because you still have your uterus; you may get endometriosis if the estrogen is given unopposed by progesterone."

    c. "It is important for you to bleed each month so we know that you are not pregnant."

    d. "This combination decreases the potential for adverse effects such as a heart attack."

3. Your 66-year-old patient comes to the clinic for a checkup after a CVA. She is actively involved in rehabilitation and uses a cane to ambulate. The patient tells you she is concerned that she might "break something" if she should fall and wishes to take estrogen and progesterone to reduce her osteoporosis risk. Which of the following statements would be most appropriate?

   a. "You are really doing your homework. It sounds like a good idea."

   b. "You should really finish your rehab before we consider any new drugs."

   c. "With your history of stroke, these medications are not suggested for use."

   d. "I think you should take only progesterone because you had a stroke."

4. Your 14-year-old patient comes to the clinic after a therapeutic abortion. The patient states she still plans to have intercourse and can't always remember to take her contraception. For this patient, what would be an appropriate form of birth control?

   a. intrauterine device (IUD)

   b. condoms and foam

   c. medroxyprogesterone (Depo-Provera)

   d. cyclic birth control pills

5. Your 19-year-old patient comes to the clinic for a routine checkup. She states she had an intrauterine progesterone insert placed approximately 4 months ago. She is concerned that her normal 2-day flow has been increased to 5 days. Which of the following statements would be most appropriate?

   a. "It sounds like the device may have perforated the uterus."

   b. "This is an expected change with use of the insert."

   c. "This may be the beginning of endometriosis."

   d. "You probably have a pelvic infection."

6. Your 42-year-old patient comes to the clinic requesting birth control pills. The patient states she has been divorced for 2 years and is now ready "to do some serious dating." Which of the following statements from this patient's health status history would contraindicate the use of birth control pills?

   a. first pregnancy at age 16 years

   b. smoked 1 pack per day until 2 years ago

   c. COPD

   d. deep vein thrombosis

7. Your 16-year-old patient has been prescribed triphasic birth control pills. The patient calls the clinic and states that she has forgotten to take her pill for 2 days. Which of the following statements is most appropriate?

   a. "Take all three pills today and continue your pack."

   b. "Take two pills today and two pills tomorrow and continue your pack."

   c. "Stop taking the pack and start a new pack in 4 days."

   d. "Take one pill a day and don't forget any more."

8. Your patient has just had a progesterone IUD placed. Patient education should include:

   a. "This needs to be replaced in 1 year."

   b. "This does not need to be replaced for 5 years."

   c. "Should you become pregnant, this will just fall out."

   d. "This should stop your monthly menstrual cycle."

9. Your patient took mifepristone (Mifeprex) 3 weeks ago. She comes to the clinic because of continued vaginal bleeding. With your knowledge of this drug, which of the following is appropriate?

   a. Tell the patient this is normal and to return if bleeding continues more than 2 weeks.

   b. Obtain orthostatic vital signs. If normal, send her home.

   c. Obtain a CBC and have her evaluated by the health care provider.

   d. Call for paramedics.

10. Your patient is taking alendronate (Fosamax) for the prevention of osteoporosis. Patient education should include:

    a. "Take it first thing in the morning with a glass of orange juice."

    b. "Take it at bedtime with a glass of milk."

    c. "Take it first thing in the morning, with water, before you eat or drink anything else."

    d. "Lie down after taking the medication for 30 minutes."

NURSING MANAGEMENT: EVERY GOOD NURSE SHOULD …

Multiple Choice

Circle the option that best answers the question or completes the statement.

1. You are the nurse working in the gynecology department of an outpatient center. Patients frequently ask you what you think about estrogen use and if they are candidates to take estrogen. Which of these patients may be appropriate candidates for estrogen use?

    a. a 20-year-old woman with primary ovarian failure

    b. a 30-year-old woman after bilateral salpingo-oophorectomy (removal of fallopian tubes and ovaries) secondary to multiple bouts of pelvic inflammatory disease

    c. a 55-year-old woman who reports hot flashes and vaginal dryness

    d. all of the above

    e. none of the above

2. Your premenopausal, adult female patient has been prescribed estrogen HRT because of primary ovarian failure. Teaching for this patient should include:

    a. "Take the drug for 3 weeks, then stay off the drug for 1 week."

    b. "Sun exposure will promote the effectiveness of the estrogen."

    c. "X-rays will need to be taken every 6 months."

    d. "Sudden, severe headaches may occur and are not serious."

3. Your patient is a 19-year-old woman who is to receive progesterone for treatment of primary amenorrhea. To maximize the therapeutic effect and to minimize the adverse effects from drug therapy, you should

    a. assess the patient for thrombophlebitis before and during therapy.

    b. verify that the patient is not pregnant before beginning drug therapy.

    c. administer the progesterone daily for 6 to 8 days per order.

    d. do all of the above.

    e. do none of the above.

4. You are teaching a class on birth control to women who are 6 weeks' postpartum. Which of the following statements should be included?

    a. Levonorgestrel implants prevent pregnancy for up to 2 years.

    b. Intrauterine progesterone inserts have no serious adverse effects.

    c. Estrogen-progestin combination oral contraceptives are the best choice for women older than 35 years who smoke cigarettes.

    d. all of the above

    e. none of the above

5. You are the nurse practitioner working in a practice with OB-GYN physicians in the United States. A patient has come to see you because she is concerned that she became pregnant after she was raped 4 weeks ago. You confirm that she is pregnant, and because she wishes to terminate this pregnancy, you prescribe mifepristone. Patient education for this patient must include

    a. a discussion of the facts contained in the FDA Medication Guide, after she has obtained a copy and read it.

    b. verification that she can return to the office for two follow-up appointments.

    c. instruction that she will need to take three tablets in the presence of the nurse practitioner.

    d. all of the above.

    e. none of the above.

CASE STUDY

A 20-year-old patient is 6 weeks' postpartum after vaginal delivery. She has come for her checkup. She questions you about resuming birth control. Her record indicates that she was on Ortho-Norvum 7/7/7, a triphasic oral contraceptive, before becoming pregnant. She has been breast-feeding but is planning to stop when she returns to work in the next week. She has not yet had a menstrual period since she delivered.

Consider this patient's core patient variables. What advice would you give her regarding resuming birth control?

CRITICAL THINKING CHALLENGE

The patient described above asks if there is a better form of birth control than the Ortho-Novum 7/7/7 oral contraceptives. She says, "I got pregnant while I was using those pills. I really wasn't planning on becoming pregnant right now. I definitely want to wait awhile before I get pregnant again."

What questions might you want to ask this patient to more completely assess her?

CHAPTER 56

Drugs Affecting Uterine Motility

TOP TEN THINGS TO KNOW ABOUT DRUGS AFFECTING UTERINE MOTILITY

1. Drug therapy may be used to induce labor, augment (improve) labor, or stop labor that begins preterm.
2. Oxytocin, a synthetic form of an endogenous hormone, is given by intravenous (IV) infusion to initiate or augment labor when clinically indicated. Oxytocin is also used intramuscularly (IM) to control postpartum bleeding, and through a nasal spray to initiate milk let-down before pumping or breast-feeding. There is a three-phase response to oxytocin therapy: incremental phase, stable phase, and hyperstimulation.
3. Adverse effects of oxytocin are dose related. Most common maternal adverse effects are nausea, vomiting, uterine hypertonicity, and cardiac ~~Water~~ intoxification is uncommon but ~~most common fetal adverse~~ ~~lia.~~
   ~~l vital signs, length of~~ ~~e between contractions, fetal~~ ~~novement, and maternal fluid~~ ~~ng oxytocin. Always administer~~ ~~nd piggyback the diluted drug~~ ~~V line.~~
5. ~~Tocolytic~~ ~~s~~ are given to stop preterm labor long enough (24 to 48 hours) to give the woman corticosteroids, which assist in preparing fetal lungs before delivery, and allow the woman to be transported to another facility if needed (e.g., to a facility with a neonatal intensive care).
6. Terbutaline is used off label to control preterm labor in pregnancies of 20 weeks to 34 weeks. Using terbutaline to control preterm labor, although a widespread practice, is still considered controversial (the effectiveness of the drug for this use has never been clearly demonstrated). Terbutaline has also been used to prevent additional preterm labor after an episode of preterm labor has been stopped. This use is also considered controversial (the effectiveness has never been demonstrated by positive perinatal or neonatal outcomes). Terbutaline is approved for use as a bronchodilator.

7. Terbutaline is a beta-receptor agonist (stimulant) that selectively prefers the beta-2 receptors over beta-1 receptors. Stimulation of these receptors inhibits contractility of uterine smooth muscle, and induces bronchial dilation, vasodilation, and hepatic glycogenolysis and gluconeogenesis. Some beta-1 receptors are also stimulated, altering cardiac function.
8. Adverse effects of terbutaline are dose related and secondary to beta stimulation; they are present in the woman and the fetus. The most common adverse effects are tachycardia (maternal and fetal), cardiac arrhythmias (maternal), palpitations (maternal), and tremor (maternal). The antidote for overdose is a beta blocker. Always administer on a IV pump to control the rate.
9. Magnesium sulfate is the drug of choice to treat or prevent seizures associated with preeclampsia, eclampsia, and pregnancy-induced hypertension. It is widely used off label to control preterm labor; its effectiveness as a tocolytic remains a matter of controversy. Magnesium sulfate acts as a central nervous system (CNS) and muscular depressant, producing peripheral neuromuscular blockade. It prevents or controls convulsions. Magnesium sulfate also relaxes smooth muscle, decreasing uterine contractions and blood pressure. It appears to inhibit myometrial contractility but does not prolong pregnancy much. It can help prevent labor long enough to allow corticosteroids to be administered to the woman to protect the fetal lungs.
10. Adverse effects of magnesium sulfate are dose related and occur in the woman and the fetus. The most common maternal adverse effects are headache, hyporeflexia, weakness, thirst, flushing, and burning at the infusion site. The most common fetal/neonatal adverse effects are heart rate changes, neonatal hypotonia, and neonatal respiratory depression (possibly serious). Monitor blood levels carefully to

prevent overdose; calcium gluconate is the antidote. Administer by IV pump.

KEY TERMS

Anagrams

Use the following anagrams to explain the key terms in this chapter.

1. Pregnancy before labor starts

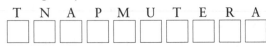

2. Uterine relaxants used to stop labor

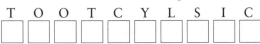

3. After delivery of the fetus

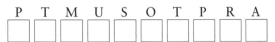

4. Fibrillation and prolonged contraction of the uterus

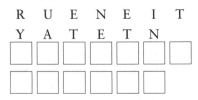

5. Uterine stimulants used to initiate or augment contraction

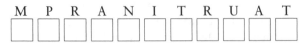

6. Onset of labor

M	P	R	A	N	I	T	R	U	A	T

PHYSIOLOGY AND PATHOPHYSIOLOGY: THE BODY HUMAN

Essay

1. In the uncomplicated pregnancy, when should labor begin?

2. In addition to stimulation of the uterus, what are the actions of endogenous oxytocin?

3. What are the regulatory processes involved in the control of uterine motility?

4. In the intrapartal period, what adaptations are required by the cardiovascular system?

5. In the intrapartal period, what changes occur in the respiratory system?

6. In the intrapartal period, what major change occurs in the hemopoietic system?

7. In the intrapartal period, what are the expected changes in the renal system?

8. In the intrapartal period, what occurs in the gastrointestinal (GI) system?

CORE DRUG KNOWLEDGE: JUST THE FACTS

Multiple Choice

Circle the option that best answers the question or completes the statement.

1. What methods of administration are appropriate for inducing labor with oxytocin (Pitocin)?
   a. oral
   b. intramuscular
   c. intravenous
   d. all of the above

2. What is the initial dose of oxytocin (Pitocin) to stimulate labor?
   a. 0.5 to 1 mU/minute
   b. 5 to 10 mU/minute
   c. 2 to 3 mU/minute
   d. 4 to 8 mU/minute

3. Maximum effect from oxytocin (Pitocin) administration occurs within
   a. 1 minute.
   b. 40 minutes.
   c. 2 hours.
   d. 4 hours.

4. Before oxytocin (Pitocin) therapy is initiated, which of the following should occur?
   a. 10 hours of nonprogressing labor
   b. fetal distress
   c. assessment of pelvic adequacy
   d. uterine tetany

5. Contraindications for the use of oxytocin include (*Mark all that apply.*)
   a. active genital herpes
   b. fetal distress without signs of imminent delivery
   c. maternal hypertension
   d. cord presentation or prolapse
   e. maternal dehydration
   f. uterine tetany

6. Common maternal adverse effects associated with oxytocin include
   a. nausea and vomiting.
   b. rupture of the uterus.
   c. water intoxication.
   d. hyponatremia.

7. Fetal adverse effects associated with oxytocin include
   a. congenital anomalies.
   b. structural defects.
   c. bradycardia.
   d. tachypnea.

8. The primary pharmacotherapeutics for ergonovine maleate (Ergotrate) is
   a. suppression of uterine motility.
   b. induction of labor.
   c. prevention of postpartum hemorrhage.
   d. all of the above.

9. Which of the following drugs may be used to induce an abortion?
   a. carboprost (Hemabate)
   b. dinoprostone (Prepidil)
   c. ergonovine maleate (Ergotrate)
   d. both a and b

10. Terbutaline (Brethine) works by
    a. stimulation of alpha receptor sites in the uterine smooth muscle.
    b. inhibition of alpha receptor sites in the uterine smooth muscle.
    c. stimulation of beta receptor sites in the uterine smooth muscle.
    d. inhibition of beta receptor sites in the uterine smooth muscle.

11. Terbutaline (Brethine) is contraindicated for use in patients with (*Mark all that apply.*)
    a. first-trimester pregnancy.
    b. maternal respiratory disorders.
    c. eclampsia.
    d. last-trimester pregnancy.
    e. maternal hypertension.
    f. fetal distress.

12. To maximize the therapeutic benefits from magnesium sulfate, the serum level should be
    a. 1.5 to 3 mEq/L.
    b. 16 to 25 mEq/L.
    c. 7 to 10 mEq/L.
    d. 4 to 7 mEq/L.

CORE PATIENT VARIABLES: PATIENTS, PLEASE

Multiple Choice
Circle the option that best answers the question or completes the statement.

1. Your 26-year-old patient is receiving IV oxytocin (Pitocin) to enhance labor. The patient appears lethargic, confused, and intermittently agitated. You suspect
   a. dehydration.
   b. water intoxication.
   c. stroke.
   d. bradycardia.

2. Your patient has been in labor for 6 hours. Favorable induction with oxytocin (Pitocin) is most likely to occur if this patient has a Bishop score of
   a. 1 to 2.
   b. 0 to 1.
   c. 3 to 4.
   d. greater than 5.

3. Your patient is receiving oxytocin (Pitocin) to stimulate delivery. The patient is experiencing contractions lasting 90 seconds, with resting pressure of 18 mm Hg. Which of the following interventions would be most appropriate?
   a. Continue the infusion at the current rate.
   b. Increase the infusion rate.
   c. Stop the infusion and call the health care provider.
   d. Continue the infusion and call the health care provider

4. Your patient is receiving IV oxytocin (Pitocin) to stimulate labor. To safely administer this medication, you should
   a. give the drug by rapid IVP.
   b. piggyback the drug into the primary IV line.
   c. give the drug IVP over 5 to 6 minutes.
   d. not give IV; give SC only.

5. Your patient is prescribed terbutaline (Brethine) for preterm labor. Which of the following interventions should be done to assure safe administration of this drug? Dilute with
   a. normal saline.
   b. lactated Ringer's solution.
   c. a dextrose solution.
   d. Hartmann solution.

6. Your patient has been receiving terbutaline (Brethine) for 3 days. The patient reports palpitations, tachycardia, and nervousness. Which of the following interventions would be appropriate? Advise the patient to
   a. stop the medication.
   b. contact the provider for an order to decrease the dosage.
   c. decrease her intake of dairy products.
   d. have her thyroid checked.

7. Your patient is 33 weeks' pregnant and has preterm contractions. The patient has been prescribed terbutaline (Brethine). She asks, "It's so close to my due date; why can't I just deliver?" Which of the following is the best response?
   a. "Infants born this early have difficulty breathing."
   b. "Delaying delivery gives your baby an opportunity to fully develop and avoid complications."
   c. "Maternal hemorrhaging may occur with delivery at this time."
   d. "Your baby might have brain damage if it is born this early."

8. Your patient has preeclampsia and is brought to the hospital. For prevention of seizures caused by preeclampsia, you would anticipate treatment for this patient with which of the following drugs?
   a. magnesium sulfate
   b. oxytocin (Pitocin)
   c. ritodrine (Yutopar)
   d. terbutaline (Brethine)

9. Your patient has just delivered a baby boy. She has been receiving magnesium sulfate for eclampsia for the past 24 hours. The baby should be monitored for which of the following?

   a. hypotonia

   b. heart rate changes

   c. respiratory depression

   d. all of the above

NURSING MANAGEMENT: EVERY GOOD NURSE SHOULD …

Multiple Choice

Circle the option that best answers the question or completes the statement.

1. Before initiating therapy with oxytocin, the nurse should

   a. verify that vaginal delivery is contraindicated.

   b. confirm significant cephalopelvic disproportion.

   c. assess that cervical ripening is favorable through Bishop scoring.

   d. determine if fetal distress is present but delivery is not imminent.

2. Which of the following solutions is appropriate to use to dilute oxytocin for IV administration?

   a. 5% dextrose in lactated Ringer's solution

   b. 20% dextrose in water

   c. 0.2% sodium chloride

   d. none of the above; oxytocin should not be diluted

3. Your patient is receiving oxytocin for induction of labor. Her contractions begin to occur every 1 minute 50 seconds, and last 1 minute 40 seconds. You should

   a. increase the oxytocin rate.

   b. increase the concentration of the oxytocin.

   c. shut off the oxytocin.

   d. decrease the rate of the mainline fluids.

4. Which of the following solutions would be appropriate to dilute terbutaline for IV infusion?

   a. 0.9% normal saline

   b. 5% dextrose and lactated Ringer's solution

   c. 5% dextrose and 0.9% normal saline

   d. 5% dextrose and water

5. To minimize adverse effects during terbutaline infusion, the nurse should

   a. use an IV pump.

   b. position patient on her right side.

   c. encourage high fluid intake.

   d. do all of the above.

   e. do none of the above.

CASE STUDY

Your patient is pregnant with a gestation of 40 weeks. She has been in labor for 6 hours but has not progressed in the labor. Bishop scale indicates a score of 7. Her vital signs are: pulse, 84; respirations, 18; and blood pressure, 110/70. She is started on oxytocin IV infusion 1 mU/minute. The order states to increase the rate every 60 minutes by 1 mU/minute until effective contractions occur.

1. Are these orders appropriate for this patient? Why or why not?

2. What actions of the nurse are indicated to maximize therapeutic effect and minimize adverse effects of the oxytocin?

CRITICAL THINKING CHALLENGE

The patient described above continues on the oxytocin infusion for 4 hours, with the rate being increased each hour per order. The patient now has contractions every 2 minutes 30 seconds, which last 90 seconds. She is 10 cm dilated. She says she feels like she has to have a bowel movement.

1. What is your assessment of this patient's condition?

2. What actions should the nurse take now?

Answer Key

Chapter 1

KEY TERMS

1. Desired effect of the drug
2. Changes that occur to the drug when it is inside the body
3. Effects of the drug on the body
4. When the drug should not be used or when it should be used with caution
5. Effects that are not intended or may be undesirable
6. Effects that occur when a drug is given along with another drug, food, or substance
7. Grouping of pharmacologic facts: pharmacotherapeutics, pharmacokinetics, pharmacodynamics, contraindications and precautions, adverse effects, and drug interactions
8. Assessment of patient-centered variables
9. Chronic conditions causing system or organ dysfunction
10. Age, physiologic development, reproductive state, ability to read and write, and gender
11. Amount of activity and exercise; sleep-wake patterns; occupation; use or abuse of such substances as nicotine, alcohol, and illegal drugs; use of nonprescribed, or over-the-counter (OTC) drugs; use of alternative health practices; and eating preferences and patterns
12. Location where drug therapy will be administered; physical environment that may influence aspects of drug therapy; exposure to potentially harmful substances; lighting that may affect the drug or the person receiving the drug; cost of the drug
13. Religious beliefs that may hinder the use of pharmacotherapy; ethnic or inherited genetic factors that may influence an individual's response to drug therapy
14. Anticipated therapeutic and adverse effects of a drug
15. Application of knowledge in the administration of drug therapy
16. Drug that is representative of a drug class

CORE DRUG KNOWLEDGE: JUST THE FACTS
MULTIPLE CHOICE

1. c. Theophylline is a bronchodilator that opens the bronchioles in the lungs; thus, the patient with asthma will breathe better. This makes the use of aminophylline a therapy for asthma.
2. a. Drugs have more than one effect on the body. Because hair growth is an expected event, it is a pharmacodynamic of the drug.
3. b. Because of the patient's pregnancy status, the drug must be safe for both the patient and the fetus.
4. a. Lowering the white cell count is potentially dangerous to a patient, so it is an adverse effect. Answers b, c, and d are all examples of the pharmacodynamics of the drugs.

CORE PATIENT VARIABLES: PATIENTS, PLEASE
MULTIPLE CHOICE

1. a. Medical history belongs in the health status category of patient care variables.

2. d. The patient's occupation and how that occupation may be affected by drug therapy is documented in the lifestyle, diet, and habit category.
3. d. Cigarette smoking is considered a patient's habit.
4. a. Environment includes where the drug may be administered. If the patient will self-administer the medication, the nurse teaches the patient to keep it out of the reach of children.

CASE STUDY

1. Health status: Are you allergic to any medication? Do you routinely take any other medications? Do you take any over-the-counter drugs? Do you have any history of kidney or liver disease? Do you have any other chronic illnesses? What difficulties are you having with urination?

   Life span and gender: Are you postmenopausal? Do you take hormone replacement therapy?

   Lifestyle, diet, and habits: Do you smoke cigarettes, use alcohol, or use recreational drugs? Do you drink caffeinated beverages? If yes to any of the above, how much? What is your usual diet? How many meals a day do you usually eat? Do you use herbs, vitamins, or other alternative therapies?

   Environment: Do you live alone? Do you have stairs in your home?

   Culture and inherited traits: What is your religion? Do you often have difficulty tolerating drug therapy? Do you have unusual reactions to the drugs, or is it ever hard for the doctor/nurse practitioner to find the right dose for you when you are taking medications?

2. How often do you garden? At what time of the day are you in the sun? How long do you remain in the sun? What type of protective clothing do you wear? Do you wear sunscreen when you garden?

CRITICAL THINKING CHALLENGE
ESSAY

1. Because this drug can induce photosensitivity, the patient is at risk for sunburn.
2. The nurse should teach the patient about the potential for photosensitivity and the need to limit her sun exposure. When sun exposure is unavoidable, the patient should use sunscreen and wear appropriate clothing, including a head cover.

Chapter 2

KEY TERMS
MATCHING

1. q	2. m	3. r	4. k	5. o	6. b	7. d
8. h	9. i	10. l	11. a	12. c	13. n	14. s
15. j	16. e	17. p	18. g	19. f		

CRITICAL THINKING CHALLENGE

1. Ask the patient how long he has been out of medications. Assess if the desired therapeutic effect of the drug has occurred. Assess for adverse effects. Assess the patient's financial situation. If needed, refer to a social worker to evaluate the possibility of assistance for obtaining his medications.

2. Explain that online pharmacies are not regulated like the pharmacies in the United States and Canada, and the efficacy and potency of the medications may be different; in fact, counterfeit drugs are frequently sold via the Internet. Explain the potential for adverse effects from a drug with an unknown source or the possibility of contamination from an unsafe environment. Teach the patient that pharmaceutical companies have programs to assist patients without the financial means to obtain their prescribed medications.

Chapter 3

KEY TERMS
FILL IN THE BLANK

1. Enteral
2. Intradermal
3. Parenteral
4. Topical
5. Local effect
6. Systemic effect
7. Emulsion
8. Enteric coating
9. Suspension
10. Intrathecal
11. Sublingual
12. Buccal
13. Troche
14. Tablet
15. Intravenous
16. Sustained-release
17. Capsule
18. Syrup
19. Intramuscular
20. Elixir
21. Intravenous push; intravenous piggyback
22. Subcutaneous
23. Intra-articular
24. Intra-arterial

CORE DRUG KNOWLEDGE: JUST THE FACTS
MULTIPLE CHOICE

1. d. Although the absorption of drugs may begin in the stomach, the majority of the drug will absorb within the small intestine.
2. b. Elixirs contain alcohol, which is contraindicated for use in children.
3. c. Drugs administered intramuscularly reach the vasculature via the excellent blood supply to the muscles; the drugs bypass the GI system.
4. c. Saline locks are used only in the periphery of the body.
5. a. Enteric coating on a drug delays its absorption until it reaches the part of the GI system with the right pH to dissolve the outer coating. Disrupting the outer coating allows the drug to be absorbed more quickly.

ESSAY

1. **Advantages:** provides immediate effect; allows administration of a large volume of drug; avoids tissue irritation or injury; use is acceptable when no other route is possible; circumvents impaired circulation; provides potential for prolonged, continuous administration of solution
Disadvantages: cannot be retrieved once given; distribution cannot be slowed or stopped

2. Intradermal, intra-articular, intra-arterial, or intrathecal

3. An enteric coating allows a tablet to resist the acid environment of the stomach to protect acid-labile drugs, provide a sustained-release dose, or guard against local adverse effects from a drug.

4. The layers of enteric coating dissolve in response to changes in the pH of fluids. The drug is released in a steady, controlled manner from a matrix of drug encased in a slowly dissolving substance such as wax. The drug may be bound to ion-exchange resins or chemical compounds that form insoluble complexes within the capsule.

5. Transdermal patches, ointments, creams, drops, suppositories, foams, liquid vaginal tablets, sprays, or inhalers

CORE PATIENT VARIABLES: PATIENTS, PLEASE
ESSAY

1. Vastus lateralis
2. Patient is vomiting, uncooperative, or unconscious; NPO status; patient is unable to swallow or has difficulty swallowing
3. Crush the pill and mix with a few milliliters of water. Mix in a tablespoon of jelly, applesauce, or pudding. Contact the provider to substitute a liquid formulation.
4. Verify placement of the tube. For an NG tube, elevate the head of the bed, unless contraindicated. Assess if the drug can be administered in the presence of food (tube feeding). Flush the tube with normal saline. Administer the medication. Flush the tube again with normal saline.
5. The skin is abraded or denuded. The drug is added to a specific solvent. The skin is covered by an occlusive dressing after the drug is applied.
6. Wear gloves when applying topical drugs. Use an applicator to administer. Use sterile technique when the skin is broken or denuded. Remove the patch immediately if adverse reactions occur.
7. Right patient, right drug, right dose, right time, right route, right documentation
8. Does this patient have diabetes? If so, monitor glucose levels. Assess for gingivitis. Assess for dental caries.
9. Lying on left side
10. Central access device

NURSING MANAGEMENT: EVERY GOOD NURSE SHOULD …
SITUATIONS

a. Vastus lateralis or ventrogluteal (dorsal gluteal as last resort—only if no other site possible)
b. Deltoid (preferred site), vastus lateralis, rectus femoris, ventrogluteal (dorsal gluteal as last resort—only if no other site possible)
c. Vastus lateralis, rectus femoris, ventrogluteal (dorsal gluteal as last resort—only if no other site possible)
d. Vastus lateralis or rectus femoris
e. Back of arms, abdomen, anterior medial midthigh

CASE STUDY

1. Does he have difficulty swallowing his medications? Does he have more difficulty with some of the oral forms than other forms (e.g., he might have great difficulty with the dry tablets, only some difficulty with the enteric-coated tablets and the capsules, and no difficulties with the suspensions)? If he has difficulties swallowing any of his drug

therapy, does this mean that he doesn't take all of his prescribed medication? What methods assist him to swallow?

2. Do any of the drugs come in liquid form? (This is especially important for the enteric-coated tablet because it cannot be crushed or broken to promote ease in swallowing.) If not, could another drug or another brand of this same drug be substituted for the drug therapy?

3. How to crush tablets and mix with a small amount of fluid or soft food, such as applesauce or jelly. Not to crush enteric-coated tablets and the rationale for this. How to open capsules and mix with fluid or soft food to swallow. Why to mix in only a small volume of fluid or food. Necessity for shaking suspension well before measuring. The importance of using a medication cup or dosage spoon or cup, rather than household teaspoon or tablespoon, to measure the correct dose of the suspension. If he is able to swallow some or all of his drug therapies but has some difficulty (reports that they stick in his throat, for example), instructing him to take a sip of water before placing tablets or capsules in his mouth can assist in swallowing. Also, he may be more successful swallowing one item at a time, rather than attempting to swallow two or more items at one time.

CRITICAL THINKING CHALLENGE

a. Does he have the ability (cognitive ability, physical dexterity, sight) to self-administer his drugs through the gastrostomy tube? Will a family member or other caregiver be involved in administering the drug therapies to him some or all of the time? If yes, they also need to be involved in teaching.

b. How to crush tablets finely into powder that can be mixed with water to administer. Enteric tablets cannot be crushed; an alternative form of the drug must be used. Capsules may be opened and mixed with water to administer through the tube. Whether tube feedings will interfere with drug administration or absorption. If yes, how long before or after an intermittent tube feeding should the drugs be administered? If a continuous tube feeding is used, how long should the feeding be shut off before and after drug administration?

Chapter 4

KEY TERMS
MATCHING
1. m   2. d   3. o   4. c   5. e   6. k   7. q
8. b   9. l   10. f   11. n   12. a   13. p   14. j
15. g   16. h   17. i

TRUE OR FALSE
1. False, pharmacodynamics
2. False, receptor
3. False, agonist
4. False, antagonist
5. False, affinity
6. False, potency
7. False, efficacy
8. False, loading dose
9. False, maintenance dose
10. False, pharmacokinetics
11. True

CORE DRUG KNOWLEDGE: JUST THE FACTS
MULTIPLE CHOICE
1. c. Parenteral drugs bypass the GI system and first-pass effect, allowing more drug to be delivered to the bloodstream.
2. a. Intravenous drugs are delivered directly to the bloodstream, allowing the drug to reach its highest potential serum drug concentration.

3. b. Ischemia is a decreased blood flow that would keep the drugs from reaching the site of action.
4. b. Many drugs will not cross the blood–brain barrier. Drugs that are lipid soluble (i.e., benzodiazepines) or those with an active transport will diffuse into the brain.
5. c. While all these sites metabolize some drugs, the primary organ of metabolism is the liver.
6. d. Affinity is the likelihood that a drug will attach to a specific receptor; efficacy is how well a specific drug creates a response; potency is the amount of a drug required to create a response.
7. c. Metabolism is the changing of a drug into another drug or substance; thus, it is also called biotransformation.
8. d. Although a drug may stimulate one receptor more than another, at this time, selectivity of drugs is not absolute.

ESSAY
1. Sweat and salivary glands; GI tract; liver; lungs; skin
2. The point at which the dose would be effective in 50% of the population receiving that dose is called effective dose 50% (ED_{50}). The point at which the dose would be lethal in 50% of the population receiving that dose is called lethal dose 50% (LD_{50}). The therapeutic index is the difference between LD_{50} and ED_{50}. The therapeutic range is the difference between the minimum effective concentration of a drug and the level at which the patient will experience adverse effects or toxicity.

CORE PATIENT VARIABLES: PATIENTS, PLEASE
MULTIPLE CHOICE
1. b. Patient B would not be able to keep the drug in the stomach long enough for it to be absorbed. Patients A and C would have alterations in their bowel that would allow increased absorption and increase the risk for adverse effects and toxicity.
2. a. Decreasing the contact time of a drug decreases the amount of drug that will be absorbed.
3. a. Patients with decreased liver and kidney function cannot metabolize or excrete drugs efficiently; thus, the drug stays in the system longer.
4. c. Because Drug B is more highly protein bound, it will displace Drug A. When Drug A is displaced, it becomes a free drug and is pharmacologically active.
5. a. Because the drug is not metabolized or excreted appropriately in patients with liver and renal problems, the patient has an increased risk for adverse effects or toxicity. The nurse does not have the ability to change the dose of a medication without the approval of the health care provider.

NURSING MANAGEMENT: EVERY GOOD NURSE SHOULD …
MULTIPLE CHOICE
1. a. Patients who have difficulty swallowing may not be able to swallow oral medication, depending on the drug form. Circulatory impairment will not affect a patient who has difficulty swallowing, although it will decrease the distribution of the drug. Skin integrity is not relevant for orally administered drugs, only those administered topically. Visual acuity might be important to assess if the drug caused an adverse effect of visual impairment, but this is not relevant here.
2. b. A smaller dose than normal to achieve the desired effect would be expected. A patient with renal disease will have kidneys that don't work as well as someone without renal disease. If the kidneys don't work optimally, the drug

will be excreted at a slower rate. This will increase the circulating level of the drug and place the patient at increased risk of adverse effects from the drug if the dose is not decreased. A larger dose than normal would be the opposite of what you would expect because it would additionally increase the risk of adverse effects and toxicity. Giving the drug more frequently does not alter the half-life of the drug, which is related to the time required for half of the drug to be eliminated.

3. b. Risk for injury related to potentially high drug serum levels would be an appropriate nursing diagnosis and relates most directly to drug therapy.

4. b. Drug toxicity. Because her albumin (protein) levels are below normal, more drug will be free and active than would usually be expected from this dose. Therefore, she will be more likely to have adverse effects, in addition to having increased therapeutic effects from the drug. Low albumin levels are hypoalbuminemia, not hyperalbuminemia. Low potassium levels (hypokalemia) are not related to protein levels. CNS depression would be a concern only if the drug could produce CNS depression as an adverse effect.

5. c. Drug B induces the isoenzyme P-450; this will increase the metabolism of drug A. Because the drug is more rapidly metabolized, blood levels of Drug A will fall, and this may produce a decreased therapeutic effect from Drug A. The effects (both therapeutic and adverse) of Drug B are not altered by this interaction.

6. d. Potency refers to how much of a drug is needed to produce an effect. Unless the increased dose increases the size of the pill or tablet to a size that is difficult or impossible to swallow, potency is not the most important consideration when comparing different drugs designed to treat the same condition. How well the drug works, or its efficacy, is the most important consideration.

7. b. Liver disease will decrease the rate of drug metabolism. This will cause an increase in the circulating drug. Unless the dose is decreased some, the patient is likely to have adverse effects from the drug therapy. A smaller-than-usual dose given to a patient with liver disease will produce the same response as the standard dose in a patient with normal liver function.

8. a. and b. Both absorption and distribution may be impaired. Metabolism is primarily in the liver, and elimination is primarily via the kidneys; because these systems are not affected by her pathologies or surgeries, these phases of pharmacokinetics are not altered.

CASE STUDY

1. The IV route will achieve a faster onset of action than the oral route. The faster route was chosen today to quickly bring down the heart rate. The oral route can be used tomorrow, once the heart rate has decelerated some.

2. The large dose today is a loading dose. It is designed to quickly bring the drug into therapeutic level without waiting for steady state to occur. The smaller dose beginning tomorrow is the maintenance dose; it will keep the drug at a therapeutic level.

3. There is an increased risk of toxicity and adverse effects from the digoxin during digitalization with the loading dose. The nurse should monitor closely for signs of adverse effects during this time period.

CRITICAL THINKING CHALLENGE

Steady state should have been achieved in five half-lives or 7.5 hours. An assessment of effectiveness was made before

the drug was at steady state. Therefore, the drug was increased too early, causing an excessively high (very prolonged time to clot) aPTT in 8 hours.

Chapter 5

KEY TERMS

1. Interaction
2. Adverse
3. Anaphylaxis
4. Idiosyncratic
5. Additive
6. Synergistic
7. Potentiation
8. Neurotoxicity
9. Immunotoxicity
10. Hepatotoxicity
11. Nephrotoxicity
12. Ototoxicity
13. Cardiotoxicity

CORE DRUG KNOWLEDGE: JUST THE FACTS

1. Drug interaction
2. Rash, hives, redness, swelling, and itching
3. Respiratory distress, bronchospasm, laryngeal edema, marked hypotension, rash, tachycardia, cyanosis or pale, cool skin.
4. Vasopressor agents, bronchodilators, antihistamines, corticosteroids, oxygen therapy, and IV fluid administration.
5. Drowsiness, auditory or visual disturbances, restlessness, nystagmus, and tonic-clonic seizures
6. Hepatitis, jaundice, elevated liver enzyme levels, fatty infiltration of the liver
7. Tinnitus, sensorineural hearing loss, light-headedness, vertigo, nausea and vomiting
8. Drug binding, alteration in GI transit time, alteration in gastric pH, and presence of food in the stomach
9. Non-narcotic analgesic with a narcotic analgesic
10. Synergism is an interaction in which two "unlike" drugs produce an effect greater than either drug's activity alone; potentiation is an interaction between two "unlike" drugs in which only one of the drug's activity is enhanced.
11. Physical incompatibility of the two drugs

CORE PATIENT VARIABLES: PATIENTS, PLEASE
MULTIPLE CHOICE

1. d. Because the patient has a history of multiple drug allergies, it is prudent to have epinephrine on hand because it is the drug of choice for anaphylaxis.

2. c. The expected action of chloral hydrate is to induce hypnotic sedation. Because the patient's response is the opposite of the expected, it is termed idiosyncratic.

3. a. Neurotoxicity affects the central nervous system, resulting in the patient's symptoms.

4. b. Probenecid does not increase the effectiveness of penicillin. It only blocks its excretion, allowing penicillin to continue its antibacterial activity.

5. c. NTG is air, light, and moisture sensitive. These environmental interactions have caused a decrease in the potency of the NTG.

NURSING MANAGEMENT: EVERY GOOD NURSE SHOULD ...
MULTIPLE CHOICE

1. b. Intake and output levels indicate one parameter of renal function. Renal function is impaired with a nephrotoxic drug. ALT and AST levels measure hepatic function. Balance is altered when ototoxicity occurs. Cognitive function is altered in neurotoxicity.

2. c. Liver disease will decrease the metabolism of the drug, and this will increase the circulating blood levels of the drug. More circulating drug means that the patient is at higher risk of adverse effects. Although more therapeutic effect also may be evident, this is not generally a prob-

lem. When excessive therapeutic effects occur, they usually are considered an adverse effect (example: drugs to treat hypertension are supposed to lower the blood pressure; excessive lowering of the blood pressure produces hypotension, which is an adverse effect of the drug therapy). Allergic effects and idiosyncratic effects are both related to patient-specific conditions and not elevated drug levels. These effects occur with normal dosing.

3. c. Drug therapy is often prescribed using more than one type of drug class to treat one disease or pathology. The drugs will work in different ways to bring about an additive response to therapy. Almost all drugs used this way can be administered at the same time because the goal is for them to achieve their effect together.

4. d. Patients and their families need to have a thorough understanding of the risks involved in drug therapy and what they need to do to decrease these risks. They also need to understand possible drug interactions that may decrease the effectiveness of the drug therapy or produce adverse effects.

5. a. Older adults have physiologic changes in their body systems that decrease the effectiveness of organs (i.e., decreased renal and hepatic function). These changes place the older adult at increased risk of adverse effects. Decreased therapeutic effects and pharmacodynamic effects, although possible, generally are not a major concern for older adults receiving drug therapy. (See Chapter 8.) Allergic responses are not accentuated by age.

CASE STUDY

Both of these drug therapies may cause ototoxicity. Teach the patient that tinnitus and hearing loss are signs of ototoxicity. Other signs are light-headedness, vertigo, and nausea and vomiting. If these signs occur, she should contact her provider. She should take the drugs as prescribed and not take extra doses on her own—only if told to do so by the provider. Dosages should be taken at prescribed intervals. If a dose is missed, she should not double the dose. Regularly scheduled hearing tests may need to be part of health maintenance if drug therapy is prolonged, dosage is high, or the patient is unable to easily detect auditory changes.

CRITICAL THINKING CHALLENGE

Health status: Does she exhibit any other symptoms of gastric ulcer or gastric reflux? Is she taking any OTC drugs to treat the acidity? Is she taking regular aspirin or enteric-coated aspirin? Is she taking the prescribed dose of aspirin?

Lifestyle, diet, and habits: Is she taking the aspirin with an acidic beverage, such as orange juice, that may be contributing to excess stomach acidity? Is she taking the aspirin on an empty stomach?

Minimizing adverse effects: Suggest taking the aspirin on a full stomach or with food. Enteric forms of aspirin may help decrease gastric distress. Avoid drinking large amounts of acidic beverages, especially when taking drug doses. Avoid self-medicating with large doses of antacids, especially sodium bicarbonate because acid rebound may occur. If these suggestions do not eliminate the problem, she should see her physician or nurse practitioner because she may be experiencing a gastric ulcer from the aspirin.

Chapter 6

KEY TERMS
MATCHING

1. c   2. d   3. e   4. b   5. a

CORE DRUG KNOWLEDGE: JUST THE FACTS

1. Immature body systems; greater fluid composition; smaller size
2. Appropriate drug dosages
3. $BSA = \dfrac{\text{weight in kg} \times \text{height in cm}}{3,600}$
4. 1 year
5. Water content; fat content; immature liver function; immature blood–brain barrier
6. Generic and trade names of drugs; rationale for therapy; anticipated therapeutic effects; route; frequency and duration of therapy; potential adverse effects; precautions or restrictions

MATCHING

1. b   2. c   3. d   4. a   5. e

CORE PATIENT VARIABLES: PATIENTS, PLEASE
MULTIPLE CHOICE

1. b. $11.9 \times 50 = 595 \div 4 = 148.75$. Round to 150 mg per dose.
2. c. Because the daughter is only 9 months old, her skin is thinner and more permeable than that of her brothers. If the same amount were used on the 9-month-old girl, too much of the drug would be absorbed, risking adverse effects.
3. c. A water-soluble drug moves to areas of water throughout the body, not just the vasculature, so the serum drug concentration may be subtherapeutic.
4. b. A 6-year-old child has fewer fat stores than does an adult, so fat-soluble drugs are not widely distributed and remain in the blood. If given the same dose as an adult, the child would be at risk for toxicity.
5. d. Preschoolers are often afraid of body mutilation. Showing the patient how the injection will be given may overcome this fear.

NURSING MANAGEMENT: EVERY GOOD NURSE SHOULD …
MULTIPLE CHOICE

1. c. In this case, a 25 gauge would be appropriate. The correct site is the vastus lateralis because it is the most developed at birth. The ventral gluteal site is difficult to find on an infant. The needle length should be 5/8 inch or shorter. Aspiration should always occur before an IM injection is administered to prevent accidental administration into the vein.
2. d. Use the measuring dropper, found with the medicine, to measure an accurate dosage of this drug. Avoid mixing the drug into an infant's formula to prevent rejection of future feedings because of memory of bad taste. Infants are not cognitively developed enough to be able to understand explanations and willingly comply with drug administration. However, infants will respond to a soothing voice and calm attitude.
3. b. This will prevent the toddler from playing with the pump settings and accidentally increasing the dose received. A pump should always be used to regulate IV infusions; they should not run by gravity. Enough volume

should be placed in the microdrip calibrated chamber (e.g., Metriset, Buretrol, or Volutrol) to last for 1 hour only to prevent overdosage if the pump malfunctions. In pediatric patients, IV insertion sites should be checked every hour for patency.

4. a. This offers preschoolers a true choice and allows them to have some control. They are therefore likely to be co-operative. Asking preschoolers if they want to take the medicine at all is not an appropriate choice because the child might say no. You would then have to coax or force the child to take the prescribed drug therapy. Children should never be threatened regarding taking their drug therapy. Preschoolers fear punishment and bodily harm. Threatening them makes them fearful and uncooperative. Children should not be called "bad" if they are hesitant to take the drug therapy. This creates more unpleasant feelings and anxiety and reduces cooperation.

5. c. The adolescent needs to be involved in the therapy and have an accurate understanding of it. Understanding will promote cooperation. Although the parents need to be involved, the adolescent needs to have an active role in the therapy, unlike with younger children, for whom the parent is the primary person responsible for answering questions and voicing concerns. Adolescents need support but should not be treated like younger children. The nurse needs to relinquish some control to the adolescent, as appropriate. The sense of control and ability to make choices promote cooperation in the adolescent.

6. b An accurate weight should be obtained prior to adminis-tration of any medication. The other nursing actions may be necessary for *some* drugs, but an accurate weight is required for *all* drugs.

CASE STUDY

To maximize therapeutic effect, assess the child's lifestyle, diet, and habits. It is important to determine if he smokes either cigarettes or marijuana. If he uses these substances after discharge, he will likely have a drop in theophylline levels and thus will not achieve therapeutic effects from the theo-phylline drug therapy. To minimize adverse effects, assess an-other aspect of the child's lifestyle, diet, and habits: his use of caffeine. How many caffeinated sodas does he drink in a day? Does he drink coffee or tea? Does he drink hot chocolate regularly? How much chocolate candy does he eat? Because theophylline is similar to caffeine, it produces similar CNS stimulant effects. A high intake of caffeinated products in-creases the risk of tachycardia, palpitations, insomnia, and other CNS effects.

CRITICAL THINKING CHALLENGE

The newborn is at risk of CNS depression and toxicity from the morphine his mother receives. This is because the blood–brain barrier is not fully developed in the newborn. In addi-tion, the newborn's liver and kidneys are not yet functioning optimally. Drugs are not metabolized or excreted as fast as they are in an older child, so more drug is available to cause adverse effects.

Chapter 7

KEY TERMS
FILL IN THE BLANK
1. Preeclampsia
2. Organogenesis

3. Hyperemesis gravidarum
4. Fetal alcohol syndrome
5. Lactation

6. Eclampsia
7. Gestational diabetes
8. Teratogenic
9. Fetal hydantoin syndrome

CORE DRUG KNOWLEDGE: JUST THE FACTS
MULTIPLE CHOICE
1. c. Absorption, distribution, and excretion are all altered during pregnancy.
2. b. Increased cardiac output and decreased arterial blood pressure may alter the pharmacodynamics of a drug.
3. a. Heart rate, cardiac output, venous and arterial blood pressures, blood volume, circulation, and coagulation are all hemodynamic changes that occur during preg-nancy.
4. c. Breast milk contains a high percentage of fat, so lipophilic drugs enter breast milk without difficulty.
5. c. Less than 2% of a mother's total dose enters fetal circulation.

MATCHING
1. c   2. e   3. b   4. a   5. d

CORE PATIENT VARIABLES: PATIENTS, PLEASE
MULTIPLE CHOICE
1. a. The major fetal organs form in the period of conception to approximately 60 days after conception.
2. d. Hydralazine, one of the drugs of choice for preeclamp-sia, is a direct vasodilator. The drug is used to decrease blood pressure.
3. d. Most antiepileptic drugs have the potential to induce teratogenic effects on the fetus.
4. a. Acetaminophen is the only analgesic recommended for use during pregnancy.

NURSING MANAGEMENT: EVERY GOOD NURSE SHOULD …
MULTIPLE CHOICE
1. d. Metabolic needs vary during the course of the preg-nancy, so insulin requirements also vary. Oral hypo-glycemics are contraindicated during pregnancy because they cross the placenta. Insulin is used to keep the blood glucose levels in a normal range because elevated glu-cose levels may cause fetal deformities. Patients who ex-perience gestational diabetes may have a return to nor-mal glucose levels after delivery, so insulin may be needed only during the pregnancy.
2. b. Piperazines have not been found to be teratogenic. The patient has concerns that injury may occur to her baby while taking a drug, and the correct information needs to be provided to reduce anxiety. The greatest risk for fetal injury from drug therapy is in the first trimester, not sec-ond. Because this drug has not been found to be terato-genic, an effective dose should be taken. Hyperemesis gravidarum has deleterious effects on the mother and fetus because of the risks for dehydration and fluid and electrolyte imbalance.
3. d. All of the above are necessary before giving the first dose.
4. d. Instructing the patient to rest with her feet elevated sev-eral times a day is a nonpharmacologic intervention for swelling, a common occurrence during pregnancy. Drug therapy should be avoided if possible to reduce the risk of adverse effects to mother and fetus. Extra sodium in the diet causes fluid retention, so recommending a diet high in sodium is not an appropriate response. Although caffeine produces a mild diuresis, large doses of caffeine are not recommended during pregnancy.

5. b. Patient education should include that heroin and cocaine are contraindicated in breast-feeding because they are transferred in breast milk to the infant. Because the patient abuses both of these drugs, this is critical information to share with the patient. Breast milk has significant advantages over commercial formula (not the other way around), among them being that antibodies are passed to the child from the mother and breast milk is easily digested. However, because of the possibility the mother may continue to abuse drugs, encouraging the use of commercial formula may be more prudent in this situation. The mother also needs to be referred to treatment for her drug abuse. Because breast-feeding is not the best choice for this patient, teaching positions for breast-feeding is not appropriate. Although postpartum rest is important, it is not the priority in this situation.

CASE STUDY

This patient needs to have blood levels of aminophylline drawn at regular intervals during infusion of the drug and after dose increases. This is because aminophylline can reach toxic levels, causing adverse effects in both the mother and the fetus. Breath sounds and vital signs should be assessed at regular intervals to determine the effectiveness of the drug. In addition, the patient should be assessed for signs of adverse effects (tachycardia, insomnia, GI distress). Use of aminophylline should be discontinued as soon as possible to help minimize risk to the fetus. However, therapeutic effect should be attained.

CRITICAL THINKING CHALLENGE

Although it is unknown whether ipratropium is excreted in breast milk, it is unlikely to be of concern. Little of the drug is absorbed systemically when it is administered through an inhaler. Assess the patient's lifestyle to determine if she smokes because this may be contributing to her bronchitis. Smoking cigarettes also would counteract the effect of the inhaler. Assess her home environment. Does another person who smokes live with her? Second-hand smoke is also irritating and can cause respiratory problems for the patient and her baby. In addition, consider whether environmental pollutants may be contributing to her bronchitis.

Chapter 8

KEY TERMS
TRUE OR FALSE

1. False, risk-benefit ratio
2. True
3. False, paradoxical
4. True
5. False, polypharmacy
6. False, frail elderly

PHYSIOLOGY AND PATHOPHYSIOLOGY: THE BODY HUMAN
ESSAY

1. Increased gastric pH levels; slowed blood flow; decreased GI motility; reduced surface area of the GI tract
2. Decreased body mass; reduced levels of plasma albumin; less effective blood–brain barrier; declining cardiac output; extreme changes in body weight; poor nutrition or dehydration; inactivity or extended bed rest
3. Decreased size of the liver; decreased number of metabolically active hepatocytes; decreased blood flow to the liver; decreased ability to remove many by-products; overall efficiency of the liver is reduced
4. Decreased glomerular filtration rate; decreased renal tubular secretion; decreased renal blood flow

CORE DRUG KNOWLEDGE: JUST THE FACTS
MULTIPLE CHOICE

1. a. In the elderly, the onset of action is delayed and the intensity of peak reaction is blunted because the rate of absorption is slowed; however, the extent of absorption is the same as a younger adult.
2. b. As we age, we have a higher percentage of fat than lean muscle. Thus, a fat-soluble drug will bind to tissues and prolong the distribution phase, half-life, and duration of action.
3. a. In the elderly, phase 1 metabolism slows, resulting in the extended half-lives of many drugs.
4. c. Creatinine production declines in the older patient because muscle mass decreases. This can give a "false" normal reading of creatinine.
5. a. In the elderly, the liver and kidneys are "mature" and do not work as efficiently as a younger adult's. This allows for accumulation of drugs in the blood, risking overdose, toxicity, and adverse effects.

CORE PATIENT VARIABLES: PATIENTS, PLEASE
MULTIPLE CHOICE

1. c. In the elderly, the liver may not be functioning effectively, including the production of clotting factors. When using an anticoagulant such as heparin, the activity of the drug may be enhanced because of the decreased liver function.
2. c. In an elderly patient, the onset of action is delayed only when taking a drug intermittently. Once the drug has reached steady state, by taking it daily, the onset of action does not change.
3. a. Chloral hydrate is a lipophilic drug. Because of the "maturity" of the blood–brain barrier, it is not as effective in the elderly as it is in a younger adult.
4. d. All of these questions reflect changes in the functioning of an elder adult.

ESSAY

- Identify the etiology of the nonadherence first.
- Advocate with the provider to keep the medication regimen as simple as possible.
- Coordinate the orders of all providers to minimize the number of drugs needed.
- Create memory aids.
- Facilitate the ability to open medications.
- Write all instructions in simple terms.
- Print in large letters as needed.
- Coordinate with social services or pharmaceutical companies to assist the patient when there is a financial burden that may prohibit the patient from obtaining the medication.

NURSING MANAGEMENT: EVERY GOOD NURSE SHOULD ...
MULTIPLE CHOICE

1. d. This patient can swallow, but large pieces of food pose difficulty for him. Therefore, it may be assumed that he may have trouble with large pills, tablets, or capsules. Crushing the medication or providing it in a liquid oral form will make the medications easier to swallow. It is not necessary to avoid the oral route as long as he can swallow without choking. Drug absorption and elimination are not affected by his difficulty swallowing.
2. b. How this patient usually obtains prescriptions and refills. Is there a regular plan in place, such as a relative, neighbor, or friend who takes her to the store, or does she

drive herself? Does she walk to a neighborhood store? Buy her prescriptions by mail? If she is unsure how she will obtain the prescription, she may have trouble obtaining it and being adherent with the drug regimen. Although knowledge about her ability to get out of the house and her fluid intake may provide more data about her, neither directly relates to potential adherence problems. Renal and hepatic disease may alter pharmacokinetics, but they don't have an effect on her adherence with drug therapy.

3. b. The renal function of an older adult is most likely not as good as the renal function of a younger adult. This patient is receiving a drug that may cause renal damage. A smaller dose would be expected, and possibly also given at less frequent intervals, to decrease the risk of renal damage from the gentamicin.

4. d. These are signs of adverse effects from the drug therapy. Older adults are more sensitive to the CNS effects of drugs that depress the CNS, such as phenytoin. Excessive sleepiness and difficulty concentrating are signs of CNS depression. Although normal aging may include some of these symptoms, the new onset of the symptoms tends to dispute that they are age-related changes.

5. a. Begin drug dosage with the minimal effective dose and titrate upward with older adults. This is especially important with drugs that depress the CNS. In addition, she has received anesthesia, also a CNS depressant, and may still be having some CNS effects from that.

CASE STUDY

No, he is missing some doses. (He was missing one dose of nicardipine every day.) All of the drugs should have their first dose of the morning taken early in the day, such as 8 AM, because a dose would not have been taken since the previous evening. Instruct the patient to take the first dose "with breakfast" to be a memory aid. The captopril, being dosed three times a day, will need a second dose in the late afternoon to distribute the day's dosing. A recommended time would be 4 PM. Ideally, the second dose of furosemide, nicardipine, and potassium would be early evening, such as 6 PM, with dinner. Administration of furosemide, a diuretic, should be avoided in the late evening because it will create nocturia. If taking a drug at 4 PM and others at 6 PM proves to be too difficult to remember, the furosemide, captopril, nicardipine, and potassium could all be given together at 4 PM. The theophylline is due at 8 PM. To limit the dosage times, consult with the prescriber to confirm that the second dose may be given at a different time. Pharmacokinetics of the theophylline, a sustained-release drug, indicate that a 2-hour swing either way most likely should not cause significant problems with therapeutic blood levels. Therefore, ask the provider if the theophylline may be taken at 6 PM with the second dose of furosemide, nicardipine, and potassium. Or, if those drugs were given at 4 PM, consider giving the theophylline at 10 PM, with the last dose of the captopril.

Written instructions should be given regarding the dosing of each medicine. Having dosages given around mealtime and bedtime will be memory prompts to take the drugs as prescribed. In addition, a daily pill organizer, in which all of the doses for the day are placed, can be helpful. An egg crate also could be used. If the patient has a watch with an alarm setting, he could set the alarm to go off when his doses are due. The 4 PM dose especially is likely to be forgotten because it is not taken at a time when an activity (eating, going to bed) will help jog his memory. Other aids, such as pictures that show a clock, the time of the dose, and the correct drug also could be used.

CRITICAL THINKING CHALLENGE

Health status: Does he have a clear understanding of why he takes these drugs for his health problems? Does he understand why they need to be taken regularly? Does he have adequate short- and long-term memory to take the different drugs at the correct times and remember taking them? Does he have arthritis or any trouble with the fine hand movement needed to open the bottle caps? If yes, are his drugs being dispensed in a child-resistant package? Does he have physical difficulty getting to the drugstore?

Lifestyle, diet, and habits: Is he having adverse effects from one or more of the drugs that affect his life? Does he have the income or health insurance to afford the drug therapies?

Culture and inherited traits: Are there any cultural issues that may be causing him to be hesitant or resistant to taking the prescribed drug therapies?

If the answer is "yes" to any of the above, he may not be taking the drug therapies as prescribed.

Chapter 9

KEY TERMS

```
 1                          2
 A  B  S  T  I  N  E  N  C  E
                            R
          3
          P  S  Y  C  H  O  L  O  G  I  C  A  L
                   S
             4
             S  U  B  S  T  A  N  C  E
                   D
 5
 P  S  Y  C  H  O  A  C  T  I  V  E
                      6               7
                      P  H  Y  S  I  C  A  L
                      E              D
 8                                   D
 H  A  B  I  T  U  A  T  I  O  N      9
                      N               W  I  T  H  D  R  A  W  A  L
                      D               C
       10                             T
       T                              I
 11                                   O
 C  R  O  S  S  T  O  L  E  R  A  N  C  E
       L                      C       N
       E      12
       E      P  S  Y  C  H  E  D  E  L  I  C
       R
       A
       N
       C
       E
```

PHYSIOLOGY AND PATHOPHYSIOLOGY: THE BODY HUMAN

MATCHING

1. d   2. b   3. c   4. a

MATCHING

1. c   2. b   3. a   4. d

CORE DRUG KNOWLEDGE: JUST THE FACTS

TRUE OR FALSE

1. False   2. True   3. False   4. False   5. True
6. True   7. False   8. True   9. True   10. False

CORE PATIENT VARIABLES: PATIENTS, PLEASE

MULTIPLE CHOICE

1. a. Alcohol is metabolized by way of the MEOS in the endoplasmic reticulum. Use of this pathway produces acetaldehyde and free radicals, which damage liver cells.
2. b. Esophageal varices is a complication of alcohol abuse caused by increased pressure in the portal circulation.
3. c. Cocaine is a stimulant drug that increases both the blood pressure and heart rate.
4. b. To achieve the highest response to the use of heroin, it is most commonly abused using the IV route.
5. d. Lability is the hallmark of hallucinogenic drugs such as LSD.

6. c. Inhalants initially give the abuser a "high" but have a very short duration of action, leaving the abuser tired mentally and physically.
7. a. These are symptoms of fetal alcohol syndrome (FAS).
8. c. These are symptoms of neonatal narcotic abstinence syndrome.

NURSING MANAGEMENT: EVERY GOOD NURSE SHOULD …

MULTIPLE CHOICE

1. d. Nicotine (in cigarettes), alcohol, and street drugs are all substances that may be abused and may interact with prescribed drug therapy.
2. c. Disulfiram interacts with alcohol, producing feelings of acute illness and unpleasant sensations. Any alcohol intake will produce this response. This would include alcohol found in elixirs (such as some cough and cold medicines). The drug needs to be taken regularly. It does not decrease craving.
3. c. Staying with the patient and speaking in a calm and soothing manner will help alleviate fear and anxiety from the "bad trip." Patients should be placed in a quiet room to decrease sensory stimulation, not the middle of a busy emergency room. Phenothiazines should not be administered because they cause hypotension, confusion, or increased panic reactions. Contact the physician for

orders for tranquilizers, barbiturates, or benzodi-azepines. Although a referral for substance abuse counseling would be important after the crisis of the "bad trip" is over, referral to an inpatient psychiatric hospital would not be the initial action of the nurse, and depending on the situation, may not be the most appropriate action. The immediate concern is keeping the patient safe and maintaining normal physiologic status.

4. b. Patients who have intoxication from inhalants may experience hypoxia from CNS depression; therefore, oxygen may be required. Maintenance of respiratory function is a priority. The child is already short of breath. Epinephrine is contraindicated because this is not an allergic reaction, and the cardiac stimulation from the epinephrine (a vasopressor) may interact with the inhalant, causing cardiac arrhythmias. A defibrillator should not be needed as long as vasopressors have not been administered, although significant overdosage may produce cardiac arrest secondary to CNS depression. An emesis basin is not a priority item in this situation.

5. b. Naltrexone (Vivitrol) is an IM injection given once monthly to assist the patient to maintain sobriety. Disulfiram (Antabuse) is an oral drug that is given daily. The patient should not be drinking alcohol with either of these drugs, thus a serum alcohol level is not indicated. Many alcoholics may seek counseling, in addition to pharmacotherapy. However, it is not the role of the nurse to refer to a psychiatrist.

CASE STUDY

This patient abuses alcohol. It is likely that there was still alcohol in his system when he underwent surgery. This may have created an additive CNS effect with the anesthesia and narcotics he received. He may have also required a larger dose of anesthesia and analgesia because of a cross-tolerance to the CNS depressant effects of these drugs from his alcohol abuse.

CRITICAL THINKING CHALLENGE

1. He may be demonstrating signs of alcohol withdrawal. He needs to be monitored carefully for additional changes. The physician should be notified regarding these findings. Consult with the physician regarding drug orders to prevent complications of withdrawal.

2. He is well educated and a professional. He does not meet the image of an alcoholic being a "skid row bum." The documentation that he "drinks socially on weekends" is vague and can be interpreted in different ways. Alcohol use is an accepted practice in the United States. The difficulty in arousing him after surgery may have been attributed to individual variation from anesthesia and analgesia if additional questions had not been asked regarding his drinking.

Chapter 10

KEY TERMS

1. Alternative therapies and complementary therapies include supplements of basic food elements, vitamins, and minerals, as well as the use of herbs and botanicals. Initially they were called alternative therapies because they were viewed as "non-Western." Today they are viewed as augmentations or supplements to Western health care, thus the term "complementary."

2. Herbal and botanical preparations are those substances derived from a plant source used either as a dietary supplement or as a medication.

3. The major mineral cations are calcium, magnesium, potassium, and sodium.

4. Phytomedicinals are therapeutic agents derived from plants or a preparation derived from a plant.

5. The most important trace elements are chromium, copper, iron, selenium, and zinc.

6. A vitamin is an organic compound needed by the body to maintain health, regulate metabolism, assist in the biochemistry of food digestion, and act as a co-factor for enzymes.

CORE DRUG KNOWLEDGE: JUST THE FACTS
MULTIPLE CHOICE

1. c. The appropriate diet consists of protein 15% to 20%; carbohydrates 50% to 60%; and fat 25% to 30%.

2. c. These are the physiologic processes affected by potassium.

3. a. Water-soluble vitamins are stored in the body only to a limited extent, whereas lipid soluble vitamins are maintained in the body much longer.

4. c. Iron is the principle element used to form hemoglobin.

CORE PATIENT VARIABLES: PATIENTS, PLEASE
MULTIPLE CHOICE

1. b. Excess magnesium causes CNS changes, hypotension, and cardiac toxicity, which induces changes on the electrocardiogram.

2. d. Diuretics, such as furosemide, cause electrolyte loss.

3. c. Homeless people, especially those who must choose between food and alcohol because of finances, frequently are malnourished, resulting in hypoalbuminemia.

NURSING MANAGEMENT: EVERY GOOD NURSE SHOULD …
MULTIPLE CHOICE

1. d. It is important to consider all nutritional supplements that the patient is taking because these may interact with current drug therapy or therapy that will be prescribed. It is also important to ask if the patient is taking the supplement on his/her own or on a prescriber's recommendation because patients may self-medicate without knowing of potential drug interactions.

2. d. Older adults with chronic health problems and who take multiple medications are more at risk of having drug-induced nutritional deficiencies. Asking what is the patient's typical daily diet provides some information as to whether any foods or beverages taken may interact with drug therapy. Knowing when the patient normally takes his medications may indicate if drug absorption might be impaired from taking a drug with food when it should be taken on an empty stomach, or vice versa.

3. c. Echinacea is an immune stimulant. Taking it with drug therapy designed to suppress the immune system will counteract the purpose of the drug therapy. As the intended effect is not achieved from the drug, the patient may have disease-related complications. Although vitamin C may be helpful in preventing infections, it should not be taken with echinacea. The nurse should encourage patients to buy herbs from a reputable source because purity and strength can vary; however, this patient should not be encouraged to buy echinacea.

CASE STUDY

Because he is malnourished, this patient likely has low serum albumin (protein) levels. Heparin is a highly protein-bound drug that binds to albumin. The low protein level will cause him to have higher-than-expected blood levels of heparin because of the decreased amount of albumin available to bind with heparin. When heparin is not bound to a protein molecule, it is free to exert additional effects on the body. This would cause the additional anticoagulant effect from the heparin.

A blood test measuring his protein levels would confirm this.

CRITICAL THINKING CHALLENGE

The chamomile and the garlic may both potentiate the action of anticoagulants, such as warfarin. Taken together they have significantly increased the coagulation time.

Chapter 11

KEY TERMS
MATCHING
1. d   2. a   3. c   4. e   5. b

CORE DRUG KNOWLEDGE: JUST THE FACTS

1. Acute care hospitals, acute rehabilitative units, transitional care units, outpatient units, long-term care facilities, and the home or community environment
2. In addition to the setting, other major considerations include trained personnel, and the ability to safely monitor the patient.
3. Heat, light, moisture, and sudden temperature changes
4. Industrial solvents, polycyclic aromatic hydrocarbons, pesticides, and ethanol
5. Smoking and diet

CORE PATIENT VARIABLES: PATIENTS, PLEASE
MULTIPLE CHOICE

1. a. Hepatic enzyme inducers increase metabolism, resulting in decreased serum concentration of the drug. For a drug to be effective, it must maintain a sufficient serum concentration to evoke its desired response.
2. c. Driving may be contraindicated, even with only one pill, if the medication sedates the patient too much.
3. b. The goal is to get the patient to sleep. Decreasing the environmental stimuli would be the first step to reach that goal. If unsuccessful, the nurse may then have to contact the physician for additional orders.
4. c. Because the patient is leaving the hospital, the nurse must assure that the patient understands how to safely and effectively continue pharmacotherapy in the home environment.

NURSING MANAGEMENT: EVERY GOOD NURSE SHOULD ...
MULTIPLE CHOICE

1. d. How long the patient is outdoors and in the sunlight will determine how much risk the patient has to develop a photosensitivity reaction. Assessing if there is refrigeration, where medications are usually stored, and other people in the house to assist the patient can be important questions to ask concerning other drug therapies interacting with the environment, but they are not especially relevant here.
2. b. Heat from hot water in a hot tub will cause vasodilation. Because the patient is prescribed a vasodilator, hypotension may occur from excessive vasodilation. You would not recommend that a hot tub be used every day, and patients need to be aware of this interaction with the environment.
3. a. Exposure to polychlorinated biphenyls, among other environmental pollutants and chemicals, is known to alter drug metabolism occurring in the liver. If the drug is not metabolized as well, more drug may be circulating than

would normally be expected, placing the patient at increased risk of adverse effects from drug therapy. The patient should be well aware of the potential adverse effects and notify the physician if they occur. Telling a patient he cannot work because of a potential drug–environment interaction would not be appropriate.

4. c. Medication reconciliation is required in JCAHO-accredited facilities and involves obtaining the patient's medication history and reviewing the health care provider's orders; however, the purpose in doing these actions is to protect the patient from injury, thus improving patient outcomes.

CASE STUDY

No, the obstetrician would not begin administering oxytocin to induce labor in her office suite, even if she has a nurse to be with the patient. Oxytocin needs to be administered in an environment in which the patient and fetus can be continuously monitored, specifically a labor and delivery unit of a hospital.

CRITICAL THINKING CHALLENGE

You need to refuse to accept this patient for admission to your floor. A general medical-surgical unit is not equipped to adequately monitor a woman and fetus during induction of labor. Contact the nurse manager, nursing supervisor, and the attending obstetrician for assistance, if necessary. The induction may have to be postponed for a short time until the labor and delivery suite can attend to the patient.

Chapter 12

KEY TERMS
1. Pharmacogenetics
2. Biocultural ecology
3. Stereotyping
4. Culture
5. Ethnocentrism
6. Ethnicity
7. Cultural competence
8. Cultural blindness
9. Pharmacogenomics

CORE DRUG KNOWLEDGE: JUST THE FACTS
MULTIPLE CHOICE

1. a. It is impossible to know the medical practices of every ethnicity, and it is inappropriate to expect an individual to "normalize" himself/herself to Western medicine. The best practice is to provide appropriate care and integrate ethnic or religious beliefs whenever possible.
2. c. Acceptance and respect are the most important concepts of being culturally competent.
3. b. This definition is from Burnell and Paulanda (2003).
4. a. The philosophy of yin and yang is associated with Chinese Americans.
5. c. There is no known cultural accommodation needed with the administration of penicillin.

ESSAY

1. Overview (heritage and residence); communication; family roles and organization; workforce issues; biocultural ecology; high-risk health behaviors; nutrition; pregnancy and childbearing practices; death rituals; spirituality; health care practices; health care practitioners
2. Genetic variations that have a low incidence in the population (<1%) are termed mutations, whereas genetic variations that have an incidence of 1% or greater in the population are polymorphisms.
3. Pharmacogenomics has the potential role of creating drugs that are individualized to optimally meet each patient's needs while minimizing risks for adverse effects.

CORE PATIENT VARIABLES: PATIENTS, PLEASE
MULTIPLE CHOICE
1. c 2. c 3. b 4. b 5. a 6. c

NURSING MANAGEMENT: EVERY GOOD NURSE SHOULD …
MULTIPLE CHOICE
1. d. All of the above are important reasons to consider a patient's culture.
2. b. Evenly spaced daily doses will help to maintain an effective blood level. Teaching with present-oriented people should emphasize current or present situations, as opposed to possible complications that may occur in the future.
3. d. Ask the patient about other herbs he uses regularly. These may have an interaction with prescribed drug therapy. Teasing, verbal "put downs," and insistence that Western medicine is the only correct approach are examples of ethnocentrism.
4. a. The white American is more likely to be a slow metabolizer of isoniazid than are the men of the other cultural backgrounds. Thus, he is more at risk for adverse effects from the drug. To prevent this, the doses are likely to be spaced further apart, providing less drug in a 24-hour period.
5. b. In order for the drug to be effective, it must have an adequate concentration in the blood. Ultra-rapid metabolizers will metabolize drugs with that isoenzyme more rapidly and thus may be at risk for subtherapeutic system levels of a prescribed drug. If a drug level has been ordered by the health care provider, the nurse evaluates the results and reports abnormalities to the provider. The nurse does not have the ability to order the test, or the frequency of testing. While the drug may not be sufficient to treat the disorder, it would be inappropriate to refuse to administer the drug.

CASE STUDY
Chinese Americans tend to have thalassemia, an inherited disorder of hemoglobin metabolism, more often than do other cultures. This makes the Chinese-American woman more at risk for anemia. Sulfonamides have the possible adverse effect of anemia. The risk of anemia developing from sulfonamide use is increased in Chinese Americans with thalassemia. In addition, Chinese Americans may have G6PD deficiency, which results in anemia; again the risk of anemia developing is increased by the use of sulfonamides.

CRITICAL THINKING CHALLENGE
Health status: Low or low-normal hemoglobin before the start of drug therapy.
   Life span and gender: Her hemoglobin may be normally low because of loss of blood from menstruation.
   Lifestyle, diet, and habits: Diet may be poor in iron-rich foods.

Chapter 13
KEY TERMS
FILL IN THE BLANK
1. Central nervous system
2. Peripheral nervous system
3. Autonomic nervous system
4. Agonists
5. Antagonists
6. Neurotransmitters

7. Synaptic transmission
8. Nonselective-acting drugs
9. Selective-acting drug
10. Sympathetic nervous system; parasympathetic nervous system
11. Adrenergic nervous system
12. Shock

PHYSIOLOGY AND PATHOPHYSIOLOGY: THE BODY HUMAN
MATCHING
1. c 2. a 3. d 4. a 5. b
6. c 7. a 8. a 9. d 10. d

CORE DRUG KNOWLEDGE: JUST THE FACTS
MULTIPLE CHOICE
1. a. Phenylephrine stimulates only alpha-1 receptors.
2. c. Phenylephrine is contraindicated in hypertension, pregnancy, closed-angle glaucoma and hyperthyroidism, not hypothyroidism.
3. e. Epinephrine is a nonselective agonist in the sympathetic nervous system that stimulates all of the adrenergic receptors except for the dopamine receptor.
4. b. Alpha and beta receptors stimulate the cardiovascular and respiratory systems.
5. c. Dopamine is used to correct the hemodynamic imbalances present in shock.
6. c. Dopamine does not exert effects to alpha-2 or beta-1 receptor sites.
7. b. Inhibiting alpha-1 results in decreased peripheral vascular resistance, thus lowering blood pressure.
8. a. Doxazosin (Cardura) is the only alpha-1 antagonist in this list.
9. c. One of the actions of propranolol is to decrease the heart rate; therefore, it would be contraindicated for patients with bradycardia.
10. d. Propranolol may cause CNS disturbances, especially in the elderly; it may also mask the signs of hypoglycemia in type 1 diabetes mellitus, and it may induce hyperthyroidism in susceptible patients.
11. b. Radiocontrast media is difficult for the kidneys to excrete. Fenoldopam (Corlopam) promotes vasodilation to the coronary, renal, mesenteric, and peripheral arteries and protects the kidneys, especially in patients with pre-existing renal insufficiency.

CORE PATIENT VARIABLES: PATIENTS, PLEASE
MULTIPLE CHOICE
1. d. As an adrenergic agonist, phenylephrine may increase blood pressure.
2. c. Epinephrine is a nonselective adrenergic agonist; thus, it increases blood pressure.
3. d. For a quick onset, epinephrine should be given subcutaneously.
4. a. Because epinephrine stimulates both alpha and beta receptors, adverse effects such as those described are likely to occur.
5. b. Albuterol is a beta-2 selective drug, whereas isoproterenol stimulates both beta-1 and beta-2.
6. b. Prazosin may cause "first-dose syncope." The patient should be sitting or lying to minimize this effect.
7. a. Alcohol may vasodilate, thus increasing the risk for hypotension when combined with prazosin.
8. d. A patient who is "beta blocked" should have a slowed heart rate.

9. c. Propranolol is a nonselective beta blocker. Stimulation of beta-2 causes bronchoconstriction, which may induce asthma symptoms.
10. c. The action of fenoldopam is to decrease blood pressure.

NURSING MANAGEMENT: EVERY GOOD NURSE SHOULD …
MULTIPLE CHOICE
1. b. The first priority is to limit the vasoconstrictive damage done by the drug by limiting the drug that gets into the tissues. To limit the blood flow to the area, the arm should be elevated, not lowered. A tourniquet placed below the area of extravasation will cause additional venous constriction to the arm and hand. Blood pressure should be assessed because the drug was being given to treat hypotension, but this is not the priority.
2. c. Phentolamine is an alpha blocker and is the antidote for overdosage or extravasation of phenylephrine. It should be injected subcutaneously into the affected tissue. Epinephrine is not appropriate because it also causes vasoconstriction.
3. b. Changes in rhythm may occur from epinephrine use. Hypertension is possible after epinephrine administration, not hypotension. Decreased urinary output and fever are not related to epinephrine use.
4. d. Administering whole blood is the best way to correct the hypovolemia after hemorrhage. Although other fluids can be used, they are not the best method for correcting the blood loss. Hypovolemia must be corrected before a dopamine infusion is started.
5. c. The first dose of prazosin may cause sedation or syncope. To avoid dizziness and weakness related to orthostatic hypotension, the patient should avoid quick position changes, drinking alcohol, and activities that cause more vasodilation, such as hot showers. Taking the drug at night, at least the first dose, will minimize the recognition of the adverse effects of sedation and syncope.
6. b. Abruptly stopping therapy with propranolol and other beta blockers causes a reflex tachycardia, resulting in angina and possibly even myocardial infarction. Depression can be a significant adverse effect from propranolol and other beta blockers. The depression goes away when the drug therapy is stopped. An increased dose should not be given because this may worsen depression or cause other adverse effects.

CASE STUDY
1. Dopamine raises the blood pressure by increasing cardiac output. Systolic blood pressure is predominantly elevated. Dopamine also increases the blood flow to the heart, brain, and kidneys. Increased blood flow to the kidneys increases the glomerular filtration rate and urinary output. Thus, both blood pressure and urinary output will increase if the dose of dopamine is appropriate for the patient's needs.
2. The dopamine appears to have been increased too much because the patient is now hypertensive, although urinary output is satisfactory. The rate of dopamine infusion should be slowed somewhat. Continue to monitor the blood pressure and the urinary output. It is hoped that a small adjustment will return the blood pressure to the desired reading.

CRITICAL THINKING CHALLENGE
Although abrupt cessation of beta blockers can cause tachycardia and angina, skipping or delaying one dose is not the same as abrupt cessation. Although drug levels will fall, possibly to subtherapeutic levels, some of the drug will remain in circulation. The patient is expected to be able to take oral fluids after surgery, so he could receive the next dose at that time. Mark the chart to make sure the anesthesiologist is aware of the hypertension, the use of propranolol, and the dose that was withheld this morning in case the patient experiences hypertension during surgery. Plan on giving the propranolol when the patient is fully recovered from surgery and allowed oral intake.

Chapter 14

KEY TERMS
MATCHING
1. h   2. f   3. c   4. e   5. i
6. a   7. g   8. b   9. d

PHYSIOLOGY AND PATHOPHYSIOLOGY: THE BODY HUMAN
TRUE OR FALSE
1. False, constriction
2. False, decreases
3. True
4. False, hypotension
5. False, increase
6. False, retention
7. True
8. False, antagonize
9. False, high
10. True

CORE DRUG KNOWLEDGE: JUST THE FACTS
MULTIPLE CHOICE
1. a. Pilocarpine is used in the management of glaucoma.
2. d. Pilocarpine is administered as any other type of ophthalmologic drug.
3. b. Nicotine has very few pharmacotherapeutics; smoking cessation is its most common use.
4. d. Nicotine may induce many CNS effects, including headache.
5. a. Cholinesterase clears acetylcholine from the synaptic gap; thus, a cholinesterase inhibitor indirectly increases the activity of acetylcholine at the synapse.
6. b. Neostigmine is used in the management of myasthenia gravis because it increases the amount of acetylcholine available at the myoneural junction, resulting in enhanced strength of muscle contraction.
7. b. Atropine is a cholinergic antagonist that blocks the activity of acetylcholine.
8. c. PAM is the antidote of choice for irreversible cholinesterase inhibitors.
9. a. The principal actions of atropine are reductions in salivary, bronchial, and sweat gland secretions.

ESSAY
1. The major actions of atropine include a reduction in salivary, bronchial, and sweat gland secretions; mydriasis; cycloplegia; changes in heart rate; contraction of the bladder detrusor muscle and of the GI smooth muscle; decreased gastric secretion; and decreased GI motility.
2. Symptoms of a cholinergic crisis include nausea and vomiting, diarrhea, increased salivation, sweating, peripheral vasodilation, bronchial constriction, and respiratory arrest.

CORE PATIENT VARIABLES: PATIENTS, PLEASE
MULTIPLE CHOICE
1. c. Patients with cardiac disease may not be able to compensate for the transient changes in heart rhythm or hemodynamics caused by oral pilocarpine.
2. b. Nicotine may induce adverse effects in patients with preexisting cardiovascular disorders.

3. b. When taking nicotine, the patient should refrain from additional sources of nicotine, such as smoking.

4. a. In the case of a cholinergic crisis, it is likely that too much anticholinesterase has been given, whereas a myasthenic crisis may be the result of inadequate dosages failing to control myasthenic symptoms. If there is no relief or an increase in muscle weakness follows, the patient is receiving too much anticholinesterase.

5. d. Pregnancy, gender, or culture does not induce psychogenic effects.

6. c. The action of atropine is to increase the heart rate.

7. b. Elderly male patients have an increased incidence of benign prostatic hypertrophy, which predisposes them to urinary retention.

8. a. Many OTC and herbal medications have the ability to stimulate cardiovascular events.

ESSAY

Respiratory status; presence of ptosis; diplopia; ability to chew and swallow; strength of hand grip bilaterally; gait

NURSING MANAGEMENT: EVERY GOOD NURSE SHOULD …

MULTIPLE CHOICE

1. a. Pilocarpine will cause pupil constriction, which makes it difficult to see in the dark. Eye drops should be administered into the conjunctival sac rather than directly over the eyeball. Pilocarpine will increase saliva; actions to relieve dry mouth are not indicated.

2. b. Starting at the higher dose will prevent abrupt withdrawal and minimize craving. The patient already has a high tolerance to nicotine from smoking. Starting at a low dose and increasing the dose does not prevent tolerance and will not wean the patient from the drug. The patches should be used in the sequence recommended by the manufacturer. Because the drug is slowly absorbed through the skin, the patch is worn continuously to achieve a steady state and therapeutic level of the drug. Patients should not smoke while wearing a nicotine patch because this may cause them to overdose on nicotine.

3. c. Onset of action is within 75 minutes, so 1.5 hours after administration the drug will be working. Duration is as long as 4 hours after onset. After this period, the drug's effectiveness is diminished, so tiring activities should be avoided. Earlier than this period and the drug will not have taken effect, so again, tiring activities should be avoided.

4. b. Pilocarpine is a cholinergic agonist. Excessive cholinergic stimulation increases salivation (thus the drooling) and causes abdominal cramps, nausea, vomiting (from increased GI tone), flushing (vasodilation), and sweating.

5. b. Atropine, an anticholinergic, is the direct antidote to cholinergic overdose.

CASE STUDY

Health status: Does this patient have glaucoma? Does he have a history of urinary retention or difficulty voiding? Does he have constipation or signs of intestinal obstruction? Any cardiac history? All of these would be aggravated by the use of anticholinergics.

Life span and gender: How old is this patient? Older adults are more likely to be sensitive to the adverse effects of anticholinergics. Older males are more likely to have some urinary retention from an enlarged prostate.

CRITICAL THINKING CHALLENGE

This patient appears to be demonstrating excessive anticholinergic effects. Verify that he only used one patch per day because using more could lead to overdosage. Question whether he washed his hands after removing the patch. There is still drug left in the patch after it has been worn. It is likely that he removed the patch, got some scopolamine on his fingers, and then rubbed his eyes. This would have gotten scopolamine into his eyes, causing adverse effects such as blurred vision.

Chapter 15

KEY TERMS

TRUE OR FALSE

1. False, narcoanalysis
2. False, nondepolarizing
3. False, local
4. False, paralysis
5. True
6. False, anesthesia
7. False, neuroleptanesthesia
8. False, depolarizing
9. False, balanced
10. True
11. False, general

PHYSIOLOGY AND PATHOPHYSIOLOGY: THE BODY HUMAN

MATCHING

1. d   2. a   3. c   4. b

CORE DRUG KNOWLEDGE: JUST THE FACTS

MULTIPLE CHOICE

1. d. Isoflurane produces surgical anesthesia within 7 to 10 minutes and is usually administered with 50% to 70% nitrous oxide.

2. b. Isoflurane will increase cerebral blood flow, which may lead to increased intracranial pressure in a patient with head injury.

3. c. An emergence reaction is more likely to induce hallucinations in a patient with pre-existing psychiatric disorders.

4. b. The bright green urine does not cause an ill effect.

5. d. Because the propofol emulsion does not contain preservatives, it is important to limit its duration of administration to avoid bacterial growth.

6. d. General anesthesia requires systemic drugs.

7. c. The onset of muscle paralysis occurs within 2 minutes after administration and peaks at 3 to 5 minutes

8. b. The release of histamine causes dilation of peripheral vessels that may in turn cause hypotension.

9. a. ECT is a quick procedure. The pharmacokinetics of succinylcholine are quick onset and short duration of action.

10. b. Tubocurarine causes a decrease in the response of the muscle to acetylcholine, resulting in a flaccid or relaxed paralysis. Succinylcholine depolarizes the postsynaptic membrane, producing repetitive excitation of the motor end plate followed by flaccid paralysis.

ESSAY

Esters are relatively unstable in solution and are rapidly hydrolyzed in the body by plasma cholinesterase and other esterases. One of the main breakdown products is para-amino benzoate (PABA), which is associated with allergic phenomena and hypersensitivity reactions. In contrast, amides are relatively stable in solution, are slowly metabolized by hepatic amidases, and hypersensitivity reactions to amide local anesthetics are extremely rare. In current clinical practice, esters have largely been superseded by amides.

CORE PATIENT VARIABLES: PATIENTS, PLEASE
MULTIPLE CHOICE

1. a. Respiratory depression occurs with all inhaled anesthetics. Because of this patient's age and history of a pre-existing respiratory disorder, the risk for adverse effects increases.
2. d. Inhaled anesthetics can alter vital signs, GI motility, and the ability to micturate.
3. a. Propofol is delivered in a fat emulsion.
4. c. Keeping a quiet environment is adjunctive to the drug therapy.
5. c. The duration of action of subcutaneously administered lidocaine is 1 to 3 hours, depending on the strength of the lidocaine preparation used.
6. a. The patient should have an intact gag reflex before ingesting food or fluids.
7. b. The release of histamine may induce bronchospasm.
8. b. Tubocurarine does not cross the blood–brain barrier to induce sedation.
9. b. This information may change the anesthesiologist's choice of induction drugs.
10. c. Because of rapid depolarization, potassium is released, which may induce cardiac arrhythmias.

NURSING MANAGEMENT: EVERY GOOD NURSE SHOULD …
MULTIPLE CHOICE

1. d. A relaxed patient will have an easier and smoother induction into anesthesia. Active conversations will stimulate the patient, possibly causing stress, and will not promote relaxation. The environment should be quiet, not a busy hallway where noise and activity occur. Thorough preoperative teaching, including what to expect during induction of anesthesia, will decrease anxiety because the patient does not have to contend with "fear of the unknown."
2. d. Because isoflurane may cause hypotension and cardiovascular depression, vital signs need to be carefully assessed to be stable and to have returned to the patient's baseline. The patient should void before leaving the recovery room to demonstrate return of urinary function. Because isoflurane is a general, inhaled anesthetic, residual drowsiness may occur after initial recovery. For safety, the patient should not be driving or engaging in activities requiring full alertness and concentration.
3. d. While receiving tubocurarine the patient will not be able to speak, move, or breathe for himself. Turning and repositioning him will help prevent venous pooling and ulcer formation. Keeping the skin clean and dry will also prevent skin breakdown. Although the drug prevents him from speaking, he can hear and think. It is important for the nurse to speak to the patient while providing care and to offer explanations of what is being done to reduce fear and anxiety that may accompany being paralyzed by the tubocurarine.
4. c. Succinylcholine causes intense muscle fasciculations before muscle paralysis. This may produce severely sore muscles. The presence of sore muscles is not a dangerous finding or a sign that the patient was injured through negligence or drug error. Contacting the anesthesiologist is not necessary, and an incident sheet is inappropriate. Another dose of succinylcholine is inappropriate because it is used for rapid endotracheal intubation and before short procedures such as endoscopy and ECT.
5. d. Lidocaine with epinephrine is contraindicated for use in fingers, toes, the nose, and the penis because prolonged vasoconstriction from the epinephrine may damage these parts of the body. The physician determines the size of suture material required and whether Betadine will be used. It is the responsibility of the physician to explain the procedure to the patient.

CASE STUDY
The lidocaine would be administered subcutaneously to provide local anesthesia around the tissues where the chest tube is to be inserted. Lidocaine comes in several concentrations. Consult with the physician regarding the strength of lidocaine desired if such information is not in the orders.

CRITICAL THINKING CHALLENGE
This patient is showing signs of lidocaine toxicity. This may have been from a large dose, or the physician may have inadvertently administered the drug into a vessel, increasing the rate of absorption.

Chapter 16

KEY TERMS
MATCHING
1. g   2. c   3. f   4. e   5. d   6. b   7. a

PHYSIOLOGY AND PATHOPHYSIOLOGY: THE BODY HUMAN
ESSAY

1. Actin and myosin
2. When muscle contracts, the sarcomere shortens and the Z lines move closer together. The filaments slide together because myosin attaches to actin and pulls on it. The myosin head attaches to actin filament, forming a crossbridge. After the crossbridge is formed, the myosin head bends, pulling on the actin filaments and causing them to slide. The end result is the Z lines move closer together, the I band becomes shorter, and the A band stays the same.
3. Localized skeletal muscle injury from acute trauma, hypocalcemia, hypo- or hyperkalemia, chronic pain syndromes, or epilepsy
4. Spasticity is usually caused by damage to the portion of the brain or spinal cord that controls voluntary movement. It may occur in association with spinal cord injury, multiple sclerosis, cerebral palsy, anoxic brain damage, brain trauma, severe head injury, and some metabolic diseases, such as adrenoleukodystrophy, and phenylketonuria.
5. Symptoms may include hypertonicity (increased muscle tone), clonus (a series of rapid muscle contractions), exaggerated deep tendon reflexes, muscle spasms, scissoring (involuntary crossing of the legs), and fixed joints.

CORE DRUG KNOWLEDGE: JUST THE FACTS
MULTIPLE CHOICE

1. c. Although the onset of relief is 1 hour, optimal effects require 1 to 2 days of therapy.
2. d. Cyclobenzaprine has no direct action on the neuromuscular junction or the muscle involved, so it is ineffective for the spasticity of cerebral palsy.
3. a. Because of its structural similarity to tricyclic antidepressants (TCAs), cyclobenzaprine may reduce tonic somatic motor activity by influencing both alpha and gamma motor neurons.
4. b. Again, because of its similarity to TCAs, cyclobenzaprine may affect the cardiovascular system.
5. d. Baclofen is useful in multiple sclerosis (MS) and traumatic lesions of the spinal cord that result in paralysis.
6. b. Abrupt withdrawal of baclofen may result in agitation, auditory and visual hallucinations, seizures, psychotic

symptoms, or, most commonly, acute exacerbations of spasticity.

7. b. Carisoprodol and orphenadrine are similar to cyclobenzaprine; dantrolene is a peripherally acting spasmolytic drug.

8. b. Dantrolene is the only one of these drugs effective against malignant hyperthermia.

9. a. Dantrolene reduces the amount of Ca^{++} released from the sarcoplasmic reticulum, thereby relaxing muscle contraction from excitation.

10. d. For patients with cardiac disease, dantrolene can precipitate pleural effusions or pericarditis. In patients with pulmonary dysfunction, it can precipitate respiratory depression. Dantrolene may also induce liver toxicity.

CORE PATIENT VARIABLES: PATIENTS, PLEASE
MULTIPLE CHOICE

1. c. This patient's age makes her more susceptible to these adverse effects.

2. b. Long-term or high-dose use of cyclobenzaprine may induce a withdrawal syndrome if abruptly ceased.

3. a. Cyclobenzaprine should be taken around the clock for best results, and the patient should refrain from all alcohol. There are no dietary needs associated with this drug.

4. a. The blood–brain barrier is not as efficient in the elderly, and patients may have more CNS effects with cyclobenzaprine use.

5. c. Cyclobenzaprine and alcohol have an additive effect, resulting in increased sedation that increases the risk for injury.

6. d. All of these adverse effects are associated with the use of dantrolene.

NURSING MANAGEMENT: EVERY GOOD NURSE SHOULD …
MULTIPLE CHOICE

1. b. Dry mouth is a common adverse effect of cyclobenzaprine because of the anticholinergic properties of the drug. Although this adverse effect is not dangerous to the patient, it is uncomfortable, and the nurse should recommend some general strategies for dealing with a dry mouth. A dry mouth is not a sign of a drug interaction, an allergy, or a normal therapeutic response to cyclobenzaprine therapy.

2. d. To prevent withdrawal symptoms, the patient should slowly taper the drug over 2 weeks. Giving 2 pills a day initially cuts the dose by one third. Reducing the dose to 1 pill next cuts the dose in half again. Because this tablet is not scored, the dose cannot be decreased to less than one pill or less than 10 mg. Use of this drug should not be discontinued abruptly, but it does not need to be tapered over 2 months.

3. a. Baclofen causes sedation, dizziness, weakness, lightheadedness, lethargy, and fatigue, among other CNS effects, as adverse effects. Until the effects on the patient are known, he should be assisted in ambulation so he does not fall. Doing toe touches may increase feelings of dizziness or light-headedness and should be avoided. Alcohol may potentiate the CNS effects of baclofen and should be avoided, especially in the early period of drug therapy. GI distress often occurs with baclofen; smaller, frequent meals may be indicated.

4. b. This will promote ease of swallowing. The dantrolene helps to control the muscle spasms with multiple sclerosis, and its use should be continued if possible. However, because there are some choking episodes, the patient should not be forced to try to swallow the capsule because he

may choke on it. Cutting the capsule in half changes the prescribed dose and may not eliminate difficulty in swallowing; it is not an appropriate nursing intervention.

5. b. Because a major effect of these classes of drugs is sedation, the nurse must ensure the safety of the patient. Muscle strain may prolong the duration of therapy but safety is the primary goal of the nurse at this time. It is important to monitor for adverse effects and to intervene appropriately, but again, the most important role for this nurse is the safety of the patient.

CASE STUDY

1. When did the fatigue and weakness begin in relation to starting drug therapy? Was it a rapid change or a progressive deterioration? Are the fatigue and weakness getting worse or have they improved at all? These questions will help to sort out whether the fatigue and weakness are adverse effects of baclofen or signs of disease progression of the ALS. Sudden onset after the start of baclofen therapy and gradual improvement indicate drug-related effects. Are you taking the miglitol as prescribed? Are you following the prescribed diabetic diet? Elevated blood glucose levels may be responsible for the urinary frequency.

2. Assess the blood glucose levels, preferably fasting. Baclofen may increase blood glucose levels in patients with diabetes. If the levels are normal and the patient reports using drug and diet therapy as prescribed to control his diabetes, the increased urinary frequency may be an adverse effect of the baclofen.

CRITICAL THINKING CHALLENGE

1. Additive CNS depression has occurred from the combination of the antidepressant amitriptyline and the baclofen. Accommodation to these effects is likely if the patient continues to take both drugs.

2. Teach the family to assist with ambulation and to correct environmental factors that might promote falls, such as removing scatter rugs and arranging furniture so items are not in the traffic pathway. Suggest that the amitriptyline be administered at night instead of in the morning, to help minimize daytime sedation. If this is not effective in the next few days, the nurse should contact the physician regarding decreasing the dose of the amitriptyline. In addition, contact the physician regarding whether the depression could be related to the baclofen and whether this dose should be decreased.

Chapter 17

KEY TERMS
ANAGRAMS

1. Paralysis agitans
2. Bruxism
3. Bradykinetic episodes
4. Akinesia
5. Ballismus
6. Substantia nigra
7. Dopaminergic
8. Neuroleptic malignant syndrome
9. Dopamine agonist
10. Bradykinesia
11. Parkinsonism
12. On-off effect

PHYSIOLOGY AND PATHOPHYSIOLOGY: THE BODY HUMAN
ESSAY

1. Dopamine is an inhibitory neurotransmitter, whereas acetylcholine is an excitatory neurotransmitter. These two

neurotransmitters work in balanced antagonism, allowing for the initiation, modulation, and completion of smooth, coordinated movement.

2. Trauma, bacteria, viruses, and environmental factors can induce diseases. In this disease, the loss of dopamine occurs with the natural aging process and is not induced by other factors. This means all of the elderly are at risk for this disease.

3. Muscle rigidity, tremor at rest, akinesia, bradykinesia

4. Parkinsonism is a syndrome of similar characteristics of Parkinson disease. However, parkinsonism is not naturally occurring. It is secondary to other conditions that have structurally damaged the dopaminergic pathway or interfered with the action of dopamine within the basal ganglia.

5. ALS begins in the distal neurons and progresses in a centripetal but asymmetric direction. Ultimate neuronal cell death results in muscular weakness, muscle atrophy and fasciculations, spasticity, dysarthria, dysphagia, and respiratory compromise.

CORE DRUG KNOWLEDGE: JUST THE FACTS
MULTIPLE CHOICE

1. c. The symptoms of Parkinson disease are caused by an imbalance between stimulation of the dopamine and acetylcholine receptors. This drug increases the amount of dopamine available to stimulate the dopamine receptors.

2. c. When carbidopa is administered in combination with levodopa, it inhibits the destruction of levodopa in the periphery of the body, thereby increasing the amount of levodopa to cross the blood–brain barrier and be converted into dopamine.

3. a. Rarely, leukopenia may occur, but thrombocytopenia is not associated with this drug.

4. c. Concurrent use of carbidopa-levodopa and hydantoins decreases the therapeutic effects of carbidopa-levodopa.

5. c. Because there is an imbalance between dopamine and acetylcholine, one way to attempt homeostasis is to decrease the amount of acetylcholine.

6. a. Levodopa is destroyed in the periphery by COMT. Tolcapone inhibits this action.

7. b. These drugs act directly on dopamine receptors in the brain, thus reducing the amount of carbidopa-levodopa needed.

8. c. Riluzole is the only pharmacotherapeutic for amyotrophic lateral sclerosis (ALS).

9. a. The administration of riluzole with CYP1A2 inhibitor drugs, such as theophylline, has the potential to increase plasma concentrations of riluzole by decreasing the rate of clearance.

10. a. Bromocriptine is used in the management of Parkinson disease.

CORE PATIENT VARIABLES: PATIENTS, PLEASE
MULTIPLE CHOICE

1. a. Carbidopa-levodopa may not be used in patients with closed-angle glaucoma but may be used in patients with open-angle glaucoma. It is important to obtain additional information before this drug is prescribed.

2. a. Avocados contain pyridoxine (vitamin B_6), a vitamin that increases the action of decarboxylases that destroy levodopa in the periphery of the body.

3. c. COMT activity destroys levodopa in the periphery of the body and is found in people of Chinese, Filipino, or Thai descent.

4. b. Use of this drug should not be discontinued abruptly. It is best to have the prescriber discuss the adverse effects with the patient before making the decision to stop taking the drug.

5. a. Ropinirole acts directly on the dopamine receptors in the brain, thus reducing the amount of carbidopa-levodopa needed. The less carbidopa-levodopa, the less potential for adverse effects.

6. c. Riluzole does not affect the oxygen saturation level of the body, so arterial blood gases are not needed.

7. c. Riluzole prolongs the time before artificial ventilation is needed in the patient. The cost is prohibitive.

8. b. Caffeine products can inhibit CPY1A2, resulting in increased serum concentration of riluzole. Its absorption may be diminished by as much as 20% in patients who consume a high-fat diet.

NURSING MANAGEMENT: EVERY GOOD NURSE SHOULD ....
ESSAY

The patient receiving both benztropine and carbidopa-levodopa needs to receive care to maximize the therapeutic effects and to minimize the adverse effects from both of these drugs. Maximize therapeutic effects of benztropine by administering it regularly as ordered. To maximize the therapeutic effect of carbidopa-levodopa, administer it on an empty stomach (to promote absorption), limit intake of dietary protein (high protein slows or prevents absorption), and limit intake of foods high in pyridoxine (e.g., avocados, bacon, beans, beef liver, dry skim milk, oatmeal, peas, pork, sweet potatoes, tuna) because pyridoxine increases the breakdown of levodopa in the peripheries (i.e., there is less available to cross the blood–brain barrier). Constipation may occur from both benztropine (an anticholinergic) and carbidopa-levodopa, so actions to prevent constipation are essential to minimize the adverse effects of these drugs. Provide a diet high in dietary fiber with at least 2,000 cc of fluid intake per day and encourage moderate daily exercise to minimize constipation.

Benztropine, like other anticholinergics, causes dry mouth, so frequent mouth care is important. Offer the patient sugarless hard candy; chewing gum may also relieve a dry mouth, if this is appropriate for the patient. If these interventions are not sufficient, contact the health care provider to obtain an order for a saliva substitute. To minimize the other anticholinergic adverse effects, caution patients against driving, especially at night, because they may have blurred vision or enlarged pupils. If their eyes are sensitive to the light, they should be instructed to wear sunglasses. If their eyes are dry, administer artificial tears. Urinary retention from benztropine can be minimized by having male patients stand to void, and having female patients sit upright on a bedpan or commode seat. Monitor the patients' output and for any signs of retention.

Carbidopa-levodopa may cause nausea or vomiting, so the dose should be titrated upward slowly. This action also will minimize the adverse effect of orthostatic hypotension from carbidopa-levodopa.

CASE STUDY

1. a. You should do a complete physical examination to establish a baseline to monitor the progression of the disease. It is especially important to assess the patient's ability to perform activities of daily living.

   b. Drug therapy for Parkinson disease loses effectiveness over time. It is not started until the symptoms become distressing for the patient and interfere with normal activities.

2. Assess for blurred vision, dry mouth, constipation, and urinary retention. Assess for a decrease in tremors. Assess for any other signs of progression of Parkinson disease.

3. You should advise the patient that carbidopa-levodopa will not cure Parkinson disease but will help control symptoms. The onset of action is slow, and immediate results will not be evident. Take the medication exactly as prescribed and never abruptly stop taking the medication. You should provide dietary instructions to limit or avoid excessive vitamin B_6 and ingestion of alcohol. The patient should also be cautioned to take the medication with a low-protein meal. In addition, the patient should be advised to contact the clinic immediately if she experiences uncontrolled movements of the face, eyelids, mouth, tongue, neck, arms, hands, or legs. The patient should also contact the clinic if she experiences any mood or mental changes, irregular heartbeat or palpitations, difficulty urinating, severe or persistent nausea or vomiting, appetite loss, difficulty swallowing, or taste distortion. The patient should be given information about the "on-off effect" that may occur. The patient should be taught not to perform any activities that require mental alertness until the effects of the medication are known. The nurse should demonstrate how to change positions slowly to avoid falling from dizziness or fainting. The nurse should teach the patient about the potential for bradykinetic episodes and the slow decline in efficacy of anti-Parkinson drugs with long-term use. Caution the patient to sit down immediately if feelings of weakness occur to avoid injury from falls.

4. The patient should be taught about the potential for bradykinetic episodes and the slow decline in efficacy of anti-Parkinson drugs with long-term use. Caution the patient to sit down immediately if she experiences a feeling of weakness to avoid injury from falls.

CRITICAL THINKING CHALLENGE
Riluzole can elevate liver enzymes. This may be a transient effect while the body accommodates to the drug therapy. Repeated blood work will determine if accommodation has occurred (and enzymes are returned to normal or near normal levels) or if liver damage is occurring and the therapy cannot be continued in this patient.

Chapter 18

KEY TERMS
CROSSWORD PUZZLE

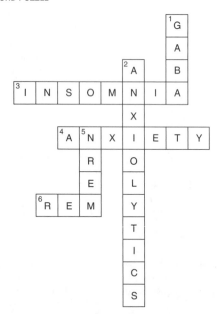

ESSAY
Panic disorder, obsessive-compulsive disorder (OCD), post-traumatic stress disorder (PTSD), social phobia, specific phobias, and generalized anxiety disorder (GAD) are the most common types of pathologic anxiety.

PHYSIOLOGY AND PATHOPHYSIOLOGY: THE BODY HUMAN
ESSAY
1. The amygdala interprets incoming sensory signals first processed by the frontal lobes of the brain.
2. The hippocampus is responsible for processing threatening or traumatic stimuli and helps encode information into memories.
3. Sleep stages 3 and 4 are also known as delta or slow wave sleep. These stages allow deep restorative sleep, during which time immune function is fortified and growth hormone is secreted.

CORE DRUG KNOWLEDGE: JUST THE FACTS
MULTIPLE CHOICE
1. d. The spinal cord affects muscle relaxation, the limbic system affects emotional behavior, and the cerebellum affects ataxic movement.
2. c. Lorazepam has been found in maternal and cord blood and can be transmitted to the fetus.
3. a. In addition to patients with psychiatric disorders, paradoxical reactions may occur in hyperactive, aggressive children.
4. c. Drugs that depress the CNS potentiate lorazepam.
5. b. Withdrawal symptoms such as nausea, vomiting, anxiety, or even seizure activity occur when long-term benzodiazepine use is stopped abruptly.
6. d. Children and elder patients require lower doses because of the potential for adverse effects in these populations. Asians require a lower dose because the half-life of lorazepam is prolonged in this population.

ESSAY
1. In addition to benzodiazepines, drugs for the management of anxiety include selective serotonin reuptake inhibitors, tricyclic antidepressants, monamine oxidase inhibitors, beta buspirone, hydroxyzine, meprobamate, and blocking agents.
2. Benzodiazepines for anxiety are generally considered pregnancy category D drugs, whereas those for insomnia are classified as pregnancy category X.

CORE PATIENT VARIABLES: PATIENTS, PLEASE
MULTIPLE CHOICE
1. d. Lorazepam is a pregnancy category D drug and should not be used during pregnancy or when breast-feeding.
2. c. Abrupt cessation of lorazepam may induce withdrawal symptoms. Tapering the dose of benzodiazepine decreases the risk for withdrawal.
3. b. The age of the patient and his ethnic background require the use of a lower dose of benzodiazepines.
4. b. Lorazepam may elevate liver enzymes and cause blood dyscrasias.
5. a. Because sedation is such a common adverse effect, the patient could be harmed if overconfident in his abilities while sedated.

NURSING MANAGEMENT: EVERY GOOD NURSE SHOULD ...
MULTIPLE CHOICE
1. d. Initial use of lorazepam may cause drowsiness, so driving should be avoided until the effects of the drug on the

individual patient are known. Alcohol and other CNS depressants cause additive CNS depressant effects and so should be avoided. Lorazepam is a pregnancy class D drug and may cause birth defects. Because the patient is in child-bearing years, this information is important to include.

2. c. Older adults generally have age-related deterioration of the liver, which can slow metabolism of lorazepam. They tend to be more sensitive to the CNS depressant effects, so the dosage should be started with a low dose and titrated upward if needed.

3. d. Because sedation and ataxia are common adverse effects from lorazepam, the patient is at risk for falling when going down the stairs of her house, so she should be instructed to hold the hand railing. Taking the evening dose at bedtime will allow the sedation that occurs from the drug to be beneficial and promote sleep. If she is having significant daytime sedation from the drug, the 24-hour dose should be divided in unequal halves (if possible), and the larger half taken at night so the sedation is helpful rather than an adverse effect. Women may metabolize lorazepam differently and have different adverse effects, but exactly what effects will occur are not currently known.

4. d. Tapering the dose slowly will prevent withdrawal symptoms. Withdrawal symptoms are likely if the drug is stopped suddenly. Because alcohol potentiates the CNS depression from lorazepam and other benzodiazepines, it should not be used with the drug, especially when trying to wean the patient from the lorazepam.

5. b. Low serotonin levels are known to be present in severe stress and in many mood and anxiety-related disorders. SSRI drugs block the reuptake of serotonin, thus it remains active for a longer period of time.

6. a. Zaleplon is a non-benzodiazepine sleep agent that is most useful for patients who have difficulty falling asleep. It has a short half-life so the patient should not feel "hungover" in the morning when discharged home. Lorazepam is a very close second choice because the patient states her mind is "racing" which could be a symptom of anxiety. However, lorazepam has a longer half-life and may cause daytime sedation when the patient does not routinely take the medication. Morphine is not indicated because the patient does not complain of pain.

CASE STUDY

Tell the patient not to be concerned. The IV lorazepam often causes amnesia of events that occurred after receiving the drug. This is a temporary effect and will not alter his permanent memory.

CRITICAL THINKING CHALLENGE

This patient may be experiencing digoxin toxicity because of a drug interaction with lorazepam. Check his blood level of digoxin to determine if it is elevated. See Table 18.2 for a list of drug interactions with lorazepam and Chapter 30 for more information about digoxin.

Chapter 19

KEY TERMS
ANAGRAMS

1. Antidepressants
2. Depression
3. Mania
4. Mood stabilizers
5. Psychotropics
6. Mood
7. Bipolar disorder
8. Dysregulation
9. Neurotransmitters
10. Serotonin syndrome

PHYSIOLOGY AND PATHOPHYSIOLOGY: THE BODY HUMAN
ESSAY

1. Changes in appetite; changes in weight, sleep, or energy; decrease in concentration; and recurring death wishes or thoughts of suicide

2. Grandiosity, distractibility, decreased sleep, more goal-directed activities or psychomotor agitation, belief that there is pressure to keep talking, subjective expression of racing thoughts, and excessive involvement in pleasurable activities that have a high potential for painful consequences

3. Flu-like (for example, fatigue, myalgia, loose stools, nausea); light-headedness, dizziness, or both; uneasiness, restlessness, or both; sleep and sensory disturbances; and headache

CORE DRUG KNOWLEDGE: JUST THE FACTS
MULTIPLE CHOICE

1. a. SSRIs are generally tried first because they are so effective and have a safe adverse effect profile.
2. b. Bulimia is not an FDA or off-label use of sertraline.
3. d. Antidepressant effects can take anywhere from 10 days to 4 weeks.
4. c. SSRIs do not have a high affinity for muscarinic, histaminergic, and alpha-adrenergic receptors.
5. a. There are no special considerations for patients with chronic heart failure or those with renal insufficiency.
6. d. Seizure activity is associated with doses greater than 300 mg per day.
7. c. Blocking alpha receptors may decrease the blood pressure.
8. d. Because of their lack of specificity, TCAs may induce cardiovascular toxicity.
9. b. Nortriptyline is useful in a variety of conditions that cause pain.
10. c. Although these are the most frequently reported, they are usually transient.
11. d. Phenelzine's primary pharmacotherapeutic is depression, although there are some off-label uses as well.
12. b. All of these adverse effects are possible; however, hypertensive crisis is the most serious. It is more likely to occur with the ingestion of tyramine-rich foods.
13. a. Lithium is the drug of choice; however, carbamezepine, valproic acid, and gabapentin may be combined with lithium for a greater therapeutic effect.
14. b. Lithium is not biotransformed into metabolites, so hepatic insufficiency is not an issue; it does not lower the seizure threshold as antidepressants do, and it is easily absorbed through the GI tract.
15. d. Be sure to note the decimal point in this range. The answer "5 to 12 mEq/L" is 1,000 times the actual range; "0.5 to 2.0 mEq/L" is the range for digoxin; and "10 to 20 mEq/L" is the range for Dilantin.

CORE PATIENT VARIABLES: PATIENTS, PLEASE
MULTIPLE CHOICE

1. b. All of the SSRIs, including nortriptyline, require 10 days to 4 weeks before they are fully effective.
2. a. Concern exists that sertraline may increase depression and risk for suicide in children. Whether the increased risk for suicide is related to the drug itself or to an increase in energy that enables action on suicidal thought is unclear.
3. b. Sertraline may cause sexual dysfunction, and many patients are hesitant to discuss this personal subject.
4. d. Because of the potential cardiovascular adverse effects, you should verify the order with the health care provider.

5. b. Dehydration must be avoided in patients taking lithium; foods containing tyramine are contraindicated in patients taking MAOIs; and nortriptyline causes sedation, rather than insomnia.

6. d. Weight gain is not generally associated with phenelzine, and OTC weight-loss products may contain sympathomimetics that interact with phenelzine.

7. a. These are early symptoms of lithium toxicity. Late symptoms include seizures, coma, arrhythmias, and neurologic impairment.

8. b. Patients should have serial evaluations of neuromuscular, GI, cardiovascular, kidney, and thyroid function. Cardiac enzymes do not need to be evaluated unless the patient has specific complaints of chest pain.

NURSING MANAGEMENT: EVERY GOOD NURSE SHOULD …
MULTIPLE CHOICE

1. a. Cured meats and aged cheeses are high sources of tyramine, which can precipitate hypertensive crisis when taking MAO inhibitors such as phenelzine; they should be avoided. Semolina pasta, apples, and orange juice are not food with high tyramine levels and do not cause an adverse effect when taken with phenelzine.

2. b. A dry mouth is one anticholinergic effect that is common with use of tricyclic antidepressants. Most patients will develop a tolerance to this adverse effect with time, and it will be less bothersome. Tricyclic antidepressants require several weeks to months to be fully effective. She needs to tolerate the adverse effects for a while, until the therapeutic effects are known. Coping strategies, such as sucking on hard candies, might be suggested. Dry mouth is not a sign of an allergic response, and the drug therapy should not be stopped.

3. a, b, c, d. Sertraline and other SSRIs often cause sexuality problems and changes. This adverse effect is a common reason patients stop taking their antidepressant. The changes to their sexuality become more bothersome to them after they have been on the drug a while and their mood has improved. If the patient cannot afford the medication, this will be a reason to stop taking the drug. If the prescription has run out and the patient has no refills, this will also contribute to nonadherence. While relieving the depression may encourage some patients to continue with an antidepressant, some patients may stop taking the drug because they no longer feel bad and don't think they need the medication any more.

4. b. Depressed patients will regain energy before their mood is fully lifted by antidepressant drug therapy. This is the time when they are at risk of committing suicide because they still have the mindset, and now they have the ability. Children and adolescents may be at special risk from SSRIs such as sertraline because the drug itself may induce suicidal thought or action. This risk appears to be greatest when therapy has recently been started.

5. b. The patient is stating that he is considering suicide because of his depression. Large overdosages of a tricyclic antidepressant such as nortriptyline may be life threatening. Therefore, it is important that the number of pills in the prescription the patient receives is limited. Several weeks of drug therapy are needed to fully lift the depression. Psychotherapy will be of assistance in helping this patient cope and work through his depression; it should be encouraged during drug therapy.

6. a. Lithium is a drug with a narrow therapeutic index, meaning that the effective dose and the dose that causes severe toxicity and potentially death are not greatly dif-ferent. Patients receiving lithium should have their lithium blood levels monitored at the beginning of therapy, at each dose change, and whenever they appear to have signs of lithium toxicity.

CASE STUDY
Health status: Is he taking an anxiolytic or antipsychotic with the lithium? These are needed to control some of the symptoms until the lithium achieves its desired effects.

Lifestyle, diet, and habits: Does the patient take a caffeinated beverage (coffee, tea, hot chocolate, cola) in the morning? The caffeine may be decreasing the effectiveness of the lithium and aggravating mania. Is he abusing drugs or alcohol? These may also reduce the effectiveness of lithium. Does he eat breakfast? Does he take his lithium on an empty stomach? If yes, have him take it with food to minimize GI upset.

CRITICAL THINKING CHALLENGE
This patient is showing signs of lithium toxicity, based on symptoms and elevated blood levels. His significant decrease in salt (sodium) content has contributed to the toxicity. Because the body interprets a lithium ion to be similar to a sodium ion, it treats them the same way. When his sodium level declined from its usual state, the body tried to conserve sodium. Unfortunately, it mistakenly conserved lithium, leading to increased drug levels in the blood.

Chapter 20

KEY TERMS
FILL IN THE BLANK

1. Dementia
2. Extrapyramidal symptoms
3. Tardive dyskinesia
4. Neuroleptic malignant syndrome
5. Delirium
6. Alzheimer disease
7. Psychosis
8. Schizophrenia
9. Vascular dementia

PHYSIOLOGY AND PATHOPHYSIOLOGY: THE BODY HUMAN
ESSAY

1. The frontal lobes control voluntary body movement, expression of feelings, perceptual interpretation of information, and thinking.

2. The extrapyramidal system is responsible for muscle coordination; the limbic system is responsible for the emotions of anger, anxiety, fear, pleasure, sorrow, learning and memory; and the reticular activating system is responsible for consciousness, and filtering and stimulus alert.

3. The primary neurotransmitter related to thought processing is believed to be dopamine. Dopamine is secreted by neurons originating in the midbrain that function in coordination, emotion, and voluntary decision making. Many areas of the brain secrete acetylcholine; reductions in the amount of this neurotransmitter cause cognitive changes. Acetylcholine has a number of functions, including arousal, coordination of movement, memory acquisition, and memory retention. Research is also being conducted on the extent to which norepinephrine and serotonin might be involved in thought processes.

4. Blockade of dopaminergic receptors produces a decrease in movement disorders, relief of hallucinations and delusions, relief of psychosis, worsening of negative symptoms, and a release of prolactin. Dopamine blockade also quiets the chemoreceptive trigger zone in the brain that produces

nausea and vomiting. Blockade of alpha receptors produces many of the cardiac adverse effects of haloperidol treatment, such as tachycardia, hypertension or hypotension, and EKG changes. Blockade of serotonin receptors produces adverse effects such as alterations in mood, such as depression or euphoria. Blockade of histamine produces adverse effects such as sedation. Blockade of dopamine receptors actually creates the net effect of too much cholinergic stimulation because the delicate balance between these two systems is altered.

5. "Positive" symptoms of schizophrenia "add" a dimension to the patient. These symptoms include delusions and hallucinations. "Negative" symptoms take away from the patient's personality. Flat or blunted emotions, lack of pleasure or interest in things, and limited speech are examples of negative symptoms. Disorganized behavior may make the patient do things that do not make sense, such as repeated rhythmic gestures or ritualistic movements.

CORE DRUG KNOWLEDGE: JUST THE FACTS
MULTIPLE CHOICE
1. a. Haloperidol is not effective in the management of depression.
2. c. Although all of these adverse effects are possible, extrapyramidal syndromes (EPS) are most common.
3. a. Haloperidol blocks dopamine, alpha, serotonin, and histamine receptors.
4. c. Patients with Parkinson disease have excessive cholinergic stimulation that will worsen with haloperidol use.
5. b. Clozapine (Clozaril) is rarely used today because of its ability to cause agranulocytosis.
6. d. Although the occurrence is rare, olanzapine may cause tardive dyskinesias and neuroleptic malignant syndrome.
7. a. Olanzapine is well tolerated; however, symptoms such as drowsiness, sedation, insomnia, agitation, nervousness, hostility, and dizziness may occur.
8. d. Olanzapine may substantially elevate blood glucose levels.
9. b. Antipsychotic agents (typical or atypical) are not indicated for use in Alzheimer disease.
10. a. Rivastigmine inhibits acetylcholinesterase, resulting in an increased concentration of acetylcholine.
11. c. Because of its increased cholinergic activity, rivastigmine may induce bronchoconstriction.
12. b. Gastrointestinal adverse reactions include nausea, vomiting, anorexia, and weight loss.
13. c. Memantine is used to treat moderate to severe Alzheimer disease. Because it has a different mechanism of action than rivastigmine, the two drugs may be used together for better control of cognition.

MATCHING
1. d   2. b   3. a   4. c

CORE PATIENT VARIABLES: PATIENTS, PLEASE
MULTIPLE CHOICE
1. c. These are typical symptoms of tardive dyskinesia. Older adult women have the highest risk for tardive dyskinesia.
2. d. These are signs of impaired liver function. Refer the patient to the health care provider immediately.
3. c. Haloperidol decreases the seizure threshold, thus seizure activity may occur, especially in patients with pre-existing seizure disorders..
4. c. Haloperidol may induce photosensitivity. Teach the patient interventions to minimize sun exposure.

5. a. The anticholinergic effects of chlorpromazine may cause dry mouth, blurred vision, constipation, and urinary retention.
6. d. Olanzapine may induce dizziness and orthostatic hypotension, so the patient should not be in the hot tub alone.
7. d. Olanzapine increases serum glucose.
8. c. Carbamazepine increases the clearance of olanzapine, resulting in low serum concentration of olanzapine. This may allow the symptoms of schizophrenia to recur.
9. a. Nicotine increases the oral clearance of rivastigmine by 23%.
10. d. The cholinergic activity of rivastigmine may induce bronchoconstriction and bradycardia. Rivastigmine is associated with nausea, vomiting, and anorexia, which would lead to weight loss.
11. b. The goal of rivastigmine therapy is to improve cognition.

NURSING MANAGEMENT: EVERY GOOD NURSE SHOULD …
MULTIPLE CHOICE
1. b. Sugarless hard candies or gum help promote formation of saliva to reduce dry mouth. Drinking extra water is also helpful. Hydrogen peroxide rinses will not decrease dryness of the mouth; neither will increased sodium intake.
2. a. Haloperidol causes photosensitivity, and protective measures need to be used to prevent severe sunburn. The goal of antipsychotic drug therapy is to have the patient's affective behavior stabilized so that he can interact appropriately in society. If he is well enough, he should work. Urine will not discolor during use of haloperidol.
3. d. Taking the drug at bedtime will help eliminate daytime sedation. The patient should stand up more slowly and gradually to prevent orthostatic hypotension, not stand up quickly. Increased appetite and weight gains are common adverse effects of chlorpromazine. Eating six large meals a day will make this problem worse and not correct daytime sedation. Increasing the dose of chlorpromazine is not an appropriate response of the nurse because it is not an independent action of the nurse and will most likely make adverse effects worse.
4. c. Atypical antipsychotics such as olanzapine can produce significant hyperglycemia. So it is important to monitor blood glucose levels, perhaps several times a day. Liver (SGOT, SGPT), kidney (BUN), and sodium levels are not affected by olanzapine.
5. c. Patients with akathisia have uncontrollable feelings of restlessness and the need to move. Actions that might promote rest and relaxation (sleep, quiet music) will do nothing to help the patient manage the akathisia. Telling the patient to accept that these feelings will occur is also not helpful in managing the symptoms.
6. b. c. This patient is presenting with neuroleptic malignant syndrome. Large volumes of normal saline infused as rapidly as the patient can tolerate will help to flush the drug out of the patient's system and correct any dehydration that is often present with this syndrome. Acetaminophen is administered to bring down the patient's fever. The rectal route is used because the patient has an altered level of consciousness and may not be able to swallow safely. Use of haloperidol should be stopped at this time; another dose should not be given. The patient needs to be watched but should be in a quiet environment, not in the middle of the ER, which is loud and busy.

7. a. Uncorrected hearing problems or vision problems may exacerbate the confusion the patient is exhibiting. These factors should be corrected first so that the full effect of rivastigmine can be determined. Eyeglasses should not be taken from the patient because this will contribute to confusion if the patient doesn't see well. Patients with Alzheimer disease have memory loss and are not reliable to be in charge of their own medication schedule. The memory loss is the reason drug therapy is prescribed.

8. c. Anorexia and weight loss are a common problem associated with rivastigmine therapy. High caloric supplements, such as Boost or Ensure, help add calories and needed nutrients. Encouraging higher water intake may fill the patient without providing any calories. Roughage and fiber are not usually well tolerated by those with anorexia. Withholding solid foods decreases caloric intake further. Small frequent meals would be a better answer.

CASE STUDY

This patient is demonstrating pseudoparkinsonism, one of the EPS effects. This is an adverse effect of the typical antipsychotics and is caused by the relative imbalance of dopamine and acetylcholine in the body from blocking dopamine receptors. This patient might benefit from a decrease in the haloperidol dose to minimize the EPS effect. If the dose cannot be decreased and still control the psychotic symptoms, an anticholinergic drug such as diphenhydramine, benztropine, or trihexyphenidyl might be prescribed orally.

CRITICAL THINKING CHALLENGE

The patient is experiencing acute dystonia, another EPS effect. Stopping and starting antipsychotic therapy can increase the risk of acute EPS. Diphenhydramine or benztropine given either IM or IV would be the expected treatment to quickly correct the imbalance. In addition to being given a drug antidote to correct the acute dystonia, the patient needs to be monitored closely for respiratory complications. A crash cart with airway management supplies should be at hand.

Chapter 21

KEY TERMS
FILL IN THE BLANK
1. Convulsion
2. Generalized seizure
3. Postictal
4. Absence
5. Seizure
6. Partial seizure
7. Tonic-clonic seizure
8. Epilepsy
9. GABA
10. Status epilepticus
11. Glutamate

PHYSIOLOGY AND PATHOPHYSIOLOGY: THE BODY HUMAN
1. GABA
2. When the activity from a focus spreads to other areas of the brain causing other neurons to join in the hyper-activity, seizures result.
3. Tonic-clonic (grand mal), absence (petit mal), atonic, myoclonic, status epilepticus, and febrile

CORE DRUG KNOWLEDGE: JUST THE FACTS
MULTIPLE CHOICE
1. b. Phenytoin reversibly binds to sodium channels while they are in the inactive state, which delays the return of the channel to an active state.
2. b. Phenytoin is used for generalized and other psychomotor seizures, status epilepticus, severe preeclampsia, trigeminal neuralgia, and for specific types of arrhythmias.
3. a. Although this is the therapeutic index for phenytoin, it is important to remember that it is a guideline only.
4. d. This type of integumentary symptom could be the beginning of Stevens-Johnson syndrome or exfoliative or purpuric dermatitis, all of which are potentially life threatening.
5. c. CNS symptoms include nystagmus, ataxia, dysarthria, slurred speech, mental confusion, dizziness, insomnia, transient nervousness, numbness, tremor, and headache.
6. a. Phenytoin affects ventricular automaticity, so it is contraindicated in patients with slow heart rhythms.
7. a. Carbamazepine is used in treating several psychiatric disorders.
8. b. Potentially fatal blood dyscrasias, such as aplastic anemia, thrombocytopenia, and agranulocytosis, can occur.
9. a. Liver toxicity appears to be more of a risk in children younger than 2 years who are receiving multiple AED therapy.
10. b. Patients with decreased sweating and elevated temperature should seek medical attention.
11. c. In addition to weakness (asthenia), levetiracetam may cause somnolence.
12. b. The incidence of aplastic anemia is more that 100 times the incidence found in the general population.
13. b. Ethosuximide controls the action potentials in the hypothalamic neurons responsible for absence seizures.
14. b. Answers a, c, and d do not meet the minimum serum concentration necessary to control seizures.
15. d. In addition to blood dyscrasias, ethosuximide may induce SLE.
16. c. Diazepam and Ativan are the benzodiazepines used for status epilepticus. Although clonazepam and clorazepate are also benzodiazepines, they are used as a maintenance drug for very specific types of seizures. Phenytoin is used for status epilepticus, but only after a benzodiazepine has already been administered.
17. d. These are all benefits of gabapentin.
18. c. Respiratory depression is most likely to occur when the drug is taken with other CNS depressant drugs, especially alcohol.
19. a. Children and older adults are prone to these paradoxical effects of phenobarbital therapy.
20. d. Although all of the answers may occur with some AEDs, only teratogenic effects may occur with all AEDs.

In the following table, identify which AED drugs are used for partial seizures, generalized seizures and status epilepticus. Drugs may be used in more than one column.

Partial Seizures	Generalized Seizures (except status epilepticus)	Status Epilepticus
carbamazepine	carbamazepine	diazepam
clonazepam	clonazepam	fosphenytoin
clorazepate	ethosuximide	lorazepam
ethotoin	ethotoin	midazolam
felbamate	felbamate (lennox-gastaut syndrome)	pentobarbital
gabapentin	lamotrigine	phenobarbital
lamotrigine	levetiracetam	phenytoin
levetiracetam	methsuximide	propofol
oxcarbazepine	oxcarbazepine	
phenytoin	phensuximide	
pregabalin	phenytoin	
tiagabine	topiramate	
topiramate	valproic acid	
valproic acid	zonisamide	
zonisamide		

CORE PATIENT VARIABLES: PATIENTS, PLEASE

MULTIPLE CHOICE

1. b. Phenytoin may cause gingival hyperplasia, so good oral care is important.
2. c. You need more information before you tell the patient to take or not take the additional medication. It is best to refer back to the prescribers.
3. d. Pregnancy is a complex discussion that should be done by the provider. It is important that the patient does not abruptly stop taking the medication in the meantime.
4. c. Ethosuximide may cause liver problems, so it would be prudent to know if the patient's liver had been damaged by his bout of hepatitis.
5. c. Ethosuximide may induce anemia, which would increase the risk of infections. The CBC will indicate the WBC count.
6. a. Diazepam should be administered undiluted, no faster than 5 mg per minute.
7. d. Although the patient may need to speak with a psychiatrist, it is more important at this moment to ensure his safety by telling him the potential for seizures should he stop the medication abruptly.
8. c. These are potential signs of infection and, because carbamazepine can induce serious blood dyscrasias, it is important to be seen as soon as possible.
9. a. Tablets should never be broken or chewed because of a bitter taste if broken.
10. b. Primidone is converted to PEMA and phenobarbital. To assess long-term use of primidone, you should obtain a phenobarbital level.

NURSING MANAGEMENT: EVERY GOOD NURSE SHOULD …

MULTIPLE CHOICE

1. c. Phenytoin interacts with a long list of drugs. Before initiating any new drug therapy, the nurse should assess if there is a potential drug interaction. Administering the drugs on opposite days is not an acceptable practice; it will decrease the effectiveness of both therapies considerably and may precipitate seizures. Antacids, although they may be helpful adjuncts to cimetidine therapy, should not be administered with phenytoin because of interference with absorption, so there is no need to seek an order for antacids.
2. a. As metabolism of phenytoin is increased because of the introduction of theophylline, there is less active phenytoin available for the patient. If blood levels fall below therapeutic range or the patient shows increased seizure activity, contact the prescriber.
3. c. Before the patient attempts to become pregnant, she should consult with her provider about the possibility of being weaned from the drug because she has been seizure free for 5 years. Phenytoin is a pregnancy category D drug and causes teratogenic effects in the fetus. Fetal phenytoin syndrome is not related to dose toxicity and may occur with normal therapeutic drug levels, although most women receiving this drug deliver healthy infants. She should not abruptly stop taking phenytoin because this may bring about recurring seizures or status epilepticus. In addition, fetal injury may occur if she stops and thus induces seizures.
4. c. Tube feedings interfere with the absorption of phenytoin. Phenytoin should not be mixed with tube feedings. Daily doses of phenytoin cannot be combined; overdosage may result.
5. b. Too rapid administration of IV phenytoin may produce cardiovascular collapse, hypotension, and life-threatening arrhythmias. Have resuscitation equipment nearby when administering phenytoin IV. Status epilepticus is an emergency situation, and drug therapy needs to be instituted immediately. Blood levels would be expected to be below the therapeutic range if the patient is experiencing status epilepticus. Gingival hyperplasia is a long-term adverse effect of phenytoin. Oral hygiene is important with long-term use. Warning the patient that he may be drowsy from therapy is inappropriate during emergency use of the drug while the patient continues to have seizures.
6. a. CNS depressant effects are common adverse effects from ethosuximide and other AEDs. However, fever and other signs of infection may indicate that a blood dyscrasia is occurring. Fatal blood dyscrasia, although not common, has occurred. Doses should never be doubled because of the likelihood of inducing overdosage. There are no known drug–food interactions with ethosuximide; fried foods do not need to be avoided.
7. a. Because carbamazepine can cause fatal blood dyscrasias (aplastic anemia and agranulocytosis) it is very important that a complete blood count be obtained regularly. Carbamazepine does not alter urinary elimination, requiring additional fluid intake. Like all AEDs, carbamazepine may cause CNS depression, including drowsiness when therapy is first started. The patient should avoid driving and other potentially dangerous activities for which alertness is needed until it is known how the carbamazepine affects the patient.

CASE STUDY

1. The child has a toxic level of phenytoin.
2. Question the mother closely about dosing. Was the drug given exactly as prescribed? Were there any double doses? What type of spoon is used to measure the dose? (A household "teaspoon" may be larger than 5 cc.) Was there a change in the measuring spoon? Is there any chance that the child took doses on her own? Did anyone other than the mother give doses? Overdosage may have occurred from these methods. Was the suspension shaken well before each dose? If not, the early doses may have had little or no active drug in them, leading to the low blood levels, and the last doses were pure drug, leading to the overdosage.

CRITICAL THINKING CHALLENGE

1. This patient appears to be having adverse effects and is possibly showing signs of early toxicity to the phenytoin.
2. Although most people need a drug level between 10 and 20 mcg/mL to be in the therapeutic range, this patient apparently was receiving a therapeutic dose for him when the blood levels were at 8 mcg/mL. Increasing the dose to achieve a "normal" range induced toxicity. Drug blood levels are only one parameter of therapeutic effect from drug therapy. In this case, they were misleading. The dose should have been maintained at the original level because it was effectively controlling seizures.

Chapter 22

KEY TERMS

FILL IN THE BLANKS

1. Attention deficit hyperactivity disorder
2. Cataplexy
3. Narcolepsy
4. Sleep paralysis
5. Obesity
6. Hypercapnia
7. Analeptic
8. Anorectic
9. Hypnagogic hallucinations
10. Overweight

PHYSIOLOGY AND PATHOPHYSIOLOGY: THE BODY HUMAN

MULTIPLE CHOICE

1. c   2. b   3. d   4. b

CORE DRUG KNOWLEDGE: JUST THE FACTS

ESSAY

1. Advanced arteriosclerosis, symptomatic cardiovascular disease, moderate to severe hypertension, hyperthyroidism, previous idiosyncratic reactions to sympathomimetic drugs, glaucoma, history of drug abuse, concurrent use of MAOI drugs, pregnancy
2. Restlessness, dizziness, insomnia, agitation
3. Palpitations, tachycardia, increased blood pressure. Sudden death may occur in patients with underlying serious heart problems or defects, and stroke and heart attack in adults with certain risk factors.
4. Cachexia and hypoproteinemia may alter the pharmacokinetics of other drugs, thus increasing the risk for adverse reactions, subtherapeutic levels, or toxicity.
5. Acidic juices and fruits must be limited. Foods containing caffeine, such as cola, tea, coffee, and chocolate, must be limited.
6. Sibutramine inhibits the central reuptake of dopamine, norepinephrine, and serotonin. It is thought that the serotonin mechanism enhances satiety, whereas the norepinephrine mechanism raises the metabolic rate.
7. The most common adverse reactions are anorexia, constipation, insomnia, headache, and xerostomia.
8. This combination may result in "serotonin syndrome" characterized by CNS irritability, motor weakness, shivering, myoclonus, and altered consciousness.

CORE PATIENT VARIABLES: PATIENTS, PLEASE

MULTIPLE CHOICE

1. d. MAOI therapy may predispose the patient toward a hypertensive crisis. Amitriptyline would require close supervision of the patient because of the potential for cardiac arrhythmias should the patient attempt suicide by overdosing on this medication.
2. b. Monitoring children's growth is important because dextroamphetamine may cause growth retardation.
3. a. Caffeine-containing drinks such as tea, coffee, and cola may increase the adverse effects associated with dextroamphetamine.
4. d. Children with ADHD require behavior modification in addition to drug therapy. It is impossible to predict the amount of weight loss an individual patient may experience. Dextroamphetamine should not be given at night because it causes insomnia.
5. c. Dry dilated eyes may cause blurred vision, which, in turn, may contribute to an injury to the patient.
6. a. Metabolic reasons for obesity should be ruled out before starting sibutramine therapy.
7. c. Sibutramine is a pregnancy category C drug. There are no conclusive studies that indicate that it is safe during pregnancy. It is not known if it enters breast milk.
8. d. Grapefruit juice increases the effects of caffeine.

NURSING MANAGEMENT: EVERY GOOD NURSE SHOULD …

MULTIPLE CHOICE

1. d. Symptomatic cardiovascular disease will be aggravated by the use of CNS stimulants such as dextroamphetamine. In hyperthyroidism, the CNS is already stimulated; adding a CNS stimulant may cause significant adverse effects. A patient with a history of drug abuse is more at risk for abusing dextroamphetamine.
2. b. Caffeine is also a CNS stimulant and may produce signs of CNS overstimulation when taken with dextroamphetamine. To minimize insomnia from dextroamphetamine, take in the morning or at least 6 hours before bedtime. Sustained-release capsules should never be chewed or crushed. Never take double doses because signs of CNS overstimulation may develop.
3. d. Insomnia and restlessness are signs of CNS overstimulation. Sleeping aids will treat her symptoms but not address the real issue of overstimulation. Contact the health care provider concerning decreasing the dosage to avoid adverse effects.
4. c. An increase in activity levels or exercise will assist in raising metabolism and promoting the weight loss effects from sibutramine. In addition, diet changes that incorporate a low-calorie and low-fat approach will increase the effectiveness of sibutramine. This may not be what the patient is currently following. Additional assessment is needed here. Peak levels of the drug are achieved when the drug is taken on an empty stomach, not a full stomach. Because the drug may cause insomnia, it should not be taken at bedtime.
5. d. All of these questions are appropriate to ask; however, the most important is whether or not the patient is being medicated for her depression. Both SSRI and MAOI drugs interact with sibutramine and are contraindicated for concurrent use.

6. d. Signs of intolerance or overdose from caffeine in newborns include tachypnea (rapid breathing), fever, and hyperglycemia.

CASE STUDY

Prescription anorexics are indicated when the patient is clinically obese and other methods have been unsuccessful. This patient does not meet these requirements. Over-the-counter anorexiants do help to suppress the appetite by stimulating the satiety center in the brain. However, these agents are not recommended during breast-feeding because they will enter breast milk and thus the infant. Safety has not been established in children.

CRITICAL THINKING CHALLENGE

This patient would be best advised to use nonpharmacologic methods to lose weight. She should drink plenty of fluids to promote breast milk production. Drinking water will also help promote feelings of satiety and help with weight loss. She should also be advised to cut down on calories while maintaining balanced nutrient intake and to increase her exercise to lose weight.

Chapter 23

KEY TERMS
MATCHING

1. d 2. c 3. h 4. a 5. g 6. f 7. b
8. e 9. j 10. k 11. m 12. i 13. n 14. l

PHYSIOLOGY AND PATHOPHYSIOLOGY: THE BODY HUMAN
ESSAY

1. CNS depressants may provoke a decreased release of neurotransmitters or an increased reuptake and inhibition of the postsynaptic enzymes.
2. Delta fibers are fast-traveling, myelinated, and responsive to mechanical stimuli. They sense sharp, stinging, cutting, or pinching pain. C fibers are slow-traveling, unmyelinated, and responsive to mechanical, chemical, hormonal, or thermal stimuli. They sense dull, burning, or aching pain.
3. Anxiety, fear, apprehension, attention, motivation, and cognitive processes
4. The areas of the brain involved in interpreting pain include the contralateral insula and anterior cingulate cortex, frontal inferior cortex, posterior cingulate cortex, bilateral thalamus and premotor cortex, and cerebellar vermis. These brain regions are functionally diverse and involved with sensation, motor control, affect, and attention.
5. Unrelieved pain can affect the patient's psychological, social, physiologic, and spiritual health and can prevent productive work and enjoyment of personal relationships.

CORE DRUG KNOWLEDGE: JUST THE FACTS
MULTIPLE CHOICE

1. d. Morphine is the standard measure of pain relief.
2. c. Decreasing substance P modulates pain perception.
3. a. Morphine causes sedation which would mask changes in the level of consciousness. The level of consciousness is the most sensitive indicator of neurologic compromise.
4. c. Morphine causes respiratory depression, especially in combination with other drugs that are CNS depressants.
5. c. Codeine acts directly on the medullary cough center to depress the cough reflex.
6. d. Codeine does not affect the diameter of the bronchioles, nor does it decrease respiratory secretions.
7. b. When codeine is co-administered with H2 antagonists, the narcotic actions are enhanced, resulting in potential toxicity and an increased risk for respiratory depression.
8. c. Pentazocine has agonist effects at the kappa receptors and antagonist effects at the mu receptors.
9. a. When pentazocine is given intravenously, it elevates systemic and pulmonary arterial pressures systemic vascular resistance, and left ventricular end diastolic pressure. These effects increase the workload of the heart.
10. c. All of these adverse effects are possible, but these are the ones most likely to occur.

CORE PATIENT VARIABLES: PATIENTS, PLEASE
MULTIPLE CHOICE

1. a. These symptoms are the exact opposite of what you expect in a patient receiving morphine.
2. c. In the elderly, the blood–brain barrier is less efficient, so CNS-depressant drugs cross the blood–brain barrier more freely.
3. b. It is important to assess the use of alcohol because it is a CNS depressant that interacts with all opioids.
4. a. All opioids cause constipation. Bulk laxatives are the type of laxatives that mimic the body's action to expel feces.
5. c. It is important to assess potential risks for injury as well as other drugs that may potentiate the action of codeine.
6. a. Excessive doses of propoxyphene, either alone or in combination with other CNS depressants (including alcohol), are a major cause of drug-related death. For this reason, propoxyphene and products that include it should not be prescribed to suicidal patients or those with addictive tendencies.
7. b. The most serious complications of "T's and Blues" are pulmonary disease and neurologic events.
8. b. The fentanyl iontophoretic transdermal system is a transdermal route of patient-controlled analgesia (PCA) for hospitalized patients. It is used to treat acute postoperative pain in adults but not intended for home use
9. d. Naloxone has a very short half-life. Careful monitoring of the patient beyond initial response is warranted because the duration of action of the methadone may be longer than the duration of naloxone.
10. a. Morphine and other opioid medications cause respiratory depression, constipation, and nausea and vomiting. In addition to these adverse effects, tramadol may induce seizure activity.

NURSING MANAGEMENT: EVERY GOOD NURSE SHOULD …
DECISION TREE

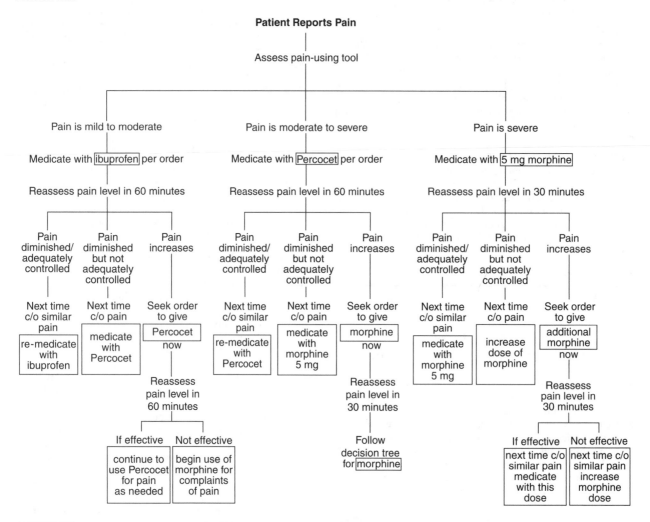

CASE STUDY

1. Yes. Pain is subjective, and the patient reports he has severe pain. It is not unexpected that he has pain because he has undergone surgery.
2. Does he obtain any relief from the one Percocet? How long does the relief last? What does the pain level become when the drug is working? What nonpharmacologic methods are effective for this patient in dealing with pain and reducing sensation of pain?
3. Medicate him with two Percocet tablets now, repeat the dose in 4 hours, not 6 hours. (One tablet was not effective; do not repeat an ineffective dose.) If two are not effective, begin use of morphine 8 mg IM every 3 hours.

CRITICAL THINKING CHALLENGE

The first patient has a history of opioid and alcohol abuse, which may have created a cross-tolerance to the opioid analgesics, requiring him to have a higher dose for pain relief. His tolerance for substances that depress the CNS will minimize the sedation, an adverse effect, of morphine. The second patient does not have a history of substance abuse and thus may be more sensitive to the CNS depressant effects of the morphine. In addition, because it is only 2 hours since his surgery, the anesthetics, which are also CNS depressants, may have created an additive effect with the morphine.

Chapter 24

KEY TERMS
MATCHING

1. f	6. h
2. j	7. b
3. g	8. a
4. e	9. d
5. c	10. i

PHYSIOLOGY AND PATHOPHYSIOLOGY: THE BODY HUMAN
ESSAY

1. Swelling, heat, redness, pain, and loss of function
2. Initial vasoconstriction of the surrounding vessels, then vasodilation to allow increased blood flow to the area; increased capillary permeability and release of chemical mediators
3. Margination, emigration, chemotaxis, phagocytosis
4. NSAIDs work by the inhibition of prostaglandins. There are many different types of prostaglandins, many of which have opposing function. When NSAIDs inhibit prostaglandins, they not only inhibit the cells that cause inflammation, but they also inhibit the cells that provide the body's protective mechanisms.

CORE DRUG KNOWLEDGE: JUST THE FACTS
MULTIPLE CHOICE

1. d. Aspirin has analgesic, anti-inflammatory, antipyretic, and antiplatelet activity.
2. c. With a history of peptic ulcer disease, this patient would have an increased risk for GI bleeding from aspirin therapy.
3. b. Aspirin has a short half-life and thus must be taken frequently.
4. b. The lethal dose of aspirin is 5 to 8 g for a child and 10 to 30 g for an adult.
5. a. These symptoms can progress to more serious symptoms if the toxicity continues.
6. c. Because most NSAIDs are nonselective to both COX-1 and COX-2, the protective prostaglandins are inhibited, especially in the GI tract.
7. c. Ibuprofen is quickly and extensively absorbed in the GI tract.
8. b. Because of their extended half-life, NSAIDs do not need to be taken as frequently as aspirin.
9. d. Ketorolac (Toradol) is the only NSAID that is administered IM.
10. c. Celecoxib is a COX-2 selective drug. Although it may still cause GI adverse effects, it is less likely to do so because it has a decreased effect on the protective prostaglandins of the body.
11. a. Celecoxib has the same actions as the nonselective NSAIDs, with the exception of antiplatelet activity.
12. d. Acetaminophen is a weak inhibitor of prostaglandins. It does not have any antiplatelet or anti-inflammatory effects but it has excellent analgesic and antipyretic effects.
13. c. Acetaminophen is associated with hepatic injury, especially in overdose events.
14. d. An alcoholic is most likely to have pre-existing hepatic injury. The patient with a history of hepatitis should also have LFTs checked if the acetaminophen therapy will be lengthy; however, hepatitis is less likely than alcohol to leave persistent hepatic damage.
15. b. Sumatriptan is selective for 5-HT$_{1B/1D}$ receptors located on cranial blood vessels and sensory nerves of the trigeminal vascular system. Stimulation of these receptors decreases the throbbing sensation in the head and vascular inflammation.
16. c. Sumatriptan vasoconstricts, so it should not be given to anyone with a cardiovascular disorder that would be exacerbated by decreased blood flow.
17. a. Frequently occurring cardiovascular adverse effects include hypotension or hypertension, palpitations, or syncope.
18. b. Sumatriptan is ineffective for nonmigraine headaches.

CORE PATIENT VARIABLES: PATIENTS, PLEASE
MULTIPLE CHOICE

1. c. Age, smoking, and intake of alcohol all have the potential to induce gastric and hepatic damage.
2. a. Aspirin is an irreversible platelet inhibitor. The patient should have coagulability tests done to assure the combination does not induce bleeding.
3. a. There is a drug–drug interaction between corticosteroids and aspirin. Corticosteroids may decrease the effectiveness of aspirin.
4. d. Patients with asthma and nasal polyps have an increased risk for bronchospasm that will induce an asthma attack.

5. c. Ibuprofen inhibits renal prostaglandin synthesis, allowing unopposed pressor systems to produce hypertension. It also impairs the antihypertensive effects of beta blockers.
6. b. Ibuprofen may reduce the renal elimination of lithium, necessitating a close watch on lithium levels.
7. a. Although ibuprofen may not alleviate this patient's pain, it is too early to change medications. If the patient is still experiencing pain after a couple of weeks, the patient should be referred to the prescriber for a recheck.
8. b. It is generally accepted that people older than 60 years should take a prophylactic aspirin daily to prevent cardiovascular and cerebrovascular events. Ibuprofen may block aspirin's antiplatelet activity, diminishing its protective effects against cardiovascular and cerebrovascular events. COX-2 inhibitors do not affect platelet activity.
9. d. Acetaminophen overdose can be lethal. Many OTC drugs contain acetaminophen, and the patient should be cautious not to accidentally overdose.
10. d. Acetaminophen may cause adverse effects in the hepatic, renal, and hematologic systems. Patients on high-dose or long-term therapy should have these systems monitored periodically throughout therapy.
11. a. The drugs of choice for depression are SSRIs. These will interact with sibutramine and potentially cause adverse effects. The patient with diabetes may have problems with sibutramine, but more information is needed.
12. b. Sumatriptan should be taken at the first sign of migraine. Patients should never double a dose. The history of smoking has more to do with an increased risk for adverse effects than the efficacy of the drug.

NURSING MANAGEMENT: EVERY GOOD NURSE SHOULD …
MULTIPLE CHOICE

1. c. Aspirin may cause bleeding disorders because of the inhibition of platelet aggregation. Agranulocytosis and aplastic anemia are also possible. In addition, aspirin may cause hepatic or renal toxicity. Laboratory blood work on a regular basis will help to detect early signs of these problems. Because of its gastric-irritating effects, aspirin should not be taken on an empty stomach. Moisture causes aspirin to lose its effectiveness. Because there frequently is a good bit of steam in bathrooms, the bathroom medicine cabinet is usually not the best choice as a storage location for aspirin. Crushing coated tablets intended for extended release will cause the aspirin to be released more rapidly into the bloodstream, possibly causing excessively high levels and adverse effects. The action also will be for only a short duration if the tablets are crushed.
2. a. Unusual bruising. This is a sign of excessive interference with platelet aggregation. Tachycardia is a sign of serious adverse effects because it relates to internal bleeding. Upset stomach and slight dizziness are common adverse effects and are not significant problems that need to be reported immediately.
3. b. Administer acetylcysteine. This is the only antidote for acetaminophen and should be administered as soon as possible. Acetylsalicylic acid is aspirin and would not be given. Acetaminophen does not have an effect on platelet aggregation. CT scan of the abdomen would not be relevant.
4. b. The child is demonstrating flu-like symptoms and should not be treated with aspirin because of the

[handwritten notes at top: "worst 12-24 hrs B4 surgery High molecular weight"]

possibility of Reye syndrome developing. Dosage of acetaminophen for children is based on height and weight. The most appropriate dose can be calibrated with a children's formula.

5. c. Because of the patient's history of GI ulceration and age she is at risk for GI complications from aspirin or ibuprofen. Neither of these should be substituted for the celecoxib, although they are effective in treating arthritis pain. Celecoxib works in a different way than do aspirin and ibuprofen. It is not the same as aspirin or a prescription-strength aspirin.

6. a, b, d. Sumatriptan should be taken with a full glass of water at the first sign of a migraine headache. Dizziness, weakness, and light-headedness are all common adverse effects of sumatriptan. Sumatriptan should not be crushed because that would alter the onset and duration of the drug's activity.

CASE STUDY

1. Ibuprofen was ordered for its analgesic and anti-inflammatory effects.
2. Yes, it is safe to receive both ibuprofen and oxycodone. The ibuprofen acts on the peripheral nervous system, and the oxycodone acts on the central nervous system. Combined use of an opioid and NSAID is recommended by the U.S. Department of Health and Human Service's Clinical Practice Guidelines. This combination provides more pain relief, while minimizing the dose of the opioid and thus the adverse effects from the opioid.
3. Round-the-clock dosing maintains a therapeutic blood level and prevents pain from escalating. Round-the-clock dosing should be used during periods when acute pain can be anticipated, such as immediately after surgery.

CRITICAL THINKING CHALLENGE

1. This patient may be having water retention and acute renal failure related to his use of ibuprofen.
2. This patient's age puts him at higher risk for adverse effects from the ibuprofen. He may also have had some renal insufficiency or diminished renal blood flow, possibly also related to his age.
3. Hold the next dose of ibuprofen and contact the physician. Monitor intake and output and blood pressure closely. Assess for signs of fluid overload.

Chapter 25

KEY TERMS
MATCHING
1. f	7. g
2. h	8. d
3. e	9. k
4. i	10. j
5. a	11. c
6. b	

PHYSIOLOGY AND PATHOPHYSIOLOGY: THE BODY HUMAN
ESSAY

1. Rheumatoid factor (RF) interacts with IgG or other antibodies to form immune complexes that activate the complement system, resulting in an inflammatory response. Leukocytes, monocytes, and lymphocytes are attracted to the area and phagocytize the immune complexes. When the immune complexes are destroyed, lysosomal enzymes are released. These enzymes are capable of destroying joint cartilage, resulting in an inflammatory process that starts the cycle again.

2. Symptoms include morning stiffness that lasts more than 1 hour, symmetric involvement of joints, and rheumatoid nodules over bony prominences or extensor surfaces.
3. Gout occurs when the hyperuricemia forms monosodium urate crystals, which precipitate into the synovial fluid and initiate an inflammatory response.

CORE DRUG KNOWLEDGE: JUST THE FACTS
MULTIPLE CHOICE

1. b. Methotrexate was originally approved by the FDA for the treatment of various malignancies.
2. a. Although methotrexate may induce photosensitivity, it does not cause these serious integumentary complications, and it does not affect the cardiovascular system or create kidney stones.
3. d. Methotrexate is contraindicated in patients with immunosuppression, pre-existing blood dyscrasias, bone marrow impairment, and during pregnancy and lactation.
4. b. A baseline chest x-ray should be done, but it is not a serial requirement. An EKG is not required because methotrexate does not have effects on the cardiovascular system.
5. a. Methotrexate is a pregnancy category X drug because of documented fetal abnormality.
6. c. Etanercept blocks the biologic activity of TNF that could potentially affect the patient's defense against infections .
7. a. The patient needs to keep away from anyone who is ill to prevent infection. Vaccinations need to be completed before the patient begins TNF therapy. Infliximab is another TNF inhibitor with the same risk for infection as etanercept. Administration of two TNF inhibitors does not have any clinical benefit but does increase the risk for infection, so these two drugs should not be taken concurrently.
8. d. Before each injection, a urinalysis and CBC are performed. Therapy must stop if the patient develops hematuria, proteinuria, or blood dyscrasias. A UA, rather than renal function tests, is required to check for proteinuria.
9. c. Patients may experience anaphylactic shock, syncope, bradycardia, difficulty swallowing, and angioedema after an injection of aurothioglucose.
10. a. Because of its unique mechanism of action, it may be used in conjunction with other drugs such as NSAIDs and other DMARDs.
11. b. Etanercept binds specifically to circulating TNF, prevents it from binding to TNF receptors on the cell membranes, and prevents the TNF-mediated cellular response.
12. c. Colchicine is not used in the treatment of chronic gout because of its adverse effect profile.
13. c. These symptoms may indicate toxicity. The patient should be evaluated if these symptoms occur.
14. b. Allopurinol is used when patients have recurring bouts of gout.
15. c. Probenecid may be used to prolong the activity of penicillin or cephalosporin antibiotics.

ESSAY

Symptoms of infection—fever or chills, cough, sore throat, pain, or difficulty passing urine; symptoms of decreased platelets or bleeding—bruising, pinpoint red spots on the skin, black, tarry stools, blood in the urine; symptoms of anemia—

Warfarin can be given
b/c of ⊖ pill
interacts c drugs/food

Answer Key 329

unusual weakness or tiredness, fainting spells, light-headedness, diarrhea, difficulty breathing, a nonproductive cough, mouth and throat ulcers; redness, blistering, peeling or loosening of the skin, including inside the mouth; skin rash, hives, or itching, changes in vision, vomiting

CORE PATIENT VARIABLES: PATIENTS, PLEASE
MULTIPLE CHOICE

1. c. It is important to assess whether the patient is experiencing any other symptoms of blood dyscrasias.
2. b. Methotrexate should be given cautiously to patients who take other drugs, such as acetaminophen, that are potentially hepatotoxic. The nurse cannot change the frequency of an order.
3. b. Serial testing is imperative when etanercept is used. When noncompliance is known before the initiation of therapy, the provider may choose to use a different drug.
4. d. Etanercept, like most of the DMARDs, takes time for the patient to feel its full effect.
5. c. A nitritoid crisis is called such because the symptoms resemble those of a patient taking nitroglycerin.
6. b. Live vaccines should be avoided during etanercept therapy because definitive clinical data on potential effects are not completed.
7. b. Penicillamine can cause serious integumentary complications. The patient should be seen as soon as possible.
8. c. Patients taking anakinra (Kineret) have an increased risk for infections.
9. a. Allopurinol is not recommended for use during an acute gout attack because the decrease in plasma uric acid levels mobilizes urate deposits in the body, resulting in exacerbation of the acute attack.
10. a. Foods such as organ meats, oily fish, seafood, beans, peas, oatmeal, spinach, asparagus, cauliflower, and mushrooms should be avoided, as these foods are high in purines.
11. b. Probenecid should not be administered to patients with medical conditions in which uric acid production can increase acutely, such as those undergoing cancer chemotherapy or radiation therapy.
12. d. Monitoring for ketones in the urine or using Clinitest strips are not accurate ways of assessing blood glucose.

NURSING MANAGEMENT: EVERY GOOD NURSE SHOULD …
MULTIPLE CHOICE

1. c. The full therapeutic effects of methotrexate will take some time to occur. Diarrhea is not a common adverse effect. Some serious adverse effects, such as bone marrow suppression, GI ulceration, hepatitic fibrosis, or pneumonitis can occur from methotrexate.
2. b. Taking this drug at the first sign of a gout attack will most minimize the pain from the attack. Taking colchicine when the pain is most severe will not control as much pain. Taking colchicine near the end of the gout attack will offer minimal decrease of pain. Colchicine is taken on an as-needed basis; it does not prevent gout attacks.
3. b. Take the allopurinol after a meal to minimize GI distress. Probenecid may cause gastric upset, and this will minimize it. Water intake should be encouraged, at least 10 glasses a day, to help reduce the risk of kidney stones forming while the patient is taking allopurinol. Alcoholic beverages should be avoided because they can cause stomach problems and increase uric acid in the blood, predisposing the person to a gout attack.

4. a. High consumption of meat products and seafood confer a high risk of hyperuricemia and resultant gout. Purine-rich vegetables do not increase the risk for hyperuricemia and a high dairy intake is actually protective

CASE STUDY
Combination therapy of nonsteroidal anti-inflammatory drugs (NSAIDs), such as ibuprofen, and disease-modifying anti-rheumatic drugs (DMARDs), such as methotrexate, has been found to be highly effective and well tolerated. By combining the drugs, the dosages of each individual drug can be kept to a minimum, preventing more adverse effects. Methotrexate, like other DMARDs, is capable of arresting the progression of rheumatoid arthritis (RA) and can induce remission in some patients. Ibuprofen relieves many of the symptoms of RA. Before initiating the therapy, the following lab values need to be evaluated: CBC, renal and hepatic function tests, urinalysis, and a chest x-ray. The CBC, renal function, and liver function tests should be repeated 2 weeks after therapy begins, again at 1 month, and then every 2 months thereafter throughout therapy because of the potential serious adverse effects on the bone marrow, liver, and kidneys. Assess the patient's willingness to adhere to this series of lab tests.

CRITICAL THINKING CHALLENGE
Methotrexate is a pregnancy category X drug. It is important that the patient not become pregnant while taking this drug. Because of a prolonged washout period after methotrexate is stopped, the patient needs to wait at least 3 months after stopping before attempting to become pregnant.

Chapter 26

KEY TERMS
ESSAY

1. Atherosclerosis is a narrowing of the arterial interior caused by buildup of hard, thick deposits, and a loss of elasticity of the arterial wall.
2. This is another name for atherosclerosis.
3. Hyperlipidemia is an elevation of blood lipid levels.
4. Serum lipids are the fats found in the bloodstream. These lipids include cholesterol, cholesterol esters (compounds), phospholipids, and triglycerides.

PHYSIOLOGY AND PATHOPHYSIOLOGY: THE BODY HUMAN
ESSAY

1. Chylomicrons; very low-density lipoproteins (VLDLs); intermediate-density lipoproteins (IDLs); low-density lipoproteins (LDLs); and high-density lipoproteins (HDLs)
2. Low-density lipoprotein (LDL) is the major cholesterol carrier in the blood. LDL has a structure that can vary, based on its size and density. LDL includes VLDL and IDL. (IDL is considered an abnormal lipoprotein.) Lp(a) is a type of LDL and is considered a genetic variation. About one third to one fourth of blood cholesterol is carried by HDL. Chylomicrons are the largest and least dense of the lipoproteins. Triglycerides are transported primarily by the chylomicrons and VLDL, a subgroup of LDL.
3. It has been hypothesized that triglyceride-rich lipoproteins move into macrophages in the bloodstream and then interact with small, dense LDL and HDL particles to form arterial thromboses.
4. Lowering serum lipid levels decreases the risk for atherosclerosis, hypertension, and coronary heart disease. Lowering cholesterol levels can stop or reverse atherosclerosis in all vascular beds.

5. The antihyperlipidemics are composed of the HMG-CoA reductase inhibitors, the fibric acid derivatives, nicotinic acid, the bile acid sequestrants, and the cholesterol absorption inhibitors.

CORE DRUG KNOWLEDGE: JUST THE FACTS
MATCHING
1. c   2. d   3. a   4. b

MULTIPLE CHOICE
1. b. The elevation in hepatic enzyme levels is an adverse effect that may occur fairly frequently and is usually dose related.
2. d. Fetal harm is likely caused by the decrease in cholesterol synthesis and possibly other products in the cholesterol biosynthesis pathway.
3. c. Rhabdomyolysis has the potential to induce acute renal failure and even death. Elevated liver enzymes are also common; however, liver failure is very rare and may not be directly related to lovastatin use. Myalgias are common symptoms such as nonspecific muscle pain, weakness, or cramping. They are not associated with muscle damage. Lovastatin does not cause blood dyscrasias.
4. c. Patients with partial biliary obstruction have an increased bile acid concentration, so by decreasing circulating bile acid, bile acid deposits in the skin tissues are reduced, with a resultant decrease in pruritus.
5. b. The constipation can be severe and may lead to fecal impaction.
6. a. Like lovastatin, gemfibrozil may induce liver failure and rhabdomyolysis, despite the fact that the mechanism of action is different.
7. d. Ezetimibe is contraindicated for patients with active liver disease because it has the potential to cause hepatitis.
8. c. In addition to hypercholesterolemia, cholestyramine and colestipol are indicated for patients with pruritus. Colesevelam does not have this indication.

CORE PATIENT VARIABLES: PATIENTS, PLEASE
MULTIPLE CHOICE
1. a. Drug and alcohol abuse frequently results in liver damage.
2. a. Severe muscle pain may be a symptom of rhabdomyolysis.
3. a. Immediate-release lovastatin should be administered after the evening meal; extended-release lovastatin is administered at bedtime without food to be most effective.
4. b. Gemfibrozil produces a moderate hyperglycemic effect; special monitoring will be necessary for patients with diabetes who are receiving gemfibrozil.
5. d. The vasodilation and increased blood flow from niacin administration are caused by histamine release. Flushing is usually transient.
6. d. All of the bile acid sequestrants should be taken prior to a meal.
7. d. These are symptoms of rhabdomyolysis. Diagnosis of rhabdomyolysis is made when the CK is greater than 10,000 U/L regardless of whether the patient has experienced a change in renal function.

NURSING MANAGEMENT: EVERY GOOD NURSE SHOULD …
MULTIPLE CHOICE
1. c. Lovastatin should not replace a low-fat diet but supplement it to achieve the greatest effect in lowering cholesterol levels. Dosages of lovastatin should not be randomly increased by the patient because adverse effects may occur. The goal is to lower dietary fat intake, not to raise it. Raising fat intake will not prevent adverse effects from lovastatin but will counteract some of its therapeutic effect.
2. b. Lovastatin is metabolized by the hepatic enzyme CYP3A4. Many drugs interact with this pathway. Because the patient receives multiple drug therapies, it is likely that one or more of the drugs may interact with lovastatin and inhibit this hepatic enzyme pathway. This will slow metabolism of lovastatin, increasing circulating blood levels, and increasing the risk for adverse effects. Older adults are also more likely to have adverse effects. An increase in therapeutic response, rather than a decrease, is also possible. Anaphylactic reactions and electrolyte imbalances are not adverse effects from lovastatin.
3. a. Lovastatin will raise liver enzymes, especially when the drug therapy is first started. Although this elevation is not normally serious, it is important to monitor the enzymes carefully to verify that liver function is not being impaired. Photosensitivity may occur from lovastatin, and patients should minimize their sun exposure until they know how the drug will affect them. Serious skeletal muscle effects (rhabdomyolysis) may result from lovastatin. Although this is rare, it may be fatal. The patient should report muscle pain or weakness immediately. Constipation is not a common adverse effect of lovastatin; it can be serious with cholestyramine, a bile acid sequestrant.

CASE STUDY
1. The lovastatin was showing therapeutic effect because the LDL cholesterol level had dropped. Although the liver enzymes (AST and ALT) are elevated, they are not considered significantly elevated at this time.
2. The patient needs to return so the effect of the drug on the LDL levels and liver enzymes may be further evaluated.

CRITICAL THINKING CHALLENGE
The nurse should contact the physician or nurse practitioner and inform them of the elevated liver enzymes. At this point, the enzymes are more than three times the upper range for normal and may indicate liver damage. Consult with the prescriber about decreasing the dose. It is also possible that use of the drug will be discontinued, but because this patient has no other noted complications from the drug therapy, this is not as likely. If the dose is decreased, the patient should return in 6 weeks for additional evaluation. If the dose is not decreased, he will still need to return for additional evaluation, but the interval may be longer, as determined by the physician or nurse practitioner.

Chapter 27
KEY TERMS
ANAGRAMS
1. Glomerular filtration
2. Tubular secretion
3. Oliguria
4. Edema
5. Diuresis
6. Hypervolemia
7. Tubular reabsorption
8. Hypertension
9. Hypokalemia
10. Osmolality
11. Diuretic
12. Hyperkalemia

PHYSIOLOGY AND PATHOPHYSIOLOGY: THE BODY HUMAN
ESSAY
1. The kidneys are responsible for filtering and purifying the body; ridding the body of impurities and waste by produc-

ing urine, and excreting water, electrolytes, and other substances; regulating the body's acid-base balance; maintaining blood pressure; influencing circulating fluid volume; assisting in the production of red blood cells; and contributing to calcium metabolism.

2. Kidneys, ureters, and bladder
3. Glomerular filtration, renal tubular reabsorption, and renal tubular secretion
4. Less than 2 L in 24 hours
5. Excretion of hydrogen ions or reabsorbing bicarbonate
6. Synthesis, storage, and release of renin
7. Secretes erythropoietin, which stimulates bone marrow to produce red blood cells
8. Chemically transforms precursors of vitamin D to an active form

CORE DRUG KNOWLEDGE: JUST THE FACTS
MULTIPLE CHOICE

1. b. Although the onset of HCTZ is 2 hours, full effects take 2 to 4 weeks.
2. c. Thiazide diuretics may elevate BUN and creatinine.
3. c. HCTZ has many drug interactions that affect electrolyte balance. It also increases the serum concentration of many drugs and has its own serum concentration increased by many drugs.
4. a. Thiazide drugs are structurally similar to sulfonamides.
5. c. The dosage does not reflect the term "high-ceiling."
6. c. Furosemide may induce a gout attack.
7. a. Miscellaneous adverse affects include hyperuricemia, hyperglycemia, and activation of SLE.
8. a. Triamterene spares potassium, so administering it with other drugs that also may cause hyperkalemia may lead to cardiac arrhythmias.
9. c. Hyperkalemia does not cause constipation or affect LDH or triglycerides.
10. b. Mannitol increases osmotic pressure and pulls fluid into the vascular space, thereby decreasing intracranial pressure.
11. a. Pulling fluid into the vascular space puts an additional stress on the heart to pump the fluid efficiently. Patients with pulmonary edema already have pump failure.
12. d. An in-line filter is used because mannitol is a sugar and may crystallize.
13. c. Inhibition of carbonic anhydrase decreases aqueous humor formation and consequently decreases intraocular pressure.
14. c. Acetazolamide has adverse effects that affect most body systems.
15. b. Tolterodine is a competitive cholinergic muscarinic antagonist with relative selective preference for the muscarinic receptors in the bladder. Blockade of these muscarinic receptors decreases the ability of the bladder to contract. Tolterodine is used in treating overactive bladder, to help manage the symptoms of urinary frequency, urgency, and urge incontinence.

CORE PATIENT VARIABLES: PATIENTS, PLEASE
MULTIPLE CHOICE

1. c. HCTZ may cause electrolyte imbalances.
2. a. Sodium holds on to water. There are many hidden forms of sodium in our everyday foods, especially canned foods and condiments.

3. b. Rapid loss of plasma volume and the resulting hemoconcentration are likely to cause thromboembolic episodes.
4. b. IV furosemide should be given over 1 to 2 minutes to decrease the risk for ototoxicity.
5. a. Type 2 diabetes mellitus occurs frequently in the elderly. Because the patient is aging and furosemide may induce hyperglycemia, this test is most appropriate.
6. d. Since this is a potassium-sparing diuretic, the patient should monitor the amount of potassium ingested. These instructions may be modified in the patient taking a potassium-sparing diuretic who continues to have a potassium level at the lower end of the normal range.
7. c. Diuretics should be taken so that their peak action occurs while the patient is awake. If the patient works the night shift, the instructions need to be modified.
8. b. Mannitol pulls fluid back into the vasculature. The most common cause of CHF is left ventricular pump failure. If the increased circulating fluid exacerbates the patient's CHF, the fluid will back up into the lungs first.
9. a. To accurately assess fluid loss, an indwelling catheter should be inserted.
10. d. Patients with adrenocortical insufficiency are susceptible to electrolyte imbalances.
11. c. Hydrochlorothiazide may be given for a variety of disorders. It is used most commonly for edematous states or hypertension. It may also be used for prophylaxis of nephrolithiasis. Understanding the reason the patient is receiving the medication helps the nurse develop a plan of care that incorporates appropriate assessments and interventions.
12. b. Furosemide increases the net loss of fluid from the body resulting in weight loss. An acute exacerbation of CHF does not always change the patient's blood pressure or the level of consciousness. Long-term therapy with furosemide may induce hyperglycemia. Giving IV furosemide will not lower the blood glucose.
13. b. Warning signs of dehydration and significant electrolyte imbalance are dryness of mouth, thirst, anorexia, weakness, lethargy, drowsiness, restlessness, muscle pains or cramps, muscle fatigue, tetany (rarely), hypotension, oliguria, tachycardia, arrhythmia, and GI disturbances (e.g., nausea/vomiting).
14. c. Ototoxicity can occur with rapid IV therapy, especially in patients with poor renal function, and in those patients receiving high doses of furosemide, either oral or IV. Furosemide is associated with the potential development of digoxin toxicity because of its potential to cause hypokalemia, but it does not have any direct cardiotoxic effect.
15. b. Hyperkalemia is more likely to occur in patients with renal impairment and diabetes (even without evidence of renal impairment), and in the elderly or severely ill.

NURSING MANAGEMENT: EVERY GOOD NURSE SHOULD.....
DECISION TREES

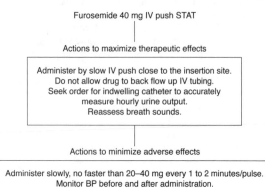

Furosemide 40 mg IV push STAT

Actions to maximize therapeutic effects

> Administer by slow IV push close to the insertion site.
> Do not allow drug to back flow up IV tubing.
> Seek order for indwelling catheter to accurately
> measure hourly urine output.
> Reassess breath sounds.

Actions to minimize adverse effects

> Administer slowly, no faster than 20–40 mg every 1 to 2 minutes/pulse.
> Monitor BP before and after administration.
> Check serum potassium level.

Reassess/Evaluate Effectiveness of Furosemide

> Reassess breath sounds — they should be clear and be less labored.
> Reassess BP — it should go down to normal
> Reassess P and R rate — they should be in normal range.
> Assess hourly urine output — it should be > 30 cc/hour.
> Weigh the patient daily.

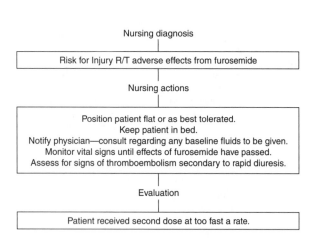

Nursing diagnosis

> Risk for Injury R/T adverse effects from furosemide

Nursing actions

> Position patient flat or as best tolerated.
> Keep patient in bed.
> Notify physician—consult regarding any baseline fluids to be given.
> Monitor vital signs until effects of furosemide have passed.
> Assess for signs of thromboembolism secondary to rapid diuresis.

Evaluation

> Patient received second dose at too fast a rate.

CASE STUDY
1. The vial of mannitol should be warmed in a warm water bath to dissolve the crystals. The drug should be no warmer than body temperature. An IV administration set with a filter should be used.
2. Mannitol is not absorbed via the GI route, so it must be given IV.
3. Hourly urinary output should be measured to see if the mannitol is effective. Output should increase and be at least 30 cc per hour. An indwelling urinary catheter is needed to accurately determine hourly output.
4. Elderly patients are at increased risk for the development of dizziness, disorientation, and confusion caused by rapid fluid loss when receiving mannitol.

CRITICAL THINKING CHALLENGE
1. You should administer a test dose of 0.2 g/kg in 3 to 5 minutes before beginning the main infusion. If urine output remains less than 30 cc/hour after the test dose, the infusion should be held and the physician contacted. A second test dose may be ordered.
2. This patient's age was a risk factor for decreased renal function.

Chapter 28

KEY TERMS
FILL IN THE BLANKS AND WORD SEARCH
1. Sympathomimetic
2. Sympatholytic
3. Systolic blood pressure
4. Diastolic blood pressure
5. Primary hypertension
6. Essential hypertension
7. Hypertensive crisis
8. Hypertension
9. Hypotension
10. Secondary hypertension
11. Renin-angiotensin-aldosterone system

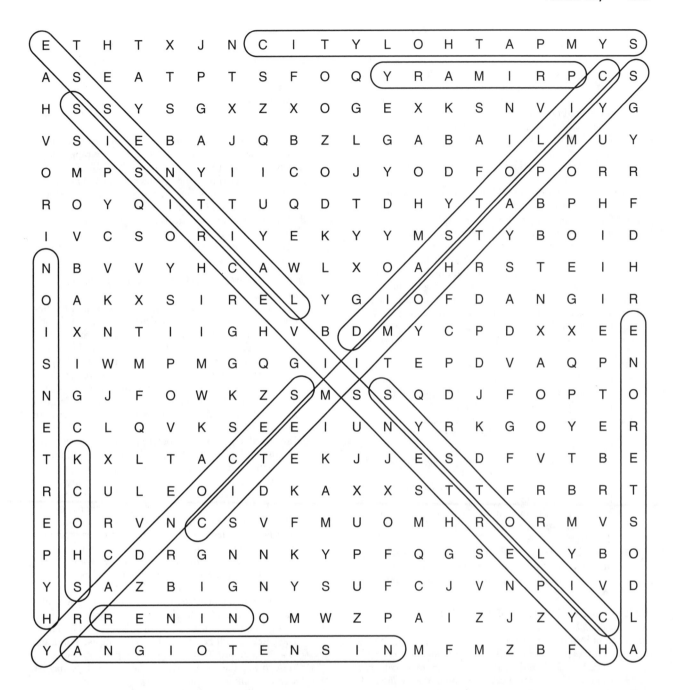

E	T	H	T	X	J	N	C	I	T	Y	L	O	H	T	A	P	M	Y	S
A	S	E	A	T	P	T	S	F	O	Q	Y	R	A	M	I	R	P	C	S
H	S	S	Y	S	G	X	Z	X	O	G	E	X	K	S	N	V	I	Y	G
V	S	I	E	B	A	J	Q	B	Z	L	G	A	B	A	I	L	M	U	Y
O	M	P	S	N	Y	I	I	C	O	J	Y	O	D	F	O	P	O	R	R
R	O	Y	Q	I	T	T	U	Q	D	T	D	H	Y	T	A	B	P	H	F
I	V	C	S	O	R	I	Y	E	K	Y	Y	M	S	T	Y	B	O	I	D
N	B	V	V	Y	H	C	A	W	L	X	O	A	H	R	S	T	E	I	H
O	A	K	X	S	I	R	E	L	Y	G	I	O	F	D	A	N	G	I	R
I	X	N	T	I	I	G	H	V	B	D	M	Y	C	P	D	X	X	E	E
S	I	W	M	P	M	G	Q	G	I	I	T	E	P	D	V	A	Q	P	N
N	G	J	F	O	W	K	Z	S	M	S	S	Q	D	J	F	O	P	T	O
E	C	L	Q	V	K	S	E	E	I	U	N	Y	R	K	G	O	Y	E	R
T	K	X	L	T	A	C	T	E	K	J	J	E	S	D	F	V	T	B	E
R	C	U	L	E	O	I	D	K	A	X	X	S	T	T	F	R	B	R	T
E	O	R	V	N	C	S	V	F	M	U	O	M	H	R	O	R	M	V	S
P	H	C	D	R	G	N	N	K	Y	P	F	Q	G	S	E	L	Y	B	O
Y	S	A	Z	B	I	G	N	Y	S	U	F	C	J	V	N	P	I	V	D
H	R	R	E	N	I	N	O	M	W	Z	P	A	I	Z	J	Z	Y	C	L
Y	A	N	G	I	O	T	E	N	S	I	N	M	F	M	Z	B	F	H	A

PHYSIOLOGY AND PATHOPHYSIOLOGY: THE BODY HUMAN
ESSAY
1. Systolic
2. Generally speaking, decreased cardiac output would result in a decreased blood pressure. However, other factors, such as peripheral resistance, stimulation of the adrenergic system, or stimulation of the renin-angiotensin-aldosterone system, could mediate that response.
3. Alpha-1 and beta-1 generate a sympathomimetic response, whereas alpha-2 and beta-2 generate a sympatholytic response.
4. Alpha-1 is in the vasculature, alpha-2 in the brain, beta-1 in the heart, and beta-2 in the bronchial and vascular musculature.
5. This system vasoconstricts and increases circulating volume by retention of sodium and water. These actions result in an elevation of blood pressure.

CORE DRUG KNOWLEDGE: JUST THE FACTS
MULTIPLE CHOICE
1. d. Orthostatic hypotension is a potential adverse effect with any drug that decreases blood pressure.
2. a. ACE inhibitors are used in combination with beta blockers and diuretics in the management of CHF.
3. c. Captopril therapy may induce hyperkalemia and hyponatremia.
4. b. Captopril inhibits the degradation of endogenous bradykinin, resulting in a nonproductive cough.

5. a. Black Americans may be "low-renin hypertensive patients." In this population, captopril is less effective.

6. c. In contrast to ACE inhibitors, angiotensin II blockers act directly on the angiotensin receptors.

7. b. Both ACE inhibitors and angiotensin II blockers are pregnancy category C drugs because of the potential for fetal abnormalities.

8. b. Eplerenone binds selectively to the mineralocorticoid receptors, thereby blocking aldosterone from binding to these receptors.

9. c. Eplerenone may induce hyperkalemia, which can lead to fatal arrhythmias.

10. a. The ratio of alpha-beta blocking is 1:3 orally and 1:7 intravenously.

11. a. Stimulation of alpha-2 receptors blocks the release of norepinephrine. It is important to remember that clonidine is a sympathetic agonist.

12. b. When stimulated (agonist effect), it blocks the release of norepinephrine (decreases blood pressure).

13. b. When norepinephrine is no longer being inhibited, its release will induce a rebound of the blood pressure.

14. a. The reduction of symptoms and increase in urine flow rate are attributed to relaxation of smooth muscle from the alpha-1 blockade in the bladder neck and prostate gland.

15. d. In addition to its direct smooth muscle relaxation, it alters cellular calcium, with resultant interference with calcium movement within the vascular smooth muscles responsible for venous contraction and dilation.

16. b. Peripheral vasodilation stimulates a reflexive sympathetic response that includes an increase in the heart rate.

17. a. Minoxidil, packaged as "Rogaine," can be purchased over the counter for this indication.

18. b. It is the drug of choice when an immediate reduction of blood pressure is indicated.

19. c. Its onset is less than 5 minutes, which makes it an excellent drug for treating hypotension associated with shock states.

20. d. Unlike dopamine, dobutamine has almost no effect on alpha receptors to cause vasoconstriction. Dobutamine does not cause the release of endogenous norepinephrine that dopamine causes.

CORE PATIENT VARIABLES: PATIENTS, PLEASE
MULTIPLE CHOICE

1. c. Captopril therapy decreases aldosterone, which, in turn, increases potassium levels. Thus, a potassium-sparing diuretic would place the patient at risk for hyperkalemia.

2. b. Captopril is contraindicated for use in the second and third trimesters of pregnancy. Patients should be warned about increasing potassium intake; exercising will help with potential constipation, and women have a higher risk for cough than do men.

3. d. The beta-blocking effects of this drug may induce bronchoconstriction, leading to an asthma attack.

4. a. It is important to contact the prescriber immediately should any signs of CHF occur to initiate further treatment of drug-induced CHF.

5. c. Oral labetalol should be administered with food to increase absolute bioavailability.

6. a. Forty percent to 60% of clonidine is excreted unchanged by the kidneys, so the drug is given cautiously in patients with chronic renal failure.

7. c. Abrupt cessation of clonidine may induce severe rebound hypertension.

8. b. Alpha-1 blockade in the bladder neck and prostate gland decreases the symptoms of BPH.

9. c. Hydralazine increases plasma renin activity, leading to production of angiotensin II. Angiotensin II increases aldosterone production, which increases sodium and water retention.

10. c. These are symptoms of a too-rapid reduction of blood pressure.

11. a. Nitroprusside is light sensitive. The diluted solution should be placed in an opaque sleeve or wrapped in aluminum foil to ensure stability of the solution.

12. a. Low-dose dopamine therapy increases renal blood flow, whereas moderate- and high-dose therapies decrease renal blood flow.

13. d. Dopamine does not disturb the oxygen-carrying capacity of the blood.

14. b. One of the most common adverse effects of eplerenone is hyperkalemia.

NURSING MANAGEMENT: EVERY GOOD NURSE SHOULD …
MULTIPLE CHOICE

1. b. Hypotension can occur during the 2 hours after the first dose of captopril. Taking the drug at bedtime will minimize the effects of the hypotension because the patient will be lying down during this time. Captopril should be taken on an empty stomach to promote absorption. Position changes should be gradual to minimize any orthostatic hypotension or dizziness felt from the drug therapy. Sodium intake should be kept the same or limited. Increased sodium intake would be counterproductive to the drug action.

2. c. Tachycardia (a sign of hypoglycemia) is not experienced because of the beta-blocking actions of labetalol; therefore, patients need to rely not on how they feel but on their blood glucose levels to determine if they are experiencing hypoglycemia. Hyperglycemia is also possible. Beta blockage reduces insulin release in response to elevated blood glucose. Increasing dietary sugar is not appropriate in patients with diabetes. Hot baths or showers increase peripheral vasodilation and promote orthostatic hypotension. These should be avoided during labetalol therapy. Rapid discontinuation of use of the drug may cause angina, myocardial infarction, or ventricular arrhythmias in patients with cardiovascular disease. Use of the drug should be slowly stopped.

3. a. This promotes a constant therapeutic level of clonidine. The patch should be applied to a new site each time and to a site that has minimal hair. If the patch becomes loose during the 7 days, extra adhesive overlays may be used to maintain a seal.

4. a, b, c, d. Most patients do require at least two drugs to adequately control hypertension. Each of the drugs works differently. Beta blockers such as atenolol reduce blood pressure by slowing heart rate and decreasing cardiac output. They also may decrease the release of renin. Diuretics, such as hydrochlorothiazide, promote excretion of sodium and water from the body, thus decreasing the volume of circulating fluid. This results in a decrease in peripheral resistance and lowers blood pressure. Hydralazine produces peripheral vasodilation, decreased peripheral resistance, and a decrease in blood pressure. Beta blockers are used to prevent the reflex tachycardia and increase in cardiac output that can occur after vasodilation from hydralazine. Hydralazine also causes an increase in angiotensin II, which increases sodium and water retention, so a diuretic is helpful. Telling a patient

he/she is to blame for needing drug therapy is not therapeutic or appropriate teaching.

5. d. Nitroprusside can be inactivated by reactions with trace contaminants that will cause the nitroprusside to appear blue, green, or red or brighter than its normal faint brown appearance. It should not be used if this discoloration is seen. Nitroprusside is never given directly by IV push; it must be diluted and administered by IV infusion. Nitroprusside should be protected from light after dilution.

6. a. Patients of childbearing age should be cautioned about becoming pregnant. Losartan is associated with fetal and neonatal deaths and morbidity. Dietary sodium should not be increased with hypertension because this can cause retention of fluid and increase peripheral resistance. Fluid loss is not a problem with losartan, although fluid retention may occur. Losartan is used to treat hypertension; it does not cause hypertension.

CASE STUDY

1. The nurse should slow the infusion rate. If symptoms do not disappear, the infusion may need to be stopped for a while.
2. Abdominal pain and nausea are two signs that the blood pressure has been reduced too quickly. These symptoms will disappear if the infusion is slowed or stopped.

CRITICAL THINKING CHALLENGE

1. It appears he is experiencing cyanide poisoning.
2. The infusion should be stopped, and the physician should be notified immediately. The nurse should consult with the physician regarding new orders to counteract the cyanide poisoning, usually sodium nitrate followed by sodium thiosulfate. Additional blood work, such as blood gases to assess whether acidosis has occurred and cyanide level assay, also may be ordered.

Chapter 29

KEY TERMS

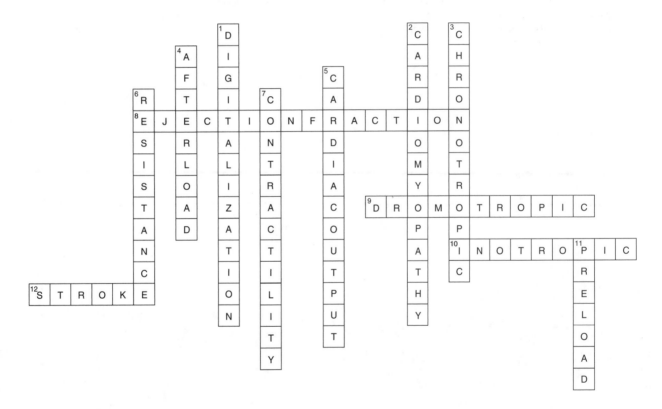

PHYSIOLOGY AND PATHOPHYSIOLOGY: THE BODY HUMAN
ESSAY

1. Blood flows from the vena cava to the right atrium, through the tricuspid valve to the right ventricle through the pulmonary valve to the pulmonary artery to the lungs to the pulmonary vein to the left atrium, through the mitral valve to the left ventricle and through the aortic valve to the aorta.
2. Preload, contractility, and afterload
3. Right-sided failure induces systemic symptoms, i.e., edema, jugular vein distention, and a third heart sound. Left-sided failure induces pulmonary symptoms, i.e., rales, rhonchi, and shortness of breath.

CORE DRUG KNOWLEDGE: JUST THE FACTS
MULTIPLE CHOICE

1. d. CHF is not an arrhythmia; therefore, antiarrhythmics are not indicated.
2. c. Serum drug levels are not affected significantly by changes in fat tissue weight, so dosing is best calculated on lean (ideal) body weight, rather than actual weight, if the patient is obese.
3. b. These actions allow for an increased contractility and a slowing of the heart rate to allow the ventricles to completely fill, thus increasing cardiac output.
4. a. Digoxin toxicity is related to hypokalemia, hypomagnesimia, and hypercalcemia.

5. c. This is the only drug approved as an antidote.
6. a. It is important to remember that this is a guideline. Toxicity may occur at lower doses.
7. b. Inamrinone has a direct relaxant effect on the vascular smooth muscle, creating vasodilation.

CORE PATIENT VARIABLES: PATIENTS, PLEASE
MULTIPLE CHOICE

1. c. In untreated hypothyroidism, digoxin requirements are reduced; in thyrotoxic patients, larger doses of digoxin may be necessary. In compensated thyroid disease, the dose is unchanged.
2. c. This is well over the upper limit of the therapeutic index. Evaluate the patient for signs of toxicity, then notify the prescriber prior to administering any additional medication (even if the patient is asymptomatic).
3. a. The symptoms of CHF have diminished. The drug is working appropriately.
4. d. It is important to assess the apical pulse for a full minute to assure there is a regular rate and rhythm.
5. c. Nausea, vomiting, and anorexia are early signs of digoxin toxicity. Electrolyte imbalances, especially hypokalemia are a frequent cause of digoxin toxicity, thus, electrolyte levels should also be evaluated.
6. c. Digoxin is not affected by light.

NURSING MANAGEMENT: EVERY GOOD NURSE SHOULD .....

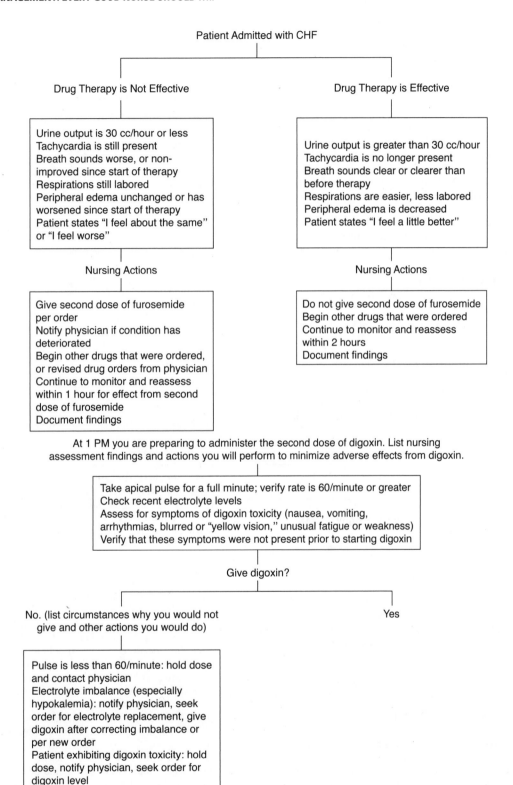

Patient Admitted with CHF

Drug Therapy is Not Effective

Drug Therapy is Effective

Urine output is 30 cc/hour or less
Tachycardia is still present
Breath sounds worse, or non-improved since start of therapy
Respirations still labored
Peripheral edema unchanged or has worsened since start of therapy
Patient states "I feel about the same" or "I feel worse"

Urine output is greater than 30 cc/hour
Tachycardia is no longer present
Breath sounds clear or clearer than before therapy
Respirations are easier, less labored
Peripheral edema is decreased
Patient states "I feel a little better"

Nursing Actions

Nursing Actions

Give second dose of furosemide per order
Notify physician if condition has deteriorated
Begin other drugs that were ordered, or revised drug orders from physician
Continue to monitor and reassess within 1 hour for effect from second dose of furosemide
Document findings

Do not give second dose of furosemide
Begin other drugs that were ordered
Continue to monitor and reassess within 2 hours
Document findings

At 1 PM you are preparing to administer the second dose of digoxin. List nursing assessment findings and actions you will perform to minimize adverse effects from digoxin.

Take apical pulse for a full minute; verify rate is 60/minute or greater
Check recent electrolyte levels
Assess for symptoms of digoxin toxicity (nausea, vomiting, arrhythmias, blurred or "yellow vision," unusual fatigue or weakness)
Verify that these symptoms were not present prior to starting digoxin

Give digoxin?

No. (list circumstances why you would not give and other actions you would do)

Yes

Pulse is less than 60/minute: hold dose and contact physician
Electrolyte imbalance (especially hypokalemia): notify physician, seek order for electrolyte replacement, give digoxin after correcting imbalance or per new order
Patient exhibiting digoxin toxicity: hold dose, notify physician, seek order for digoxin level

CASE STUDY

The furosemide is a diuretic to pull excess fluid out of the lungs and the periphery. This will help her to breathe more easily and keep her heart from working so hard. It is a powerful diuretic and works quickly, especially when given by IV push. The ACE inhibitor (captopril) blocks the creation of a substance that constricts the blood vessels.

Constricted blood vessels mean the heart works harder to pump the blood. Thus, the ACE inhibitor allows the blood vessels to become relaxed and allows the blood to leave the heart more easily. The diuretic that is a pill (hydrochlorothiazide) is not as strong and does not work as fast as the furosemide. Once the excess fluid has been quickly eliminated, this will keep the circulating volume low to make an easier workload for the heart. The digoxin slows the rate the heart beats but makes each contraction stronger, so more blood is pushed out with each beat. Because it takes a while for the full effect of the digoxin to occur, a loading dose is given. This is a larger-than-normal dose, given in three increments. This helps the drug to reach a therapeutic level faster. A smaller, maintenance dose is then given daily.

CRITICAL THINKING CHALLENGE

Additional doses of furosemide IV may be ordered until edema has resolved completely and the breath sounds are clear. A potassium supplement might be added because potassium is lost with loop diuretics, and low potassium levels increase the risk for digoxin toxicity. Because she is no longer tachycardic, the digoxin dose is apparently effective. You would not expect to see that dose changed. The dose of the ACE inhibitor and the thiazide diuretic might also be increased. If the blood pressure remains elevated once the CHF is controlled, a beta blocker, such as carvedilol, is likely to be added. This will have therapeutic effects for both the hypertension and the CHF.

Chapter 30

KEY TERMS
MATCHING
1. c   2. g   3. f   4. a   5. b   6. d   7. e

PHYSIOLOGY AND PATHOPHYSIOLOGY: THE BODY HUMAN
ESSAY
1. Angina occurs when the oxygen demands of the heart exceed the oxygen supply available to the heart. This can be because of blockage, increased workload of the heart, or vasospasms.
2. Cardiac troponin T and cardiac troponin I, CK-MB, C-reactive protein, and B-type natriuretic peptide
3. Three main drug groups are used to treat angina—beta blockers, calcium channel blockers, and nitrates.
4. Antianginal drugs work by slowing the heart rate, depressing AV conduction, decreasing cardiac output, or reducing systolic and diastolic blood pressure at rest and during exercise.

CORE DRUG KNOWLEDGE: JUST THE FACTS
MULTIPLE CHOICE
1. b. Nitroglycerin relaxes vascular smooth muscle and dilates both arterial and venous vessels.
2. d. This is the only one of the choices that has an immediate onset of action that is required for acute anginal pain.
3. d. Vasodilation induces an immediate decrease in the blood pressure. As the blood pressure decreases, the body's compensatory response is to increase the heart rate in order to sustain cardiac output.
4. b. 40%–80% of nitroglycerin migrates into many plastics, including IV administration tubing made of PVC. Using

note

the non-PVC IV administration tubing that comes with the nitroglycerin increases the amount of drug delivered to the patient.
5. a. If no response after three pills, the patient should receive NTG by an IV route, or another drug should be used.
6. c. Because of nitroglycerin's ability to relax vascular smooth muscle and dilate both arteries and veins, the patient is prone to hypotension.

CORE PATIENT VARIABLES: PATIENTS, PLEASE
MULTIPLE CHOICE
1. b. This provides a nitroglycerin-free period, which reduces tolerance to the medication.
2. c. Nitroglycerin may increase intracranial pressure.
3. a. Intravenous nitroglycerin can be titrated to decrease chest pain and keep the patient's blood pressure at an acceptable level.
4. b. Because the patient may experience hypotension, it is best to sit or lie down. Also, just the action of sitting or lying decreases the oxygen demand of the heart. NTG should be kept in its original bottle to decrease its exposure to light, air, and moisture.
5. d. The tablet should be placed between the cheek and gum to promote slow dissolving and extended absorption. NTG should never be chewed.
6. a. Placing a NTG patch over an area of the skin that is abraded will increase its absorption, resulting in an increased risk for adverse effects. Absorption is best when worn on the trunk of the body. The patient should have a nitrate-free period each day, and patch placement should be rotated among sites.

NURSING MANAGEMENT: EVERY GOOD NURSE SHOULD …
MULTIPLE CHOICE
1. c. Nitroglycerin given sublingually (SL) is administered under the tongue so it is absorbed by the vascular system there. For chest pain, administer as many as three doses, each 5 minutes apart, if the previous dose is not effective. Administering the tablet into the patient's mouth does not allow for rapid absorption of the drug because it will be dissolved and some of it swallowed, losing effectiveness. Although three doses may be administered, they are not administered all at one time. There is no need to contact the physician immediately. The patient was admitted with chest pain and has orders to treat chest pain. Notify the physician if three tablets do not relieve chest pain.
2. c. Pulse and blood pressure indicate how the heart is functioning during the chest pain, and also show the effect from the nitroglycerin. They should be measured before and during therapy. In addition, hypotension and tachycardia are possible from nitroglycerin, and you should assess for these adverse effects. Lung sounds are not a priority assessment during an episode of acute chest pain. Although urinary output gives some information about cardiac output, this is also not the priority at this time.
3. d. A patient with a history of stable chronic angina who experiences acute chest pain should be treated with the quick-acting sublingual form of nitroglycerin. Nitrol ointment is not used in acute situations. Furthermore, you would not want to administer a standing dose, which is to be given every 6 hours, 4 hours early. Excessive vasodilation may occur from this short interval of dosing. This also would mean that 10 hours would elapse until the next dose, and the patient may experi-

ence chest pain from altered scheduling. Nitrol ointment is not applied to the foot because this is the most distal point from the heart. The chest wall or upper arm is normally used. The patient who has experienced acute chest pain should not be left untreated for 4 hours because this may be an MI and not angina.

4. d. Active ingredient remains in the used patches, which can be very harmful to small children or to pets. It is important to safely dispose of patches to prevent accidental poisoning. Patches should be folded with the medicated side inward and flushed down the toilet. Transdermal patches of nitroglycerin are impregnated with active drug; the patient does not need to measure the dose. To minimize the risk of nitrate tolerance, the patient should not wear the patch 24 hours a day but should remove it for 10 to 12 hours a day. Transdermal patches of nitroglycerin are used routinely to manage chronic angina, not for acute episodes of angina.

5. a. Nitroglycerin tablets lose their potency when exposed to light, moisture, and air. Keeping them in the original brown bottle minimizes light exposure. The bottles should not be left with the cap off because this exposes the tablets to moisture and air, which decrease the effectiveness of the nitroglycerin. Activity should not be encouraged during an episode of chest pain; rather, the person should sit or lie down to decrease the oxygen demands on the heart. Because she has a diagnosed history of angina and is prescribed nitroglycerin for it, she should take her tablets immediately. If three pills in 15 minutes offer no relief of chest pain, she would call 911 because she might be having an MI.

6. d. All of the above are necessary. The patient needs to have blood pressure and pulse continuously monitored during IV infusion of nitroglycerin. The use of IV glass bottles and non-PVC tubing, supplied by the manufacturer, prevents the loss of active drug during infusion.

CASE STUDY

A family history of coronary artery disease, his gender, and diabetes are significant risk factors for this patient's cardiovascular disease progressing and causing a second MI. It is important to treat him aggressively with multiple drug therapies at this time.

The transdermal nitroglycerin will provide vasodilation and decrease peripheral resistance and blood pressure, decreasing the workload on the heart. The propranolol will slow the heart rate, depress AV conduction, decrease cardiac output, and reduce blood pressure. These effects decrease the oxygen demands of the heart and thereby decrease angina. The antianginal effects will be compounded because the different drugs work in different ways. Aspirin is used for its anticoagulant effects. This prevents thrombus formation and the occurrence of another MI. The sublingual nitroglycerin is to treat any acute episodes of chest pain that may develop.

CRITICAL THINKING CHALLENGE

If this patient had asthma, beta blockers would not be used because they constrict the bronchioles, worsening asthma. Instead, a calcium channel blocker, such as verapamil, would be used.

Chapter 31

KEY TERMS

TRUE OR FALSE

1. False, dysrhythmia
2. False, arrhythmia

3. True
4. True
5. False, transmembrane potential
6. False, depolarization
7. True
8. False, automaticity
9. False, repolarization
10. False, reentry phenomena
11. False, atrial fibrillation
12. False, proarrhythmia
13. False, ectopic foci
14. False, action potential
15. False, ventricular tachycardia
16. True
17. False, resting membrane potential

PHYSIOLOGY AND PATHOPHYSIOLOGY: THE BODY HUMAN

ESSAY

1. The progression of the electrical impulse that produces the heartbeat starts in the SA node. The action potential leaves the SA node traveling through the atria, causing them to contract. The impulse is slowed at the AV node so that the atria and the ventricles do not contract simultaneously. The impulse then travels through the bundle of His to the bundle branches and then through the Purkinje fibers.

2. Phase 0: Depolarization occurs rapidly, and "fast sodium channels" open, and sodium rushes into the cell, changing the inside of the cell to a positive charge.

    Phase 1: Immediately after the interior positive charge is achieved, the movement toward repolarization begins. The initial downward movement toward zero is phase 1 of the action potential.

    Phase 2: In this plateau phase, the calcium channels open slowly. These "slow channels" allow calcium ions to enter the cell. The positively charged calcium channels close, potassium channels open, and potassium again moves into the cell.

    Phase 3: When potassium moves into the cell, a rapid acceleration of repolarization begins.

    Phase 4: Full polarization is achieved, and the cell is capable of depolarization again.

3. The plateau phase allows for a slower repolarization of cardiac muscle and is considered a protective mechanism of the heart muscles to promote effective contractions.

4. Initially after depolarization, the cell is in the absolute refractory period and cannot be stimulated to fire, no matter how great the stimulus. As repolarization continues, the cell enters the relative refractory period and is able to respond to a stimulus, although the intensity of the stimulus needs to be much greater than when the cell is in the resting state.

5. Imbalances of electrolytes may produce changes in the action potential and cause various cardiac arrhythmias. Contractility of the heart is also affected.

CORE DRUG KNOWLEDGE: JUST THE FACTS

MULTIPLE CHOICE

1. c. Antiarrhythmics are used to restore appropriate electrical activity to the heart.
2. a. Quinidine is the only class 1A drug listed. Lidocaine is a class 1B, flecainide is a class 1C, and propranolol is a class II.
3. b. In addition to depressing myocardial excitability, they also depress conduction velocity and contractility.
4. c. In addition to its antiarrhythmic uses, it is also used in the treatment of malaria.
5. b. Lidocaine is indicated for ventricular arrhythmias.
6. d. Class II drugs are beta-blocking agents.

7. a. Blocking adrenergic receptors decreases heart rate and contractility.
8. c. Amiodarone has 3 major Black Box warnings: pulmonary toxicity, hepatotoxicity, and exacerbation of the arrhythmia being treated.
9. d. It shares some structural similarities to thyroid hormones, and one molecule of amiodarone contains two iodine atoms.
10. b. Class IV antiarrhythmic agents are composed of calcium channel blockers.
11. a. These drugs are known as beta blockers.
12. a. Although there are several common adverse effects associated with verapamil, constipation is the most prevalent.

CORE PATIENT VARIABLES: PATIENTS, PLEASE
MULTIPLE CHOICE
1. c. Myasthenia gravis is a listed contraindication for this use of this drug.
2. d. These are symptoms of cardiotoxicity, so use of the drug should be discontinued.
3. a. The patient's potassium level must be reviewed because potassium enhances the effect of quinidine, and hypokalemia will reduce the effectiveness.
4. c. Lidocaine has a short half-life. To prevent recurrence of the arrhythmia, the drug should continue to be administered by an infusion.
5. b. Blocking the adrenergic receptors may induce bronchoconstriction that may trigger an asthma attack.
6. d. Amiodarone contains iodine atoms and affects thyroid function.
7. a. One of the most serious adverse effects of amiodarone is pulmonary toxicity.
8. b. The use of polyvinyl chloride tubing is required because this is the type of tubing that was used to determine the appropriate dose during clinical trials.
9. c. Sick sinus syndrome, severe CHF, and third-degree heart block are all contraindications to the use of verapamil.
10. b. Constipation can be severe. If the patient bears down to have a bowel movement, the vagus nerve is stimulated, and the patient may experience bradycardia.

NURSING MANAGEMENT: EVERY GOOD NURSE SHOULD …
MULTIPLE CHOICE
1. c. Serum levels of quinidine are needed to determine that a therapeutic and nontoxic drug level has been reached and maintained. Blood tests for potassium levels, liver enzymes, renal function, and complete blood counts are needed to monitor for adverse effects. Potassium levels need to be in normal range to prevent decreased effectiveness and increased adverse effects of quinidine; thus, dietary intake should not be limited. Oral quinidine should be taken with food to minimize GI upset. Sustained-release tablets should never be chewed because this alters the absorption time, allowing more drug to be active at a time, which may cause adverse effects and overdosage.
2. b, c, d, e. Hypotension is possible, especially during the initiation of amiodarone IV therapy, so blood pressure needs to be monitored. The drug should be mixed in polyolefin bags of D5W because this is the manner that dosing was established. Because pulmonary toxicity is a possibility, assessing for changes in respiratory function, such as oxygen saturation measured through pulse oximetry, is an important aspect of care. Because exacerbation of the underlying arrhythmia is possible and may be fatal, the patient receiving IV amiodarone must be constantly monitored for cardiac changes. Ambulating the patient with a difficult-to-treat, life-threatening arrhythmia is inappropriate.
3. b. Beta blockers and verapamil both suppress contractility and AV conduction of the heart and thus should not be given together because significant decreases in cardiac output may occur. Digoxin is used with verapamil in atrial flutter to prevent the ventricles from developing tachycardia. Potassium and diuretics have no known interaction with verapamil.
4. a, b, d. A cleansing enema will clear the tract of stool so that when the drug is administered into the rectum, the exchange of sodium for potassium ions will be facilitated. The potassium-removing resin needs to be mixed into a suspension, and 100 mL sorbitol or 20% dextrose is recommended. The suspension is administered by gravity, not a pump. The tube will need to be clamped and left in place to prevent the patient from expelling the enema. The longer the time the drug is in contact with the mucous membranes of the rectum, the more potassium will be pulled into the bowel tract from the vascular space. Pulse and ECG should be monitored for adverse effects of hyperkalemia. Electrolyte levels should be drawn. Liver enzymes are not affected by the drug therapy or hyperkalemia.
5. c. Beta blockers constrict the bronchioles, making it even more difficult for the patient to breathe. Beta blockers are used to treat hypertension and angina, as well as arrhythmias.
6. b. This patient appears to be demonstrating lidocaine toxicity because confusion and disorientation are some of the first symptoms. This assessment needs to be confirmed with a lidocaine blood level. Treating the symptoms of confusion is not appropriate treatment, and neither is increasing the lidocaine level because this will worsen the toxicity.

CASE STUDY
1. Assess the pulse and blood pressure. Verapamil also reduces blood pressure and thus should be monitored, as well as pulse for rhythm.
2. Renal disease causes the drug to be excreted more slowly. Blood levels may build up, creating an increased risk of adverse effects.

CRITICAL THINKING CHALLENGE
Any drug used to treat an arrhythmia may also induce an arrhythmia. This patient has renal disease and thus doesn't eliminate verapamil as rapidly as do other people, which may have contributed to the development of a secondary arrhythmia, although arrhythmias may occur with normal doses and blood levels of antiarrhythmics.

Chapter 32

KEY TERMS

CROSSWORD PUZZLE

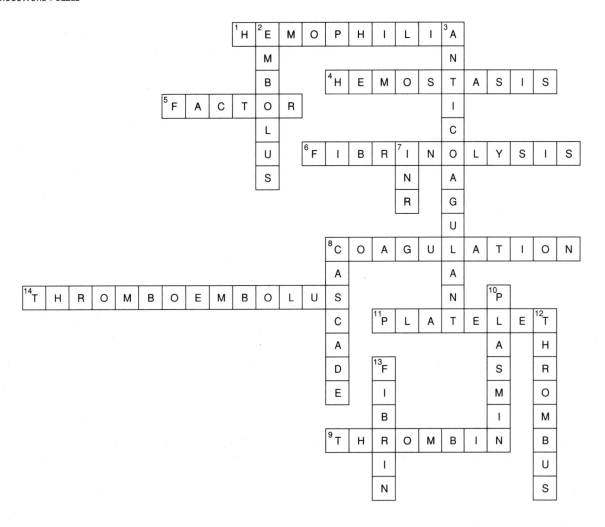

PHYSIOLOGY AND PATHOPHYSIOLOGY: THE BODY HUMAN
ESSAY

1. Anticoagulant drugs "thin" the blood by interrupting the clotting cascade. Antiplatelet drugs decrease the ability of the blood to clot by interfering with platelet membrane function and platelet aggregation. Hemorheologics reduce blood viscosity, increase the flexibility of the RBC, and decrease platelet aggregation. Thrombolytics have the ability to dissolve existing clots.
2. The clotting cascade is initiated by the tissue damage and platelet activation, which mobilize the clotting factors circulating in the blood. Once active, these clotting factors work with calcium to form fibrin. At this point, blood coagulation is completed and blood loss stops.
3. Factors are plasma components that are an integral part of the clotting cascade.
4. Plasmin is the substance that lyses a blood clot.

CORE DRUG KNOWLEDGE: JUST THE FACTS
MULTIPLE CHOICE

1. d. Heparin, along with antithrombin III, rapidly promotes the inactivation of factor X, which, in turn, prevents the conversion of prothrombin to thrombin.

2. a. The monitoring test for heparin is the aPTT. The PT is more helpful for warfarin, the bleeding time for thrombolytics, and a CBC is not helpful for any of the anticoagulant drugs.
3. a. Whenever you alter coagulation factors, bleeding is a potential adverse effect.
4. b. The PT is 1.4 to 1.7 times the control, and the INR is 2 to 3.
5. c. The predictability of low-molecular-weight heparin is one reason some prescribers do not always order aPTT testing.
6. a. Warfarin works by competitively blocking vitamin K at its sites of action. Thus, it prevents the activation of factors II (prothrombin), VII, IX, and X.
7. c. The INR is 2 to 3; the aPTT should be 1.5 to 2 times the control; and the PT is 1.4 to 1.7 times the control.
8. d. This is the time required for the drug to reach a steady state in the blood.
9. d. Pentoxifylline (Trental) is classified as a hemorheologic drug. It increases the flexibility of RBCs by increasing cAMP levels. In turn, this decreases platelet aggregation and promotes vasodilation.

10. c. Inhibiting ADP binding decreases the subsequent ADP-mediated activation of the glycoprotein GPIIb/IIIa complex and thus inhibits platelet aggregation.

11. d. In these procedures, the blood is thinned, but not as much as with anticoagulants.

12. a. Dipyridamole increases functional levels of adenosine, which produces vasodilation.

13. d. These drugs may be used alone or in combination with low-molecular-weight heparin.

14. d. Pentoxifylline increases the flexibility of RBCs by increasing cAMP levels. In turn, this decreases platelet aggregation and promotes vasodilation.

15. a. Pentoxifylline's adverse effects occur primarily in the central nervous, cardiovascular, and GI systems.

16. c. Anticoagulants do not have the ability to dissolve clots.

17. a. Alteplase, recombinant binds to the fibrin in a clot and converts the trapped plasminogen to plasmin. Fibrinolysis, or breakdown of the clot, then occurs.

18. b, c, d, e. These are all symptoms of active bleeding that may occur with therapy.

19. c. Patients with sepsis are prone to clot development. Drotrecogin alfa (activated) prevents processes that are involved in creating stable clots.

20. c. Factor VIII is required for the conversion of prothrombin to thrombin.

21. d. This is necessary to prevent bacterial growth.

22. c. Hemostatics stop blood loss by enhancing blood coagulation.

23. a. Aminocaproic acid induces anorexia and nausea.

CORE PATIENT VARIABLES: PATIENTS, PLEASE
MULTIPLE CHOICE

1. b. Patients with peptic ulcer disease may have an increased risk for bleeding because of the alteration in the stomach lining.

2. c. Aspirating and massaging the area increase the risk for bleeding

3. d. Protamine sulfate is the antidote for heparin overdose.

4. c. This patient should be on long-term anticoagulation therapy because of a prosthetic heart valve.

5. c. Low-molecular-weight heparin does not significantly prolong bleeding.

6. d. INR is the standard of care; however, some providers still do both tests.

7. a. Drugs metabolized through the P-450 2C9 pathway may increase the potential for bleeding.

8. a, d, e. Bleeding time and platelet function assess its antiplatelet action, and the CBC assesses the neutrophil count.

9. c. Smoking is a potent vasoconstrictor that counters the vasodilation effects of pentoxifylline.

10. a. Patients with a recent obstetric delivery have an increased risk for bleeding.

11. d. During the reperfusion process, arrhythmias may occur.

12. c. Protamine sulfate is the antidote for heparin; vitamin K is the antidote for warfarin; and pentoxifylline is an antiplatelet drug.

13. d. Using a thrombolytic in a patient with a hemorrhagic stroke would increase bleeding.

14. b. Glycoprotein IIb/IIIa inhibitors decrease platelet aggregation, which may occur on the rough endothelium of the stented area of the vessel.

15. b. Therapeutic effects occur in 2 to 4 weeks

16. a. Although the medication is refrigerated before use, it should be room temperature when it is infused.

17. d. Hyperfibrinolysis causes life-threatening hemorrhage.

NURSING MANAGEMENT: EVERY GOOD NURSE SHOULD …
MULTIPLE CHOICE

1. d. Intravenous heparin infusions should not be stopped to run other drugs through the IV site because this lowers the blood level of heparin and alters the therapeutic response. Many other drugs are incompatible with heparin, and they should not be piggybacked or added to heparin infusions. Use of a separate IV site for the antibiotics allows continuous infusion of heparin and appropriate dosing of the antibiotics.

2. b. Research has shown that a 3-cc syringe produces less hematoma formation than a 1-cc syringe. To further prevent hematomas, do not aspirate before injection and do not massage the insertion site after injection. The scapula is not a recommended site for heparin administration.

3. c. Warfarin causes a known pattern of fetal changes, known as fetal warfarin syndrome. Precautions should be taken to prevent pregnancy during warfarin therapy. Vitamin K is the antidote to warfarin, and increases in dietary sources, such as green leafy vegetables, should be avoided. Potassium does not have an effect on warfarin. The symbol for potassium is "K," but it is not the same thing as vitamin K. Doses should be taken regularly; however, a double dose should not be taken because it may produce bleeding.

4. a, b, d, e. Clopidogrel may cause GI distress; taking the drug with food will minimize this effect. Lab tests to evaluate bleeding time and white blood cell count (neutropenia is possible) need to be done throughout therapy. The home environment needs to be modified if necessary to minimize the risk of falls in the home. Scatter rugs and loose carpeting are primary causes of falls in the home. This drug lengthens the bleeding time, not shortens it. Patients need to apply extra pressure if they bleed from a minor cut.

5. c. Although onset of therapeutic effect begins in 2 to 4 weeks, full effect is delayed. Patients need to realize this and be encouraged to be patient to see results. Drug therapy needs to be continued until full therapeutic effect is achieved. There is always individual variation in response to drug therapy; however, the patient needs to hear reinforcement regarding the delayed onset of action to prevent discouragement and premature cessation of drug therapy.

6. a. Vital signs should be assessed frequently throughout therapy with recombinant alteplase because bleeding is possible from therapy. Recombinant alteplase is always administered with an infusion pump, never by gravity flow, to prevent overdosage. Avoid IM injections because this may cause internal bleeding. Coffee-ground emesis is a sign of internal bleeding and the infusion should be stopped.

7. b, c, d. This drug is kept refrigerated but must be allowed to come to room temperature before dilution. Diluted drug is rotated, not shaken, to prevent gel formation in the antihemophilic factor. The drug is administered by the IV route to deliver it directly into the bloodstream where it can act. IM routes are avoided to prevent bleeding into the muscle. Coagulation studies are monitored during therapy to assess for therapeutic effect of the drug. Additional antihemophilic factor may be needed if bleeding is not controlled or coagulation studies show subtherapeutic levels of the factor.

8. b. The fresh incision is a likely source for bleeding. Checking the incision frequently will help to determine that an appropriate amount of aminocaproic acid has been administered to control bleeding. Aminocaproic acid is administered by the IV route. It should not be mixed with other drugs. The patient should be connected to a cardiac monitor throughout therapy to detect any cardiac arrhythmias that may occur.

CASE STUDY

1. Heparin is an anticoagulant used to treat DVT. It is safe to use during pregnancy because it does not cross the placenta.
2. Some heparin is ordered to be given by IV push as a bolus of the drug. This brings about a quick rise in blood levels and helps to achieve a therapeutic level more quickly.
3. The aPTT done before the heparin is started is the baseline measurement. Repeated measurements will determine if the drug has reached therapeutic levels. If the blood level is not in the therapeutic range, the nurse needs to seek an order to increase the heparin dosage. If the blood level is above the therapeutic range, the nurse needs to seek an order to decrease the heparin dosage.
4. Heparin does not break down the formed clot. It prevents additional clots from forming while the body naturally walls off the clot and allows it to be broken down. Heparin also prevents the extension of the clot. Ambulating before the clot has lysed makes it more likely that the clot will break off from the vein wall and travel, lodging perhaps in the heart, lungs, or brain.

CRITICAL THINKING CHALLENGE

The nurse should immediately turn off the infusion and disconnect the pump from the infusion tubing. The nurse should then contact the physician and seek orders for STAT aPTT levels. Because the patient is stable and is not showing any evidence of bleeding, protamine sulfate is not indicated immediately, although the nurse may obtain an order for the drug at this time to be given later if needed. This patient must be monitored closely for signs of bleeding. In another 6 to 8 hours, the aPTT should be reassessed to determine if she has recovered from the overdosage. The heparin infusion may be restarted after it is determined that blood levels have returned to a preoverdose level. A different IV pump should be used, and the defective pump should be returned for servicing. The nurse should write an incident sheet detailing the pump's malfunction and the effect on the patient. Additional protocols may need to be followed, depending on the institution's policies for equipment malfunctions, and the nurse should check her hospital's policies.

Chapter 33

KEY TERMS
WORD SEARCH

PHYSIOLOGY AND PATHOPHYSIOLOGY: THE BODY HUMAN
ESSAY

1. The essential components of the immune system are hematopoietic cells, barrier defenses, the nonspecific immune response, the specific immune response, and immunity.
2. Skin, mucus, and the GI tract
3. Granulocytes, monocytes, and lymphocytes
4. T cells and B cells

CORE DRUG KNOWLEDGE: JUST THE FACTS
MULTIPLE CHOICE

1. b. Blood pressure may rise during therapy, especially during the early phase of treatment, when the hematocrit is rising.
2. d. Anemias caused by iron or folate deficiency, hemolysis, or GI bleed should be treated with other modalities.
3. a. It is important to gradually increase the hematocrit to avoid adverse effects.

4. c. Iron is needed to develop RBCs.
5. c. Filgrastim stimulates and mobilizes the cells that are the progenitor cells for neutrophils.
6. a, d. The vial should never be shaken to avoid damaging the protein; administration with saline may cause a precipitate; and iron is not necessary for the development of white cells.
7. c. Filgrastim is discontinued at this point to avoid an excessively elevated white blood cell count.
8. c. It is also used to reduce the need for platelet transfusions after myelosuppressive chemotherapy. Epoetin alpha stimulates production of RBCs and filgrastim stimulates production of WBCs.
9. b. In addition to weight gain, fluid retention may be responsible for cardiovascular effects such as tachycardia.
10. c. Oprelvekin is generally given for 10 to 21 days, but the drug therapy is begun at least 6 hours after chemotherapy is completed.

CORE PATIENT VARIABLES: PATIENTS, PLEASE

MULTIPLE CHOICE

1. b. The dose should not be adjusted more than once a month.
2. c. The prescriber should be notified when the hematocrit is greater than 36%.
3. d, f. Adding albumin to a 5% dextrose solution prevents absorption of the medication into plastic materials. Diluting with saline may cause a precipitate; shaking the vial may damage the protein. The medication should be kept refrigerated; however, allow the medication to reach room temperature before administration.
4. b. One of the most common adverse effects of oprelvekin is fluid retention and weight gain. As the patient's circulating volume increases, the blood pressure rises.
5. c. These are all appropriate interventions for the patient receiving sargramostim. Answers a, b, and d minimize the pain that is associated with administration. Although rare, some patients will have a first-dose effect that may include respiratory distress, hypoxia, flushing, hypotension, syncope, or tachycardia. This effect occurs within the first 20 minutes of the initial dose of sargramostim.

NURSING MANAGEMENT: EVERY GOOD NURSE SHOULD …

MULTIPLE CHOICE

1. d, e, f. Epoetin alfa is administered subcutaneously. It can also be administered IV. Shaking will denature the protein in epoetin alfa and make the drug less effective, so shaking should be avoided. The single-dose, 1-mL vials have no preservative in them and any remaining drug should be discarded.
2. d. Patients with decreased white blood cell counts are at increased risk of contracting an infection. Frequent hand washing by the patient and family members is an important method of preventing infection. The patient needs to avoid crowds and people with illnesses to minimize the risk of infection. Filgrastim will make the neutrophil count rise 1 to 2 days after starting therapy, but this is a transient increase. The use of filgrastim must be continued until the full nadir (lowest point) of marrow-suppressing activity from the antineoplastic has occurred. This varies by the antineoplastic used. Medullary bone pain occurs in about one fourth of the patients receiving filgrastim.
3. c. When giving epoetin to patients with cancer who are receiving chemotherapy, give the initial dose for 8 weeks. After that period, seek orders to adjust the dose, if needed. If patients still do not experience a response to therapy, they are unlikely to have a response to higher doses.
4. b, c, d. Oprelvekin should be administered at least 6 hours after the chemotherapy is administered, not before the chemotherapy. All of the other responses are correct.

CASE STUDY

1. Yes, this was an appropriate order. This patient is anemic secondary to chronic renal failure. The hematocrit, hemoglobin, and red blood cell counts are all below normal.
2. Yes, the epoetin alfa is beginning to have the desired effect in the patient. The first sign of this positive response is a rise in the reticulocyte (new RBCs) count. This should occur within 10 days and has occurred within 7 days. It is too soon for the erythrocyte, hematocrit, or hemoglobin to rise.
3. No, it is too soon to seek a change in the epoetin alfa dose.

CRITICAL THINKING CHALLENGE

1. The rise in the patient's blood pressure may be related to a too-rapid increase in the hematocrit. It is not recommend to raise the hematocrit more than 4 points in 2 weeks; this patient experienced a 6-point increase. The epoetin alfa therapy and the rapid rise in RBCs can also contribute to thrombotic episodes. This patient appears to have a deep vein thrombosis.
2. This patient should have her clotting times assessed carefully. She may need additional heparin to prevent the artificial kidney in dialysis from becoming clotted.

Chapter 34

KEY TERMS

CROSSWORD PUZZLE

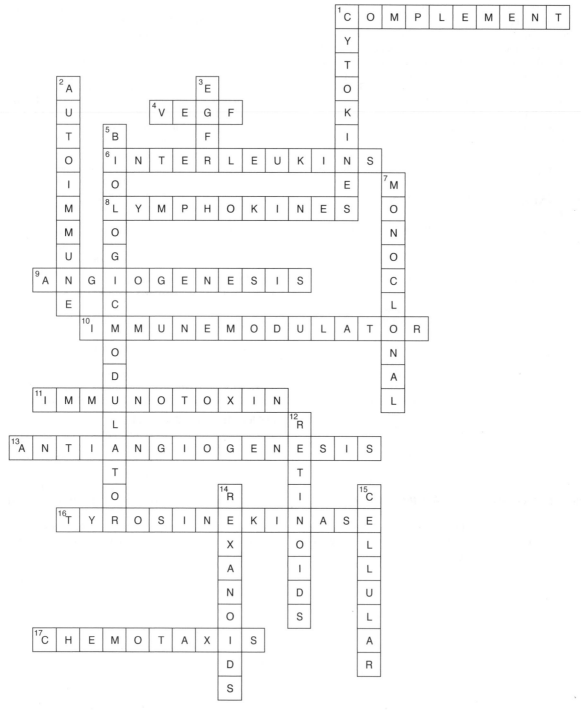

PHYSIOLOGY AND PATHOPHYSIOLOGY: THE BODY HUMAN
ESSAY

1. T cells are divided into T-4 helper cells, suppressor T cells, and effector or cytotoxic T cells. Cytotoxic T cells are found in various areas of the body and aggressively attack nonself cells by releasing chemicals called lymphokines. T-4 helper cells stimulate other lymphocytes' suppressor T cells slow immune responses.

2. B cells react with their specific antigen and change into a plasma cell that produces antibodies or immunoglobu-lins. B cells locate the antigen to which they are sensitized and form an antigen–antibody complex. This binding activates a series of plasma proteins in the body called complement. Complement proteins can destroy the antigen by altering the membrane and allowing osmotic in-flow of fluid that bursts the cell. The complement proteins also can induce

an attraction of phagocytic cells to the area (chemotaxis) and increase the activity of phagocytes. In addition, they can release histamine, which causes vasodilation, increases blood flow to the area, and brings together all the components of the inflammatory reaction to destroy the antigen.

CORE DRUG KNOWLEDGE: JUST THE FACTS
MULTIPLE CHOICE

1. a. Interferon alfa-2a is approved to treat Kaposi sarcoma, chronic myelogenous leukemia in selected patients, chronic hepatitis, and metastatic renal cell carcinoma.
2. d. Interferon alfa-2a must be given parenterally.
3. b, d, e. The most common adverse effects of interferon alfa-2a are dizziness, confusion, lethargy, flu-like symptoms, anorexia, nausea, and changes in taste.
4. d. Kidney function should be evaluated with a BUN and creatinine.
5. a. As many as 80% of patients receiving rituximab experience an infusion-related adverse effect.
6. a, c, f. Rituximab should be mixed with saline or dextrose, but in a plastic bag because it sticks to glass, decreasing the amount of drug delivered. Antihypertensives should be held for an additional 12 to 24 hours after the infusion. The infusion should be stopped if any adverse
   effects occur; however, after they have resolved, the infusion may be restarted at a slower rate.
7. c. The exact mechanism of action is not known, but experimental evidence suggests it is caused by specific, reversible inhibition of immunocompetent T lymphocytes by targeting their cytotoxic effects to lymphocytes in the G0 and G1 phases of the cell cycle.
8. d. The patient should be monitored for signs of renal toxicity.
9. c. Interferon alfa-2a carries a Black Box warning regarding potential neuropsychiatric effects such as severe emotional distress, extreme sadness or depression, or they or family perceive that they are confused.
10. b. Within the Black Box warning for aldesleukin, there's a warning that mild lethargy during administration can rapidly progress to coma even after discontinuation of the drug.
11. c. Bevacizumab is a humanized monoclonal antibody that binds to VEGF so that it is unable to attach to its receptor site on cells, which decreases its ability to stimulate new blood vessel formation.

ESSAY

1. The most common symptoms of an infusion reaction with rituximab include fever, flushing, chills, and rigors. Other symptoms include nausea, urticaria, fatigue, headache, pruritus, bronchospasm, dyspnea, hypotension, angioedema, dyspnea, rhinitis, vomiting, flushing, pain at disease sites, and throat swelling.
2. False. Monoclonal antibodies are specific to a particular pharmacotherapy. Although many of the monoclonal antibodies are approved for use in specific types of cancers, others in this class do not have any antitumor function.

CORE PATIENT VARIABLES: PATIENTS, PLEASE
MULTIPLE CHOICE

1. a. As many as 10% of patients receiving interferon alfa-2a experience hypothyroidism.
2. b. Diphenhydramine not only makes the patient sleepy so the patient can sleep through the worst of the adverse effects, but it also decreases the intensity of the flu-like symptoms.

3. c. Although these are expected symptoms, the infusion should be stopped until they are resolved. When restarting the infusion, start at a lower rate.
4. d. Antihypertensive medications should be withheld both before and after the infusion.
5. c. It is important to remember that these drugs are not interchangeable, and each has a specific pharmacotherapy.
6. b. Grapefruit juice changes the drug's metabolism.
7. b. Renal dysfunction is a common adverse effect to cyclosporine.
8. c. Rituximab may cause a rare but potential fatal neurologic adverse effect called progressive multifocal leukoencephalopathy (PML) that may cause coma and seizures.
9. a. These are the most common symptoms associated with infusion reaction syndrome
10. b. Patient teaching for rituximab includes the need to consume large amounts of water to enhance renal excretion of tumor lysis products.

NURSING MANAGEMENT: EVERY GOOD NURSE SHOULD …
MULTIPLE CHOICE

1. d. Interferon alfa-2a is administered only by injection. The patient is at risk for infections because of possible bone marrow suppression. Bone marrow depression, hypothyroidism, and elevated liver enzyme levels can occur as adverse effects, and blood work should be monitored carefully to prevent serious problems.
2. b. Rituximab is administered by slow IV infusion. Using an IV pump will regulate the infusion rate and keep it at the prescribed rate. Antipyretics, such as acetaminophen, should be administered before the first dose. Because infusion reactions appear to be dose related, the infusion should be started with a fairly small dose and titrated upward.
3. d. Turn off the infusion because she is experiencing an infusion reaction. Keep the infusion off until the symptoms resolve; then resume the infusion at half the rate that produced the reaction. Turning down the infusion may be helpful, but it is not the best choice. Blankets and ice chips are not the priority initial action. The patient should have been premedicated with acetaminophen; another dose would not be the priority now.
4. c. Elevated BUN levels indicate that kidney function is impaired. This is a concern because cyclosporine has a significant risk of causing nephrotoxicity. The damage to the kidney may persist even if use of the cyclosporine is discontinued. Hyperkalemia may occur from cyclosporine, but a small elevation is not a sign of significant problem. A slightly lower white cell (neutrophil) count would be expected; only significant neutropenia would be a concern.
5. c. The IV dose of Sandimmune is $1/3$ that of the oral dose, so no medication error has occurred. Neoral is not bioequivalent with Sandimmune and cannot be substituted without adjusting the dose.
6. c. Rituximab has such potential for infusion reactions that concomitant administration of other agents that may cause severe allergic or anaphylactic reactions should be avoided during and within 2 hours before or after infusion. Agents to avoid include amphotericin, blood products, or first doses of antibiotics.

CASE STUDY

1. This patient needs to know how to reconstitute the interferon alfa-2a, draw up the proper dose in the syringe, locate injection sites, administer by correct technique, rotate

sites of injection, and store the reconstituted drug. Although the patient has had diabetes for years, the nurse needs to assess the patient's ability to do these skills and not just assume that the patient has appropriate technique.

2. Concerns would be related to this patient's eyesight. Can she see well enough to read the labels? Read the syringes? Locate an appropriate injection site? Is there lipoatrophy or lipohypertrophy at any injection site from receiving insulin long term (those with type 1 diabetes require insulin) that would alter the absorption of the interferon alfa-2a? Is she capable of performing the injection herself? If not, does her husband's arthritis preclude him from being able to help her? Would the daughter be available to help with the administration of the drug if necessary?

CRITICAL THINKING CHALLENGE

• Is there a refrigerator to store the reconstituted drug?
• Is there a place to safely store the needles and syringes? How about used syringes?
• Are there environmental risks for falls in the home? (Are there stairs? Is a handrail present on the stairs? Are there scatter rugs? Is there adequate lighting in hallways and stairwells?)

Chapter 35

KEY TERMS
FILL IN THE BLANKS

1. Mineralocorticoid
2. Addison disease
3. Adrenal insufficiency
4. Salt-losing adrenogenital syndrome
5. Aldosterone
6. Hyperaldosteronism
7. Glucocorticoid
8. Addisonian crisis
9. Cushing syndrome
10. Cortisol
11. Steroid hormone inhibitors

PHYSIOLOGY AND PATHOPHYSIOLOGY: THE BODY HUMAN
ESSAY

1. Epinephrine and norepinephrine
2. Glucocorticoids and mineralocorticoids
3. Increase blood glucose concentrations; anti-inflammatory, antiallergenic, and immunosuppressant actions
4. The metabolic effects of the glucocorticoids result in an increase in circulating amino acid levels, an overall depletion of muscle protein, a negative nitrogen balance, and a mobilization of fatty acids, converting cell metabolism from using glucose for energy to using fatty acids for energy.

    Other physiologic effects of the glucocorticoids include an antagonistic effect on antidiuretic hormones to maintain water balance, a lowering of the threshold for electrical excitation in the brain, and a reduction in the amount of new bone synthesis.
5. Suppression of the HPA-axis, resulting in adrenocortical atrophy and impaired glucocorticoid biosynthesis
6. Aldosterone
7. Cortisol and cortisone

CORE DRUG KNOWLEDGE: JUST THE FACTS
MULTIPLE CHOICE

1. b. The water and electrolyte balance is controlled by mineralocorticoids.
2. c. This may result in infection, sepsis, and death.
3. a. Complications of prednisone therapy affect every other system of the body.

4. d. Prednisone has drug–drug interactions with many drugs.
5. b. Alternate-day dosing does not minimize the risk of osteoporosis or cataract formation.
6. a. The hypothalamic-pituitary-adrenal (HPA) axis is depressed during therapy. If use of the drug is abruptly stopped, the patient could experience addisonian crisis.
7. c. Fludrocortisone produces marked sodium retention.
8. b. Because sodium retention is an adverse effect of this drug, patients should avoid ingestion of sodium.
9. a. Fludrocortisone enhances the excretion of potassium.
10. c. Hypercortisolism is an excess of steroids, so use of a steroid hormone antagonist is appropriate.
11. b. This drug may cause orthostatic hypotension.
12. c. In addition, the following tests should be done: serum electrolyte levels, kidney and liver function, glucose tolerance test, electrocardiogram, x-ray films of spine and chest, and tuberculin skin test.
13. a. The most common symptoms of corticosteroid withdrawal syndrome are malaise, myalgia, nausea, headache, and low-grade fever. In addition, if the corticosteroid is withdrawn too quickly the patient may experience an exacerbation of asthma.

CORE PATIENT VARIABLES: PATIENTS, PLEASE
MULTIPLE CHOICE

1. d. Postoperative patients have an increased risk for infection.
2. b. Because of the child's age, growth suppression may occur.
3. b. The patient's diet plan should include low sodium and high potassium.
4. b. Long-term therapy may induce both of these adverse effects.
5. d. Normal cortisol production follows a diurnal cycle. Levels peak in the early morning hours and decline throughout the day, with a second, lower peak in the late afternoon, so the most opportune time for administration of daily doses of glucocorticoids is early in the morning.
6. a. Normally, cortisol secretion increases in response to stress (physical or emotional). Because the patient's body cannot do this on its own, an increased dose may be required.
7. a. Fludrocortisone retains sodium. Because of the sodium retention, water will also be conserved and may increase the blood pressure.
8. c. Meperidine is too strong for an occasional headache, and salicylates may not be effective because of an interaction with fludrocortisone.
9. a. Many foods are high in sodium and the patient already has sodium retention.
10. b. Aminoglutethimide may cause drowsiness and hypotension.

NURSING MANAGEMENT: EVERY GOOD NURSE SHOULD ...
MULTIPLE CHOICE

1. b. Prednisone is irritating to the GI tract and can cause peptic ulcer, which may hemorrhage or perforate. Milk or food given with the drug will decrease the gastric irritation from the prednisone. Proton pump inhibitors and H_2 antagonists also are used to decrease the risk of ulcer development. Administering prednisone on an empty stomach would increase the risk of ulcer formation. Additional prednisone may be needed in times of physical stress, such as illness, injury, or surgery, to prevent adrenal crisis.

2. a. Intrinsic cortisol secretion is highest early in the morning. Taking prednisone at this time will stimulate this intrinsic cycling of cortisol levels and allow the body to use the drug in the most physiologic manner.

3. e. Hypokalemia, hypertension, and weight gain are signs of excessive fludrocortisone dosing.

4. d. Wear or carry a Medic Alert bracelet or card. Information as to whether the patient is taking corticosteroids is important if emergency care is needed. This information can also help emergency personnel in determining whether an adrenal crisis is occurring. Potassium intake should be increased somewhat and sodium intake decreased somewhat to offset the mineralocorticosteroid effects of the fludrocortisone. Drug therapy should not be stopped during illness; this may induce an adrenal crisis. The dosage may need to be increased during illness to meet the increased need for glucocorticoids.

5. d. Thyroid function may be decreased (hypothyroidism) during aminoglutethimide therapy. Blood pressure may drop because of suppression of aldosterone release secondary to aminoglutethimide use. Although this drug is used for hypercortisolism (excess production of corticosteroids by the adrenals), adrenal insufficiency may occur if the dose is too high or if the need for corticosteroids is increased because of stress or illness.

CASE STUDY

1. A glucocorticosteroid was ordered for its anti-inflammatory effect to counteract the inflammation of the respiratory tract, which occurs in chronic asthma.

2. This patient needs to learn what the drug is for, how it will work, when it should be taken, the dose, and possible adverse effects. This patient also needs to be instructed in how to use a metered-dose inhaler properly and the importance of rinsing the mouth after use of the inhaler to prevent oral candidiasis.

CRITICAL THINKING CHALLENGE

1. It appears this patient is experiencing adrenal crisis.

2. Some stressor placed on the body, such as an infection, may have increased the need for glucocorticosteroids. Because of drug-induced suppression of the adrenals, the patient's body was not able to produce additional glucocorticosteroids, and the dose from the prednisone was inadequate to meet the current, elevated needs. Elderly patients are more prone to adrenal suppression from prolonged prednisone administration. Elderly patients may require lower doses because of physiologic changes resulting from aging, such as decreased muscle mass and plasma volume or impairment of hepatic or renal functions. This patient had lost weight from the time the medication dose was originally determined.

   Alternately, this patient may have stopped taking the prednisone abruptly, and this precipitated the adrenal crisis. When the crisis is passed and the patient is in stable condition, the nurse should question the patient about discontinuing use of the drug. Alternately, the family members may know this information now. Knowing about the patient's limited income, be sure to explore whether financial reasons contributed to the cessation of drug use, if the patient did indeed stop taking the drug suddenly.

Chapter 36

KEY TERMS

CROSSWORD PUZZLE

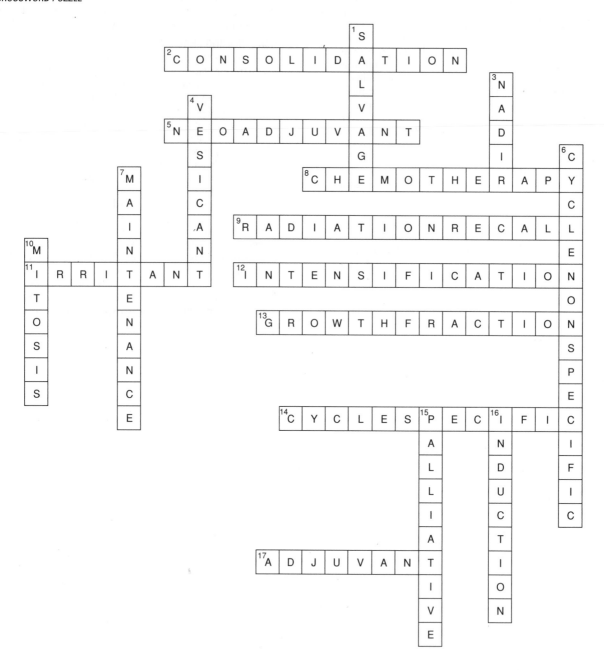

PHYSIOLOGY AND PATHOPHYSIOLOGY: THE BODY HUMAN

MATCHING

1. d
2. b
3. e
4. c
5. a

ESSAY

1. Prophase, metaphase, anaphase, and telophase
2. Actual division of the cytoplasm into new daughter cells

3. The length of time needed to complete the cell cycle
4. Uncontrolled cell proliferation; decreased cellular differentiation; inappropriate ability to invade surrounding tissue; ability to establish new growth at ectopic sites
5. The number of tumor cells killed by an antineoplastic drug is proportional to the dose used.

CORE DRUG KNOWLEDGE: JUST THE FACTS

MULTIPLE CHOICE

1. d. During the S phase, 5-FU exerts its maximum cytotoxic effects. It acts as a "false" antimetabolite, causing a thymine deficiency.

2. d. Because 5-FU is known for its toxicity, patients who are poor risks should be monitored vigilantly. Toxicity can cause death even in patients who are in relatively good condition.

3. b. It is effective against solid tumors, especially those in the GI tract.

4. c. Discontinue use of the drug if stomatitis, esophagopharyngitis, leukopenia, thrombocytopenia, intractable vomiting, diarrhea, GI ulceration or bleeding, or bleeding from any site occurs.

5. c. Vincristine is also used in combination therapy for Hodgkin's disease, non-Hodgkin's malignant lymphomas, sarcoma, breast cancer, small-cell lung cancer, rhabdomyosarcoma, neuroblastoma, and Wilms tumor.

6. b. Vincristine is an extremely acidic drug that may cause substantial tissue damage when accidental infiltration occurs.

7. b, d. Vincristine should be kept refrigerated, and the patient should have a CBC before each administration.

8. b. Rapid administration may cause hypotension.

9. d. Radiation recall is characterized by erythematous rash in the previously irradiated area.

10. b. It is also used in the management of Kaposi sarcoma.

11. d. These are all common adverse effects of paclitaxel.

12. a. The fluid retention is cumulative and is believed to be caused by increased capillary permeability and by the vehicle used to increase docetaxel's solubility, Tween 80.

13. a. The enzyme topoisomerase-I causes nicks and breaks along DNA strands, relieving stresses that build up as the DNA molecule unwinds in preparation for cell division and protein synthesis.

14. c. There are no known drug–drug interactions that affect the potency of topotecan; however, when given with other cytotoxic drugs, myelosuppression may occur, which is serious.

15. d. Hydroxyurea is well absorbed from the GI tract, so it is given orally.

16. b. Hydration is important for hydroxyurea's therapeutic effect.

ESSAY

1. CBC with differential, liver function, renal function, and platelet count

2. Practice good body and oral hygiene; eat a nutritious diet and drink plenty of fluids; avoid injury, especially cuts to the skin; avoid possible sources of infection, such as animal excrement or people with colds, chickenpox, and herpes; and pace activities of daily living to provide adequate rest and exercise.

MATCHING

1. f, h
2. c, i
3. b
4. b, d, e
5. b, e
6. a, b, g, j

CORE PATIENT VARIABLES: PATIENTS, PLEASE

MULTIPLE CHOICE

1. c. Myelosuppression is the dose-limiting adverse effect of 5-FU.

2. b. These assessments should be made because of the potential cutaneous changes associated with 5-FU.

3. a. Because myelosuppression is the limiting factor of this drug, the CBC should be routinely assessed before administration.

4. b. These are symptoms that the neurologic system has been affected by the drug.

5. c. These symptoms can be ameliorated by stopping the infusion and giving the patient IV fluids, corticosteroids, antihistamines, and volume expanders, as ordered.

6. a. The cytotoxicity from these two drugs is sequence dependent; for optimal results, paclitaxel should be given first.

7. b. Measure and closely monitor the patient's baseline vital signs during the first 15 minutes of the infusion, and continue monitoring the patient for the first hour.

8. d. Prophylactic measures include the use of corticosteroids, such as dexamethasone, 8 mg orally twice daily for 5 days before docetaxel, with or without H_1- and H_2-receptor antagonists given IV 30 minutes before the drug; these measures appear to be effective in reducing the fluid retention.

9. c. Because of clinical trial data, administration of a minimum of four courses of topotecan is required.

10. c. As with other chemotherapeutic drugs, myelosuppression is the dose-limiting adverse effect of hydroxyurea.

11. d. Vomiting can be a serious adverse effect and should be investigated.

12. c. Each drug has a different nadir. This is the time the patient is most susceptible to infection.

NURSING MANAGEMENT: EVERY GOOD NURSE SHOULD ...
MULTIPLE CHOICE

1. c. Soft, cool, bland foods such as these will be less irritating. Hot beverages are usually too irritating. Commercial mouthwash is too astringent and will irritate mouth sores. Aspirin should be avoided because it may promote bleeding as the platelet count is decreased from the 5-FU.

2. b. While all of these systems require ongoing assessment, 5-FU has been associated with cardiac events such as angina, palpitations, sweating and /or syncope. Electrocardiogram (ECG) changes, arrhythmias, pulmonary edema, myocardial infarction, (rarely) cardiac arrest, and severe but reversible cardiogenic shock have been noted to occur within the first 72 hours of the initial round of chemotherapy.

3. d. This is a sign of infiltration and extravasation. An antidote is needed immediately to prevent serious tissue damage. Hair should be brushed carefully because hair and skin become weak from the drug therapy, although this doesn't occur until 2 or 3 weeks after treatment. Patients need a high-fiber diet with plenty of fluids to prevent constipation. Heart rate is not significantly affected by vincristine.

4. a. It appears that the IV line has infiltrated and that the vincristine has extravasated. Shutting off the infusion will minimize the amount of drug that enters the tissues and the damage that may occur. Hyaluronidase is the antidote for vincristine extravasation, not isotonic sodium thiosulfate. Warm compresses should be used on the extravasation site after vincristine extravasation.

5. b. Hypersensitivity reactions to etoposide are related to infusing the drug too rapidly. The drug is administered by IV infusion, not IV push, which would be an extremely concentrated and rapid delivery rate. The nurse should stay with the patient during the infusion due because of severe consequences of hypersensitivity reaction. It is not appropriate to leave the patient alone or to expect family members to be responsible for the patient.

6. b. Support the patient emotionally on this issue and discuss the use of wigs, hats, and scarves to cover her head

during the period of alopecia. Hair loss may be severe and include eyebrows, eyelashes, axillary hair, and pubic hair. Although myelosuppression, neurotoxicity, and hypersensitivity reactions pose more significant risks to the patient's physical health, hair loss is what concerns the patient, and the nurse should not minimize the patient's feelings.

7. d. CBC should be checked for the presence of anemia, leukopenia, and low platelet counts. Drug therapy should begin before radiation therapy but then may continue throughout therapy. BUN and creatinine levels may increase because of deterioration of renal function secondary to drug therapy.

8. c, e. To prevent accidental skin exposure to a hazardous drug, you should use a sterile gauze pad around the connecting site when disconnecting IV tubing. Also use a gauze over the tip of the syringe when purging air from a chemotherapy-filled syringe, when opening chemotherapy vials and ampules, when removing syringes from IV lines after IV push administration, and when removing empty chemotherapy bags or bottles from IV spikes. Eye protection is necessary to keep hazardous drugs, such as chemotherapy, out of the eyes. IV tubings should be purged with normal saline, not the antineoplastic drug. All chemotherapy waste should be disposed of in an impervious, leak-proof container, not open trash cans. Avoid all eating, drinking, smoking, chewing gum, and applying makeup when preparing hazardous drugs. You should wash your hands before and after working with antineoplastic drugs.

CASE STUDY

1. 5-Fluorouracil (5-FU) interferes with the synthesis of DNA and RNA. It is clinically effective in treating solid tumors, including colorectal cancers. Levamisole is a T/B cell modulator that restores depressed immune function, stimulates antibody formation, enhances T-cell response, and potentiates monocyte and macrophage activity. Levamisole is adjunct therapy in the treatment of colorectal cancers. Because it stimulates the immune function of the body, it is helpful in preventing adverse effects from the antineoplastic drug 5-FU.

2. The patient's CBC count needs to be monitored before, during, and after therapy. 5-FU should not be given if the WBC is less than $3500/mm^3$ because this indicates leukopenia. Bone marrow depression from levamisole is rare but potentially serious. Also monitor for nausea, vomiting, stomatitis, and diarrhea because these can be adverse effects of both drugs. GI ulceration and hemorrhage can occur with 5-FU use. Headache can be an adverse effect of either drug therapy. However, if caused by levamisole, other CNS effects of dizziness, depression, and paresthesia may be present. If the headache is related to 5-FU use, it indicates the development of acute cerebellar syndrome. This syndrome would also have disorientation and nystagmus as symptoms; photophobia and ocular changes also may be present.

CRITICAL THINKING CHALLENGE

1. Dark, tar-colored or black stools are a sign of old GI bleeding. GI bleeding is a serious complication of 5-FU therapy.

2. Report these findings to the physician at once. Consult with the physician regarding decreasing the dose of 5-FU. Assess for bright red bleeding, which would indicate active bleeding. Assess the patient's hematocrit and hemoglobin for information regarding severity of bleeding. Closely monitor the patient.

Chapter 37

KEY TERMS
FILL IN THE BLANKS
1. Radiomimetic
2. Hormones and hormone antagonists
3. Combination therapy
4. Alkylating agent
5. Nitrosoureas
6. Antitumor antibiotics
7. Disease flare
8. Cell cycle–nonspecific
9. Liposomes
10. Acute emesis
11. Delayed emesis
12. Tumor burden
13. Emetogenic

CORE DRUG KNOWLEDGE: JUST THE FACTS
MULTIPLE CHOICE
1. d. Cyclophosphamide is effective for hematologic malignancies as well as solid tumors, such as those associated with breast cancer, small-cell lung cancer, endometrial cancer, and with ovarian tumors.
2. d. This occurs more frequently with high-dose cyclophosphamide therapy.
3. a. This risk is associated with long-term, low-dose therapy.
4. c. This will help metabolites of the drug to be excreted and not stagnate to erode the bladder wall.
5. b. Cisplatin is belongs to a group of antineoplastic drugs called emetogenics.
6. b. Carmustine is a nitrosourea used in the palliative therapy of brain tumors, multiple myeloma, Hodgkin's disease, and non-Hodgkin's lymphoma.
7. c. Bone marrow suppression and pulmonary fibrosis are associated with its use.
8. d. Extravasation is especially problematic with doxorubicin because it binds to nucleic acids, causing destructive and prolonged tissue injuries.
9. d. This toxicity is cumulative and may manifest weeks or months after the initial treatment.
10. b. In addition, it is the only drug approved for the prevention of breast cancer in high-risk women and for reduction of the risk of contralateral breast cancer.
11. d. Tamoxifen competes with estrogen for binding sites in tissues high in estrogen receptors, such as breast tissue.
12. c. Most patients taking tamoxifen experience no toxicity.
13. a. All of these drugs have the potential to cause myelosuppression.

MATCHING
1. a, b, h, k, l
2. b, c, g, i
3. e, m
4. f, j, d

CORE PATIENT VARIABLES: PATIENTS, PLEASE
MULTIPLE CHOICE
1. b. GI distress is very common with cyclophosphamide therapy.
2. c. These are symptoms of rapid infusion.
3. a. Hemorrhagic cystitis is caused by acrolein, a metabolic by-product of cyclophosphamide that irritates the bladder wall. These interventions decrease the risk for hemorrhagic cystitis.
4. b. Carmustine may cause pulmonary fibrosis.

5. d. The standard of care is to use a large vein to diminish the intense discomfort associated with this infusion, but in some patients they may still experience intense discomfort.

6. c. The phenomenon can occur weeks or months—even years—after radiation but appears more frequently with shorter time intervals and high-dose chemotherapy.

7. c. Dexrazoxane is a potent intracellular chelating drug that interferes with iron-mediated free radical generation thought to be responsible for anthracycline-induced cardiotoxicity.

8. b. Reassure the patient that reddish urine after doxorubicin injection is a harmless and expected response to the drug. This reaction may happen within 1 to 2 days after the infusion.

9. a. Carmustine has a delayed nadir that is 4 to 6 weeks after administration. It is too soon to adequately evaluate its affect on this patient's blood count.

NURSING MANAGEMENT: EVERY GOOD NURSE SHOULD …
MULTIPLE CHOICE

1. b. Prehydration is important to flush the kidneys well during and after therapy to minimize renal toxicities. Oral prehydration may also be used. Diuretic drugs cause dehydration and would not be appropriate. Limiting potassium and magnesium is not relevant. Aminoglycoside antibiotics also cause nephrotoxicity, as does cyclophosphamide, and should be avoided because of the additive effects.

2. a, b, c, d. Amenorrhea, nausea, and vomiting are all possible adverse effects. Secondary malignancies are possible after cyclophosphamide therapy, and adolescents are at most risk for this adverse effect. High fluid intake prevents hemorrhagic cystitis, which may contribute to the development of bladder cancer later in life.

3. c. These are signs of chronic heart failure. Because doxorubicin is a vesicant, a large vein should be used. Aspirin should be avoided because it may induce bleeding when platelet counts are low. Aspirin is also avoided in children because of the risk of Reye syndrome. Reddish urine is a normal effect from doxorubicin and is not an adverse effect.

4. c. Administer the next dose of tamoxifen as ordered. Bone pain and pain at the site of the tumor are signs of disease flare, which occurs with tamoxifen therapy. They are actually signs of tumor response to the drug. Although the physician should be aware of disease flare, there is no need to contact him or her immediately because a problem does not exist.

5. c. Thrombocytopenia can occur at 6 weeks after carmustine treatment. Adequate platelet function needs to be determined before administering another dose of carmustine. Weight, blood pressure, and BUN are not critical measurements that must be assessed before a dose of carmustine can be given.

6. a. Because doxorubicin is a vesicant, it is important to prevent extravasation. Verifying that the IV is patent and running well is one important step in this process. Although ice might be applied after an extravasation has occurred, it is not done before drug administration. Use of a tourniquet likely would cause extravasation because it would impede circulation. Massaging the vein is not helpful or indicated.

CASE STUDY

1. Although both doxorubicin and cyclophosphamide are cell cycle–nonspecific drugs, using two drugs, or combination therapy, has advantages. Combination therapy maximizes cell kill, has a broader range of kill, and minimizes the emergence of cancer cells resistant to chemotherapy. Dosage of each drug can be kept to a minimum, thus decreasing serious toxicities from each drug.

2. This patient may have nausea and vomiting, an adverse effect from doxorubicin, and the same may also occur with cyclophosphamide. Abnormal blood cell levels are also possible because cyclophosphamide causes leukopenia, and doxorubicin causes bone marrow depression. Cardiotoxicity is a significant risk because both drugs cause this adverse effect. Alopecia also may occur with either drug. Hemorrhagic cystitis, syndrome of inappropriate antidiuretic hormone, hypersensitivity, reproductive effects, cutaneous problems, mucositis, extravasation injury, and radiation recall are all possible, although the risk is minimized because combination drug therapy minimizes the dose of each drug used.

CRITICAL THINKING CHALLENGE

1. The combined chemotherapy has been effective so far, and there are no adverse effects from the drug therapy as of today. All blood work is within normal ranges, and the ECG is normal.

2. Yes, you should administer the next prescribed doses of cyclophosphamide and doxorubicin.

Chapter 38

KEY TERMS
TRUE OR FALSE

1. True
2. False, bactericidal
3. False, postantibiotic
4. True
5. False, selective toxicity
6. False, Gram stain
7. False, spectrum
8. False, pathogens
9. False, empiric therapy
10. True
11. False, microbe
12. False, culture, sensitivity
13. True

CORE DRUG KNOWLEDGE: JUST THE FACTS
ESSAY

1. Antimicrobials are classified by susceptible organism or by mechanism of action.

2. Antibacterial drugs, antiviral drugs, antifungal drugs, antiparasitic drugs, anthelmintic drugs

3. Inhibition of bacterial cell wall synthesis, inhibition of protein synthesis, inhibition of nucleic acid synthesis, inhibition of metabolic pathways, disruption of cell wall permeability, inhibition of viral enzymes

4. Methicillin-resistant *Staphylococcus aureus* (MRSA), penicillin-resistant *Streptococcus pneumoniae,* vancomycin-resistant *Enterococci* (VRE), and multiple drug–resistant *Mycobacterium tuberculosis* (MDR-TB)

5. Identification of the pathogen, drug susceptibility, drug spectrum, drug dose, duration, site of infection, patient assessment

6. The nurse must use aseptic technique for all procedures, obtain culture specimens appropriately, communicate culture and sensitivity results in a timely manner, adhere to isolation procedures, document improvement or worsening of symptoms of infection, and most importantly, wash his or her hands between contact with patients.

7. Nosocomial infections occur because the hospital setting has a high prevalence of pathogens, a high prevalence of compromised hosts, and an efficient mechanism of transmission from patient to patient.

CORE PATIENT VARIABLES: PATIENTS, PLEASE
ESSAY

1. Immune status, previous allergic reactions, previous hypersensitivities
2. Drug toxicity is more likely to happen in infants and the elderly because of immaturity or dysfunction of the kidney and liver.
3. Complete entire course of therapy, take prescribed dose, take at prescribed intervals
4. The most important nursing action to limit nosocomial infections is consistent cleaning of hands between patient contact, using either soap and water or alcohol-based hand antiseptics.
5. Some antimicrobial agents have the ability to induce toxic adverse effects. Serum drug levels are monitored to assure sufficient drug remains in the bloodstream to eradicate the bacterial (trough level) but it not too high to induce these severe adverse effects (peak level). Blood for a peak level is generally drawn 1 hour after IV or IM administration. Trough levels are drawn 30 minutes before the next dose of medication.

Chapter 39

KEY TERMS

MATCHING

1. a
2. d
3. f
4. e
5. b
6. c

CORE DRUG KNOWLEDGE: JUST THE FACTS

MULTIPLE CHOICE

1. c. Although all antibiotics may induce an allergic response, penicillin allergies occur most frequently.
2. a. Only a few gram-negative bacteria respond to penicillin G.
3. b. Penicillin may be given by the oral, intramuscular, and intravenous routes.
4. b. Patients may have forgotten to report that they have a penicillin allergy. It is prudent to ask before initiation of therapy.
5. b. 5% to 10% of patients allergic to penicillins will also be allergic to cephalosporins.
6. a. Aminopenicillins have an altered side chain that makes them effective against many gram-negative microorganisms.
7. c. The extended penicillins are also known as "antipseudomonal penicillins" because they are effective against *Pseudomonas*.
8. c. Beta-lactamase can inactivate the beta-lactam ring, which is responsible for the activity of these antibiotics. Beta-lactamase inhibitors stop the inactivation of the beta-lactam ring, thus allowing the penicillin to eradicate the microbe.
9. b. The structure of aztreonam differs substantially from those of other beta-lactam antibiotics; thus, there is little cross-sensitivity, and this drug may be given safely to patients allergic to penicillin.

10. d. Imipenem is rapidly inactivated by renal dehydropeptidase 1. Therefore, imipenem is always administered with cilastatin, a drug that inhibits this enzyme. This does not occur with other carbapenems.
11. b. One of the major differences between the generations is their spectrums of activity, especially against gram-negative bacteria.
12. a. Optimal duration for complete eradication of the microbe is 7 to 10 days.
13. d. Hypersensitivity presents most frequently as a maculopapular rash that develops several days after the onset of therapy.
14. c. Vancomycin is used primarily for systemic infections that have not been resolved by less toxic antibiotics.
15. b. Ototoxicity can take the form of cochlear toxicity or vestibular toxicity. Nephrotoxicity is more likely to occur in patients receiving other nephrotoxic drugs.

CORE PATIENT VARIABLES: PATIENTS, PLEASE
MULTIPLE CHOICE

1. d. Penicillin should be taken on an empty stomach.
2. b. BUN and creatinine are the appropriate lab tests to evaluate renal function.
3. a. These drugs must be given at least 2 hours apart to avoid inactivating each other.
4. b. Patients allergic to one penicillin are allergic to all penicillins. The nurse does not have the authority to change a prescriber's order to another type of antibiotic.
5. d. Unusual behaviors such as those described indicate a procaine reaction. Allergy to penicillin usually manifests in shortness of breath, rash, hives, urticaria, etc.
6. c. Reconstitution of this drug yesterday makes it "outdated," so it should not be used.
7. c. It is important to get an appropriate order from the physician as soon as possible to get the infection under control. Some hospital policies may direct the nurse to continue the cephalosporin until the prescriber discontinues the medication.
8. b. Peak levels of the drug circulate 1 hour after the completion of the infusion.
9. b. This rate will diminish effects such as flushing, tachycardia, hypotension, or rashes that occur when administration is too fast.
10. a. Vancomycin is poorly absorbed, so it has a local effect when given orally.

NURSING MANAGEMENT: EVERY GOOD NURSE SHOULD …
MULTIPLE CHOICE

1. d. This helps to ensure that all of the organisms have been killed so that a re-infection does not occur. Administer oral penicillin G on an empty stomach. Doses should be evenly spaced throughout the 24-hour period. Take IV forms of penicillin G out of the refrigerator for 15 minutes before administering.
2. d. Alcoholic beverages and products containing alcohol should be avoided because a disulfiram-like reaction (or alcohol intolerance) may occur, making the patient feel quite ill. Elixirs always have alcohol in them, and OTC cough medicines frequently have alcohol in them.
3. b. Vancomycin should be administered over at least 60 minutes to decrease the risk of ototoxicity and red man syndrome. IV push would be too concentrated and too fast and would produce adverse effects. Vancomycin is extremely irritating to the tissues and should never be given SC. Poor absorption occurs from the oral route; this route is seldom used and is not appropriate for serious infections outside of the GI tract.

4. d. Before beginning antibiotic therapy, a culture and sensitivity should be obtained, if at all possible, to determine the exact organism present and which drug therapy will be effective in eradicating the organism. A sputum culture would be appropriate for pneumonia. It is important to always verify with patients that they are not allergic to a medication when you administer the first dose. This is especially true with penicillins because anaphylactic reactions are possible drug allergy responses. Because of possible drug allergies, observe the patient closely during the first 30 minutes of drug administration for signs of adverse effects.

5. c. Procaine penicillin is administered by IM injection. As with all penicillins, it is important to identify an injection site accurately to prevent accidental administration into a vein or nerve. Accidental injection into a vein may precipitate a reaction with the procaine that is in the drug. Procaine penicillin, like all penicillins, should be administered deep into a large muscle. The deltoid is too small to be appropriate. Because procaine penicillin is thick and viscous, it is administered more easily if it is removed from the refrigerator about 15 minutes before administration.

6. c. BUN (blood urea nitrogen) is a measurement of kidney function. Nephrotoxicity is more likely to occur when the patient takes more than one drug that may cause nephrotoxicity; in this case, those drugs are cefazolin and gentamicin. The nurse should also monitor creatinine levels to assess renal function. Hematocrit is not affected by cefazolin therapy. Blood coagulation time, aPTT (active partial thromboplastin time), is altered only if the patient is receiving oral anticoagulants, such as warfarin, and cefazolin. Cefazolin is not a drug that the blood levels indicate a therapeutic or toxic level, and cefazolin levels are not measured. However, gentamicin levels are monitored.

7. c. Daptomycin is excreted mostly unchanged through the urine. Patients with renal disease need to have a decreased dose for this reason. Daptomycin, unlike other antibiotics, is used to treat VRE infections.

CASE STUDY

1. It appears that this patient is demonstrating signs of ototoxicity from the vancomycin. The fall and the comment about being tipsy indicate ataxia, or possibly vertigo. The cricket sound may be the onset of tinnitus.

2. You should check the peak and trough levels of the drug. If such levels have not been obtained recently, an order should be sought for them, and the physician should be informed of these adverse events. It would also be important to check the patient's renal function by examining the BUN and creatinine levels. Nephrotoxicity may also be occurring from the vancomycin.

CRITICAL THINKING CHALLENGE

1. The peak and trough are both higher than the normal therapeutic range and support your assessment that ototoxicity is occurring. In addition, it is possible that some nephrotoxicity is occurring because the vancomycin trough levels are elevated and the BUN and creatinine are somewhat elevated. However, these levels may reflect normal aging. You have to compare them to the baseline levels (before vancomycin administration) for accurate assessment.

2. Contact the physician regarding these results; consult with the physician regarding decreasing the dose or discontinuing use of the drug. In some institutions, the pharmacist doses vancomycin based on drug levels, so consult with the pharmacist, as appropriate. An audiogram also may be indicated.

Chapter 40

KEY TERMS
MATCHING
1. f
2. d
3. h
4. b
5. i
6. c
7. j
8. a
9. e
10. g

CORE DRUG KNOWLEDGE: JUST THE FACTS
MULTIPLE CHOICE
1. b. These two adverse effects occur frequently with aminoglycosides.
2. d. A trough level indicates the lowest circulating level of drug; thus, it should be drawn 30 minutes before administration of the next dose.
3. a. There are many potential drug–drug interactions; the most serious include ototoxicity, nephrotoxicity, and respiratory depression.
4. a. Neomycin is too toxic to administer by any parenteral route.
5. c. Clindamycin has potentially severe adverse effects and is not used for empiric therapy.
6. c. Clindamycin's potential adverse reactions do not occur with topical application.
7. b. Pseudomembranous colitis should be considered for patients receiving clindamycin who have severe diarrhea. Hearing loss, azotemia, and migraines are not associated with the use of clindamycin.
8. b. Erythromycin, the prototype for the macrolide class, is the drug of choice for patients with allergy to penicillin.
9. d. GI distress, nausea, and vomiting are adverse effects associated with the use of erythromycin.
10. a. Clarithromycin has a longer half-life than does erythromycin and can be taken twice a day.
11. c. To minimize the risk for the development of resistance, linezolid is not used for less serious infections.
12. b. Because of its 100% bioavailability, oral linezolid is interchangeable with IV linezolid.
13. c. GI complaints are linezolid's most frequent adverse effects.
14. d. Like linezolid, quinupristin/dalfopristin is not used for less serious infections.
15. c. Pseudomembranous colitis, superinfection, and hepatotoxicity are associated with the use of quinupristin/dalfopristin.
16. a. Because of the risk for hepatotoxicity, liver function tests should be monitored.
17. a. Concurrent administration with antacids forms an insoluble chelate, which decreases absorption.
18. c. Chloramphenicol passes the blood–brain barrier, so it is used for brain abscesses.
19. a. Gray baby syndrome may occur in neonates receiving chloramphenicol.
20. d. Chloramphenicol suppresses bone marrow, resulting in aplastic anemia.

CORE PATIENT VARIABLES: PATIENTS, PLEASE
MULTIPLE CHOICE

1. b. Peak and trough levels are an important tool in minimizing the risk for adverse effects for patients receiving gentamicin.
2. a. Gentamicin may interact with neuromuscular blocking agents, which are frequently used during surgical procedures.
3. a. Clindamycin should always be given on an empty stomach unless the patient experiences GI distress.
4. c. Topical clindamycin is drying to the skin. Hydration and moisturizing cream will be helpful.
5. d. Blood-tinged diarrhea may indicate pseudomembranous colitis.
6. c. Diabetic gastroparesis is a decrease in gastric transit. Because of its ability to increase peristalsis, erythromycin can help.
7. a. Theophylline reduces the bioavailability of erythromycin and increases its renal clearance.
8. c. Diluents containing preservatives or organic salts should not be used with erythromycin.
9. d. Linezolid may interact with foods rich in tyramine.
10. c. Hypertensive crisis is a potential result when patients consume foods rich in tyramine, caffeine, and alcohol.
11. a. Quinupristin/dalfopristin is not compatible with saline or heparin.
12. b. Quinupristin/dalfopristin is irritating to the veins, so it should be administered slowly.
13. a. Tetracycline is contraindicated during pregnancy and lactation.
14. c. Tetracycline can cause mottled permanent teeth in the baby if given during pregnancy.
15. a. Both chemotherapy and chloramphenicol may induce bone marrow suppression.
16. b. Telithromycin is also contraindicated for patients taking Class Ia or Class III antiarrhythmics because coadministration may increase peak plasma concentrations of these drugs, resulting in clinically important increases in the QT interval.

NURSING MANAGEMENT: EVERY GOOD NURSE SHOULD …
MULTIPLE CHOICE

1. a, b, c, d. Do all of the above. Gentamicin has adverse effects of nephrotoxicity and ototoxicity. Output will decrease with nephrotoxicity. Tinnitus demonstrates damage to the cochlear branch of the 8th cranial nerve. Loss of balance demonstrates damage to the vestibular branch of the 8th cranial nerve. Monitoring BUN and creatinine levels will identify renal toxicity.
2. c. Burning and irritation to the vein are common with erythromycin administration. Slowing the rate will help to minimize the discomfort. Iced compresses may be used if pain persists. Burning is not a sign of drug allergy with erythromycin. Unless the IV is infiltrated or not patent, it should not be removed because of the burning sensation.
3. b. This patient may be experiencing pseudomembranous colitis, a serious adverse effect of clindamycin. The stool should be examined for WBCs, mucus, and blood. Antidiarrheals may treat the symptom; however, if pseudomembranous colitis is present, antidiarrheals may mistakenly lead the nurse and physician to believe that the diarrhea is not serious, thus delaying needed diagnosis and treatment of the disorder. A high-roughage diet will further irritate the inflamed bowel and is not appropriate.

4. d. Tetracycline causes mottling and discoloration of teeth in children. Tetracycline should be taken with water, not milk, because milk chelates with tetracycline, preventing absorption. Tetracycline, like all antibiotics, should be taken for the full course of therapy to prevent recurrence of the infection. Tetracycline causes photosensitivity, placing the patient at increased risk for sunburn. Patients should avoid direct sun exposure.
5. d. Bruising and fatigue are signs of anemia and bone marrow depression. Elevated hepatic enzymes are signs of liver damage. These are all serious adverse effects of chloramphenicol.
6. b. Quinupristin/dalfopristin must be flushed with D5W because it is incompatible with both normal saline and heparin. Quinupristin/dalfopristin can be administered only IV. It is preferable that quinupristin/dalfopristin be administered either through a PICC (peripherally inserted central catheter) line or a central line. Although diazepam will have a drug interaction with quinupristin/dalfopristin because of P-450 inhibition and diazepam levels will rise, drugs that are needed for seizure control cannot be easily discontinued. Administer the drug, but monitor the patient for signs of adverse effects from the diazepam. It is possible that a lower dose of diazepam will need to be ordered.
7. a. Bleu cheese is an aged cheese that is high in tyramine. Because linezolid is a nonselective MAO inhibitor, a hypertensive crisis can occur if foods with high tyramine content are eaten. Strawberries, graham crackers, and carrots do not have high tyramine levels. (Hint: Need help? See Chapter 19 for a discussion of MAO inhibitors used as antidepressants.)
8. a, b, c, d. All of these are advantages of telithromycin and should be included in patient education. Telithromycin is the only drug in a new class of drugs; it is significantly different from other macrolides, such as erythromycin.

CASE STUDY

1. Health status: This patient's diabetes may have contributed to his renal dysfunction. The renal impairment puts him more at risk for the development of nephrotoxicity from the gentamicin. In addition, diabetes impairs circulation throughout the body, and blood supply to the infection may be hindered, making it more difficult to treat the infection.
2. Trough levels are ordered to determine whether therapeutic levels are maintained by the dosing schedule. Peak levels are ordered to determine whether blood levels are too high, placing the patient at risk for adverse effects. Pharmacists frequently monitor these blood reports because they have the most knowledge of pharmacokinetics and pharmacodynamics of drugs, such as gentamicin. You should see that the trough is drawn no more than 30 minutes before the next dose. It is important to administer the drug on time after the trough has been drawn. The peak should be drawn 30 to 45 minutes after the infusion is completed. Monitor the infusion carefully and note the exact time the infusion is complete.

CRITICAL THINKING CHALLENGE

1. It is important to give the antibiotics on time and to document the exact time of each dose. This information will be needed for accurate laboratory interpretation of the peak and trough levels.
2. Because this patient's wound is infected with bacteria that are resistant to many antibiotics, it is important to place him on wound and skin isolation, follow those protocols, and to wash your hands thoroughly after providing care to him to prevent the spread of these difficult-to-treat bacteria.

Chapter 41

KEY TERMS
FILL IN THE BLANKS
1. Fluoroquinolone
2. Quinolone
3. Arthropathy
4. Cyclic lipopeptides

CORE DRUG KNOWLEDGE: JUST THE FACTS
MULTIPLE CHOICE
1. b. The action of ciprofloxacin is to inhibit DNA replication.
2. d. Ciprofloxacin is available as an oral, parenteral, or topical drug.
3. c. Fourth-generation fluoroquinolones, not second-generation drugs such as ciprofloxacin, are effective against anaerobic bacteria.
4. a. Many adverse effects are associated with ciprofloxacin; however, GI distress is the most common.
5. a. Nalidixic acid is a first-generation quinolone that is approved only for the management of urinary tract infections.
6. a. Because of its long half-life, levofloxacin is given once daily.
7. d. In addition to nephrotoxicity, polymyxin B may also cause neurotoxicity.
8. c. Rapid depolarization of the membrane potential leads to inhibition of protein, DNA, and RNA synthesis and, eventually, bacterial cell death.

CORE PATIENT VARIABLES: PATIENTS, PLEASE
MULTIPLE CHOICE
1. c. Nurses have the responsibility of knowing which drugs are acceptable for children and which formulations are approved for children.
2. a. Ciprofloxacin may bind to birth control pill receptor sites, thus increasing the risk for conception.
3. b. GI absorption of ciprofloxacin may be decreased if given concurrently with aluminum, calcium, or magnesium (all components of antacids).
4. d. Parenteral ciprofloxacin should be administered over 60 minutes through a large vein to minimize discomfort and reduce the risk for venous irritation.
5. c. Superinfection occurs when the normal flora of the body is eradicated by the antibiotic, allowing other microbes to grow unabated.
6. d. Daptomycin is not compatible with dextrose-containing solutions.
7. b. These are signs of potentially severe adverse effects and should be communicated to the provider immediately.

NURSING MANAGEMENT: EVERY GOOD NURSE SHOULD ...
MULTIPLE CHOICE
1. a. Ciprofloxacin may cause photosensitivity. Sunscreen will help prevent serious burns if the patient must be outdoors. Fluid intake should be increased to help offset complications from GI effects. Small meals will minimize GI upset. A dose may be taken late if it is forgotten, but a double dose should not be taken.
2. b. Ciprofloxacin inhibits the hepatic metabolism of theophylline and may result in elevated theophylline levels. Tachycardia and insomnia are adverse effects of theophylline. New onset of these problems may indicate theophylline toxicity. Insomnia may also be an adverse effect of ciprofloxacin. The patient has a severe infection and respiratory compromise; exercise is most likely not desirable at this time and may not be tolerated well.

Ciprofloxacin may cause photosensitivity, so the patient should not be exposed to excessive sunlight. Both theophylline and ciprofloxacin need to be administered regularly throughout the day for optimum effectiveness.
3. d. GI distress is a frequent adverse effect of ciprofloxacin. Eating small, frequent meals may help to manage these effects. Nausea and abdominal pain are not signs of drug allergies. Dairy products, such as yogurt, contain a large amount of calcium and impair the absorption of ciprofloxacin. Avoid taking these at the same time.

CASE STUDY
Teach the patient to take the drug on an empty stomach every 12 hours. Teach what the drug is for and possible adverse effects. Instruct the patient on what to do if she experiences possible adverse effects. Verify that she is not pregnant before starting the drug therapy. If she uses oral contraceptives, teach her to also use a backup method of contraception while taking ciprofloxacin. Teach the importance of taking the full prescription and not to stop taking the drug just because she feels better.

CRITICAL THINKING CHALLENGE
Ask when she takes her medicine in relationship to eating. Is she taking it on an empty stomach as she should? Does she take it on an empty stomach but then immediately eats so that the drug is not broken down or absorbed before food is placed in the stomach? This would also decrease the absorption of the ciprofloxacin. Does she take dairy products near the time of her medicine? Does she use antacids? Does she take a vitamin supplement at the same time that she takes her ciprofloxacin? All of these things may decrease the absorption of the ciprofloxacin. If none of these are true, consult with the prescriber about increasing the dose or changing the prescription.

Chapter 42

KEY TERMS
ANAGRAMS
1. Reinfection
2. Cystitis
3. Urethritis
4. Pyelonephritis
5. Relapse
6. Recurrent
7. Prostatitis
8. Crystalluria
9. Sulfonamides
10. PABA

PHYSIOLOGY AND PATHOPHYSIOLOGY: THE BODY HUMAN
ESSAY
1. Kidney, ureter, bladder, and urethra
2. Mucin layer of the urinary bladder; washout phenomenon; immunoglobulin A; phagocytic blood cells
3. Most UTIs occur because of ascending bacteria from the outside of the body up through the urethra. Protective mechanisms of the body have more ability to abate the ascension of bacteria because of the length of the urethra in men.

CORE DRUG KNOWLEDGE: JUST THE FACTS
MULTIPLE CHOICE
1. c. Histoplasmosis is a fungal infection that requires an antifungal drug to eradicate it.
2. b. By interfering with folic acid synthesis, sulfonamides stop bacterial replication of DNA.
3. d. All of these suggestions decrease the risk for adverse effects.

4. a. Sulfonamides have poor solubility in water and may crystallize in the renal tubules.

5. a. Sulfonamides may promote kernicterus in the newborn by displacing bilirubin from plasma proteins.

6. c. Fosfomycin is not metabolized; it is given as a one-time dose.

7. a. Urinary tract antiseptics are drugs that work by local action because high serum levels are not achievable.

8. c. Acute pulmonary reactions are manifested by sudden onset of fever, cough, chills, myalgia, and dyspnea.

9. a. Phenazopyridine is an azo dye, which will discolor the patient's urine orange or red.

10. b. Phenazopyridine is a urinary tract analgesic used to provide symptomatic relief of pain, burning, frequency, and urgency caused by bladder irritation.

CORE PATIENT VARIABLES: PATIENTS, PLEASE
MULTIPLE CHOICE

1. c. Patients who abuse alcohol have an increased risk for abnormal liver function and low folate, albumin, and thiamine levels.

2. a. Taking the medication on an empty stomach enhances the absorption of the drug.

3. c. To avoid crystalluria, patients should be advised to increase fluid intake.

4. d. A CBC is done to monitor for hematologic effects. Kidney function is monitored because of the potential for damage from crystalluria, and liver function is monitored to avoid accumulation.

5. b. Fatigue, sore throat, and easy bruising are all signs of anemia.

6. a. The package contents should be dissolved in 4 ounces of water and the liquid consumed immediately.

7. c. In acidic urine, methenamine is hydrolyzed to ammonia and formaldehyde in the bladder. This process cannot occur if the urine exits the body immediately through an indwelling catheter.

8. a. Phenazopyridine is a urinary tract analgesic used to provide symptomatic relief of pain, burning, frequency, and urgency caused by bladder irritation.

NURSING MANAGEMENT: EVERY GOOD NURSE SHOULD …
MULTIPLE CHOICE

1. d. Although this drug is normally recommended to be taken on an empty stomach, GI upset is common, and patients may need to take the drug with food to minimize this discomfort. Extra water should be encouraged to dilute the urine and decrease the risk of crystalluria and bacterial multiplication. Sulfamethoxazole-trimethoprim causes photosensitivity, and patients need to protect themselves from ultraviolet light.

2. a. A CBC should be monitored because blood dyscrasias are possible from SMZ-TMP. These adverse effects are more likely to occur if the patient has a folate deficiency or is immunocompromised. As an older adult, this patient is more likely to be both immunocompromised and folate deficient. None of the other factors are adverse effects related to sulfamethoxazole-trimethoprim use.

3. d. Patients who are immunocompromised, such as patients with AIDS, are more at risk for adverse effects, and long-term therapy also places the patient at greater risk for crystalluria. Assessing intake and output provides some knowledge regarding how well the kidney is functioning. Acidic urine increases the risk of crystalluria. The presence of crystals would indicate the formation of crystalluria.

4. e. SMZ-TMP should be infused slowly over 60 to 90 minutes. It is never given rapidly, as a bolus, or as an IM injection. All lines should be flushed to remove residual drug. Once reconstituted in preparation for IV infusion, the drug should not be refrigerated.

5. c. The patient should not consume any alcohol while taking SMZ-TMP because alcohol might cause a disulfiram-like reaction. The patient would experience nausea, vomiting, and intense abdominal pain.

CASE STUDY
An allergic reaction has occurred. Pruritus (itching) and maculopapular rashes (reddened areas with some raised spots) are types of cutaneous allergic reactions to SMZ-TMP.

CRITICAL THINKING CHALLENGE
You failed to consider that an allergy to hydrochlorothiazide may produce cross-allergies to SMZ-TMP. This is because hydrochlorothiazide, like all thiazides, has a chemical structure that is similar to that of sulfa. This similarity in chemical structure allows for cross-allergies.

Chapter 43

KEY TERMS
TRUE OR FALSE

1. True
2. False, *M. tuberculosis*
3. False, Ghon complex
4. False, chemoprophylaxis
5. True
6. False, *M. avium*
7. False, leprosy
8. False, *Mycobacterium avium* complex
9. False, *M. leprae*

CORE DRUG KNOWLEDGE: JUST THE FACTS
MULTIPLE CHOICE

1. c. INH is the drug of choice for TB.

2. b. INH works by disrupting the synthesis of the bacterial cell wall.

3. d. Because of INH's ability to induce hepatitis, its use is limited in patients older than 35 years. To decrease the incidence of peripheral neuritis, INH is given with vitamin B_6.

4. c. Isoniazid interacts with a variety of drugs, including antiseizure drugs, aluminum-based antacids, benzodiazepines, disulfiram, enflurane, ketoconazole, meperidine, oral anticoagulants, and rifampin.

5. b. Pyridoxine (B_6) does not have any effect on TB; it only decreases the incidence of peripheral neuropathy.

6. a. Patients receiving ethambutol should have baseline and periodic eye exams because of the drug's ability to induce optic neuritis.

7. c. Ethambutol may also cause hyperuricemia; therefore, patients with a history of gout should be closely monitored for exacerbations.

8. c. Rifampin works by inhibiting bacterial and mycobacterial RNA synthesis.

9. b. Rifampin may cause adverse effects similar to those of INH, especially hepatic injury.

10. c. Rifampin is a potent inducer of the cytochrome P-450 hepatic enzyme system and its subsets, so it has many potentially serious drug–drug interactions.

11. c. Spectinomycin is an aminoglycoside antibiotic that is not efficacious in the treatment of leprosy.

12. a. Dapsone can induce serious adverse effects, including hemolytic anemia, aplastic anemia, agranulocytosis,

methemoglobinemia, acute tubular necrosis, and hepatotoxicity.

CORE PATIENT VARIABLES: PATIENTS, PLEASE
MULTIPLE CHOICE
1. c. INH is the drug used for TB exposure prophylaxis. This drug requires monitoring liver function tests, especially in patients over the age of 35.
2. a. These are all signs of hepatitis.
3. b. Rifampin has the ability to turn all body fluids, including tears, red.
4. d. Rifampin is a potent inducer of the cytochrome P-450 hepatic enzyme system and its subsets. It interacts with many of the drugs used for these disorders.
5. a. Both INH and rifampin have the ability to induce hepatotoxicity.
6. b. Patients receiving ethambutol should have baseline and periodic eye exams because of the drug's ability to induce optic neuritis.
7. c. You should administer IV rifampin by slow infusion over 3 hours.

NURSING MANAGEMENT: EVERY GOOD NURSE SHOULD …
MULTIPLE CHOICE
1. d. Triple-drug therapy is the standard for TB treatment, because the TB bacillus can easily become resistant to one drug. Thus, using multiple drugs helps to eradicate the disease and prevent relapse with strains of bacteria that are resistant to common antitubercular drugs. Information about the reason behind therapy and the importance of multidrug therapy should help to gain patient acceptance toward therapy. Because of the concerns about multidrug-resistant TB, you should never administer the drugs sporadically or give only one of the ordered drugs. You cannot force the patient to take ordered drug therapy because patients have the right to refuse therapy.
2. d. Avocados and chocolate are high in tyramine and may cause hypertension. Tuna fish is high in histamine and may cause headache, palpitations, hypotension, or other reactions.
3. a. AST and ALT are liver enzymes and indicate liver functioning. Because hepatitis and other liver problems frequently are adverse effects of INH, these enzymes should be monitored closely. Creatinine clearance and BUN indicate renal function and are not a major concern with INH. Vital capacity is not altered by INH.
4. c. Giving patients all of their pills and watching them swallow them is an important aspect of direct observational therapy short course (DOTS). This confirms that patients are taking all of their medicine, eliminates TB in the patient, and helps prevent multidrug-resistant TB from developing in the patient because all of the medicines are not taken for the full course of treatment. Although the patient needs encouragement to adhere with therapy, this is not the most effective way to achieve adherence. All drugs need to be taken in multidrug therapy, not just one, to help prevent resistance. Although most patients may be a reliable source as to whether they have taken their medication, some will not be reliable.

CASE STUDY
1. Because of his age, his drinking, and prescribed drug therapy, he is at increased risk of liver damage and hepatitis.
2. This patient will need to be seen regularly and checked for elevated liver enzymes or symptoms of liver disease. He should be encouraged to stop drinking alcohol. Referral to

Alcoholics Anonymous might be appropriate. Visits to him at the shelter where he often stays might be appropriate to assess him for liver problems if he doesn't come to the clinic daily.

CRITICAL THINKING CHALLENGE
1. Disulfiram and isoniazid have a drug interaction that induces excess dopaminergic activity. Impulsivity, affective instability, and anxiety are characteristics of excessive dopaminergic activity. Individuals with a tendency toward impulsivity tend to externalize their problems and overreact to environmental events. Individuals with affective instability are characterized by rapidly occurring shifts in affect, changing from anger to disappointment to excitement in a matter of hours or minutes. They are also sensitive to shifts in the environment, such as separation or frustration. Individuals with high anxiety have a greater readiness to anticipate punishment or aversive consequences of their behavior and often show concomitant autonomic arousal associated with their fearfulness.
2. The physician needs to be notified at once of these changes.

Chapter 44
PHYSIOLOGY AND PATHOPHYSIOLOGY: THE BODY HUMAN
ESSAY
1. Budding from the parent cell into identical daughter cells
2. Long, hollow, branching filaments of a mold
3. Cutaneous level of the body
4. A dermatophyte cannot grow at the body's core temperature. A systemic mycosis is a serious, deep-tissue infection by a fungus capable of growth at the body's core temperature.

KEY TERMS
1. c
2. e
3. b
4. a
5. d

CORE DRUG KNOWLEDGE: JUST THE FACTS
1. c. Amphotericin B is an antifungal agent.
2. a. Altering the fungal cell membrane forms pores or channels and results in increased cell permeability, cell leakage, and death.
3. d. Amphotericin B affects many body systems, so monitoring these laboratory results is mandatory.
4. c. Erythropoietin is necessary for the production of red blood cells. The occurrence of decreased red cells results in anemia.
5. b. Nystatin is not used for systemic infections because of the risk for toxicity.
6. d. Flucytosine can induce hematotoxicity, nephrotoxicity, and hepatotoxicity, so it should be used cautiously in patients receiving other drugs that may induce these effects.
7. a. Fluconazole is used for primary fungal prophylaxis in immunocompromised patients with a CD4+ T-cell count of less than 200.
8. b. The most common adverse effects of fluconazole are diarrhea, nausea, vomiting, abdominal pain, headache, and dizziness.

CORE PATIENT VARIABLES: PATIENTS, PLEASE
1. a. Amphotericin B may induce hypokalemia, hypomagnesemia, hypochloremia, and hypocalcemia.
2. c. Nephrotoxicity occurs in more than 80% of patients receiving IV amphotericin B.

3. b. Patients should understand the potential for an infusion reaction so they do not believe they are experiencing an unforeseen event.
4. c. Griseofulvin decreases the effectiveness of birth control pills.
5. b. Fluconazole should be administered with an infusion pump at a rate not to exceed 200 mg/hour.
6. b. Diflucan may increase the hypoglycemic effects of sulfonylureas, so it is prudent to monitor blood glucose.

NURSING MANAGEMENT: EVERY GOOD NURSE SHOULD …

1. d. Amphotericin may cause infusion reactions. The vital signs should be monitored first to serve as a baseline. A test dose should be given to assess for an infusion reaction. Antipyretics, such as ibuprofen or acetaminophen, are helpful in preventing or minimizing the infusion reaction. Other drugs that might be given are corticosteroids, antihistamines, meperidine, and possibly dantrolene.
2. e. This patient is demonstrating signs of infusion reaction. The infusion should be stopped and the physician notified. Increasing the infusion rate would worsen the reaction. Amphotericin B should be administered through a large vein, preferably a central vein because of its irritant properties. Slowing the infusion has not been demonstrated to decrease the infusion reaction.
3. b. Diarrhea is common but not a serious adverse effect of fluconazole. The fluconazole therapy should not be discontinued because the patient needs this drug to prevent potentially fatal infections. The diarrhea is not a sign of infection; no culture is needed.
4. c. Swishing the suspension in the mouth will provide topical application of the antifungal to the affected area. The suspension should be shaken, but it should not be applied to the hip wound, mixed with water, or administered to the back of the throat.
5. c, d, f. Posaconazole is an oral solution. It is important to shake the medication before pouring it into the spoon that is supplied with the medication. It should not be taken on an empty stomach.

CASE STUDY

1. The medications digoxin and hydrochlorothiazide, a thiazide diuretic, are both risk factors. The amphotericin B may induce hypokalemia, which increases the risk of digitalis toxicity. The thiazide diuretic also increases potassium loss, so the effect of hypokalemia may be intensified. Again, this places the patient at increased risk of digoxin toxicity and for the adverse effects associated with hypokalemia (such as possibly fatal arrhythmias).
2. You should check the potassium level before and then throughout the therapy. If the patient is hypokalemic before starting therapy, a potassium supplement should be administered. Hydrate as much as possible, but do not push excessive fluids because this may precipitate CHF. Monitor for signs of fluid overload.

CRITICAL THINKING CHALLENGE

1. The oral corticosteroid, prednisone, made this patient immunocompromised. Without the body's normal ability to ward off infection or keep it as a minor infection that could be eradicated, the serious infection of *Aspergillus* was able to develop.
2. Yes, you should give the amphotericin B. Although amphotericin B is not recommended to be given with digoxin or thiazide diuretics, amphotericin B appears to be the only drug of choice to treat an infection that could be fatal. This

is the proverbial "rock and a hard place." Because the risk of not receiving the drug could be death, the drug should be given. Monitor very carefully. Nephrotoxicity can easily send this patient into acute CHF. The dose may need to be decreased from a standard dose because of the patient's other pathologies. It is possible the other drugs could be withdrawn or their dosage decreased, but this might also precipitate acute CHF.

Chapter 45

KEY TERMS

1. c
2. d
3. e
4. a
5. b

PHYSIOLOGY AND PATHOPHYSIOLOGY: THE BODY HUMAN
ESSAY

1. Adsorption, penetration, uncoating, replication and transcription, assembly and release
2. Hepatitis A: oral–fecal transmission
   Hepatitis B: blood or body fluids. Infection may occur through having sex with an infected person, through needlesticks or sharps exposures, from an infected mother to the neonate during birth, or by sharing drugs or needles.
   Hepatitis C: the same as HBV
3. Herpes simplex is transmitted by direct contact. Herpes zoster is an acute unilateral and segmental inflammation of the dorsal root ganglia caused by infection with the herpesvirus varicella zoster, which also causes chickenpox.

CORE DRUG KNOWLEDGE: JUST THE FACTS
MULTIPLE CHOICE

1. b. Human immunodeficiency virus (HIV) requires the use of an antiretroviral drug.
2. c. Viruses do not have a cell wall; acyclovir terminates DNA synthesis after the drug undergoes phosphorylation.
3. d. Intravenous acyclovir may crystallize in the nephrons on the kidney tubules.
4. c. Antiviral agents effective against CMV include cidoforvir, ganciclovir, valganciclovir, and foscarnet.
5. d. Amantadine potentiates central nervous system dopaminergic responses.
6. d. Drugs for influenza include amantadine, rimantadine, oseltamivir, and zanamivir.
7. a. Interferon alfa-2b (Intron-A) is the only FDA-approved drug for treating hepatitis B virus, hepatitis B infection, hepatitis C virus, and hepatitis C infection.
8. d. These drugs are used in children at risk for respiratory syncytial virus.

CORE PATIENT VARIABLES: PATIENTS, PLEASE
MULTIPLE CHOICE

1. a. Many patients with diabetes also have renal dysfunction. Acyclovir can crystallize in the kidneys and cause nephrotoxicity.
2. d. Acyclovir should be given slowly. The patient should be well hydrated to avoid crystallization in the kidneys.
3. a. Oseltamivir may be used in healthy patients 50 to 64 years of age on a case-by-case basis.
4. c. Antibiotics are ineffective against a virus, and prescription drugs should be used only for the person for whom they are prescribed.
5. b. Zanamivir is an inhaled drug.

NURSING MANAGEMENT: EVERY GOOD NURSE SHOULD …

MULTIPLE CHOICE

1. c. This patient may have a secondary bacterial infection in addition to the primary viral infection. He needs to be seen to be properly assessed and treated. Taking aspirin may mask the symptoms and allow the infection to become worse. Soaking in a bathtub may spread the infection to other areas, such as areas with broken skin or mucous membranes of the rectum. Stopping the acyclovir will cause the viral infection to become worse and could possibly lead to resistance of the virus to the acyclovir.

2. a, b, c. Granulocytopenia, neutropenia, and thrombocytopenia have all occurred during ganciclovir therapy. Like acyclovir, ganciclovir is potentially nephrotoxic. Elevated liver enzymes may occur. Serial laboratory tests required during therapy include complete blood count (CBC), platelet counts, and renal and liver function tests.

3. a. If treatment with Epivir-HBV is prescribed for chronic HBV for a patient with unrecognized or untreated HIV infection, rapid emergence of HIV resistance is likely because of the subtherapeutic dose and inappropriate monotherapy.

4. b. Telbivudine is used cautiously in patients with pre-exisiting myopathy or those taking drugs that might cause myopathy because of the potential increased risk for myopathy.

CASE STUDY

1. Yes, you have a legal responsibility to care for this patient, despite the fact that he has a potentially transmissible disease. Refusing to care for your assignment is considered abandonment.

2. There are vaccines to protect you against hepatitis A and hepatitis B, but there is no vaccine for hepatitis C.

3. Hepatitis C is transmitted via blood or body fluids. You are responsible to follow universal precautions to avoid contact with the patient's blood during dialysis. Be sure that you are wearing gloves and protective eye gear when you access and discontinue the dialysis site. Do not recap the needle and drop it directly into a sharps container. Wash your hands thoroughly after removing your gloves.

CRITICAL THINKING CHALLENGE

Use therapeutic communication at all times. Speak simply and clearly and avoid statements that could be interpreted as judgmental. Encourage the patient to be open and honest with his fiancée, but also assure him that his confidentiality will be maintained.

Prior to doing your patient education, assess the following:

1. Question the patient about his knowledge of genital herpes and its treatment.

2. Obtain a medication history. Valacyclovir interacts with valproic acid, hydantoins, theophyllines, and probenecid. Assess for use of drugs that are known to be nephrotoxic.

3. Ask the patient about his lifestyle, especially the type of activities that he enjoys.

Patient education should include:

1. Correct any inaccurate knowledge about genital herpes.

2. Explain that valacyclovir decreases the frequency and intensity of outbreaks but does not "cure" the infection.

3. Review how genital herpes is transmitted. Explain the prodromal symptoms and advise the patient to refrain from sexual activity when he feels the prodromal symptoms or when active lesions are present.

4. Emphasize that transmission may still occur even when symptoms are absent and encourage him to use a condom.

5. Explain the importance of having his fiancée examined for any sign of infection. This is especially important if they plan to have children in the near future.

6. Discuss the activities that he enjoys. Explain the importance of maintaining hydration to decrease the potential for crystalluria. Encourage him to keep a water bottle handy when engaging in strenuous activities.

7. Because autoinoculation is possible with herpetic lesions, teach the patient and his fiancée to wash their hands after contact with any active lesions

8. Instruct the patient to contact the prescriber if the lesions turn red, become hot, or exude purulent material, all of which are indications of a secondary bacterial infection.

Chapter 46

KEY TERMS

TRUE OR FALSE

1. True
2. False, enzyme immunoassay (EIA) and enzyme-linked immunosorbent assay (ELISA)
3. False, progression of the disease
4. False, CD4 cells
5. True
6. False, HIV RNA
7. False, fusion
8. False, Western blot
9. False, protease inhibitors
10. False, HAART (highly active antiretroviral therapy)
11. True

PHYSIOLOGY AND PATHOPHYSIOLOGY: THE BODY HUMAN

ESSAY

1. Avoid negative effects of quality of life and drug-related toxicities, more time to understand treatment demands, preserve future treatment options, delay in development of drug resistance, decreased total time on medication with decreased risk of treatment fatigue, more time for the development of more potent, less toxic, and better studied combinations of drugs

2. Risk for irreversible immune system compromise, possible greater difficulty in viral suppression, and possible increased risk for HIV transmission

3. After multiple clinical trials, the outcome of treatment has been proven to be improved by triple- or quadruple-drug therapy.

4. In addition to the EIA or WB tests, several other laboratory tests are available. They include rapid HIV testing; oral HIV testing; radioimmunoprecipitation assay (RIPA); indirect fluorescent antibody assay (IFA); and polymerase chain reaction (PCR).

CORE DRUG KNOWLEDGE: JUST THE FACTS

MULTIPLE CHOICE

1. d. Although both drug classes work on reverse transcriptase, they have two distinct mechanisms of action.

2. a. Zidovudine reduces maternal–infant transmission of HIV by approximately 62%.

3. d. Most patients taking zidovudine experience anemia.

4. c. A high-calorie, high-fat meal can substantially increase the bioavailability of saquinavir.

5. c. Drug–drug interactions with saquinavir can increase or decrease the serum concentration of saquinavir or can increase or decrease the serum concentration of the interacting drug.

6. d. Nevirapine is commonly associated with inducing a rash. Stevens-Johnson syndrome and toxic epidermal necrosis are more serious integumentary complications that may occur with nevirapine use.

7. d. It is important to monitor the function of the immune system and the progression of the disease, as well as monitor for adverse effects that may occur with HAART therapy.

8. b. Sulfamethoxazole-trimethoprim is the drug of choice, as long as the patient does not have a sensitivity to sulfa and can tolerate the adverse effects that may occur.

9. b. The macrolide antibiotics are very effective against MAC.

10. b. At this time, enfuvirtide is used as salvage therapy for those who have experienced no response with other types of antiretroviral drugs or who have become resistant to other classes of drugs.

11. c. Enfuvirtide comes as a powder and must be reconstituted by the patient, then delivered by subcutaneous injection.

12. c. Low dose ritonavir is given frequently with other antiretroviral drugs to boost the bioavailability of the drug. In this question, ritonavir and darunavir are both protease inhibitors; however, ritonavir is also given to boost the bioavailability of drugs in other classes as well.

MATCHING

1. a, c, d, e, f, h, k
2. f
3. c, h
4. k
5. b, c, h, f
6. a, f
7. f
8. g
9. k
10. g, j
11. d, e, f

CORE PATIENT VARIABLES: PATIENTS, PLEASE

MULTIPLE CHOICE

1. b. Ganciclovir and zidovudine can independently cause significant hematologic toxicity. The patient has a higher risk when these drugs are given as combination therapy.

2. a. Fatty foods can decrease the absorption of zidovudine.

3. d. While all of these lab tests will be evaluated, hepatic enzymes are most important because all three of these drugs have the potential to cause hepatotoxicity.

4. d. When these two drugs are given together, the serum concentration of rifampin may increase, resulting in an increased risk for adverse effects, and the serum concentration of saquinavir may decrease, causing decreased efficacy of the drug.

5. b. Although the suspension of ritonavir is kept at room temperature, the capsules should be refrigerated.

6. d. Prophylaxis for opportunistic diseases begins when the T-cell count is less than 200.

7. c. Protease inhibitors frequently cause lipodystrophy. It would also be prudent to assess lipid, triglyceride, and cholesterol levels.

8. d. All of these instructions are of equal importance.

9. a. Patients with an anxiety disorder frequently experience difficulty sleeping and may be taking sleeping medication such as triazolam (Halcion). There is a potentially fatal interaction between darunavir and triazolam and midazolam (another type of benzodiazepine).

NURSING MANAGEMENT: EVERY GOOD NURSE SHOULD …

MULTIPLE CHOICE

1. c. High fat intake impairs absorption. Zidovudine should be given 1 hour before meals. The daily dose should be divided into two or three doses.

2. a. Taking on a full stomach will help to decrease the GI effects and promote absorption, especially if there is fat in the meal and the meal is high calorie.

3. b. These are signs of a hypersensitivity to abacavir. Abacavir should be discontinued immediately and never restarted, because more severe symptoms can occur within hours after restarting abacavir and may include life-threatening hypotension and death.

4. d. Oral candidiasis increases the risk for PCP pneumonia, so the patient should be treated prophylactically with sulfamethoxazole-trimethoprim (Bactrim). Isoniazid and rifampin are used to treat TB. Amphotericin B is used to treat serious systemic fungal infections.

5. d. Zidovudine should be taken on an empty stomach; saquinavir should be taken on a full stomach. GI upset can occur from both of these drugs. The patient may accommodate to these adverse effects with time but not always. The HIV virus may develop resistance to the drugs if the drugs are not taken regularly as prescribed. When drug resistance develops, the pharmacotherapy for HIV is very limited.

6. a, b, c, d. Taking drug therapy at the time of some other routine activity will help the patient to remember to take the drug, which will allow the patient to be more adherent with therapy. Because many drugs will need to be taken daily to treat HIV and AIDS and most of the drugs have specific requirements regarding when or how they should be taken, therapy is complex. Patients need assistance to see how to work the drug therapy into their daily schedules to be adherent. Because the information regarding drug therapy will be quite involved, both oral and written instructions need to be provided to the patient. Some drugs need to be taken on an empty stomach, some with food, some while avoiding fatty foods, and some with a high-fat meal, so it may be confusing to the patient as to exactly what he or she can or cannot eat.

7. a, b, d. Before being reconstituted, enfuvirtide is stable at room temperature, but it must be refrigerated after reconstitution. Different sized syringes are packaged with the drug to reconstitute and administer the drug safely and accurately. The drug is administered subcutaneously, not intramuscularly.

8. d. While all of these assessments are important in the hospitalized patient, level of consciousness is most important for this patient. Tipranavir, in combination with ritonavir, may cause fatal or non-fatal intracranial hemorrhage.

CASE STUDY

This patient may need to be taught the importance of the drug therapy for treating her infection and preventing worsening of her disease or relapses of PCP. She should know what each drug is for, why it is prescribed, and exactly when and how to take it. This is especially true of the SMZ-TMP, which will be an additional drug therapy for her at home. It is also important for her to understand what drug resistance is and how the virus becomes drug resistant with inconsistent dosing.

In addition, this patient needs to be encouraged to live a healthier lifestyle to maintain her health. She should be encouraged to refrain from substance abuse. Counseling or support groups, if available, may be helpful. She may have used substances as a coping mechanism and now will need to learn other coping skills. If she does continue with drug abuse, she should be taught to use clean needles and never share her needles with anyone else to prevent spread of infection. She also needs to receive information regarding having her partner use a condom to prevent spread of disease.

CRITICAL THINKING CHALLENGE

1. Why are you refusing to take your medications? How do the medications make you feel? What is the hardest part about taking these medications for you? What is the easiest part about taking these medications for you? Who are you close to? Who helps you cope?
2. The regimen of drug therapy for HIV is demanding and difficult for every patient, no matter his/her background or lifestyle. Drug therapy may cause people to feel sick a good bit of the day. The intensity of the regimen and the severity of the illness may make them feel overwhelmed. It is important to talk *with* this patient, not just *to* her, to understand what her concerns are, so that together you can address these concerns. The other nurse's comments that this patient is expected to be noncompliant because of her history of IV drug abuse devalue this patient as a person and an individual. It is not a therapeutic response of the nurse.

Taking the time to ask a few more questions and to be empathic creates a therapeutic nurse–patient relationship. When this patient believes her feelings are valued by the nurse, she may be more likely to accept the teaching the nurse offers.

You might learn from these questions that this patient doesn't want to take the drugs because they make her nauseous all the time or cause diarrhea. A prescription for an antiemetic or antidiarrheal might help her to adhere to her drug therapy. Maybe she tells you that she can't remember to take the pills at different times. A drug time schedule could be made up by the nurse and the patient together to help her remember exactly what to take when, based on her normal eating schedule and other daily routines. Maybe she doesn't want to take any medication during the middle of the day because she doesn't want her friends or family to know she has HIV.

Based on what you learn, your teaching plan can be tailored to be specific for this patient and her needs. Thus, the patient sees that what you are offering is helpful for her, as opposed to being "your agenda." Patient education is most effective when it begins by addressing what the patient wants to know, as opposed to what you believe the patient needs to know.

Chapter 47

KEY TERMS

CROSSWORD PUZZLE

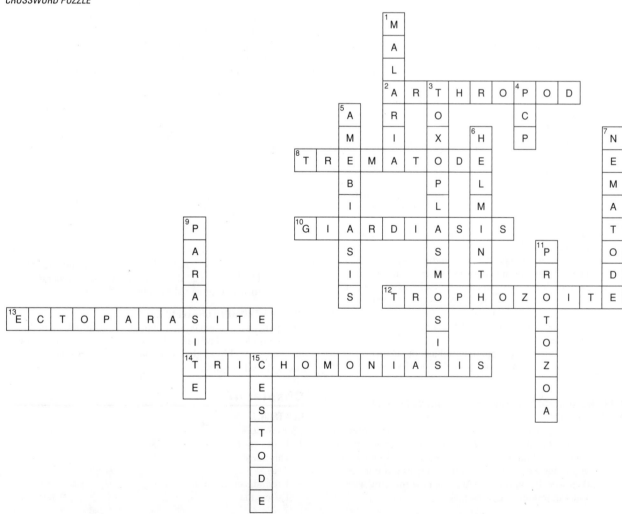

CORE DRUG KNOWLEDGE: JUST THE FACTS

MULTIPLE CHOICE

1. c. Although not a first-line drug, chloroquine may be used for RA.
2. c. Potential adverse hematologic effects include agranulocytosis, aplastic anemia, pancytopenia, neutropenia, and thrombocytopenia.
3. d. Chloroquine may cause corneal opacities.
4. d. PCP does not respond to metronidazole.
5. a. Metronidazole in combination with alcohol may induce a disulfiram-like reaction that includes nausea, vomiting, and abdominal pain.
6. b. Pentamidine is given for both prophylaxis and treatment of PCP. Cotrimoxazole is a sulfa-based drug. Atovaquone is used for the treatment, but not for prophylaxis.
7. d. Pentamidine is not available as an oral drug.
8. d. When pentamidine is mixed with saline solution, a precipitate will form.
9. c. Mebendazole is an oral medication.
10. d. Both flukes and tapeworms respond to niclosamide therapy.
11. c. The patient should wash and towel-dry the hair before using permethrin.
12. c. A second dose is advisable 24 hours after the first application.

CORE PATIENT VARIABLES: PATIENTS, PLEASE

MULTIPLE CHOICE

1. b. Chloroquine may induce the development of corneal opacities.
2. d. To ensure that malaria does not occur, the medication should be continued for an additional 4 weeks.
3. d. These are all important instructions for the patient receiving chloroquine. Chloroquine is extremely toxic to young children. It is taken on a weekly, not daily basis. One of the adverse effects associated with chloroquine is orthostatic hypotension.
4. a. The most common adverse effects of metronidazole are nausea and vomiting, dry mouth (xerostomia), altered sense of taste (dysgeusia), anorexia, and abdominal pain.
5. c. Metronidazole inhibits the metabolism of Coumadin, resulting in enhanced effects of Coumadin that could induce bleeding.
6. d. Discolored urine is an expected, harmless adverse effect to metronidazole.
7. a. Intravenous pentamidine may induce hypotension.
8. c. These are symptoms of anemia. Carbamazepine and pentamidine may independently increase the risk for anemia, and when these drugs are given concurrently, the patient has a higher risk for anemia.
9. b. Metronidazole is contraindicated during the first trimester of pregnancy.
10. b. To be sure that contamination has not occurred, the entire family should be treated at the same time.

NURSING MANAGEMENT: EVERY GOOD NURSE SHOULD ...

MULTIPLE CHOICE

1. a. Beginning drug therapy 2 weeks before travel allows the drug to become effective before the risk of exposure. Use of the drug should be continued until 4 weeks after the patient has left the malarial area. The drug should be taken weekly, on the same day. Taking the drug with food will minimize GI upset.

2. b. Over-the-counter liquid cold medications often contain alcohol. Metronidazole has a disulfiram-like reaction when taken with alcohol. Milk, rice, and antipyretics have no interaction with metronidazole.
3. d. If she has a current sexual partner, that person also needs to be treated with metronidazole. He likely also has the infection, and this will prevent reinfection of this patient after the metronidazole treatment. The drug is not recommended during the first trimester of pregnancy because the risk is unknown. Anticoagulants interact with metronidazole, producing greater anticoagulant effects.
4. b. Intravenous metronidazole contains 28 mEq of sodium per gram of metronidazole, which may promote water retention and exacerbate pre-existing chronic heart failure (CHF) or peripheral edema.
5. e. Dilute pentamidine in 5% dextrose and water. Saline solutions will form a precipitate with the pentamidine. Blood pressure, not temperature, should be monitored throughout the infusion. IM injections should not be used because of the risk of thrombocytopenia from pentamidine.
6. b. To avoid serious, life-threatening adverse effects, leucovorin MUST be given concurrently with trimetrexate and continue for 3 days after the completion of trimetrexate therapy. It is important to schedule the serial CBC test and to perform a urine dip for blood, but those actions are done *during* drug therapy to monitor for possible adverse effects. While assessment of the patient's lung sounds is an appropriate nursing action, it will not alter whether or not the drug is administered.
7. a. Nitazoxanide contains 1.48 grams of sucrose per 5 mL. Patients with diabetes should increase the frequency of blood glucose monitoring while taking this medication.
8. d. Chewing the tablets will best promote effectiveness. Taking the tablets with something fatty, such as milk, cheese, or ice cream, also will promote effectiveness. Other family members are likely to be infected and should be treated at the same time to prevent reinfection.

CASE STUDY

1. The nurse should monitor the blood pressure carefully while administering the drug. The other vital signs should also be monitored. A set of vital signs should have been taken just before the infusion to provide a baseline comparison.
2. The patient's respiratory status should be assessed throughout therapy for evidence of bronchospasm. The patient should be kept in bed during the transfusion. Emergency resuscitation equipment should be handy.

CRITICAL THINKING CHALLENGE

This patient may be having a hypoglycemic attack related to the pentamidine. The nurse should check the patient's blood glucose with a blood glucose monitor. The nurse should also check the vital signs.

Chapter 48

KEY TERMS

TRUE OR FALSE

1. False, antitussives
2. False, histamine
3. True
4. False, decongestants
5. False, cilia

6. False, expectorants
7. False, common cold
8. False, pharyngitis
9. False, sinus
10. True
11. True
12. False, laryngitis
13. True

PHYSIOLOGY AND PATHOPHYSIOLOGY: THE BODY HUMAN
ESSAY
1. Nose, mouth, pharynx, larynx, trachea, and bronchial tree
2. Produce mucus and entrap dust, foreign substances, or microorganisms
3. Particles are projected toward the throat by cilia.
4. Cough, sneeze

CORE DRUG KNOWLEDGE: JUST THE FACTS
MULTIPLE CHOICE
1. a. Dextromethorphan is chemically related to opiate agonists so they have a similar mechanism for suppressing cough.
2. c. Dextromethorphan is rarely problematic, but may cause some GI or CNS effects.
3. b. The decongestants vasoconstrict engorged vessels in the nares.
4. a. Pseudoephedrine is used to treat the common cold, allergic rhinitis, and sinusitis.
5. c. Because of its sympathomimetic effects, tachycardia may occur.
6. a. Because oxymetazoline (Afrin) is a topical drug, the effects are local and the potential for adverse effects decreases.
7. d. The "one" generic suffix gives the clue that this is the steroid drug.
8. b. Antihistamines are the drugs of choice for allergic symptoms because they block the release of histamine, which causes many of the symptoms.
9. b. Fexofenadine has less of an anticholinergic effect than does diphenhydramine because it binds to lung receptors substantially more than it binds to cerebellar receptors, resulting in a reduced sedative potential.
10. a. Guaifenesin enhances the output of respiratory tract fluids by reducing the adhesiveness and surface tension of the fluids, thus allowing the patient to cough up the less viscous secretions.
11. a. Although there are no known drug–drug interactions, patients taking guaifenesin should be advised to refrain from alcohol use because both agents are CNS depressants and may increase sedation when taken together.
12. c. Cromolyn sodium provides a protective layer that shields mast cells lining the nasal passage and prevents them from breaking down and releasing histamine.

CORE PATIENT VARIABLES: PATIENTS, PLEASE
MULTIPLE CHOICE
1. d. These symptoms could be associated with serotonin syndrome.
2. d. Because this drug is an opiate, it depresses the CNS and causes sedation.
3. c. This drug is a sympathomimetic and may increase the blood pressure.
4. d. For maximum results, drug therapy should be coupled with nonpharmacologic interventions.
5. a. Fexofenadine crosses into breast milk and may sedate the baby.

6. a. This is the only one of these drugs approved for a 5-year-old child.
7. c. Regardless of the etiology of this cough, after 4 weeks the patient should be evaluated.
8. a. It is important to assess how sedated the patient feels before doing anything that requires mental alertness.
9. b. Many OTC drugs contain other sympathomimetic drugs that will increase the risk for adverse events.
10. d. Antihistamines may cause dry mouth.

NURSING MANAGEMENT: EVERY GOOD NURSE SHOULD …
MULTIPLE CHOICE
1. d. Because dextromethorphan may cause drowsiness, driving and operating machinery that requires alertness should be avoided until it is known if drowsiness will occur. Alcohol and other CNS depressants may increase sedative effects and should be avoided. It is not recommended for use in children and should be kept out of their reach to prevent accidental overdosage or poisoning.
2. b. Drinking plenty of fluids will keep mucous membranes moist. Dietary fiber has no effect on pseudoephedrine. Hot, steamy showers will have a similar effect as using a humidifier and will also keep mucous membranes moist, which would be beneficial. To minimize adverse effects, do not take for more than 4 days; 14 days is too long.
3. c. GI distress is a common adverse effect and is minimized if the drug is taken with food. There is no indication the patient should stop taking the drug. Decreasing the dose will prevent full therapeutic effect from being achieved and may not relieve GI upset. The use of other antihistamines should be avoided during therapy with this drug.
4. d. Both Benylin (dextromethorphan) and Robitussin (guaifenesin) are not to be used if the patient has chronic asthma or emphysema, or if the cough is from smoking. Dextromethorphan interacts with several other drugs, whereas guaifenesin does not. This information may indicate which preparation would be preferred for this patient.
5. b. In excessive doses, dextromethorphan may induce symptoms similar to phencyclidine (PCP). Dextromethorphan abuse has become a serious problem with adolescents.

CASE STUDY
Lifestyle, diet, and habits: Do you drive? Do you do other skills/activities that require concentration? Environment: Do you have stairs in your house? Do you have railings on your stairways? Do you have loose rugs in the halls?

Because of this patient's age, he is at increased risk of drowsiness from fexofenadine. If he drives or does other activities that require concentration and alertness, such as using power tools and saws or using a riding lawn mower on hills, he should limit these activities until he knows how he will respond to the fexofenadine. If he does become drowsy, he may be at increased risk of falling. Stairs without railings and scatter rugs increase his risk of a fall.

CRITICAL THINKING CHALLENGE
1. The patient has likely taken another antihistamine, such as diphenhydramine (Benadryl). The patient is likely experiencing drowsiness as an adverse effect of drug therapy.
2. Taking two antihistamines together has likely intensified the CNS depression, causing drowsiness. Diphenhydramine is readily available over the counter and is commonly used for itching. As a first-generation antihistamine, diphenhydramine causes considerable sedation. Because this patient is an older adult, he is more sensitive to this adverse effect.

Chapter 49

KEY TERMS

MATCHING
1. c
2. e
3. i
4. f
5. d
6. h
7. a
8. g
9. b
10. j

PHYSIOLOGY AND PATHOPHYSIOLOGY: THE BODY HUMAN
ESSAY
1. Paired lungs, bronchi, alveoli, blood vessels
2. No. The act of breathing in and out is actually ventilation. The passage of gas across the alveolar membrane is respiration.
3. The vagus nerve stimulates diaphragm contraction and inspiration. It also induces bronchoconstriction.
4. In the respiratory system, stimulation of the sympathetic nervous system results in bronchodilation.

CORE DRUG KNOWLEDGE: JUST THE FACTS
MULTIPLE CHOICE
1. c. Acetylcysteine splits disulfide bonds that are responsible for holding the mucous material together. The result is a decrease in the tenacity and viscosity of the secretions.
2. b. In this disorder, the thick, sticky mucus accumulates in the lungs, plugging the bronchi and making breathing difficult.
3. a. In acetaminophen overdose, it normalizes hepatic glutathione levels and binds with a reactive hepatotoxic metabolite of acetaminophen.
4. a. Albuterol is a beta-2 agonist. In the sympathetic nervous system, stimulation of beta-2 relaxes bronchial smooth muscle, resulting in bronchodilation.
5. d. When given by MDI or nebulizer, the onset is 5 minutes. When given PO, the onset is 30 minutes.
6. b. Albuterol is a beta-2 selective drug; however, some stimulation of beta-1 may also occur, resulting in these symptoms.
7. d. An anticholinergic drug blocks the action of the cholinergic (parasympathetic) nervous system.
8. a. Ipratropium aerosols can produce a paradoxical acute bronchospasm that can be life threatening in some patients. This rare problem, when it occurs, is usually seen with the first inhalation from a newly opened MDI.
9. b. The recommended dose is 2 to 3 puffs 3 to 4 times a day, with a maximum of 12 puffs per day.
10. c. Although the exact mechanism of action is unknown, the resultant effect occurs directly on the smooth muscle of the respiratory tract.
11. a. Keeping the level within this therapeutic range decreases the risk of adverse effects.
12. c. Theophylline interacts with many significant drugs. It can increase the serum concentration of other drugs and other drugs can increase the serum concentration of theophylline.
13. b. Theophylline elimination is increased by a low-carbohydrate, high-protein diet and by charcoal-broiled beef.
14. d. Flunisolide also increases the number of beta receptors.
15. c. Steroids depress the immune system, so serious adverse effects may occur if they are given to patients with an active respiratory infection.
16. a. Because of its route of administration, no important drug–drug interactions occur.
17. d. Cromolyn sodium inhibits the rupture of mast cells.
18. b. Cromolyn sodium is another type of maintenance drug and is ineffective for an acute asthma attack.
19. a. Like inhaled glucocorticosteroids, there are no significant drug–drug interactions.
20. b. Zafirlukast blocks receptors for the leukotrienes bound to the amino acid cysteine. The cysteinyl leukotrienes are potent bronchoconstrictors, approximately 100 to 1,000 times more potent than histamine.
21. c. Although such effects are rare, zafirlukast may elevate hepatic enzymes, cause symptomatic hepatitis, or cause hepatic failure.
22. b. Zafirlukast is not approved for children younger than 5 years.
23. d. Albuterol is a short-acting beta-2 agonist. It is the only drug that has a quick onset to abate acute symptoms.
24. a. This is especially true in patients with a history of neoplasm.

CORE PATIENT VARIABLES: PATIENTS, PLEASE
MULTIPLE CHOICE
1. d. Using a beta-2 agonist drug will open the bronchial tree and allow acetylcysteine to penetrate deeper into the lungs.
2. b. Patients with serious hepatic disease have a higher serum concentration of acetylcysteine than do other patients.
3. b. Overuse of a beta-2 agonist drug results in rebound. The more you use, the more you need.
4. d. Assess the patient's intake of caffeine, including coffee, tea, soda, cocoa, candy, and chocolate. Caffeine has sympathomimetic effects that may increase the risk for adverse effects.
5. c. Maintenance drugs should be taken without regard to symptoms for the drug to reach an adequate level in the bloodstream.
6. d. Ipratropium aerosol inhalation is contraindicated in patients who have soya lecithin hypersensitivity, including patients with a history of peanut oil hypersensitivity or hypersensitivity to related foods and legumes, such as soybeans and peanuts.
7. b. The newest recommendations suggest an inhaled steroid (ICS) for maintenance and the use of oral medications only when the ICS is not sufficient.
8. a. Smoking cigarettes may decrease serum theophylline levels. In fact, some patients who smoke require an increase in theophylline dosage of up to 50%.
9. a. Rinsing the mouth after use will decrease the potential for thrush, as well as decrease the amount of drug swallowed. Although drinking water is always good for patients with asthma, this intervention is not specific to inhaled steroids.
10. c. When using the agent for prophylaxis of asthma, the patient needs to take the medication daily.
11. d. This drug interferes with the release of inflammatory mediators and cytokines released from an antigen–antibody reaction.
12. b. Use of the beta-2 agonist opens the bronchial tree, allowing the other drugs to be distributed farther into the lungs.

NURSING MANAGEMENT: EVERY GOOD NURSE SHOULD …

MULTIPLE CHOICE

1. d. This sticky residue should be removed with water after drug administration. Diluted acetylcysteine should be refrigerated, not left at room temperature. Nebulization of acetylcysteine causes an unpleasant, transient smell. The purpose of the therapy is to loosen thick secretions so that they may be expelled via cough. Therefore, coughing is expected and to be encouraged, not discouraged.

2. d. Breath sounds should clear if therapy is effective; assessment throughout therapy is important. Insomnia, tachycardia, and irritability are signs of adverse effects and should be assessed. Blood will need to be drawn so blood levels of theophylline can be measured to determine if therapeutic or toxic levels have been achieved.

3. d. All of the above are true and should be included in patient education.

4. a. Because this patient has a history of lactose intolerance, she may have the same type of problems with the use of cromolyn sodium. She needs to contact the prescriber if she has any of these symptoms of lactose intolerance. Cromolyn sodium is used as prophylaxis, not to treat an acute episode of asthma. Metered-dose inhalers require the patient to exhale, trigger the release of medication, and then inhale. (Irregular menstrual periods pose no additional risk for adverse effects from cromolyn sodium, and no special teaching is required.)

5. c. Iced tea contains caffeine. Caffeine, like theophylline, is a xanthine. Adverse effects from the theophylline are more likely if caffeine is taken also. If the patient drinks several glasses a day, he needs to avoid it, although an occasional glass would be acceptable. Sprite soda does not contain caffeine. Although lemon meringue pie and fettuccine alfredo are high in carbohydrates, eating these occasionally is acceptable, as long as his protein intake is normal. Overall, he should avoid a high-carbohydrate, low-protein diet because this can decrease urinary elimination of theophylline. One particular food item does not alter the overall dietary pattern: Cheerios cereal would have no effect on theophylline.

6. c. A yellowing of the whites of the eyes is a sign of jaundice and may indicate that hepatitis or hepatic failure is developing. These are serious adverse effects of zafirlukast. Absence of wheezing is a positive effect from the drug, indicating that the therapeutic effect is being achieved. A mild headache and an upset stomach can be common adverse effects from zafirlukast, not signs of serious problems.

CASE STUDY

1. This patient is showing symptoms of theophylline toxicity. His blood levels are elevated above the therapeutic range, and he is showing CNS excitation as an adverse effect. Cigarette smoking increases the metabolism of theophylline. Because this patient has ceased smoking after the dose of theophylline has been adjusted, the metabolism of theophylline was no longer stimulated. Thus, the metabolism rate of theophylline slowed, allowing more theophylline to circulate in the bloodstream and be active.

2. Contact the physician or nurse practitioner who had prescribed the theophylline. Inform him or her of the current blood levels, adverse effects, and that this patient was no longer smoking cigarettes. A dose adjustment of theophylline is needed.

CRITICAL THINKING CHALLENGE

1. This patient appears to be having toxicity from the theophylline, most likely because of a drug interaction with the ciprofloxacin.

2. To confirm this assessment, a blood level of theophylline is needed. If the level is in a toxic range, the theophylline needs to be decreased, or the ciprofloxacin needs to be changed to another antibiotic (this is the more probable action).

Chapter 50

KEY TERMS
CROSSWORD PUZZLE

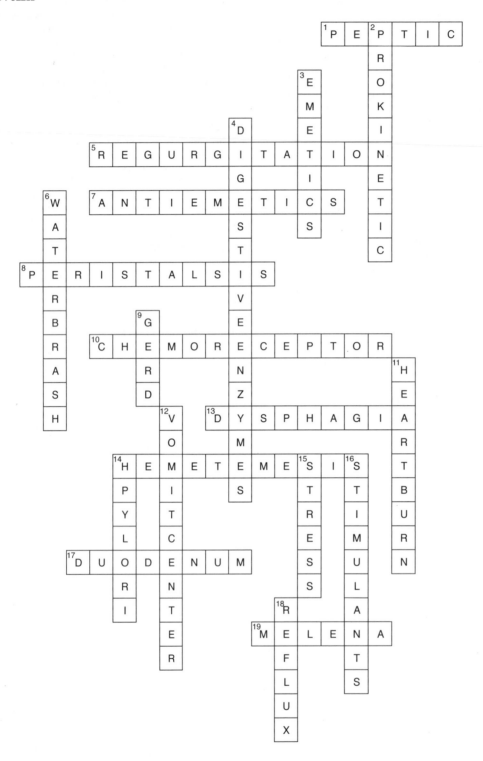

PHYSIOLOGY AND PATHOPHYSIOLOGY: THE BODY HUMAN

ESSAY

1. Mouth, oropharynx, esophagus, stomach, duodenum
2. Mucosa: forms folds and projections that increase the surface area of the intestine

Submucosa: contains blood vessels that provide nutrients and oxygen to the tissues and remove the products of digestion

Muscularis externa: contains muscles that are responsible for peristalsis

Serosa: contains secretory cells that keep the outer surface of the tract moist and lubricated
3. Mucous, chief, and parietal
4. Parasympathetic
5. Amylase: splits starch or glycogen into disaccharide
   Lipase: hydrolyzes fats to fatty acids
   Trypsin, chymotrypsin, and carboxypeptidase: split proteins into amino acids

CORE DRUG KNOWLEDGE: JUST THE FACTS
MULTIPLE CHOICE
1. c. Additionally, it may be used to treat duodenal and gastric ulcers, erosive esophagitis chronic hypersecretory conditions, multiple endocrine adenomas, and systemic mastocytosis.
2. b. Omeprazole suppresses the last phase of gastric acid production by suppressing the H^+/K^+ ATPase enzyme system.
3. a. Omeprazole is generally well tolerated.
4. d. A basically nonabsorbent paste forms and adheres to the ulcer lesions, protecting the lesion from acid, pepsin, and bile salts.
5. c. Pharmacotherapeutics of the agent are similar to those of omeprazole.
6. c. By blocking histamine at the parietal cells, this drug inhibits gastric acid secretion in all phases.
7. d. This drug is generally well tolerated but has the potential for serious adverse effects.
8. a. Ranitidine does not inhibit the cytochrome P-450 system, reducing the potential for drug interactions.
9. a. It is a synthetic form of prostaglandin E and is used to prevent NSAID-induced gastric ulcers in high-risk patients, such as older adults, patients with other debilitating diseases, and patients with a history of gastric ulcers.
10. d. Ranitidine is an H_2 blocker used for the management of GERD and peptic ulcers. Misoprostol is a synthetic form of prostaglandin E and given to prevent ulcer formation. Sucralfate is used to manage duodenal ulcers.
11. b. Antacids that contain aluminum alone can cause constipation, whereas antacids that contain magnesium alone can cause diarrhea.
12. b. The onset of action is rapid. Duration of action varies according to when the drug was taken in relation to meals. If it is taken on an empty stomach, the duration is 20 to 60 minutes; if it is taken following a meal, the duration is 3 hours.
13. c. Sodium bicarbonate is the only antacid that is systemically absorbed.
14. c. It has the cholinergic-like effect on the upper GI tract of stimulating motility but does not stimulate gastric, pancreatic, or gallbladder secretions.
15. c. Metoclopramide interacts with several drugs because it increases gastric motility, thereby altering absorption.
16. b. Note the patient's age and gender because older adults, especially older women, are more likely than others to experience the adverse effect of tardive dyskinesia.
17. a. Ranitidine is an H_2 blocker used for the management of GERD and peptic ulcers. Metoclopramide is a GI stimulant. Sucralfate is used to manage duodenal ulcers.
18. c. Pancrelipase is contraindicated in patients who are hypersensitive to pork protein or enzymes because the drug is derived from pork.
19. d. Orlistat (Xenical) is used to manage obesity by promoting weight loss and weight maintenance.

20. b. GI symptoms are oily spotting, flatus with discharge of stool, fecal urgency, fatty or oily stool, oily evacuation, increased defecation, and fecal incontinence.
21. d. Serotonin receptors, of the 5-HT$_3$ type, are located peripherally on the vagal nerve terminal and centrally in the chemoreceptor trigger zone (CTZ). Ondansetron blocks these receptor sites, thus preventing nausea and vomiting.
22. b. The most common adverse effects are annoying, but a few serious adverse effects are associated with this drug.

CORE PATIENT VARIABLES: PATIENTS, PLEASE
MULTIPLE CHOICE
1. d. Omeprazole is a well-tolerated drug.
2. c. Sucralfate needs to be administered to an acid medium to work effectively.
3. a. Hospitalization, stress, illness, and surgery increase gastric secretions and increase the risk for ulcers.
4. d. These drugs should be taken at least 2 hours apart to allow ranitidine to absorb appropriately.
5. b. This drug is a pregnancy category X because it may cause spontaneous abortion.
6. a. Antacids have a very quick onset of action.
7. b. Magnesium antacids should not be given to patients with chronic renal failure because these drugs increase the risk of magnesium toxicity in such patients.
8. c. Seizures may increase with this drug.
9. c. Give oral doses 30 minutes before each meal to allow for onset of action and give an IM injection near the end of surgery to prevent postoperative nausea and vomiting. Administer IV metoclopramide over at least 15 minutes, 30 minutes before the start of chemotherapy to prevent chemotherapy-induced vomiting.
10. a. See above.
11. d. Extrapyramidal symptoms are manifested primarily as acute dystonic reactions. They occur more commonly in children and young adults during the first 24 to 48 hours of treatment.
12. b. It should not be used by patients with acute pancreatitis or acute exacerbations of chronic pancreatitis.
13. b. Inhaling the powder irritates the nasal mucosa and the respiratory tract, triggering an asthma attack in those susceptible.
14. b. Weight loss decreases the need for oral hypoglycemics. In fact, a sufficient amount of weight loss may allow the patient to control diabetes by diet alone.
15. a. Because orlistat impairs fat absorption, the absorption of fat-soluble vitamins (A, D, E, beta-carotene) will decrease if taken at the same time.
16. d. Patients receiving radiation therapy should be administered this drug orally.

NURSING MANAGEMENT: EVERY GOOD NURSE SHOULD …
MULTIPLE CHOICE
1. a. Shaking the bottle will disperse the drug evenly in the suspension. Administer the drug 1 hour after a meal for maximum effectiveness. Do not mix the drug with water. When aluminum hydroxide and magnesium hydroxide are given as tablets, they should be chewed and then followed with water to promote dissolving.
2. a. It is necessary to stagger oral aluminum hydroxide with magnesium hydroxide and oral ranitidine because the antacid will decrease the absorption of the cimetidine. Giving the ranitidine immediately before a meal and the antacid immediately after the meal will not separate the ingestion of the two drugs enough to prevent alterations

of the absorption of ranitidine. Also, if three meals are taken, this is not the proper dose for either drug.

3. d. Administering metoclopramide 30 minutes before each meal will allow time for the drug to become effective before eating. Depression may be a serious adverse effect of metoclopramide and should be assessed. Drowsiness and fatigue are common adverse effects of metoclopramide, and patients should be warned of this.

4. b. Asthma attacks can occur after sniffing pancrelipase powder. Pancrelipase is administered with every meal and snack. Steatorrhea stools are a sign that insufficient digestive enzymes are present. Steatorrhea stools should greatly diminish, if not disappear, while taking pancrelipase if the dosage is sufficient.

5. c. *H. pylori* organisms are normally responsible for gastric ulcers; the antibiotics will eradicate the organisms, and the omeprazole will decrease gastric acid, relieving pain and helping to eradicate the *H. pylori* organisms. Eradication of *H. pylori* is needed to prevent or minimize recurrence of the gastric ulcer. Bismuth therapy is not used in this patient because of his allergy to salicylates.

6. b. Gastric pH elevates as a natural process of aging. PPIs also elevate gastric pH. An elevated pH decreases the absorption of calcium which increases the risk for fractures. Milk does have calcium but is not as well absorbed as calcium citrate. PPIs should not be taken at the same time as antacids. This patient may require a CBC as an outpatient, but if it required daily testing, the patient would not be stable enough to discharge.

7. d. Pneumonia is a potential adverse effect associated with all PPIs because bacterial colonization of the stomach and respiratory tract increases when gastric acidity is reduced.

8. b. For orlistat to be most effective, the total daily fat intake should be evenly divided throughout the day at different meals. Orlistat needs to be taken with meals that contain fat. Because this patient often skips breakfast,

telling him to take the drug in the morning (as opposed to with meals) may cause the patient to take the drug on an empty stomach, thus losing the effectiveness of the drug. The patient might need to take the dose with a snack if it contains fat, or the patient should skip a dose if he doesn't eat breakfast that day. A diet to promote weight loss and promote health should have no more than 30% of its calories from fat. Orlistat does not replace the need to exercise or modify the diet.

9. a. Ondansetron should be administered 30 minutes before starting chemotherapy. The drug is not administered by IV push but should be infused over 15 minutes. Additional doses should be used after treatment.

CASE STUDY

General teaching about the drug (what it does, how it works, its proper dose, when to take the drug, adverse effects) should be included. In addition, instruct the patient to take the drug exactly as prescribed for the entire prescribed length of therapy, even if symptoms disappear. The patient should be told that smoking, drinking alcohol, drinking caffeinated drinks, and eating spicy food may aggravate an ulcer and be encouraged to stop smoking and avoid these other items.

CRITICAL THINKING CHALLENGE

1. Have you stopped smoking? Because smoking antagonizes the effect of cimetidine, if the patient had stopped smoking, this would have an effect similar to increasing the ranitidine dose. Are you taking OTC medications that treat excess acid? If this patient has been taking an OTC form of ranitidine or other H_2 receptor antagonist in addition to the prescription drug, the patient may have caused an overdosage.

2. What are the SGOT and SGPT? These tests will show functioning of the liver. Although hepatic adverse effects are rare from ranitidine therapy, the patient's history of chronic alcohol use may have affected liver function, placing the patient at greater risk for adverse effects from ranitidine.

Chapter 51

KEY TERMS

WORD SEARCH

```
F  I  D  E  F  G  L  N  O  I  T  A  P  I  T  S  N  O  C  D
L  K  H  T  F  V  Q  X  U  R  H  S  J  F  S  J  L  J  I  L
A  S  L  P  G  E  D  G  K  Q  H  Q  C  B  R  H  S  A  K  A
T  D  H  Y  N  X  C  C  Z  U  O  U  V  L  F  I  R  B  X  U
U  E  C  C  J  Y  P  A  W  N  P  I  E  Y  T  R  D  O  X  U
S  L  H  I  B  M  X  P  L  R  M  R  M  I  H  B  Q  U  G  H
C  X  N  P  W  Z  T  D  F  I  S  H  L  E  T  D  L  S  A  V
Y  M  Z  Q  S  S  F  E  K  E  M  O  A  Y  A  R  Z  X  Q  J
T  U  D  Y  I  W  O  Q  P  V  C  P  G  S  J  L  E  C  S  O
B  L  Q  G  O  Z  X  L  T  E  P  E  A  R  H  K  U  O  F  L
D  O  B  K  E  B  Y  N  V  E  N  R  L  C  R  N  W  X  L  G
X  W  T  C  A  H  D  I  R  D  C  Y  T  B  T  G  Y  F  B  P
Y  D  L  B  D  K  T  I  M  O  Y  B  S  Z  A  I  U  Y  C  X
T  M  F  C  S  A  S  Y  T  Y  I  Z  L  M  H  T  O  C  J  S
G  D  S  J  R  T  W  S  L  F  P  W  O  K  C  L  I  N  U  Q
P  B  N  E  A  C  L  F  M  W  F  H  T  G  B  D  G  R  Q  H
I  I  C  L  X  J  Q  Z  F  I  K  A  F  Q  X  Z  K  E  R  A
N  L  S  R  F  N  L  L  H  J  A  Z  T  C  M  X  S  B  I  I
U  I  L  X  N  Q  U  N  Y  R  O  T  A  M  M  A  L  F  N  I
S  D  F  L  M  X  T  M  E  S  A  E  S  I  D  N  H  O  R  C
```

PHYSIOLOGY AND PATHOPHYSIOLOGY: THE BODY HUMAN
ESSAY
1. Cecum, appendix, colon, rectum, and anal canal
2. Ascending, transverse, descending, and sigmoid
3. Relaxation of the internal and external sphincters
4. Dead bacteria, fat, inorganic matter, protein, dried digestive juices, and indigestible components of food
5. Vitamin K, vitamin B_{12}, riboflavin, and thiamine

CORE DRUG KNOWLEDGE: JUST THE FACTS
MULTIPLE CHOICE
1. b. This is the only antiflatulent in the group.
2. a. No substantial adverse reactions have been reported with this drug.
3. b, c, d. Magnesium hydroxide is a saline laxative.
4. c. The drug acts on the smooth muscle of the intestine to slow intestinal motility and prolong intestinal transit time, allowing for the reabsorption of fluid.

5. b. Because the drug slows intestinal motility, it allows time for the bacteria to replicate.

6. d. It works in the small intestine and large intestine by attracting and retaining water in the intestinal lumen, thereby increasing pressure within the intestine, which stimulates peristalsis.

7. c. Fluid and electrolyte imbalance can occur with large doses given frequently.

8. c. In the colon, lactulose is metabolized by bacteria into acids and carbon dioxide. These products increase the oncotic pressure in the colon and draw water into the stool. The acids formed also draw ammonia into the stool.

9. c. This occurs with long-term use.

10. a, c, e. Alosetron is reserved for patients with diarrhea-predominant IBS with severe symptoms.

11. c. Alosetron decreases chloride and water secretion, which helps control diarrhea but may induce constipation.

12. b. The chemical structure of 5-ASA is similar to that of aspirin.

13. d. It is used to treat moderate to severe Crohn disease and fistulizing Crohn disease.

CORE PATIENT VARIABLES: PATIENTS, PLEASE
MULTIPLE CHOICE

1. b. Chewing the tablet promotes dispersion of the drug.

2. a. Both drugs promote sedation, so an additive effect may occur.

3. b. Children with Down syndrome are at special risk for atropine sulfate toxicity, even in recommended doses.

4. b. Diphenoxylate is similar chemically to meperidine, which interacts with MAOIs.

5. c. Magnesium hydroxide decreases the effects of hydantoins such a phenytoin.

6. d. Many of the bulk-forming agents contain sodium, with a resultant increase in fluid retention that can exacerbate CHF.

7. a. Bulk-forming laxatives are considered the safest because they mimic the natural physiologic action of elimination.

8. c. Dicyclomine has a nonspecific direct relaxant effect on smooth muscle.

9. c. Patients with poor liver function are likely to have increased circulating levels of alosetron, which increases the risk for adverse effects.

10. b. Effectiveness of the oral therapy is assessed after 4 to 6 weeks, and if effective, the therapy is continued for another 4 to 6 weeks.

NURSING MANAGEMENT: EVERY GOOD NURSE SHOULD …
MULTIPLE CHOICE

1. a. Chewing the tablets promotes dispersion of the drug in the intestine. Simethicone should be administered after meals and at bedtime. Cabbage, cucumbers, and onions are gas-forming foods and should be avoided. Increased belching will occur as a mechanism of passing the gas bubbles.

2. d. This patient is showing signs of atropine toxicity. This can be very serious. No additional drug should be given at this time, and the physician needs to be notified.

3. c. The magnesium may be retained in a patient with renal failure, causing hypermagnesemia. Because multiple doses are expected to be needed, this becomes a greater risk.

4. c. Fluid and electrolyte imbalances may occur if given in large doses for a prolonged period of time. In addition, chronic use of laxatives leads to dependency on laxatives for a bowel movement to occur. The use of magnesium sulfate is not intended as a dietary source of magnesium. Magnesium sulfate has both antacid and laxative effects.

5. b. PEG-ES is used to clean the GI tract of stool so the GI tract can be clearly visualized during x-ray and other types of GI examinations. It induces diarrhea to do this. It does not prevent constipation. Unlike lactulose, PEG-ES has no effect on blood ammonia levels.

CASE STUDY
Health status: postmyocardial infarction (it is important to keep the patient from being constipated)

Life span and gender: being an older adult increases the risk of constipation

Lifestyle, diet, and habits: being on bed rest and decreased activity decrease peristalsis, thereby increasing the risk of constipation; being on a bland diet after GI bleeding may contribute to constipation

Environment: being hospitalized and out of one's normal environment may influence elimination patterns, especially by being on bed rest (unable to use toilet)

CRITICAL THINKING CHALLENGE
A Valsalva maneuver (pushing against a closed glottis) is necessary to expel a bowel movement. Straining that occurs with constipation causes an extended Valsalva maneuver and stimulates the vagal nerve. Vagal stimulation causes bradycardia, which is usually undesirable after a myocardial infarction. Stool softeners such as docusate help trap water in the stool to keep it soft, prevent constipation, and promote ease of having a bowel movement.

Chapter 52

KEY TERMS

CROSSWORD PUZZLE

Crossword solution (Across):
2. LIPODYSTROPHY
3. CORRECTIONAL
6. HYPERGLYCEMIA
7. KETOACIDOSIS
8. GLYCOGENOLYSIS
10. SUPPLEMENTAL
12. TYPE 1
13. SOMOGYI
17. DAWN
18. TYPE 2
19. HYPOGLYCEMIA

Crossword solution (Down):
1. GLUCONEOGENESIS
4. GLYCOSYLATE
5. PRANDIAL
9. BASAL
11. NONKETOTIC
14. MELLITUS
15. GESTATIONAL
16. INSULIN

PHYSIOLOGY AND PATHOPHYSIOLOGY: THE BODY HUMAN

ESSAY

1. Insulin and glucagon
2. Beta cells: insulin; alpha cells: glucagon; delta cells: somatostatin; F cells: pancreatic polypeptide used in digestion
3. Promotes the uptake and storage of glucose in the form of glycogen; promotes the conversion of excess glucose into fat; suppresses the production of glucose and the breakdown of glycogen to glucose; promotes the uptake and metabolism of glucose in muscle cells
4. Plasma glucose level
5. Stress or illness; secretion of insulin-antagonistic hormones that affect glucose metabolism; the rate of gluconeogenesis or glycogenolysis; presence and levels of insulin antibodies; use of glucose by peripheral cells or tissues; and number of cellular insulin receptors

CORE DRUG KNOWLEDGE: JUST THE FACTS

MULTIPLE CHOICE

1. b. NPH's onset is delayed.
2. b. Regular insulin is short acting.
3. a. This is one of the characteristics that makes this type of insulin unique.

4. a. Because the onset of action is delayed in intermediate and long-acting insulins, there is no reason to administer by infusion.

5. c. It is important to rotate injection sites, but the patient must remember that absorption times differ for different regions of the body.

6. c. Alcohol is a carbohydrate so it can elevate the serum glucose level, but it also potentiates hypoglycemia, so it can decrease the serum glucose level.

7. b c. Insulin pumps are used to maintain tight control of glucose levels, so a rapid and short-acting insulin is required.

8. d. Glyburide peaks at this time.

9. b. Sulfonylureas are chemically related to sulfa drugs.

10. c. Oral agents are contraindicated during pregnancy.

11. d. Because of its peak action, this drug is taken according to the number of meals taken.

12. d. Metformin has all of these actions.

13. a. This will decrease GI distress.

14. c. Although it occurs rarely, metformin may induce lactic acidosis.

15. b. It inhibits alphaglucosidase enzymes in the brush border of the small intestines.

16. a. Acarbose is contraindicated for patients with any type of disease of the bowel.

17. b. This drug works on insulin receptor sites.

18. d. Because its mechanism of action differs from that of other antidiabetic drugs, this class of drugs can be given concurrently with any other antidiabetic class.

19. c. Glucagon has a short duration of action.

20. a, b, c. Glucagon is generally used when the patient is unconscious.

21. a. Incretin hormones increase insulin synthesis and its release from the pancreas

22. c. The action of pramlintide is to inhibit glucagon secretion, slow gastric emptying time, and promote satiety, with resultant weight loss.

MATCHING

1. c	6. a
2. b	7. a
3. a	8. d
4. d	9. c
5. c	

MATCHING

1. b	6. d
2. d	7. a
3. e	8. e
4. a	9. c
5. a	10. c

CORE PATIENT VARIABLES: PATIENTS, PLEASE

MULTIPLE CHOICE

1. b. These are classic symptoms of hypoglycemia.

2. c. Lispro has a quicker onset than other insulins, so it can be taken just before a meal.

3. c. The patient has the highest risk for hypoglycemia during the peak action of the drug which is 4–12 hours.

4. a. Drawing up the regular insulin first assures the integrity of the vial so that molecules in the NPH do not enter the regular insulin vial and change the pharmacokinetics of the regular insulin.

5. a. Metformin is an antiglycemic rather than a hypoglycemic drug.

6. c. The renal excretion of metformin in patients with impaired renal function is diminished, which may result in accumulation of the drugs; lactic acidosis is more likely to occur in patients with hepatic dysfunction.

7. d. The patient must be given a glucose source because the action of the drug is to delay carbohydrate absorption.

8. a. Intravenous glucose has the quickest onset; however, if an IV cannot be established, glucagon would be the next appropriate choice.

9. d. An additional dose may be administered if the patient's response is inadequate or incomplete after 20 minutes.

10. a, c, d. Medications such as propranolol decrease the patient's awareness of hypoglycemia, thus hypoglycemia may be profound. An adequate diet, at routinely scheduled times, decreases the frequency of hypoglycemia. Overuse of insulin or an incorrect amount may result in hypoglycemia. A glycosylated hemoglobin would indicate if the patient's glucose is well controlled, not hypoglycemia. Recreational drugs, smoking, and stress would not induce repeated hypoglycemia.

11. b. Insulin detemir cannot be combined with any other type of insulin because it decreases its effectiveness.

12. c. Pioglitazone has been found to increase a woman's risk of fractures in distal upper limbs or distal lower limbs. Because your patient is 66, she already has an increased risk for fractures because of the aging process.

13. b. Exenatide slows gastric emptying, which affects the absorption of other drugs. Drugs that require absorption at a certain rate in order to achieve a therapeutic level may be affected by exanatide's use.

14. c. Pramlintide and insulin are frequently taken at the same time just prior to a meal, but they should not be combined in the same syringe. The patient is correct to use aseptic technique to administer both drugs. There is a Black Box warning regarding the potential for severe hypoglycemia when pramlintide and insulin are used together. The patient is wise to make a plan to intervene should he experience symptoms of hypoglycemia.

NURSING MANAGEMENT: EVERY GOOD NURSE SHOULD …
DECISION TREE

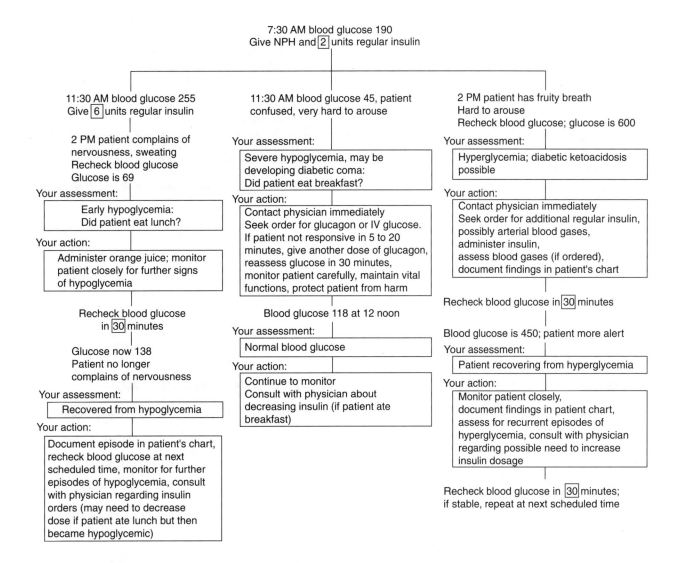

7:30 AM blood glucose 190
Give NPH and 2 units regular insulin

11:30 AM blood glucose 255
Give 6 units regular insulin

2 PM patient complains of
nervousness, sweating
Recheck blood glucose
Glucose is 69

Your assessment:

Early hypoglycemia:
Did patient eat lunch?

Your action:

Administer orange juice; monitor
patient closely for further signs
of hypoglycemia

Recheck blood glucose
in 30 minutes

Glucose now 138
Patient no longer
complains of nervousness

Your assessment:

Recovered from hypoglycemia

Your action:

Document episode in patient's chart,
recheck blood glucose at next
scheduled time, monitor for further
episodes of hypoglycemia, consult
with physician regarding insulin
orders (may need to decrease
dose if patient ate lunch but then
became hypoglycemic)

11:30 AM blood glucose 45, patient
confused, very hard to arouse

Your assessment:

Severe hypoglycemia, may be
developing diabetic coma:
Did patient eat breakfast?

Your action:

Contact physician immediately
Seek order for glucagon or IV glucose.
If patient not responsive in 5 to 20
minutes, give another dose of glucagon,
reassess glucose in 30 minutes,
monitor patient carefully, maintain vital
functions, protect patient from harm

Blood glucose 118 at 12 noon

Your assessment:

Normal blood glucose

Your action:

Continue to monitor
Consult with physician about
decreasing insulin (if patient ate
breakfast)

2 PM patient has fruity breath
Hard to arouse
Recheck blood glucose; glucose is 600

Your assessment:

Hyperglycemia; diabetic ketoacidosis
possible

Your action:

Contact physician immediately
Seek order for additional regular insulin,
possibly arterial blood gases,
administer insulin,
assess blood gases (if ordered),
document findings in patient's chart

Recheck blood glucose in 30 minutes

Blood glucose is 450; patient more alert

Your assessment:

Patient recovering from hyperglycemia

Your action:

Monitor patient closely,
document findings in patient chart,
assess for recurrent episodes of
hyperglycemia, consult with physician
regarding possible need to increase
insulin dosage

Recheck blood glucose in 30 minutes;
if stable, repeat at next scheduled time

CASE STUDY

1. This patient was not prescribed insulin initially because insulin is used only in patients with type 2 diabetes whose disease cannot be controlled with diet, weight loss, exercise, or oral antidiabetic drugs.
2. This patient was not prescribed glyburide because it is chemically related to sulfa antibiotics, to which the patient is allergic.
3. Teach this patient what metformin is, how it works, the proper dose, when to take the drug, and its adverse effects. Teaching for this patient should also include information about diabetes, diet instruction, and the importance of weight control and exercise.

CRITICAL THINKING CHALLENGE

You would expect to see that this patient begins a regimen of regular insulin, most likely on a sliding-scale basis. The insulin may be in addition to the metformin or in place of it. Elevated blood glucose levels occur with physical stress, such as infection or illness. Thus, insulin needs are greatly increased. Ad-

ministration of regular insulin will help control the elevated glucose. Sliding-scale administration of insulin is aimed at controlling blood glucose on an as-needed basis to prevent hypoglycemia from occurring from too much insulin or the combination of insulin and metformin. As the infection is controlled and blood sugar returns to normal, use of the sliding-scale insulin will be stopped.

Chapter 53

KEY TERMS
MATCHING
1. h
2. n
3. g
4. c
5. j
6. m
7. e
8. d

9. f
10. i
11. a
12. k
13. l
14. o
15. b

PHYSIOLOGY AND PATHOPHYSIOLOGY: THE BODY HUMAN
ESSAY

1. Hypothalamus
2. Temperature, catecholamine secretion, growth and development, fluid volume regulation, perspiration, GI activity, appetite and thirst regulation, blood pressure, respiration, regulation of basic body rhythms, and complex behavioral and emotional reactions
3. The releasing factors that control the anterior pituitary include:
   - Growth hormone-releasing hormone (GHRH), also known as sermorelin, stimulates anterior pituitary release of growth hormone (GH).
   - Thyroid-releasing hormone (TRH), also known as protirelin, stimulates the anterior pituitary to produce thyrotropin (thyroid-stimulating hormone), which in turn stimulates the thyroid to produce thyroxine.
   - Gonadotropin-releasing factor (GnRH) controls the release of the gonadotropins: follicle-stimulating hormone (FSH) and luteinizing hormone (LH).
   - Corticotropin-releasing factor (Xerecept) stimulates release of adrenocorticotropic hormone (ACTH).
   - There is also a small portion between the anterior and posterior lobes, known as the intermediate lobe (pars intermedia). The hormones of this lobe stimulate melanin synthesis, which affects skin pigmentation.
4. Growth hormone, thyrotropin, adrenocorticotropin, follicle-stimulating hormone, luteinizing hormone, and prolactin
5. Antidiuretic hormone and oxytocin
6. Iodine
7. The half-life of T_4 is approximately 1 week, compared with 12 hours for T_3, and T_4 is converted to T_3 (a more active hormone) at the cellular level.
8. Heat production and body temperature; oxygen consumption and cardiac output; blood volume; enzyme system activity; metabolism of carbohydrates, fats, and proteins; and regulation of growth and development
9. Parathormone
10. Membrane transport processes, nerve impulse conduction, muscle contraction, and blood clotting

CORE DRUG KNOWLEDGE: JUST THE FACTS
MULTIPLE CHOICE

1. b. Somatropin is a recombinant DNA formulation of GH.
2. c. Although rare, leukemia may occur.
3. d. Children are more likely to develop slipped-capital epiphysis.
4. c. Other adverse effects include hyperglycemia, glycosuria, and pain at the injection site.
5. a. Somatropin is a recombinant DNA formulation of growth hormone.
6. a. Desmopressin is a synthetic analogue of ADH, which is the deficient hormone in diabetes insipidus.
7. d. There are formulations for all of these routes.

8. b. Levothyroxine is a synthetic T_4 that acts as replacement for natural T_4.
9. d. The half-life of levothyroxine is long, thus it takes 1 to 3 weeks for maximal effects.
10. a. Levothyroxine increases the basal rate of the body. In therapeutic overdosage, the patient may experience hypertension, arrhythmias, anxiety, headache, nervousness, GI irritation, sweating, and heat intolerance in addition to tachycardia.
11. b. To keep up with the metabolic demands of the body during pregnancy, the levothyroxine dose may need to be increased.
12. c. Methimazole (MMI) is a thionamide used for palliative treatment of hyperthyroidism.
13. d. The half-life is 5 to 13 hours, so it has a slow onset of action.
14. b. These symptoms can be decreased by spreading the total dose over the entire day.
15. b. This drug destroys thyroid tissue.
16. d. It crosses the placenta and can cause permanent damage to the fetus' thyroid.
17. a. It plays a role in the regulation of calcium and bone metabolism.
18. a. The medication should be taken before anything else, and then the patient should remain upright for 30 minutes.
19. b. Calcitriol is the active form of vitamin D.
20. d. These are early signs of vitamin D excess. Additional signs are nausea and vomiting, constipation, and bone pain.

CORE PATIENT VARIABLES: PATIENTS, PLEASE
MULTIPLE CHOICE

1. d. Others include hypothyroidism, glycosuria, and pain at the injection site.
2. b. This could be a symptom of slipped-capital epiphysis and should be evaluated.
3. b. Somatropin can induce hyperglycemia and hypothyroidism.
4. a. These are all early signs of water intoxication.
5. c. Patients who are predisposed to thrombus formation have an increased risk for thrombotic events.
6. d. The specific gravity tells you if the patient is losing excess fluids.
7. d. Levothyroxine passes into breast milk and can influence the child's thyroid function.
8. b. In combination, levothyroxine increases the anticoagulant effect, resulting in an increased risk for bleeding.
9. a. Hypofunction of the thyroid usually requires lifelong therapy.
10. a. The drug should be taken every 8 hours; dairy products do not help GI distress.
11. a. A hyperthyroid state *decreases* the vitamin K-dependent clotting factors. As the patient becomes more euthyroid, the clotting factors increase and the dose of warfarin will be less effective.
12. c. Home pregnancy kits may give a false positive. The patient should be seen immediately to confirm pregnancy rather than abruptly stop the medication.
13. b. Thyroid function is monitored to assure the patient is euthyroid; the CBC is monitored because of the potential for blood dyscrasias.
14. b. Calcitonin is metabolized primarily in the kidneys.
15. a. Paget disease requires parenteral calcitonin; heat is better than ice for bone pain.

16. a. Alendronate (Fosamax) is a bisphosphonate given to postmenopausal women for osteoporosis.
17. c. Patients receiving long-term dialysis should avoid magnesium-containing antacids while taking anti-hypocalcemic drugs.

NURSING MANAGEMENT: EVERY GOOD NURSE SHOULD …
MULTIPLE CHOICE

1. a. Somatropin is administered by SC and IM routes only. Patients and families need to learn how to safely administer the drug. Proper storage is in the refrigerator after it has been diluted. Limping and hip or knee pain are possible signs of slipped-capital femoral epiphyses or avascular necrosis of the femoral head, a serious complication that should be reported at once by the patient.
2. d. This patient will now have hypothyroidism because she no longer has a thyroid gland. If the replacement hormone dose is too high, she will have signs of hyperthyroidism (tachycardia, hypertension, increased sweating, and intolerance to heat, among others). If the replacement dose is too low, she will show signs of hypothyroidism (bradycardia, decreased blood pressure, decreased sweating, and intolerance to cold, among others).
3. b. Nausea, vomiting, and GI distress may be minimized if the patient does not eat three large meals a day but eats small, frequent meals (such as six meals a day). Taking the drug on an empty stomach aggravates the nausea and abdominal pain. Methimazole can be taken in one daily dose, but this usually aggravates, rather than relieves, GI distress. The patient should not stop taking the drug. The drug must be used for a prolonged period of time to induce the desired effect. Instead, techniques to minimize adverse effects should be tried.
4. b. Calcitriol is designed to raise blood calcium levels. Calcium levels should be monitored to determine that they have reached normal but are not elevated above normal levels. Potassium, BUN (an indication of kidney function), and SGOT (an indication of liver function) levels are not directly related to drug therapy.
5. c. Calcitonin, salmon carries the risk of allergic reaction to the salmon antigen in this calcitonin; therefore, a skin test with 0.1 mL of a 10-IU/mL solution is given SC. If no reaction is seen in 15 minutes, the drug may be given. Calcium levels are already elevated; you would not want to give more calcium. Vitamin D is needed for calcium absorption and is not needed here. Acute severe hypercalcemia needs to be treated as an emergency. Bone deformity, which might be seen in Paget disease, is not a critical assessment at this time.

CASE STUDY
Methimazole is given to treat hyperthyroidism in preparation for subtotal thyroidectomy. By decreasing the activity of the thyroid gland before surgery, there is less chance of a serious adverse effect from sudden changes in thyroid level. Methimazole inhibits the synthesis of thyroid hormones (T_4 and T_3), so new T_3 and T_4 are not produced. It does not inactivate existing thyroxine and triiodothyronine that are stored in the thyroid, or inhibit peripheral conversion of T_4 to T_3. Thus, it takes 3 to 4 weeks to cause a depletion of T_4 levels.

CRITICAL THINKING CHALLENGE
1. A hyperthyroid state *decreases* the vitamin K-dependent clotting factors, which increases the efficacy of warfarin.

2. Prothrombin (PT) and INR tests should be checked to determine if the bleeding time is excessively lengthened. A decreased warfarin dose may be required at this time.
3. The PT/INR should be monitored closely because as the MMI works, the patient becomes more euthyroid and the clotting factors will increase, making the dose of warfarin less effective. At that time, the patient has an increased risk for thrombus formation.

Chapter 54

KEY TERMS
TRUE OR FALSE
1. False, androgens
2. True
3. False, erectile dysfunction
4. False, benign prostatic hypertrophy
5. True

PHYSIOLOGY AND PATHOPHYSIOLOGY: THE BODY HUMAN
ESSAY
1. Testosterone
2. Retention of sodium, potassium, and phosphorus; decreases urinary excretion of calcium; stimulates skeletal muscle tissue; enhances growth of long bone in prepubescent boys; ossification process of the epiphyseal growth plates; stimulates production of red blood cells
3. The parasympathetic system innervates the penile arteries. Normal erection involves the release of nitric oxide, secondary to sexual stimulation, in the erectile tissue of the penis. The nitric oxide activates an intermediary enzyme that boosts cyclic guanosine monophosphate (cGMP), a substance that mediates the action of certain hormones. By some unknown mechanism, cGMP stimulates smooth muscle, producing relaxation and an inflow of blood into the erectile tissue.

CORE DRUG KNOWLEDGE: JUST THE FACTS
MULTIPLE CHOICE
1. b. In women 1 to 5 years postmenopause, testosterone may be used as secondary treatment to slow the growth of advanced, inoperable metastatic breast cancer.
2. d. Testosterone may cause edema, which would exacerbate CHF.
3. c. Most commonly, amenorrhea may occur.
4. b. This patch should be placed on clean, dry skin every 24 hours.
5. a. This patch stays in place for 7 days before replacing.
6. a. There are potential serious adverse effects with anabolic steroids, so they should be used for medical purposes only.
7. c. Serious adverse effects include peliosis hepatitis, liver tumors, and blood lipid changes associated with an increased risk of atherosclerosis.
8. d. cGMP specific phosphodiesterase type 5 inhibitors are the drugs of choice for erectile dysfunction.
9. d. The vasodilating effects of sildenafil potentiate the hypotensive effects of nitrates.
10. c. 5-alpha reductase drugs are the drugs of choice.
11. d. When used for BPH, the trade name is Proscar; when used for male pattern baldness, the trade name is Propecia.
12. d. The drug should be applied in the morning and again at night.

CORE PATIENT VARIABLES: PATIENTS, PLEASE
MULTIPLE CHOICE
1. a. Testosterone may affect the epiphyseal centers.
2. c. The most common adverse effect in males is gyneco-mastia.
3. b. X-rays monitor bone maturation.
4. a. Monitor serum cholesterol levels, liver function, and hemoglobin and hematocrit levels throughout therapy.
5. c. Sildenafil and vardenafil are taken 1 hour before sexual activity; tadalafil's effects can occur within 30 minutes and last as long as 36 hours.
6. a. There are many drug–drug interactions with antihypertensive agents.
7. c. A high-fat meal eaten before the use of sildenafil will decrease the rate of absorption, decreasing the serum blood level.
8. c. Finasteride is a pregnancy category X drug.
9. b. This drug is generally well tolerated. These symptoms can be self-limiting.
10. c. It takes a minimum of 4 months to see fine, soft, colorless hair growth.

NURSING MANAGEMENT: EVERY GOOD NURSE SHOULD …
MULTIPLE CHOICE
1. b. X-ray films will help to document the long bone maturation and the effect of testosterone on the epiphyseal centers. Early closure of the epiphysis is to be avoided. Testosterone (short acting) is never administered IV but always by the IM route into a deep gluteal muscle. BUN and creatinine are not affected by testosterone (short acting). However, liver function tests should be monitored.
2. c. Testoderm TTS is applied to the arm, back, or upper buttocks, unlike some other testosterone products, which are applied to the scrotum. The patch should be applied to dry skin that is not irritated or damaged. It is left on the skin and changed every 24 hours. The adhesive on the patch should keep the patch in place if the system is firmly pressed into place with the palm of the hand for about 10 seconds.
3. d. Sexual activity places additional stress on the heart. Information on the signs of cardiac problems such as angina or MI is important to teach, especially to patients who have risk factors for cardiovascular disease. This patient has two risk factors: family history and elevated cholesterol levels.
4. c. A woman in childbearing years should not handle crushed or broken finasteride pills because the risk for absorption through the skin is greatest then. Finasteride is a pregnancy category X drug. If the patient has difficulty swallowing pills, forcing him to swallow all medication may lead to choking. Patients should not be forced to do anything. Finasteride must be administered orally; it cannot be administered by way of the urethra. Administering the drug just before urination has no relevancy to drug efficacy.
5. b. Fine, soft colorless hair may grow first; this will later be replaced by hair of the same color and texture as on the rest of the head. Minoxidil is available topically over the counter; no prescription is required. Topical minoxidil has no effect on blood pressure. Oral minoxidil will decrease, not raise, blood pressure. Hair growth is not seen until minoxidil has been applied topically twice a day for at least 4 months.
6. c. Sildenafil causes vasodilation of the pulmonary vascular bed, and to a lesser degree, vasodilation in the systemic circulation.

CASE STUDY
Electrolyte values should be monitored, especially sodium, calcium, potassium, chloride, and phosphates because these can be elevated from testosterone administration. Blood cholesterol levels also should be assessed because increases in cholesterol levels are possible, and this is especially problematic for this patient because of his history of coronary artery disease.

CRITICAL THINKING CHALLENGE
This patient may have edema and possibly CHF caused by testosterone's effect on fluid levels. (Increased sodium retention leads to increased water retention.) His diabetes may have narrowed vessels to his kidneys, as well as his heart, placing him at increased risk of edema secondary to testosterone use.

Chapter 55

KEY TERMS
TRUE OR FALSE
1. False, estrogens
2. False, progestin
3. False, gonadotropin-releasing hormone (GRH); follicle-stimulating hormone (FSH), and luteinizing hormone (LH)
4. True
5. False, osteoporosis
6. False, secretory phase
7. False, proliferative phase
8. True
9. False, Paget disease

PHYSIOLOGY AND PATHOPHYSIOLOGY: THE BODY HUMAN
ESSAY
1. Estrogen and progestin
2. Estradiol
3. Affect release of pituitary gonadotropins; cause capillary dilation; promote fluid retention; enhance protein anabolism; thin cervical mucus; inhibit or facilitate ovulation; prevent postpartum breast pain; strengthen the skeleton by conserving calcium and phosphorus; encourage bone formation; maintain tone and elasticity of urogenital structures; promote growth during the adolescent growth spurt; stimulate closure of epiphyseal growth plates of long bones
4. Hypothalamus secretes gonadotropin-releasing hormone → release of FSH and LH → stimulate development of ovarian follicles → release of the ovum from mature follicle → production of estrogen → increases the vascularity of uterine lining → stimulation of GRH → more LH → rupture of mature follicle and ovulation occurs. After ovulation, follicle becomes corpus luteum → produces progesterone and estrogen → prepares uterine lining for implantation → if none occurs, corpus luteum disintegrates → estrogen and progestin levels decrease → menses.

CORE DRUG KNOWLEDGE: JUST THE FACTS
MULTIPLE CHOICE
1. b. HRT replacement does not prevent cardiovascular disease or complications.
2. a, b, c, e, f. Conjugated estrogens may cause fluid retention that may exacerbate these conditions.
3. a. Estrogens are contraindicated in patients with estrogen-dependent neoplastic diseases.
4. b, c, e, f. The Women's Health Initiative proved that postmenopausal women have an increased risk for these disorders.
5. b. Shortness of breath indicates a more serious problem, such as an embolus.
6. a, c, d, f. The drug's pharmacodynamics make it effective for amenorrhea and dysfunctional uterine bleeding; it is

added to HRT to decrease the risk for endometrial cancer from estrogen therapy; and it is commonly used in birth control pills to mimic the body's menstrual cycle.

7. c. Progesterone may induce fluid retention that exacerbates asthma symptoms.

8. a, c. According to the Women's Health Initiative, breast and ovarian cancer may occur with use of these hormones in postmenopausal women.

9. a. Clomiphene is an ovulation stimulant, increasing the potential for fertility.

10. b. It inactivates and atrophies the normal and ectopic endometrial tissue.

11. a. Exactly how megestrol increases appetite in patients with AIDS who have anorexia and cachexia is unknown.

12. a. The capsules are implanted subdermally in the midportion of the upper arm, about 8 to 10 cm above the antecubital space, in a fan-like pattern.

13. c. Mifepristone inhibits the activity of endogenous and exogenous progesterone, resulting in termination of pregnancy.

14. c. The first dose should be taken as soon as possible after intercourse, but within 72 hours, and then repeated 12 hours later.

15. a, c, d. Do not place on the breast or parts of the body that will be rubbed by tight clothing.

16. d. In addition, alendronate is used in treating Paget disease.

17. c. Symptoms such as abdominal pain, flatulence, acid regurgitation, abdominal distention, gastritis, and esophageal ulcers may occur.

ESSAY

1. The three types of combination oral contraceptives are monophasic—the dose of estrogen and progestin remains the same throughout the entire cycle; biphasic—the amount of estrogen remains the same, but the amount of progestin rises in the second half of the cycle; and triphasic—estrogen amounts remain the same or may vary throughout the cycle, whereas progestin varies throughout the cycle.

2. Serious adverse effects include thromboembolism, CVA, MI, hepatic lesions, gallbladder disease, increased risk for cardiovascular and cerebrovascular events, and increased mortality in women who smoke and are older than 35 years and nonsmokers who are older than 40 years.

3. Common adverse effects include breakthrough bleeding, spotting, amenorrhea during and after treatment, breast tenderness, nausea and vomiting, steepening of the corneal curvature, contact lens intolerance, weight gain or loss, edema, migraine, elevated triglyceride levels, and depression.

CORE PATIENT VARIABLES: PATIENTS, PLEASE

MULTIPLE CHOICE

1. b. HRT is associated with an increased risk for cardiovascular and cerebrovascular adverse effects.

2. b. Unopposed estrogen may induce endometriosis.

3. c. This patient should not take any type of hormone replacement because of her stroke.

4. c. Depo-Provera is an IM injection administered every 3 months.

5. b. Additional adverse events include increased risk for pelvic inflammatory disease, device embedment in the endometrium, perforation of the uterine wall or cervix by the device, endometritis, vaginitis, midcycle spotting, pain, cramping, and amenorrhea.

6. d. Birth control pills increase the risk for thromboembolism.

7. b. Missing 3 or more pills requires the patient to start a new cycle of pills.

8. a. The levonorgestrel-releasing IUD provides birth control for as long as 5 years; the patient does not have any type of contraception should the device fall out; menstrual flow may increase with the device.

9. c. This patient may have an incomplete abortion and needs to be evaluated.

10. c. Any other type of fluid or food will decrease its absorption. The patient should remain in an upright position for 30 minutes to decrease GI distress.

NURSING MANAGEMENT: EVERY GOOD NURSE SHOULD ...
MULTIPLE CHOICE

1. d. Estrogen is used as hormone replacement with primary ovarian failure, loss of ovaries caused by surgery, and to manage the discomforts of menopause. Menopausal use is for a short duration only, and the dose should be as low as possible to be effective.

2. a. This cyclic approach to drug therapy mimics the natural cycling of estrogen. Photosensitivity may result from estrogen replacement; patients should avoid prolonged sun exposure. X-rays are taken when estrogen is given for hypogonadism before the adolescent growth spurt; they are not needed when estrogen is used after the final growth spurt has occurred. Sudden, severe headaches are signs of serious adverse effects. If they occur, they need to be reported to the physician at once.

3. d. Progesterone is avoided in patients with thrombophlebitis because this is an adverse effect of the drug. If thrombophlebitis occurs during drug therapy, use of progesterone should be discontinued. Progesterone is avoided during the first 4 months of pregnancy because it is a pregnancy category D drug. For appropriate blood levels to be obtained, progesterone needs to be administered on a regular basis for 6 to 8 days.

4. e. Levonorgestrel implants prevent pregnancy for as long as 5 years. Intrauterine progesterone inserts may have serious adverse effects, including septic abortion or congenital anomalies (if pregnancy occurs), pelvic inflammatory disease, and perforation of the uterine wall or cervix. Oral contraceptives should be avoided in women older than 35 years who smoke because these women have the highest risk for serious cardiovascular adverse effects.

5. d. Because mifepristone may cause serious harm, the patient must be aware of the potential complications and her role in reducing complications. This is the purpose of the Medication Guide. Two follow-up visits are necessary to confirm that pregnancy was completely terminated. If bleeding hasn't started by day 3 (the first visit), the patient will be given a different drug, misoprostol, which induces uterine contractions. Day 1 is the day the mifepristone tablets are taken. Because this drug is not distributed to pharmacies, but only to approved prescribers, the drug is taken in the prescriber's office, in his or her presence.

CASE STUDY

This patient may resume birth control even though she has not yet had a menstrual period. She may resume the Ortho-Novum 7/7/7 as birth control if she wishes. She should begin the oral contraceptives after she stops breast-feeding.

CRITICAL THINKING CHALLENGE

Tell me about how you take this oral contraceptive. Every day? At a certain time? Did you miss any days? How many days in a cycle did you miss? What did you do when you missed a day?

Although pregnancy is possible with the correct use of oral birth control pills, pregnancy is normally prevented with correct use. Therefore, it is likely that this patient has not been taking the drug as prescribed or that she has not used appropriate measures if she misses a pill. Alternately, confirm that the patient did not use any antibiotics while taking oral contraceptives. A drug interaction can occur from antibiotics that decreases the effectiveness of the oral contraceptives. An additional form of birth control should be used (such as a condom) if the patient must take antibiotics while taking an oral contraceptive.

Chapter 56

KEY TERMS

ANAGRAMS
1. Antepartum
2. Tocolytics
3. Postpartum
4. Uterine tetany
5. Oxytocics
6. Intrapartum

PHYSIOLOGY AND PATHOPHYSIOLOGY: THE BODY HUMAN

ESSAY
1. Weeks 38 to 42
2. Vascular constriction and increased water reabsorption from the glomerular filtrate
3. Oxytocin, cAMP, calcium, and prostaglandins
4. Fluctuations of cardiac output, heart rate, and blood pressure
5. Hyperventilation with resultant respiratory alkalosis; muscular contraction induces metabolic acidosis uncompensated by respiratory alkalosis
6. Leukocytosis
7. Concentrated urine with a trace of protein
8. Cessation of gastric motility and increase in gastric acidity

CORE DRUG KNOWLEDGE: JUST THE FACTS

MULTIPLE CHOICE
1. c. Oxytocin is administered only via the IV route.
2. a. The proper dose of oxytocin is one that achieves adequate uterine contractility while minimizing maternal and fetal adverse effects.
3. b. When the infusion is continuous, maximum contractions occur within this time frame.
4. c. Oxytocin increases the effectiveness of contraction. If the pelvic opening is not adequate, fetal injury may occur as the contraction pushes the fetus against bony structures.
5. a, b, d, f. Although the mother must be monitored carefully, maternal hypertension or dehydration is not sufficient to withhold oxytocin.
6. a. The other symptoms are serious adverse effects that are not common.
7. c. The most common fetal adverse effect is bradycardia.
8. c. This drug is used in the postpartum period to decrease uterine bleeding.
9. d. Carboprost (Hemabate) stimulates the myometrium to contract to induce abortion in pregnancies of 13 to 20 weeks.
10. c. Stimulation of the beta receptors in the sympathetic nervous system decreases uterine contractions.
11. a, c, f. The fine line here is whether the maternal hypertension is controlled.
12. d. See Table 56.3 on page 1177 in the textbook.

CORE PATIENT VARIABLES: PATIENTS, PLEASE

MULTIPLE CHOICE
1. b. Additional signs include headache, fatigue, nausea and anorexia, vomiting, seizures, and coma.
2. d. Bishop score relates to whether or not the patient's cervix is favorable for induction.
3. c. The patient is experiencing uterine hyperstimulation.
4. b. This allows for immediate discontinuation of use of the drug should adverse effects occur.
5. c. Use of other diluents may increase the risk for pulmonary edema.
6. b. These symptoms are associated with stimulation of the beta receptors of the sympathetic nervous system. The patient should not discontinue use of the drug because contractions may recur.
7. b. The respiratory system of the fetus produces sufficient surfactant after week 35.
8. a. Magnesium sulfate is the drug of choice for treating or preventing seizures associated with preeclampsia, eclampsia, and pregnancy-induced hypertension.
9. d. These are all common fetal adverse effects to magnesium therapy.

NURSING MANAGEMENT: EVERY GOOD NURSE SHOULD …

MULTIPLE CHOICE
1. c. A Bishop score of 5 or better should be present before beginning induction. Otherwise, the cervix needs to be primed with prostaglandin E2 gel. Contraindication to vaginal delivery, significant cephalopelvic disproportion, and fetal distress when delivery is not imminent are all contraindications to the use of oxytocin.
2. a. A solution of 0.9% sodium chloride could also be used. Solutions of 20% glucose in water are hypertonic and would not be used. Solutions of 0.2% sodium chloride are hypotonic and would not be used. Oxytocin is never given IV undiluted.
3. c. Contractions occurring more frequently than every 2 minutes, lasting longer than 90 seconds, or having a resting tone greater than 15 mm Hg pressure indicate a hypercontractile labor pattern caused by the oxytocin. Additional oxytocin is contraindicated. Increased IV mainline fluids are indicated.
4. d. Because of the risk of pulmonary edema, solutions with saline are not used.
5. a. This will regulate the rate to prevent overdosage. Patients should be positioned on the left side to prevent hypotension and to promote circulation to the fetus. High fluid intake is contraindicated because of the risk of pulmonary edema.

CASE STUDY

1. Yes, these are appropriate orders. Oxytocin is indicated to augment labor that is not progressing as long as cervical ripening, as measured by 5 or more on the Bishop scale, is present. Oxytocin should be started at 0.5 to 1 mU/minute and then increased by this amount every 30 to 60 minutes. This dosing pattern allows the drug to reach steady state and full therapeutic effect to occur before the dose is increased. It also mimics the natural release of oxytocin.
2. The nurse should dilute the oxytocin in 0.9% normal saline or 5% dextrose in lactated Ringer's solution. The drug should be piggybacked onto mainline fluids, and a pump or controller should regulate the infusion of the oxytocin. The nurse should monitor the patient and fetus carefully throughout drug infusion. Assess maternal vital signs, fetal heart rate, contractile rate, and fetal movement. These must be checked before increasing the infusion rate. If hyperten-

sion or other significant maternal vital sign changes occur, fetal heart rate decreases, or fetal movement stops, the nurse must notify the physician or nurse midwife immediately. If a hypercontractile pattern occurs, the oxytocin infusion should be stopped and the health care provider notified. The nurse should also assess intake and output and encourage the patient to urinate every 2 hours.

CRITICAL THINKING CHALLENGE

1. The oxytocin has been effective, and this patient has progressed through labor. She is ready to deliver and has the urge to push.
2. The nurse should have the physician or nurse midwife present, prepare for delivery of the baby, and coach or assist the patient with pushing effectively to deliver the baby.